Frazer's Foundations of Immunotherapy

Frazer's Foundations of Immunotherapy

Edited by

FERNANDO S. F. GUIMARAES
The University of Queensland, Brisbane, QLD, Australia

IAN H. FRAZER
The University of Queensland, Brisbane, QLD, Australia

WILEY

This edition first published 2026

Registered Offices
John Wiley & Sons, Inc., 111 River Street, Hoboken, NJ 07030, USA
John Wiley & Sons Ltd, New Era House, 8 Oldlands Way, Bognor Regis, West Sussex, PO22 9NQ, UK

For details of our global editorial offices, customer services, and more information about Wiley products visit us at www.wiley.com.

The manufacturer's authorized representative according to the EU General Product Safety Regulation is Wiley-VCH GmbH, Boschstr. 12, 69469 Weinheim, Germany, e-mail: Product_Safety@wiley.com.

Wiley also publishes its books in a variety of electronic formats and by print-on-demand. Some content that appears in standard print versions of this book may not be available in other formats.

Library of Congress Cataloging-in-Publication Data applied for:

Paperback ISBN: 9781394383016

Cover Design: Wiley
Cover Image: © Drs Carolina Camargo de Oliveira & Fernando Guimaraes (image), and Mr Simon Taplin (digital colouring)

Set in 10/12pt STIXTwoText by Straive, Pondicherry, India

To Jian Zhou, whose creative partnership with Ian H. Frazer turned the dream of preventing cancer through immunology into reality. His legacy continues to protect millions of lives.

Contents

About the Editors

Associate Professor Fernando S. F. Guimaraes completed his PhD in 2012 as the first graduate of the Pasteur-Paris University International PhD Program at Institut Pasteur in Paris, France. He later joined QIMR Berghofer in 2013 and the Walter and Eliza Hall Institute in 2016, where he worked on immune regulation of natural killer (NK) cells by the tumour microenvironment and immunotherapy development. He is now a Group Leader at The University of Queensland's Frazer Institute, leading a research team focused on the development of new generation immunotherapies for hard-to-cure diseases. His work bridges basic immunology and translational medicine, with over 120 publications in top tier journals. Fernando has been awarded several national and international grants, including NHMRC and MRFF funding, and his contributions have been recognised through honours such as the 2019 Cure Cancer Australia Researcher of the Year, the 2020 Queensland Young Tall Poppy Science Award, the 2022 Frazer Institute Mentor of the Year, 2023 TRI Connecting with the Clinics Award, and the 2025 Dr. Jian Zhou Foundation Award for Translational Medicine.

Emeritus Professor Ian H. Frazer is an internationally recognised immunologist and co-developer of the HPV vaccine *Gardasil*, which has greatly reduced cervical cancer rates worldwide. Born in Glasgow, he studied medicine at the University of Edinburgh and moved to Australia in 1981 to continue his research at The University of Queensland. At UQ, Ian's work on papillomavirus immunology led to one of the most significant advances in cancer prevention. He later served as founding CEO and Director of Research at Brisbane's Translational Research Institute, and he continues to contribute to immunotherapy research and education. His achievements have been recognised with numerous awards, including Australian of the Year (2006) and Companion of the Order of Australia (2012). Ian remains an active voice in science, mentoring researchers and promoting innovation in immune-based medicine. He also serves as Fernando's official mentor through the Australian Academy of Health and Medical Sciences (AAHMS).

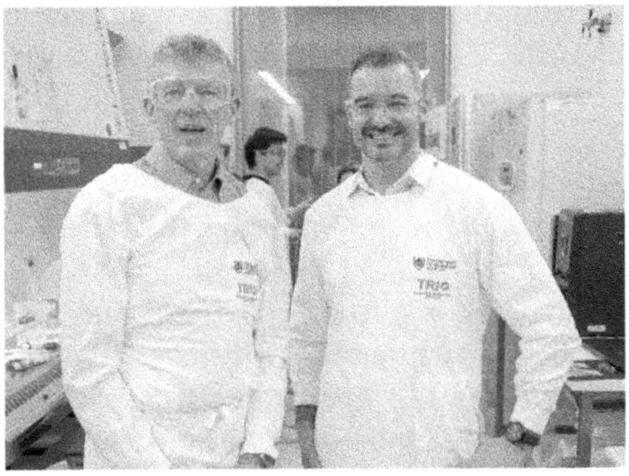

Ian H. Frazer (left) and Fernando Guimaraes (Right). Credit: Translational Research Institute (TRI) – Media and Communication's team.

List of Contributors

Marie Abitbol, VetAgro Sup Campus vétérinaire, Departement Basic Sciences, Université de Lyon, Marcy-l'Etoile, France

Rachel Elizabeth Ann Fincham, Department of Anatomical Pathology, Singapore General Hospital, Singapore, Singapore

Marion F. Barros, Frazer Institute, The University of Queensland, Brisbane, Queensland, Australia

Naomi Berrell, Queensland Spatial Biology Centre, Wesley Research Institute, The Wesley Hospital, Brisbane, Queensland, Australia; and Faculty of Health, Medicine and Behavioural Sciences, Frazer Institute, The University of Queensland, Brisbane, Queensland, Australia

Jean-Marc Cavaillon, Institut Pasteur, Paris, France

Janin Chandra, Faculty of Health, Medicine and Behavioural Sciences, Frazer Institute, The University of Queensland, Brisbane, Queensland, Australia

Zhian Chen, Frazer Institute, The University of Queensland, Brisbane, Queensland, Australia

Russell W. Cochrane, Department of Pharmacology and Immunology, Medical University of South Carolina, Charleston, SC, USA; and Hollings Cancer Center, Medical University of South Carolina, Charleston, SC, USA

Thomas J. Cole, Cancer Immunology Program, Peter MacCallum Cancer Centre, Melbourne, Victoria, Australia; and Sir Peter MacCallum Department of Oncology, The University of Melbourne, Parkville, Victoria, Australia

Phillip K. Darcy, Cancer Immunology Program, Peter MacCallum Cancer Centre, Melbourne, Victoria, Australia; and Sir Peter MacCallum Department of Oncology, The University of Melbourne, Parkville, Victoria, Australia

Riccardo Dolcetti, Peter MacCallum Cancer Centre, Melbourne, Victoria, Australia; Peter MacCallum Department of Oncology, The University of Melbourne, Melbourne, Victoria, Australia; and Department of Microbiology and Immunology, The University of Melbourne, Melbourne, Victoria, Australia

Meg L. Donovan, Queensland Spatial Biology Centre, Wesley Research Institute, The Wesley Hospital, Brisbane, Queensland, Australia; and Faculty of Health, Medicine and Behavioural Sciences, Frazer Institute, The University of Queensland, Brisbane, Queensland, Australia

Jessica A. Engel, Division of Infection and Inflammation, QIMR Berghofer Medical Research Institute, Brisbane, Queensland, Australia

Christian R. Engwerda, Division of Infection and Inflammation, QIMR Berghofer Medical Research Institute, Brisbane, Queensland, Australia

Leonardo M.R. Ferreira, Department of Pharmacology and Immunology, Medical University of South Carolina, Charleston, SC, USA; and Hollings Cancer Center, Medical University of South Carolina, Charleston, SC, USA

Marine Fidelle, Inserm UMR1367, Microbiota and Mucosal Immunity for Cancer Immunotherapy, ClinicoBiome, Université Paris-Saclay, Gustave Roussy, Villejuif, France

Ian H. Frazer, Frazer Institute, The University of Queensland, Brisbane, Queensland, Australia

Denise Goh, Institute of Molecular and Cell Biology (IMCB), Agency for Science, Technology and Research (A*STAR), Singapore, Singapore

Jingru Gong, Frazer Institute, The University of Queensland, Brisbane, Queensland, Australia

Camille Hansen, Department of Pathology, University of Utah, Salt Lake City, UT, USA; and Huntsman Cancer Institute, University of Utah, Salt Lake City, UT, USA

Behnaz Heydarchi, Inflammation Division, Walter and Eliza Hall Institute of Medical Research, Parkville, Victoria, Australia; and Department of Medical Biology, The University of Melbourne, Melbourne, Victoria, Australia

John D. Hooper, Mater Research Institute, The University of Queensland, Woolloongabba, Queensland, Australia

Alexandre Humbert, VetAgro Sup Campus vétérinaire, Departement Basic Sciences, Université de Lyon, Marcy-l'Etoile, France

Jiya Jose, Faculty of Health, Medicine and Behavioural Sciences, Frazer Institute, The University of Queensland, Brisbane, Queensland, Australia

Shannon R. Joseph, Frazer Institute, The University of Queensland, Brisbane, Queensland, Australia

Stephanie Jost, Division of Innate and Comparative Immunology, Centre for Human Systems Immunology, Department of Surgery, Duke University School of Medicine, Durham, NC, USA

Arutha Kulasinghe, Queensland Spatial Biology Centre, Wesley Research Institute, The Wesley Hospital, Brisbane, Queensland, Australia; and Faculty of Health, Medicine and Behavioural Sciences, Frazer Institute, The University of Queensland, Brisbane, Queensland, Australia

Clara Lawler, Faculty of Health, Medicine and Behavioural Sciences, Frazer Institute, The University of Queensland, Brisbane, Queensland, Australia

Jason J. Lee, Frazer Institute, The University of Queensland, Brisbane, Queensland, Australia

Graham Leggatt, Faculty of Health, Medicine and Behavioural Sciences, Frazer Institute, The University of Queensland, Brisbane, Queensland, Australia

Lixue Li, Frazer Institute, The University of Queensland, Brisbane, Queensland, Australia

Karl-Johan Malmberg, Department of Cancer Immunology, Institute for Cancer Research, Oslo University Hospital, Oslo, Norway; Precision Immunotherapy Alliance, Institute for Clinical Medicine, The University of Oslo, Oslo, Norway; and Center for Infectious Medicine, Department of Medicine Huddinge, Karolinska Institutet, Stockholm, Sweden

Cordelia Manickam, Division of Innate and Comparative Immunology, Centre for Human Systems Immunology, Department of Surgery, Duke University School of Medicine, Durham, NC, USA

Meriem Messaoudene, Inserm UMR1367, Microbiota and Mucosal Immunity for Cancer Immunotherapy, ClinicoBiome, Université Paris-Saclay, Gustave Roussy, Villejuif, France

Brett M. Paterson, Centre for Advancing Imaging, Australian Institute for Bioengineering and Nanotechnology, The University of Queensland, Brisbane, Queensland, Australia

Lakshita Patil, Faculty of Health, Medicine and Behavioural Sciences, Frazer Institute, The University of Queensland, Brisbane, Queensland, Australia

Carole Peroz, VetAgro Sup Campus vétérinaire, Departement Basic Sciences, Université de Lyon, Marcy-l'Etoile, France

R. Keith Reeves, Division of Innate and Comparative Immunology, Centre for Human Systems Immunology, Department of Surgery, Duke University School of Medicine, Durham, NC, USA

Fiona Simpson, Frazer Institute, The University of Queensland, Brisbane, Queensland, Australia

Karen Slattery, Cancer Immunology Program, Peter MacCallum Cancer Centre, Melbourne, Victoria, Australia; and Sir Peter MacCallum Department of Oncology, The University of Melbourne, Parkville, Victoria, Australia

Ng Kai Soon, Institute of Molecular and Cell Biology (IMCB), Agency for Science, Technology and Research (A*STAR), Singapore, Singapore

Fernando Souza-Fonseca-Guimaraes, Faculty of Health, Medicine and Behavioural Sciences, Frazer Institute, The University of Queensland, Brisbane, Queensland, Australia

Jenna S. Theron, Frazer Institute, The University of Queensland, Brisbane, Queensland, Australia

Lamberto Torralba-Raga, Department of Cancer Immunology, Institute for Cancer Research, Oslo University Hospital, Oslo, Norway; and Precision Immunotherapy Alliance, Institute for Clinical Medicine, The University of Oslo, Oslo, Norway

Matt VanBrocklin, Department of Surgery, Huntsman Cancer Institute, University of Utah, Salt Lake City, UT, USA

James W. Wells, Faculty of Health, Medicine and Behavioural Sciences, Frazer Institute, The University of Queensland, Brisbane, Queensland, Australia; Faculty of Health, Medicine and Behavioural Sciences, Dermatology Research Centre, The University of Queensland, Brisbane, Queensland, Australia

Ian P. Wicks, Inflammation Division, Walter and Eliza Hall Institute of Medical Research, Parkville, Victoria, Australia; and Department of Medical Biology, The University of Melbourne, Melbourne, Victoria, Australia

Joe Yeong, Institute of Molecular and Cell Biology (IMCB), Agency for Science, Technology and Research (A*STAR), Singapore, Singapore; Department of Anatomical Pathology, Singapore General Hospital, Singapore, Singapore; Department of Microbiology, Singapore General Hospital, Singapore, Singapore; and Duke-NUS Medical School, Singapore, Singapore

Arabella Young, Department of Pathology, University of Utah, Salt Lake City, UT, USA; and Huntsman Cancer Institute, University of Utah, Salt Lake City, UT, USA

Liwang Zhang, Frazer Institute, The University of Queensland, Brisbane, Queensland, Australia

Limin Zhao, Frazer Institute, The University of Queensland, Brisbane, Queensland, Australia; and Department of Otolaryngology Head and Neck Surgery, Beijing TongRen Hospital, Capital Medical University, Beijing, China

Jingchen Zhou, Faculty of Health, Medicine and Behavioural Sciences, Frazer Institute, The University of Queensland, Brisbane, Queensland, Australia

Zhu Zhu, Institute of Molecular and Cell Biology (IMCB), Agency for Science, Technology and Research (A*STAR), Singapore, Singapore; and Department of Biobank, The First Affiliated Hospital of Zhengzhou University, Zhengzhou, China

Foreword

As both a doctor and a patient, I've seen what these discoveries mean in real life. The progress in immunotherapy isn't just about science, it's about people working together, refusing to give up, and believing that we can do better.

Richard Scolyer AO, Conjoint Professor (1966 to 2026) – The University of Sydney, and internationally recognised pathologist and melanoma researcher, whose personal journey with brain cancer has brought extraordinary awareness to the potential of immunotherapy.

A timely and comprehensive resource that reflects how far immunology has come since our early understanding of immune recognition — and how much promise lies ahead.

Peter C. Doherty, AC, FRS, FAA, Nobel Laureate (1996)

Frazer's Foundations of Immunotherapy showcases the best of Australian biomedical science — rigorous, collaborative, and forward-looking. It's a prime example of how mentorship and investment in emerging clinician-scientists can shape the therapies of tomorrow. Immunotherapy is one of the most transformative achievements of modern medicine. This book highlights how scientific discovery, clinical innovation, and collaboration across disciplines come together to improve human health.

Louise A. Baur AM President, Australian Academy of Health & Medical Sciences Professor & Chair of Child & Adolescent Health, University of Sydney

Immunotherapy is the result of decades of curiosity-driven research in immunology. What once seemed abstract or theoretical has now changed how we treat cancer, infection, and autoimmunity. It's a reminder that solid scientific understanding is the foundation of medical progress and that education remains our most powerful investment in the future.

Jose A. Villadangos, PhD President, Australian and New Zealand Society for Immunology Professor of Microbiology and Immunology, The University of Melbourne

Preface

The field of immunotherapy stands at the forefront of modern medicine, offering new hope for patients with diseases once considered untreatable. From cancer and infectious diseases to autoimmune and inflammatory conditions, immunotherapy has reshaped our understanding of how the immune system can be guided to restore health. *Frazer's Foundations of Immunotherapy* was conceived to capture this transformation to bring together the scientific principles, clinical insights, and translational advances that define the current era of immune-based medicine.

This book builds on the remarkable journey that began with vaccines and evolved into targeted, cellular, and gene-based interventions. It aims to provide readers with a clear framework for understanding how these therapies work, how they are developed, and how they continue to evolve. Each chapter has been written by leading researchers and clinicians who have contributed to the progress of the field. Together, their work reflects the global and collaborative nature of immunotherapy research from fundamental immunology to bedside applications.

Our intention was not merely to compile a reference, but to create a cohesive learning resource that bridges science and practice. The book is designed for students, clinicians, and scientists alike those entering the field and those seeking to expand their expertise. It may serve as a textbook for advanced coursework or as a guide for researchers and professionals navigating the rapidly changing landscape of immunotherapy.

We have structured the book to follow a logical progression: beginning with the foundations of immune modulation and surveillance, moving through disease-specific applications in cancer, infection, and autoimmunity, and concluding with emerging technologies that are shaping the future, from engineered immune cells and precision biomarkers to microbiome-based therapies. Case studies, illustrations, and reflective questions accompany the chapters to support learning and encourage critical thinking.

This project has been made possible through the contributions of many colleagues and collaborators who share a commitment to advancing immunotherapy as a discipline. We are particularly grateful to our contributing authors and to the broader research community whose discoveries continue to expand what is possible.

Our hope is that *Frazer's Foundations of Immunotherapy* will inspire the next generation of scientists, clinicians, and innovators to continue building on these foundations, ensuring that the promise of immunotherapy translates into lasting benefit for patients around the world.

Fernando S. F. Guimaraes
Associate Professor, Frazer Institute, The University of Queensland

Ian H. Frazer
Emeritus Professor, Frazer Institute, The University of Queensland

Acknowledgements

IAN H. FRAZER

I acknowledge those who encouraged me to pursue a research career in immunology, particularly Professors John Munro, Alan Munro, Ian Mackay, and Senga Whittingham for their encouragement to study immunology in the clinic as well as the lab, Professors Harald zur Hausen, Margaret Stanley, and Denise Galloway who encouraged me to focus my research on human papillomavirus and cancer, and Dr. Jian Zhou who shared his ideas about molecular bioscience and cancer.

I commend Dr. Fernando S. F. Guimaraes for persuading me that there was an urgent need for this book to guide clinicians and clinical scientists through ten minefields of the growing field of practical cancer immunology and immunotherapy.

FERNANDO S. F. GUIMARAES

I am grateful to the Australian Academy of Health and Medical Sciences for the opportunity to participate in its mentorship program, and in particular to Emeritus Professor Ian H. Frazer for his generous guidance and steady support across many aspects of my professional development as an independent group leader at the Frazer Institute. I also acknowledge the mentors who shaped my scientific path and encouraged me to pursue my research interests, including Dorly Buchi, Edvaldo Trindade, Georgia Chenevix-Trench, Jean-Marc Cavaillon, Kiarash Khosrotehrani, Minou Adib-Conquy, Nick Huntington, Paul Clarke, Gabrielle Belz, and Seth Masters.

I sincerely thank the members of my research group, past and present, whose commitment, creativity, and resilience make this work possible. I am also grateful for the financial support that has sustained my research, provided by AEA, ANZSA, Bricks & Smiles, Cooper Rice-Brading Foundation, Cure Cancer Australia with the support of Can Too, MRFF, NHMRC, NBCF, OCRF, the Queensland Children's Foundation, Richie's Rainbow Foundation, PA Research Foundation, US DoD, The Kids Cancer Project, The Tie Dye Project, Tour de Cure, Translational Research Institute, and The University of Queensland.

Editors are grateful for the support of Allie Lam, Cui Tu, Jessica Grant, Jingchen Zhou, Josh Wong, Melissa Elliott, and all chapter contributors, who have facilitated with the development of this book project.

PART

I

Foundations of Immunotherapy

CHAPTER 1

History and Development of Immunotherapies – Key Breakthroughs and Milestones, from Early Immunology to Contemporary Immunotherapy

JEAN-MARC CAVAILLON
Institut Pasteur, Paris, France

LEARNING OBJECTIVES

- Pay tribute to key authors who contributed to the understanding of the immune response, paving the ground for immunotherapy.
- Bridge preventive vaccinations to prophylactic ones.
- Describe the evolution of serotherapy to intravenous immunoglobulins and monoclonal antibodies therapies.
- Recall how non-specific stimulation by bacterial products can favour tumour regression.
- Explain why cytokines can be harnessed or neutralised to address cancer, infectious disease, and inflammatory disorders.

1.1 KEY MILESTONES IN THE HISTORY OF IMMUNOLOGY

The history of immunology extends back before the immune response itself was properly understood. Louis Pasteur (1822–1895) set up his vaccines with an erroneous view that vaccination with attenuated microbes would deprive the host's supply of essential trace nutrients necessary for their survival and growth [1]. Pasteur's close collaborators, Émile Roux (1853–1933) (Figure 1.1) and Charles Chamberland (1851–1908), noted that: '*M. Pasteur thought that in the case of fowl cholera, the non-recurrence was due to the disappearance of some substances consumed by the microbe*'. However, they recognised that immunity was an active process developed by the host, as they showed that injecting soluble substances produced by these microbes could also induce the refractory state [2].

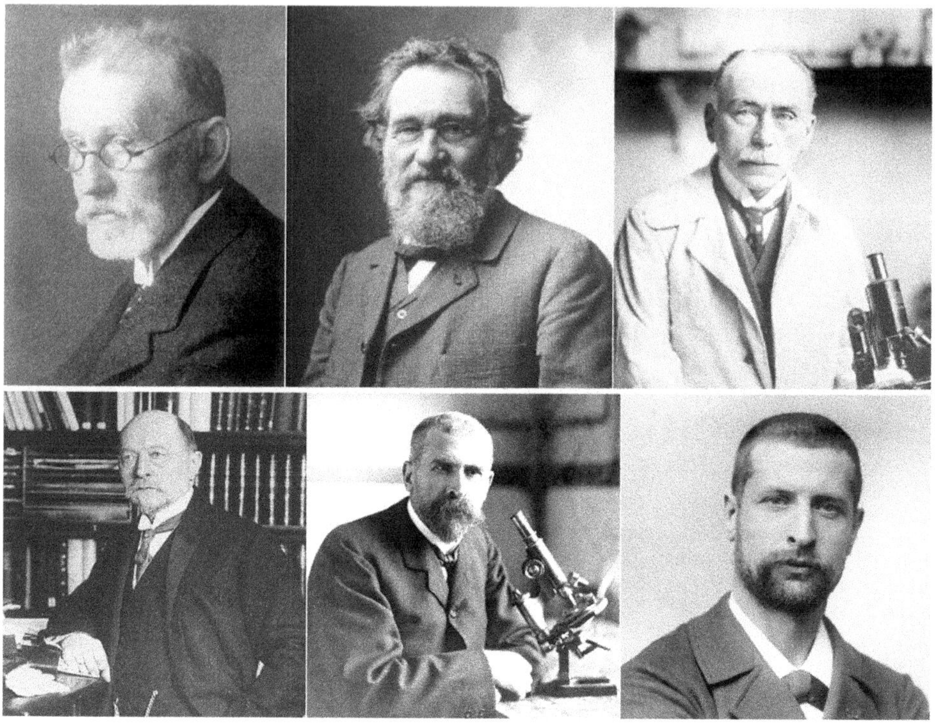

FIGURE 1.1 Some founding fathers of immunology and serotherapy. Upper row – from left to right: Paul Ehrlich, the founding father of humoral immunity. Harris & Ewing Collection / The Library of Congress / Public domain; Elie Metchnikoff, the founding father of cellular immunity. Wellcome Collection / Wikimedia Commons / CC BY 4.0; Jules Bordet, the father of the complement system, used serotherapy in Pretoria against cattle plague. Pierre Petit / Wikimedia Commons / Public domain. All three were awarded the Nobel Prize. Lower row – from left to right: Emil von Behring, the founding father of serotherapy, Nobel Prize 1901. Harris & Ewing Collection / The Library of Congress / Public domain; Émile Roux, who used horses to prepare immune sera against diphtheria (115 nominations for Nobel Prize) © Institut Pasteur; Alexandre Yersin, who discovered *Yersinia pestis* and used immune sera against plague in China. Wellcome Collection / Wikimedia Commons / CC BY 4.0.

The foundations of humoral immunity were laid by Paul Ehrlich (1854–1915) (Figure 1.1) by his discovery of antibodies which awarded him a Nobel Prize in 1908 [3]. Although Ehrlich is credited to have demonstrated the transfer of protective immunity from pregnant mothers to their newborns in 1892 [4], an earlier demonstration occurred in 1883. Hippolyte Rossignol (1837–1919), although initially very sceptical of Louis Pasteur's anthrax vaccine, welcomed his demonstration in the open field on his farm in Pouilly-Le-Fort. He reported that the immunity provided by the anthrax vaccine was transmissible from mother to foetus [5]. Ehrlich also coined the word 'complement' in 1899 [6] to describe the bactericidal capacity of the blood discovered in 1886 by the Hungarian physician and professor of epidemiology, Josef von Fodor (1843–1901) [7]. Later, Belgian medical doctor Jules Bordet (1870–1961) (Figure 1.1) further deciphered the complement system [8] and received the Nobel

Prize in 1919 [9]. Bordet, working in the laboratory of Elie Metchnikoff (1845–1916) (Figure 1.1), also investigated the relationship between the complement system and macrophages and described the process of opsonisation, a word later coined in 1903 by Sir Edward Almroth Wright (1861–1947) [10]. The identification of antibodies as immunoglobulins was discovered in 1959–1961 by Rodney Porter (1917–1985) and Gerald M. Edelman (1924–2014) [11, 12], a discovery that was recognised in 1972 with the Nobel Prize. The characterisation of the genetic mechanisms that allow antibody diversity by Susumu Tonegawa (1939–) in 1976 [13] was also awarded the Nobel Prize in 1987. Early attempts to identify the cellular origin of antibodies led to a conclusion that was later found to be false. Florence Rena Sabin (1871–1953) was a pioneering scientist who achieved many groundbreaking firsts: she was the first woman to hold a full professorship at Johns Hopkins School of Medicine, the first woman to direct a department in medical research at the Rockefeller Institute, and in 1925, the first female member of the National Academy of Sciences. In 1939, she claimed that macrophages were the source of antibodies [14]. In 1947, another woman, Astrid Fagraeus (1913–1997) from the Karolinska Institute, correctly identified plasma cells as the source of antibodies [15].

The study of cellular immunity started with the identification of blood cells. In 1674, a Dutch draper, Antoni van Leeuwenhoek (1632–1723), was the first to observe a drop of blood under a microscope and discovered red blood cells [16]. During the 18th century, two French doctors reported the presence of white blood cells. Joseph Lieutaud (1703–1780), physician of King Louis XVI, called them '*globuli albicantes*' [17] and Jean-Baptiste de Sénac (1693–1770), a chemist and a cardiologist, referred to them as 'white globules', which he had observed in both blood and pus [18]. This finding was further advanced in 1845 by William Addison (1802–1881), who first described the process of diapedesis: '*Colourless blood cells are deposited all over the interior of the vessels; [...] and at length pass into the tissue; [...] These facts are all independent of any orifices, rupture or pores in the vessels, allowing the escape of cells*' [19]. In 1865, Johann Sigismund Schultze (1825–1874) was the first to describe the main types of white blood cells which correspond to the lymphocytes, monocytes, eosinophils, and neutrophils we recognise today [20]. Although Paul Ehrlich is best known for his work in humoral immunology, he also made several key contributions to cellular immunity. With a background in chemistry, Ehrlich began his scientific career as a histologist, applying chemical dyes to stain cells selectively and was the first to identify eosinophils [21]. Metchnikoff later recognised this achievement, stating that '*The best proven result was provided by Mr. Ehrlich, who showed that the eosinophil leukocytes are mainly produced by bone marrow*'. Ehrlich's research also led to the discovery of mast cells, further enriching the understanding of immune cell types [22]. Nevertheless, Elie Metchnikoff is the one often credited as the founder of cellular immunity [23]. In 1882, he observed the process of phagocytosis by macrophages and microphages (neutrophils) and understood and demonstrated its function in defence against pathogens [24, 25]. In addition, Metchnikoff discovered the process of efferocytosis and described specific immune cell types including alveolar macrophages and 'neuronophages' (microglial cells). In 1908, both Ehrlich and Metchnikoff received the Nobel Prize for their works. Macrophages constitute a heterogeneous population, depending on the tissues in which they reside [26]. The distinction between B- and T-lymphocytes was achieved by Max Cooper (1933–) in 1965 [27], and their collaboration for antibody production was described by Jacques F. Miller (1931–) in 1968 [28]. Specific cytotoxic T cells were reported by Jean-Charles Cerottini (1938–) in 1970 [29], and the first subsets of T cells (Th1 and Th2) were mentioned in 1986 by Tim Mosmann (1949–) and Robert L. Coffman (1948–) [30]. Dendritic cells were discovered in 1973 by Ralph Steinman (1943–2011), who was awarded the Nobel Prize in 2011 [31]. Natural killer (NK) cells were first described in 1975 by Rolf Kiessling, Eva Klein, and Hans Wigzell [32]. Identified as non-T, non-B lymphocytes with the capability for 'natural' cytotoxicity, NK cells belong to a group of immune cells known as innate lymphoid cells which also exist as subsets [33].

1.2 VARIOLATION AND VACCINATION

Variolation and vaccination are not immunotherapeutic approaches *per se*, although the famous anti-rabies vaccine developed by Louis Pasteur was used therapeutically, since it was injected after the patient had been bitten by a rabid animal, and therefore administered after the infection [34]. Likewise, cancer vaccines are employed as immunotherapies [35].

To prevent smallpox, variolation was set up in China in 1014, and later introduced in Turkey (1718) and the United Kingdom (1721) by Lady Mary Wortley Montagu (1689–1762), writer and poet, and wife of the British ambassador in Constantinople. Remarkably, a similar approach was used to prevent syphilis, called 'syphilisation'. This was first suggested in Norway by Carl Wilhelm Boeck (1808–1875) and in France by Joseph-Alexandre Auzias-Turenne (1812–1870). Amusingly, the latter's book was kept hidden in a drawer of his desk by Pasteur. In 1796, Edward Jenner (1749–1823) documented his first vaccination against smallpox in a manuscript which he submitted to the Royal Society; however, the report was returned unread. Let's mention the names of those 'famous' doctors who failed to realise the importance of this discovery that would save millions of people: Joseph Banks (1743–1820), John Southey (1765–1819), and Sir Everard Home (1756–1832)! Richard Dunning (1761–1851), a friend of Jenner, coined the word 'vaccination' in his book published in 1800 [36]. Henri Toussaint (1847–1890) and Pierre-Victor Galtier (1846–1908) were the precursors of Louis Pasteur's vaccines against anthrax and rabies, respectively. In addition, Pasteur prepared a vaccine against fowl cholera and pig erysipelas. From 1880 to the severe acute respiratory syndrome-coronavirus 2 (SARS-CoV-2) vaccines developed in 2020, numerous infectious diseases have been prevented thanks to the advancement of vaccines (Figure 1.2). Only two vaccines have received a Nobel Prize: in 1951, the yellow fever vaccine developed by Max Theiler (1899–1972) and in 2023, the messenger ribonucleic acid (mRNA) vaccine against SARS-CoV-2 developed by Katalin Kariko (1955–) and Drew Weissman (1959–). Among the leaders in the field of vaccination, let's mention Maurice Hilleman (1919–2005) who was responsible for the development of 40 different vaccines; among them, 8 are a part of the 14 vaccines regularly recommended in immunisation programmes in the United States. Estimates suggest that these vaccines prevent nearly eight million deaths annually, leading many to regard Hilleman as the scientist who has saved the most lives.

Cancer vaccines were first reported in 1902, in Germany, when Ernst von Leyden (1832–1910) and Ferdinand Blumenthal (1870–1941) used an autologous tumour cell suspension as a vaccine to treat patients with advanced metastatic cancer [37]. In 1959,

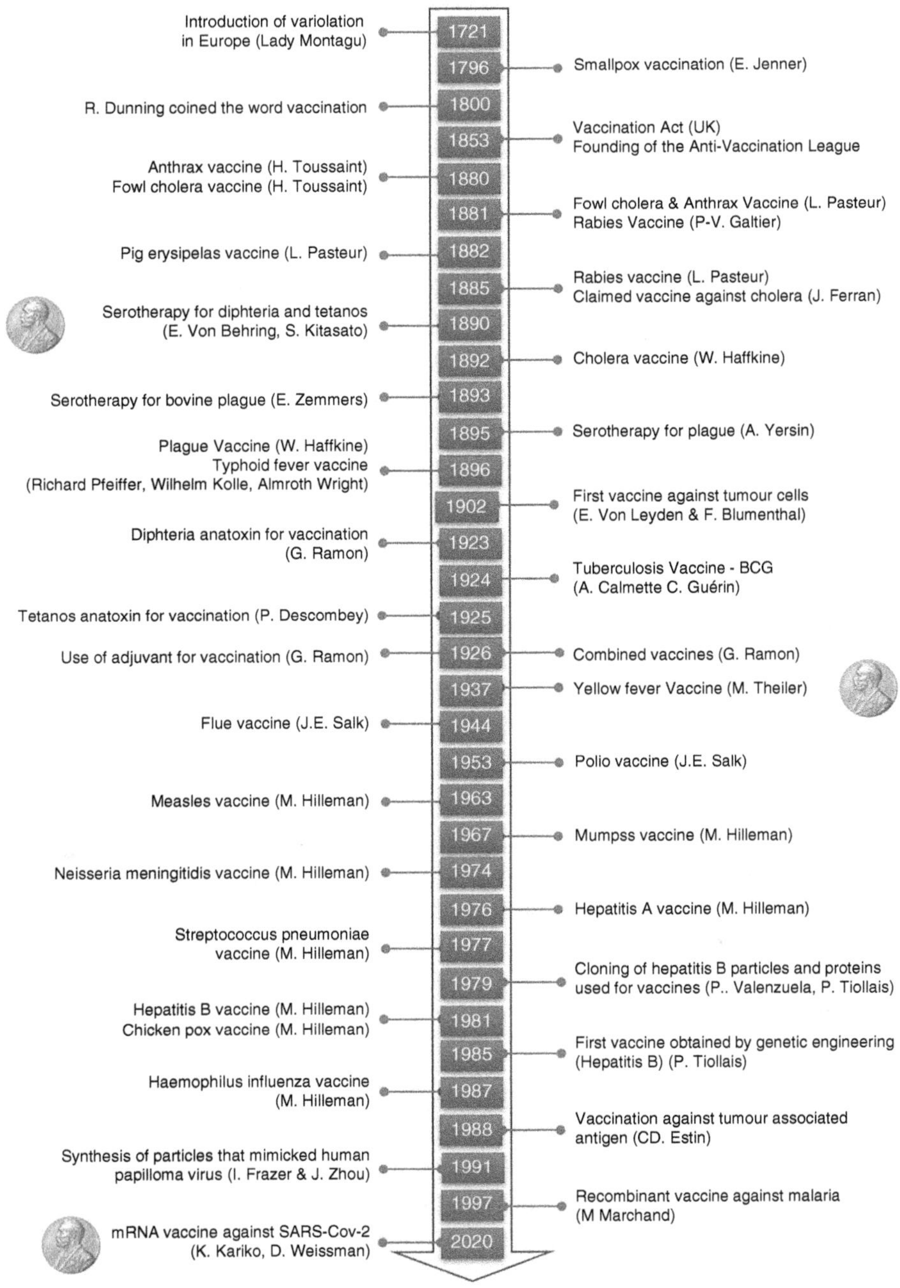

FIGURE 1.2 Timeline of immunoprophylaxis and immunotherapies by vaccination and serotherapies.

the husband-and-wife team of Ruth M. Graham (1917–1978) and John B. Graham published a cancer vaccine study on 114 gynaecologic cancer patients treated with tumour lysate associated with Freund's adjuvant [38]. In 1965, it was established that tumour cells could express specific antigens [39]. Accordingly, cancer vaccines could be designed to target tumour-associated antigens. Such an approach was achieved in 1988 using a recombinant vaccinia virus expressing human melanoma-associated antigen [40]. In the mid-1990s, tumour-specific glycopeptides, or tumour-associated carbohydrates such as gangliosides, were used in cancer vaccine formulations [41], and monoclonal antibodies (mAbs) targeting these structures were employed [42]. Of note, vaccines against certain viruses such as hepatitis B virus [43] or human papilloma virus [44] can prevent the occurrence of liver cancer and gynaecologic cancers, respectively.

1.3 SEROTHERAPY

By the late 1800s, diphtheria, nicknamed 'the child-strangling angel', killed thousands of children. A total of 1,639 children died of diphtheria in Paris alone in 1890. That same year, in Berlin, Emil von Behring (1854–1917) (Figure 1.1) and his Japanese colleague Shibasaburo Kitasato (1853–1931) showed that immune serum against the respective toxins protected against diphtheria and tetanus [45] (Figure 1.2). Later, Adolf Baginsky (1843–1918), a paediatrician who also served as Freud's mentor and established the 'Kaiser und Kaiserin Friedrich Kinderkrankenhaus' in Berlin, documented the earliest clinical trial involving diphtheria. In this study, 220 children with diphtheria were treated with intraperitoneal injections of immune serum, resulting in a 77% recovery rate [46]. In 1901, Emil von Behring earned the first Nobel Prize in Physiology and Medicine for this discovery. In France, Emile Roux, who together with Alexandre Yersin (1863–1943) (Figure 1.1) had identified the diphtheria toxin, was among the first to employ horses for producing immune serum. In 1894, working with Louis Martin (1864–1946) at the Institut Pasteur and Auguste Chaillou (1866–1915) at Necker Hospital, he reported a study treating 300 children which showed a 50% reduction in mortality [47]. This success received significant attention in the press, and 'Le Figaro' initiated a fundraising campaign that improved the poor financial status of the institute at that time. During World War I, Institut Pasteur produced a huge quantity of immune sera against diphtheria and tetanus. By the end of the war, 1,462 horses contributed to the production of 600,000 vials/month.

Serotherapy has also been applied to patients with plague. In 1894, Alexandre Yersin was sent to Hong Kong to investigate the ongoing plague epidemic. On 20 June of that year, he successfully identified and isolated the bacterium responsible, later named *Yersinia pestis* [48]. Upon returning to France, Yersin collaborated with Amédée Borrel (1867–1936) and Albert Calmette (1863–1933) to develop an anti-plague serum using horses [49]. During a subsequent outbreak in Guangzhou, China, in 1896, Yersin travelled there to administer the serum, achieving successful treatment outcomes [50]. Paul-Louis Simond (1858–1947) went to India to treat patients with the anti-plague immune serum [51].

Another successful treatment was achieved with serotherapy to treat cattle plague (Rinderpest). The disease started to spread to Africa from Egypt in 1875. By 1896, it had reached South Africa. In 1897, Robert Koch (1843–1910), the famous German microbiologist, who had isolated the bacillus of tuberculosis (1882), joined

Kimberley. He proposed a treatment with bile from convalescent animals. His colleague, Paul Kohlstock (1861–1901), applied the suggested treatment in Namibia, resulting in the death of 2,700 animals among the 6,200 treated livestock. Meanwhile, Institut Pasteur sent two of its collaborators to Pretoria, the Belgian medical doctor Jules Bordet and the Polish scientist Jan Danysz (1860–1928). There, they joined the Swiss veterinarian Arnold Theiler (1867–1936), the father of Max Theiler, who, as previously mentioned, developed the yellow fever vaccine [9]. All three of them decided to apply the serotherapy advocated by the Latvian microbiologist Eižens Zemmers (1843–1906) who had extensive expertise on cattle plague [52]. The treatment was a success, and amusingly it was referred to as 'the methods of the French doctors', even though none of them were French! Bordet and Danysz were asked by the South African government to stay to solve the problem of horse plague. However, for that specific disease, the team failed to find an appropriate treatment. Of note, on 28 June 2011, the Food and Agriculture Organization (FAO) and the World Organization for Animal Health (WOAH) declared that bovine plague was eradicated from the planet. This is the first animal disease to have been eradicated (like smallpox for humans in 1979).

1.4 ANTI-TUMOUR ACTIVITY OF BACTERIA, BACTERIAL TOXINS, AND VIRUSES

The idea that bacterial infections and bacterial-derived products could boost the immune system non-specifically and then enhance its ability to control tumour cell growth emerged when two German physicians, Wilhelm Busch (1826–1881) and Friedrich Fehleisen (1854–1924), independently noticed tumour regression in patients with erysipelas infection in 1866 and later. Two years later, Busch deliberately injected erysipelas into a patient with cancer and observed a subsequent reduction in the tumour's size. In 1882, Fehleisen replicated this approach and reported similar outcomes. The following year, he recognised *Streptococcus pyogenes* as the bacterium responsible for erysipelas [53, 54].

In 1891, William B. Coley (1862–1936) (Figure 1.3), a surgeon at the New York Cancer Hospital, began treating his cancer patients with *S. pyogenes*. He reported his first cases in 1893 [55]. He found that, in most patients, inducing erysipelas was extremely challenging, and among the few who developed an active infection, it was incredibly difficult to cure. In two cases, death resulted from widespread septicaemia rather than the patients' underlying cancers [56].

Coley later treated 140 patients with inoperable sarcoma using 'toxins' from both *S. pyogenes* and *Bacillus prodigiosus* (i.e. *Serratia marcescens*); these were most likely the supernatants of cultures from these Gram-positive and Gram-negative bacteria. For 24 cases he obtained partial regression of the tumour and complete regression for 16 patients, including one chondrosarcoma and one osteosarcoma [57] (Figure 1.4). The effects of the toxins lasted from 7 months to 6 years. Dr. Coley was viewed with suspicion by many surgeons, and his observations were largely ignored for the next 25 years, possibly because the mechanism of action of his toxins was unknown. He believed the cure was possible because sarcoma was of microparasitic or infectious origin. It was only in 1909 that Paul Ehrlich hypothesised that host immune defences could prevent the development of cancers [58], a concept now known as immunosurveillance. This concept was proposed in 1957 by Frank Macfarlane

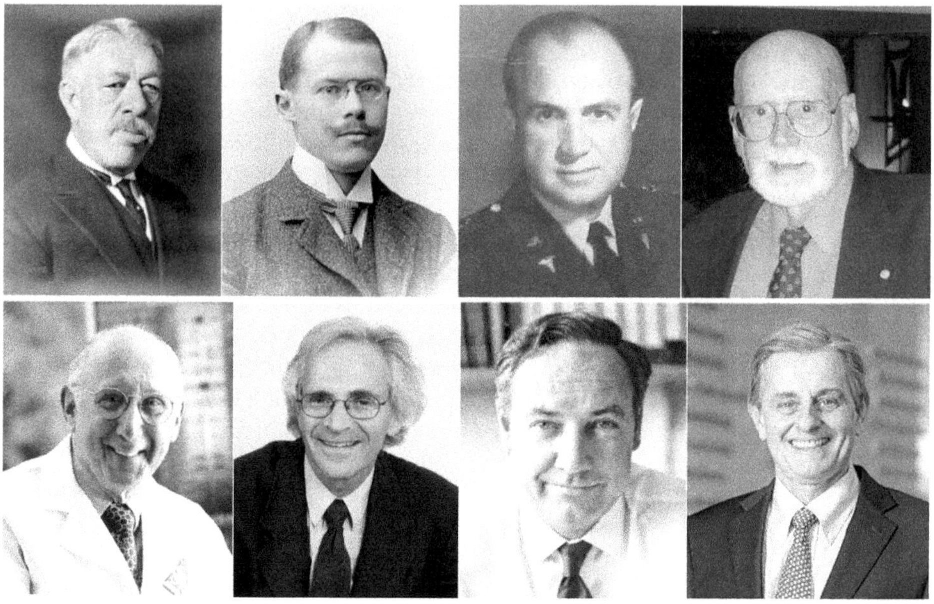

FIGURE 1.3 Some founding fathers of immunotherapy. Upper row – from left to right: William Coley (bacterial toxin to fight sarcoma). *Wellcome Collection / Wikimedia Commons / CC BY 4.0*; Israel Holmgren (BCG to treat cancer). *Gösta Florman / Västergötlands Museum / Public domain*; Ogden Carr Bruton (human immunoglobulin to treat people who have inherited antibody deficiencies). *U.S. Federal Government / Wikimedia Commons / Public domain*; Edward Donnall Thomas (anti-CD20 mAb to fight B-cell lymphoma). *Ca.garcia.s / Wikimedia Commons / CC BY-SA 4.0*. Lower row – from left to right: Steven A Rosenberg (IL-2, LAK cells, TIL for cancer therapy); Sir Marc Feldmann (anti-TNF in rheumatoid arthritis); Donald Metcalf (the discoverer of the colony-stimulating factors). *Wikimedia Commons / Public domain*; Kevin Tracey (the vagal nerve control of inflammation). *Mike Denora / Wikimedia Commons / CC BY-SA 4.0*.

Burnet (1889–1985) [59], who was awarded the Nobel Prize in 1960 for his studies on immune tolerance, jointly with Sir Peter Brian Medawar (1915–1987). It was not until 1943 that Murray J. Shear (1899–1983) recognised that the anti-tumour activity of *S. marcescens* was caused by its endotoxin (lipopolysaccharide, LPS) [60]. Regarding the anti-tumour activity of *S. pyogenes* supernatant, it has been proposed that streptococcal exotoxins are the active molecules. Known as superantigens, they could activate cytotoxic T cells, as staphylococcal superantigens do, and thereby contribute to the anti-tumour effect [61].

Attenuated *Mycobacterium bovis* in the vaccine against tuberculosis prepared by Albert Calmette (1863–1933) and Camille Guérin (1872–1961), known as the 'bacille de Calmette et Guérin' (BCG), is another bacterium used to fight cancer. The idea was derived from an observation made in 1928 by Raymond Pearl (1879–1940), working at Johns Hopkins Hospital in Baltimore, who discovered through autopsy studies that cancer occurred less frequently in individuals with *Mycobacterium tuberculosis* [62]. In 1935–1936, Israel Frithiofsson Holmgren (1871–1961) (Figure 1.3) in Stockholm administered BCG vaccine to patients with cancer [63]. He delivered

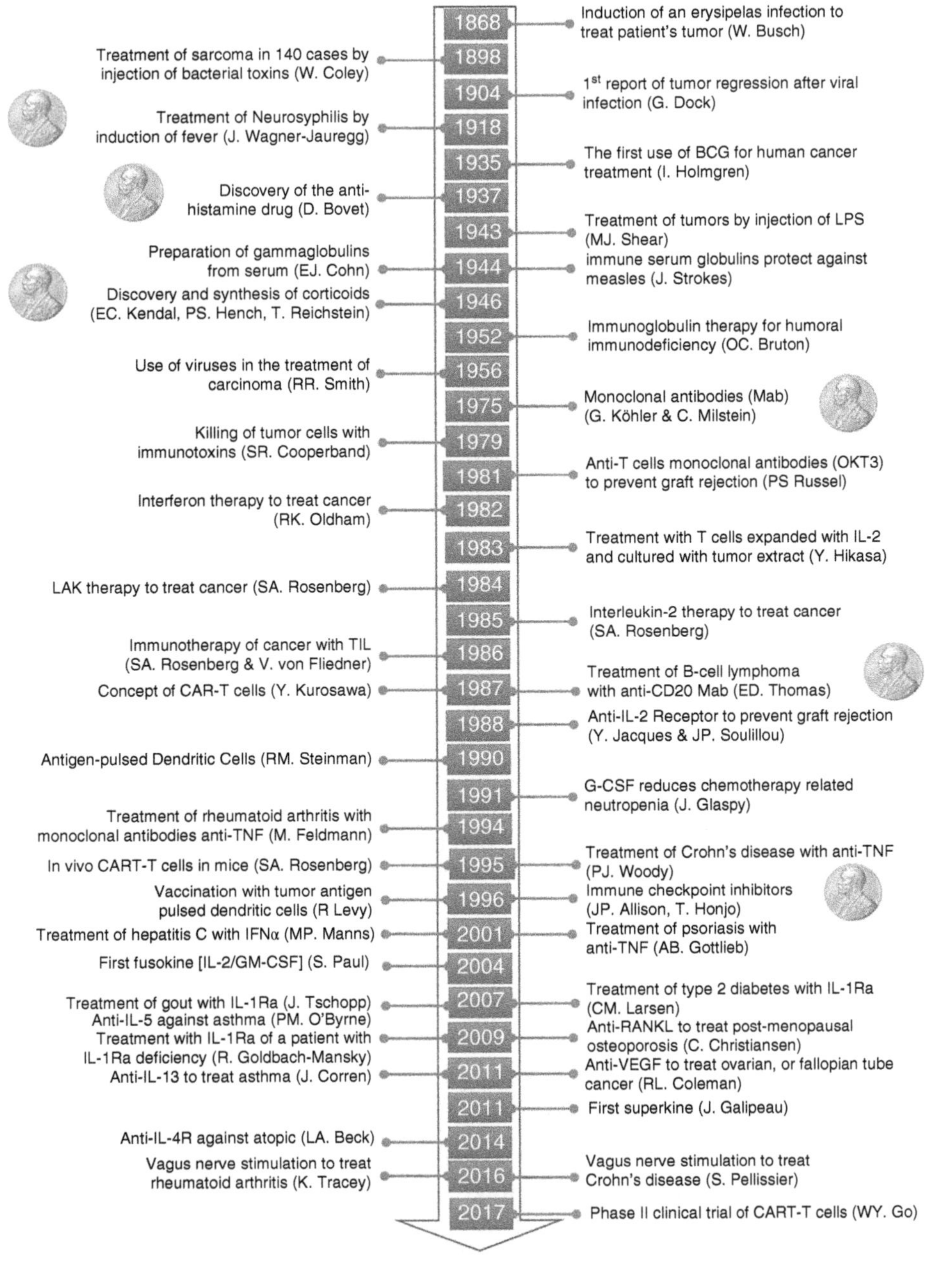

FIGURE 1.4 Timeline of the main achievements in immunotherapy.

intravenous injections of BCG to 33 individuals, most of whom had stomach cancer. One patient received as many as 37 injections, amounting to a total of 2.68 mg BCG over the course of more than a year. All patients developed fever accompanied by general malaise following treatment; however, some showed improvement in their overall condition. A similar approach was undertaken in the Philippines in the early

1960s for patients with advanced malignant disease [64] and in France in the late 1960s to treat patients with acute lymphoblastic leukaemia [65]. In 1976, Alvaro Morales (1938–) was the first to administer BCG to treat bladder cancer and reported favourable effects in reducing bladder cancer recurrence [66]. Since then, bladder cancer is still being treated with BCG.

Bacterial toxins have been engineered to offer specific tools to kill tumour cells. Diphtheria toxin or ricin (a plant toxin) has been chemically linked to purified antitumour antibodies [67] and mAbs [68]; called immunotoxins, these constructs were reported in 1976 and 1981, respectively. In 1987, another chimeric molecule combining diphtheria toxin and interleukin-2 (IL-2) was designed to target IL-2 receptor-positive cells [69] and treat cutaneous T-cell lymphoma (Denileukin diftitox). This treatment was approved by the US Food and Drug Administration (FDA) in 1999. Among other toxins employed to target tumour cells, let's mention the work of Calmette in 1933 who employed cobra venom [70].

Not surprisingly, transient improvements have also been observed in cancer patients following viral infections. The first report was published in 1904 [71], but the observation had previously been made on 29 December 1896, in a woman with leukaemia. She was the patient of a fascinating doctor, George Dock (1860–1951), when he worked at the University of Michigan Medical School. Dock wrote many articles, including some on Jenner and on vaccination. His oral notes for the students during his clinical sessions, recorded with a stenographer, resulted in 6,800 pages, gathered in 17 volumes. He noticed that '*two weeks after an attack of what was probably influenza, the leukocytes were found reduced from 367,070 to 7500, falling to 4775 in two weeks more [...] The spleen was much smaller; the liver became smaller later*'. Two months later, the disease was back, and the patient passed away 18 months after the initial observation. In the early 1950s, few reports were published on the beneficial consequences of different types of viral infection on the growth of the tumours [72–76]. A fascinating case was reported in 1950 [77]: in May 1940, a primary lesion was removed from a 32-year-old woman with malignant melanoma. Two years later, three additional cutaneous melanotic nodules were removed. Following a dog bite in September 1943, she underwent a course of 14 rabies vaccine injections. By April 1948, two further melanotic nodules were excised, but since then, there had been no further evidence of recurrence. The author indicates that on purpose, he voluntarily vaccinated 12 of his patients with the rabies vaccine with some beneficial effects. Nowadays, one refers to oncolytic viruses while the concept of virotherapy emerged [78].

1.5 IMMUNOGLOBULIN, ANTIBODIES, AND MONOCLONAL ANTIBODIES

1.5.1 IvIg

Intravenous immunoglobulins (IvIg) are the heirs of successful serotherapy. In 1944, the purification of serum gamma globulins from human plasma was achieved by Edwin Joseph Cohn (1892–1953) [79]. In the same year, Joseph Stokes (1896–1972) demonstrated that immune serum globulin (ISG) could either prevent or lessen the severity of measles in children exposed during outbreaks. He further noted that patients who had already begun to show symptoms appeared to respond better to higher ISG doses and proposed that intravenous administration at an early stage of infection might offer therapeutic benefit [80]. In 1952, Ogden Carr Bruton (1908–2003) (Figure 1.3), chief of paediatrics at Walter Reed Army Hospital (Washington), used human immunoglobulin to treat people who had inherited antibody deficiencies [81]. The first commercially available IvIg was developed in 1962 by digesting ISG with pepsin. The main component of this product was the F(ab') fragment [82]. Nowadays, IvIg therapies are prepared from a pool of polyclonal immunoglobulins (antibodies) from the plasma of thousands of healthy donors. Commercial IvIg preparations contain a wide repertoire of antibody specificities, enabling neutralisation of a broad range of antigens. They contain >95% immunoglobulin G (IgG), <2.5% immunoglobulin A (IgA), and negligible amount of immunoglobulin M (IgM). They are now far less frequently used to treat infectious diseases despite a meta-analysis suggesting that their use in sepsis could be beneficial [83]. In contrast, another meta-analysis failed to demonstrate that IvIg were of any benefit when employed in COVID-19 patients [84]. They continue to be used to treat primary humoral immunodeficiency, haematologic disorders, neurologic disorders, and autoimmune disorders [85].

1.5.2 Anti-immune Cells and Anti-tumour Cells

mAbs are widely employed for various types of immunotherapies. They were conceived by Georges Köhler (1946–1995) and César Milstein (1927–2002) [86] in 1975. mAbs are produced using hybridoma technology that fuses together myeloma cells (to give cellular immortality), and antibody-producing B cells (from which they acquire the antibody specificity). Köhler and Milstein's paper has been cited more than 15,000 times (July 2025). Both received the Nobel Prize in 1984. Of note, the term 'hybridoma' was suggested by Leonard A. Herzenberg (1934–2012) during a sabbatical in César Milstein's laboratory in 1976/1977 [87]. In 1969, Herzenberg developed the fluorescence-activated cell sorting (FACS) machine [88], while flow cytometry was invented by Mack Fulwyler (1936–2001) in 1965 [89].

The first mAbs were fully murine, resulting in the generation of human antibodies targeting the mouse IgG in patients. Thus, different technologies have since been applied to humanise mAbs using transgenic mice [90, 91] or phage display [92], making it possible to now generate fully human mAbs [93].

In 1981, OKT3 (*Muromonab-CD3*), a mouse IgG2a, became the first mAb to be applied clinically for the treatment and prevention of renal allograft rejection, and it was approved by the FDA in 1986. It was a pan-T-cell mAb, proposed by Paul Snowden Russell (1925–), professor of Surgery at the Massachusetts General Hospital (MGH) [94]. Of note, the museum at MGH has been named in honour of Paul S. Russell. Alongside Russell in 1987, Edward Donnall Thomas (1920–2012) (Figure 1.3), professor at the University of Washington, produced the anti-CD20 mAb, a specific B-cell marker which has been used to treat individuals with B-cell lymphoma with great success [95], and was the first mAb to be approved for the treatment of cancer by the FDA in November 1997 (rituximab). Thomas received the Nobel Prize in Physiology and Medicine in 1990 for his work on transplants and immune rejection mechanisms. The major role of these mAbs, once on their target cells, is to bind via their Fc moiety to the Fc-receptor on NK cells and macrophages, triggering target cell death by antibody-dependent cellular cytotoxicity (ADCC). Interestingly, glycosylation of the Fc moiety was later proposed to offer a modified mAb with enhanced affinity for receptor binding [96]. This new mAb (obinutuzumab) has now supplanted rituximab, with slightly higher efficacy [97]. Among the early mAbs used for human therapy, let's mention the anti-CD25 (IL-2Rα subunit) mAb, reported in 1988 by Yannick Jacques (1950–) and Jean-Paul Soulillou (1944–) to prevent kidney graft rejection. This anti-CD25 mAb (daclizumab) was the first humanised antibody to be approved by the FDA in 1997 for renal transplant [98, 99].

1.5.3 Immune Checkpoint Inhibitors

CTLA-4 (cytotoxic T-lymphocyte-associated protein-4) was discovered concomitantly by two independent groups in 1995 [100, 101]. CTLA-4 is constitutively expressed on regulatory T cells (Treg) and functions as an inhibitory signal upon interacting with CD80 or CD86 on the antigen-presenting cell's surface. Programmed cell death protein 1 (PD-1) was discovered in 1992 [102]. PD-1 is displayed by effector T cells, and engagement with its ligands, PD-L1 and PD-L2, inhibits immune responses. PD-L1 is typically found on activated T- and B cells, macrophages, dendritic cells, and some epithelial cells, especially during inflammation. Tumour cells can also express PD-L1 as an adaptive mechanism to evade anti-tumour immunity. mAbs aimed to neutralise CTLA-4, PD-1, or PD-L1 are called immune checkpoint inhibitors and were shown in the early 2010s to be a potential treatment for certain cancers [103, 104]. The FDA's approval of the CTLA-4 inhibitor occurred in 2011, followed by approval of PD-1 inhibitors in 2014. James P. Allison (1948–) and Tasuku Honjo (1942–) received the 2018 Nobel Prize in Medicine for discovering cancer treatments that inhibit negative regulators of the immune system.

1.6 HARNESSING AND TARGETING CYTOKINES

1.6.1 A Brief History of Cytokines

Although the discovery of type I interferon (IFN) is often attributed to Alick Isaacs (1921–1967) and Jean Lindenmann (1924–2015) in 1957 [105], the truth is that this discovery was owed to Yasuichi Nagano (1906–1998) and Yasuhiko Kojima (1928–) in 1954 [106]. Their contribution was likely overlooked because of two mistakes: they published in a French-speaking journal and failed to create a neologism. IFNα was the first human cytokine to be cloned in 1980 [107] and the first human recombinant cytokine to be used in cancer patients in 1982 [108, 109] (Figure 1.5). The second cytokine to be discovered was the macrophage migration inhibitory factor (MIF) in 1966 by Barry Bloom (1937–2026) [110]. Bax69, an anti-MIF mAb, has entered Phase I/II clinical trials focusing on cancer treatment. Because MIF was not exclusively produced by lymphocytes and could also be secreted by fibroblasts, Stanley Cohen coined the word 'cytokine' in 1974 to replace the word 'lymphokine' [111]. The discovery of IL-1 started with the efforts of Valy Menkin (1901–1960) in 1944 to identify the endogenous molecular substance responsible for fever [112]. However, his isolated 'pyrexin' from inflammatory exudates appeared to be contaminated with endotoxin [113]. The endogenous pyrogen was finally isolated in 1953 by Ivan L. Bennet Jr. (1922–1990) and Paul Beeson (1908–2006) [114] and two years later by Elisha Atkins (1921–2005) and W. Barry Wood Jr. (1910–1971) [115]. When it

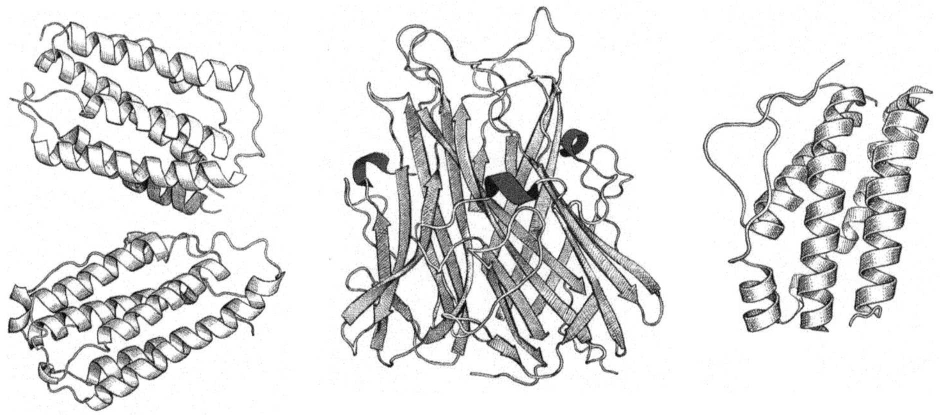

FIGURE 1.5 Cytokines used as recombinant molecules for their own properties to boost immune defences or as target of monoclonal antibodies to prevent their inflammatory properties. From left to right: Type I interferon (IFN) discovered in 1954 by Nagano, Y., & Kojima, Y.; Tumour necrosis factor (TNF) discovered in 1975 by Carswell EA, Old LJ and colleagues; and interleukin-2 (IL-2) discovered in 1976 by Morgan DA, Ruscetti FW, & Gallo R. Courtesy of Jingchen Zhou.

appeared that the endogenous pyrogen was identical to other identified molecules (namely, osteoclast activating factor, haemopoietin-1, catabolin, lymphocyte activating factor, epidermal cell-derived thymocyte activating factor), it was named 'IL-1'. In 1984, human IL-1 was first cloned by Charles Dinarello (1943–) [116] and murine IL-1 by Steven B. Mizel (1948–) [117]. While fever is an effective component of the immune response against infectious agents, inducing fever has also been used as a therapeutic approach to treat neurosyphilis. Julius Wagner-Jauregg (1857–1940) inoculated malaria to induce fever, followed by treatment with quinine. He claimed to have treated more than 150 patients using this method. In total, pyrotherapy cured about half of the patients who received the treatment, but approximately 15% died from malaria. Nevertheless, he received the Nobel Prize in 1927! IL-2 was discovered in 1976 in the laboratory of Robert Gallo (1937–) [118] (Figure 1.5). To date, there are now 41 identified ILs.

Another family of cytokines is that of tumour necrosis factor (TNF) (Figure 1.5). As mentioned earlier, LPS and BCG are microbial substances able to boost immunity against cancer cells. In 1975, TNF was identified in the serum of mice injected with BCG and LPS [119]. Ten years later, Bruce Beutler (1957–), who was awarded the Nobel Prize in 2011, showed that TNF was identical to cachectin, a molecule responsible for cachexia, isolated in the laboratory of Anthony Cerami (1940–) [120].

Among cytokines, there is a family of chemo-attractant molecules, which were named chemokines in 1992. In 1987, IL-8 was one of the first chemokines to have been characterised and extensively studied by Joost Oppenheim (1934–2022) [121].

To end this brief historical background, let's mention the amazing contribution of Donald Metcalf (1929–2014) (Figure 1.3) in Australia. Between 1965 and 1985, Metcalf's group characterised and isolated four distinct colony-stimulating factors (CSFs) which stimulate differentiation, growth, and other activities of macrophages

(M-CSF), granulocytes (G-CSF), both granulocytes and macrophages (GM-CSF), and the pluripotent multi-CSF (IL-3) [122]. The gene for GM-CSF was later cloned by Metcalf's team.

1.6.2 Cytokines Used to Restore or Boost the Immune System

Cytokines are often classified as proinflammatory or anti-inflammatory. This Yin-Yang view is far too simplistic [123] and may help to explain the side effects, or even the toxic effects, associated with their use or neutralisation. Several cytokines (IL-2, G-CSF, GM-CSF, IFN-α, IFN-β, IFN-γ, etc.) are already approved as disease therapeutics, and many other cytokines are being investigated for their anti-cancer, anti-microbial, and immunomodulatory properties in preclinical studies and trials.

IFNα was the first available recombinant cytokine and the first to be used in clinical trials in 1982, surprisingly not for viral infection, but instead in cancer patients [108, 109]. IL-2 was cloned in 1983 [124], and the first *in vivo* treatments were performed in 1984 for HIV patients [125], in 1985 in murine models of cancer [126], in 1986 in patients with hairy cell leukaemia [127], and in 1987 in patients with different types of malignancy [128]. G-CSF has been employed since the late 1980s to boost haematopoiesis to increase the number of haematopoietic stem cells for auto-transplantation [129] or to enhance haematopoiesis altered by chemotherapies during cancer treatment [130]. GM-CSF has been similarly employed, but because of its stimulatory properties, it has also been used to restore the altered immune status observed in sepsis patients [131]. A similar result was achieved in 1997 with IFN-γ [132], in 2012 with IL-7 [133], and in 2019 with anti-PD-1 [134]. Given the Yin-Yang properties of cytokines, the fact that the concept of immunosuppression in sepsis patients is largely based on analyses of circulating leucocytes (which represent only a small percentage of the total immune cells), and the compartmentalisation of the immune response during sepsis [135], we cautioned against the risks of globally boosting the entire immune cell population [136]. In fact, clinical trials of sepsis patients with IFN-γ [137] or IL-7 [138] had to be discontinued early due to safety concerns.

Despite its anti-tumour properties, TNF is difficult to use since it is a major proinflammatory cytokine. Nevertheless, it has been employed with melphalan, a chemotherapeutic medication in an isolated limb perfusion for locally advanced limb sarcomas. One hundred patients were treated, and a 36% complete remission rate was obtained [139].

When scientists wish to be smarter than nature, they invent new cytokines, named either superkines or fusokines. The concept emerged in 2012 when scientists from Zurich and Stanford universities engineered a CD25-independent version of IL-2 [140]. CD25 is the α-chain of the IL-2 receptor, which also contains a β- and a γ-chain. α-, β-, and γ-chains are displayed on Treg but cytotoxic $CD8^+$ T cells and NK cells only express β- and γ-chains. Because Tregs are negative regulators of the immune system, and CD8+ and NK cells are important players in anti-tumour immunity, it made sense to generate a superkine that fails to activate Tregs but stimulates CD8+ and NK cells. This is the role of ALKS-4230 (Nemvaleukine), a fusion protein combining IL-2 with the extracellular domain of IL-2Rα [141]. Clinical trials are now ongoing to study the molecule alone and in combination with other anti-cancer strategies. Other IL-2 superkines are under investigation including few pegylated

IL-2 (e.g. Bempegaldesleukin). Fusokines are engineered proteins created by joining two distinct cytokines into a single molecule. Compared with individual cytokines or combinations of different cytokines, these fusion proteins can offer enhanced bioavailability and therapeutic benefits, although they may also display unanticipated biological effects. The first fusokine to be reported was in 2004, which was a fusion between IL-2 and GM-CSF [142]; additional fusokines later reported were IL-2/IL-18 and IL-15/GM-CSF in 2005–2006 [143, 144]. Since then, many others have been produced and investigated (IL-4/GM-CSF, IL-7/GM-CSF, IL-9/GM-CSF, CCL2/GM-CSF, CXCL10/XCL1, and IL-21/anti-CD20) [145].

1.6.3 Neutralisation of Cytokines

In sepsis patients, a lot of efforts have been made to neutralise damage-associated molecular patterns (DAMPs), pathogen-associated molecular patterns (PAMPs) and their receptors, inflammatory mediators, and cytokines. Although therapies targeting molecules such as anti-high-mobility group box 1 (HMGB1), anti-triggering receptor expressed on myeloid cells 1 (TREM-1), anti-vascular endothelial growth factor (VEGF), anti-C5a and anti-CXC chemokines, anti-MIF, anti-IL-17, anti-IL-27, anti-IL-33, anti-IFN-γ, and anti-TNF have successfully rescued mice in sepsis models of limited clinical relevance, none of these approaches have proven effective in saving human patients [146]. While targeting cytokines might have seemed logical in a syndrome characterised by a cytokine storm, neutralisation of IL-1 or TNF (the two main drivers of the cytokine cascade) failed to display efficiency [147]. Fortunately for drug companies, success stories have been told for other patients suffering inflammatory pathologies.

I remember attending a lecture by Sir Marc Feldmann (1944–) (Figure 1.3) where he showed a film of a lady suffering from rheumatoid arthritis, sitting in a wheelchair, who after receiving the miraculous anti-TNF treatment was able to get up and go up and down stairs. That was spectacular! Since 1994, this approach has changed the lives of many patients [148]. Various antibodies have been designed and patented, humanised mAb, human mAb, and the extracellular domain of the TNF receptor connected to the Fc-portion of human IgG. In 2002, the anti-TNF adalimumab was the first fully human antibody, made via phage display, to be approved by the FDA for the treatment of rheumatoid arthritis.

Because the neutralisation of TNF is not free from side effects (e.g. increase in tuberculosis cases, cases of sepsis, increased incidence of lymphoma), other cytokines (IL-17, IL-6) have been targeted, but with limited efficiencies [149, 150]. Surprisingly, tocilizumab (anti-IL-6R gp80), which emerged from studies on rheumatoid arthritis, was used to fight SARS-CoV-2 infection with very limited rationale and has ultimately yielded unconvincing results. In 1995, the neutralisation of TNF was shown to be efficient in Crohn's disease [151, 152], and in 1997, it was found to be beneficial in psoriasis [153]. Psoriasis has also been successfully treated with anti-IL-4 [154], anti-IL-17 [155], anti-IL-17R [156], and anti-IL-12/23 p40 [157].

Other cytokines have been targeted in early studies against cancer, with, for example, mAbs against chemokines or chemokine receptors [158], VEGF [159], or IL-6 for multiple myeloma [160]. For allergies and asthma, anti-IL-5 [161], anti-IL-13 [162], IL-4Ra [163] mAbs have been proposed. Anti-IL-2R (CD25) mAbs have been used to prevent allograft rejection [164] and to treat multiple sclerosis [165]. Systemic lupus erythematosus has been addressed with anti-IFNα mAb [166]. Osteoporosis was treated with anti-receptor activator of nuclear factor kappa-B ligand (RANK-L) [167]. Following these earlier studies, a large number of mAb anti-cytokines or anti-cytokine receptors have been patented.

1.7 TARGETING THE INFLAMMATORY PLAYERS

An earlier strategy to neutralise inflammatory cytokines came from the discovery and synthesis of glucocorticoids between 1936 and 1941 by Philip Showalter Hench (1896–1965), Edward Calvin Kendall (1886–1972), and Tadeusz Reichstein (1897–1996). In 1950, these three scientists received the Nobel Prize for their work on adrenal cortex hormones, including their structure, biological effects, and therapeutic potential in patients with inflammatory disorders [168]. A total of 2,766 different genes were reported as glucocorticoid regulated [169]. The capacity of glucocorticoids to inhibit the production of inflammatory cytokines was demonstrated in the mid-1980s for IL-1 [170], IL-2 [171], IL-3 [172], IFN-γ [173], and TNF [174]. Glucocorticoids inhibit the production of most cytokines but favour the release of MIF [175] and IL-10 [176]. Glucocorticoids also inhibit a large number of cytokine functions [177].

IL-1 receptor antagonist (IL-1Ra), a natural inhibitor of IL-1, is one of the cytokines being developed for clinical use. Initial studies of recombinant IL-1Ra (anakinra) in sepsis were unsuccessful [178], but a reanalysis of the data revealed that a subgroup of patients, those displaying a macrophage activation syndrome, may have benefited from the treatment [179]. This suggests that precision medicine could in the future identify sepsis patients who might benefit from such a treatment, thanks to biomarkers allowing for the identification of different endotypes. A similar approach has been successfully performed in COVID-19 patients [180]. IL-1Ra has also been used to treat patients with type 2 diabetes mellitus [181], gout [182], Behçet disease [183], post-acute myocardial infarction [184], and young children with IL-1Ra deficiency [185]. Another means to block IL-1 is the use of specific mAbs, as done in cryopyrin-associated periodic syndromes [186].

Among the numerous inflammatory mediators, histamine plays a central role, particularly in asthma and other atopic diseases. In 1937 at Institut Pasteur, in the laboratory of Daniel Bovet (1907–1992), a Swiss-born Italian medical doctor, Anne-Marie Staub (1914–2012), his trainee, was the first scientist to save a guinea pig from an anaphylactic shock thanks to the antihistamine properties of thymoxyethyldiethyl-amine (compound 929F) and phenolic ethers [187]. Unfortunately, the drug was toxic for humans. It was Bernard Halpern (1904–1978) at Rhône-Poulenc who discovered Antergan, the first antihistamine drug for humans.

1.8 CELLULAR THERAPIES FOR CANCER

Autologous T-lymphocytes isolated from cancer patients have been widely used *in vivo* to promote the fight against cancer. In 1983, the first report was published in Japan on the injection of T cells which display increased cytotoxicity after having been expanded with IL-2 and cultured with autologous tumour extract [188]. In 1984, Steven A. Rosenberg (1940–) (Figure 1.3), a pioneer in the development of immunotherapy in cancer, took the lead in the development of 'lymphokine-activated killer' (LAK) cells, consisting mostly of NK, NK-T, and T cells [189, 190]. In 1986, Rosenberg developed the tumour-infiltrating lymphocytes (TILs) expanded in IL-2. They were tested in mice carrying micro-metastases from different tumour types. TILs demonstrated 50- to 100-fold greater therapeutic efficacy compared to LAK cells [191]. The same year, a team from the Ludwig Institute for Cancer Research, in Lausanne (Switzerland), obtained TILs from human solid tumour, but only 3 out of 22 expressed the IL-2 receptor [192]. In 1988, Rosenberg reported the first clinical trial of TIL for patients with metastatic melanoma [193]. To enhance efficacy and specificity of T cells, chimeric antigen receptor-engineered T cells (CAR-T cells) were developed. In 1987, Yoshikazu Kurosawa (1947–) and his team first described the concept of a chimeric T-cell receptor (TCR), created by fusing antibody-derived variable domains (VH and VL) with constant regions from the TCR [194]. In 1993–1995, Rosenberg then tested *in vitro* and *in vivo* the efficiency of these cells against tumours [195, 196]. A Phase II clinical trial involving 111 patients with diffuse large B-cell lymphoma reported an objective response in 82% of participants, with 54% achieving complete remission [197]. However, CAR-T cell therapy can be associated with cytokine release syndrome, a very serious and potentially life-threatening toxicity that requires careful management [198]. More recently, a comparable approach has been explored using CAR-NK cells [199].

Another cellular immunotherapy has been proposed by Steinman, who discovered dendritic cells. Steinman isolated dendritic cells and primed them with the appropriate antigen. Once injected into the patient, these dendritic cells allow for the development of antigen-responsive T cells in the draining lymphoid tissue [200]. Loaded with tumour antigens, these dendritic cells become highly effective antigen-presenting cells capable of activating tumour-specific T cells. In 1996, the first clinical trial in B-cell lymphoma-vaccinated patients with these autologous primed dendritic cells was reported [201]. Three out of four patients experienced complete or partial tumour regression. Having pancreatic cancer, Steinman applied his treatment to himself. However, he passed away a few days before the Nobel Committee for Physiology or Medicine announced he was awarded the Nobel Prize, alongside Bruce Beutler (1957–) and Jules A. Hoffmann (1941–). Although the prize is not awarded posthumously, an exception was made because the committee was unaware that he had passed away three days earlier.

1.9 NEUROMODULATION OF INFLAMMATION

Since the earlier works of Hans Selye (1907–1982), a Hungarian physician who made his career at Montreal University, it is known that stress sensed in the brain has significant consequences on the whole body including the immune system [202]. Selye wrote many books on the effect of stress on health and diseases. The crosstalk between the central nervous system and the peripheral immune system is particularly mediated by the vagal nerve. The main person to decipher the dialogue was Kevin Tracey (1957–) (Figure 1.3), a neurosurgeon, and president and CEO of the Feinstein

Institute for Medical Research (Manhasset, USA). His initial contributions were in the field of sepsis when he showed that anti-TNF could protect mice against an endotoxic shock and baboons against bacteraemia. He discovered that local inflammation is sensed in periphery by the afferent vagus nerve which transmits information to the brain. Then, the brain via the efferent vagal nerve sends signals that cause the production of acetylcholine which results in the release of epinephrine. Epinephrine acts on the β-adrenergic receptors on T cells, which then produce acetylcholine which acts on macrophages via the α7-nicotinic receptor and inhibits the production of inflammatory cytokines (e.g. IL-1, TNF) [203]. In 2016, Tracey demonstrated that an implantable device stimulating the vagus nerve reduces the production of TNF, IL-1β, and IL-6 in peripheral blood. In patients with rheumatoid arthritis, vagus nerve stimulation (administered up to four times daily) significantly suppressed TNF production for as long as 84 days and significantly improved their clinical score [204]. In July 2025, the FDA approved the SetPoint System, a groundbreaking implantable vagus nerve implant device offering a new treatment approach for rheumatoid arthritis. Furthermore, a French team using similar vagus nerve stimulation techniques obtained encouraging results in patients with Crohn's disease [205]. Vagus nerve stimulation also led to promising results in a porcine model of sepsis [206]. Transcutaneous auricular vagus nerve stimulation performed in patients with sepsis resulted in substantially lower serum proinflammatory cytokines and higher anti-inflammatory cytokines, but no differences in clinical score were obtained between the treated patients and the sham stimulation [207].

1.10 A PERSONAL CONCLUDING REMARK

Thanks to their keen observational skills, their desire to discover new therapeutic approaches, and their experimental expertise, highly motivated physicians and scientists have, over the years, offered new treatments to patients in need. Since the deciphering of the immune system and the understanding of its complex network of interactions between immune cells and molecular players, experimenters have helped improve and prolong the lives of patients with debilitating diseases or even save them. I would like to thank and congratulate specifically Edward Donnall Thomas [95], Pablo Umaña [96], and Donald Metcalf [122] whose contributions were of great use to me and allowed me to be alive and healthy to write this chapter. I would also like to thank Professor François Lemonnier and the nurses of Henri Mondor Hospital, who treated me with the most appropriate treatment, and the French Social Security system, which covered the cost of my treatment, including the obinutuzumab (€3,214 per infusion).

I would like to dedicate this text to my valued former collaborator, Dr. Minou Adib-Conquy, who supervised the thesis of Professor Fernando Guimaraes, and to Dr. Tomasz Skirecki (Warsaw), my spiritual son in the field of immunity to sepsis [208]. Both were not as lucky as I was and died of cancer at the age of 47 and 37, respectively. This illustrates how much researchers must continue their efforts and call upon their inventiveness to treat this disease which has become a major cause of mortality in developed countries, whereas 125 years ago, the main causes were tuberculosis and syphilis.

KEY TERMS & DEFINITIONS SIDEBAR

Cytokines Soluble mediators that allow the crosstalk between cells.

Immune checkpoint inhibitors Inhibitors that block key surface proteins involved in the negative regulation of the immune response.

Serotherapy Injection of immune serum to prevent infections.

Vaccination Injection of an antigen (microbial molecule, attenuated or killed bacteria or virus, etc.) to induce protective immunity against a given infection.

Variolation An injection of material sampled from a human with smallpox to prevent the infection.

LIST OF ABBREVIATIONS

BCG	bacille de Calmette et Guérin
CAR-T cells	chimeric antigen receptor-engineered T cells
CD	cluster of differentiation
CTLA-4	cytotoxic T-lymphocyte-associated protein-4
COVID-19	coronavirus disease 2019
DAMPs	damage-associated molecular patterns
FDA	US Food and Drug Administration
G-CSF	granulocyte colony-stimulating factor
GM-CSF	granulocyte-macrophage colony-stimulating factor
HMGB1	high-mobility group box 1
IFN	interferon
IgA	immunoglobulin A
IgG	immunoglobulin G
IgM	immunoglobulin M
IL	interleukin
IL-1Ra	IL-1 receptor antagonist
ISG	immune serum globulin
IvIg	intravenous immunoglobulins
LAK	lymphokine-activated killer
LPS	lipopolysaccharide
mAb	monoclonal antibody
M-CSF	macrophage-colony-stimulating factor
MIF	macrophage migration inhibitory factor
mRNA	micro ribonucleic acid
NK	natural killer
PAMPs	pathogen-associated molecular patterns
PD-1	programmed cell death protein 1

PD-L1	PD1 ligand 1
RANK-L	receptor activator of nuclear factor kappa-B ligand
SARS-CoV-2	severe acute respiratory syndrome-coronavirus 2
TCR	T-cell receptor
Th	T helper cells
TIL	tumour-infiltrating lymphocytes
TNF	tumour necrosis factor
Treg	regulatory T cells
TREM-1	triggering receptor expressed on myeloid cells 1
VEGF	vascular endothelial growth factor

REVIEW QUESTIONS

1. What were the key contributions of Ehrlich and Metchnikoff to immunology?
2. How did Coley's observations on tumour regression after bacterial infection anticipate modern cancer immunotherapy?
3. What technological advance allowed the transition from polyclonal serotherapy to the use of monoclonal antibodies?
4. Give examples of cytokines, used a tool or as a target for immunotherapy.
5. What is the aim of vagal nerve stimulation?

REFERENCES

1. Smith, K.A. (2012). Louis Pasteur, the father of immunology? *Front Immunol* 3: 68. https://doi.org/10.3389/fimmu.2012.00068.
2. Roux, E. and Chamberland, C. (1888). Immunité contre la septicémie conferée par des substance solubles. *Recueil de Médecine Vétérinaire* 5: 133–145.
3. Ehrlich, P. (1897). Die Wertbemessung des Diphterieheilserums und deren theoretische Grundlagen. *Klinisches Jahrbuch* 6: 299–326.
4. Ehrlich, P. (1892). Ueber immunität durch vererbung und säugung. *Zeitschrift für Hygiene* 12: 183–203.
5. Rossignol, H. (1883). L'immunité conférée par la vaccination pratiquée avec les virus charbonneux atténués de M. Pasteur, est-elle transmissible de la mère au fœtus. IN Les nouvelles Expériences de Pouilly-Le-Fort. Rapport. Angers, Imprimerie Lachèse et Dolbeau.
6. Ehrlich, P. and Morgenroth, J. (1899). Ueber haemolysine: zweite mittheilung. *Berl Klini Wochenschr* 36: 481–486.
7. Fodor, J. (1887). Die fahigkeit des blutes bakterien zu vernichten. *Dtsch Med Woch* 8: 745–747.
8. Bordet, J. (1895). Les leucocytes et les propriétés actives du sérum chez les vaccinés. *Ann Inst Pasteur* 9: 462–506.
9. Cavaillon JM, Sansonetti P, Goldman M. 100th anniversary of Jules Bordet's Nobel Prize: tribute to a founding father of immunology. *Front Immunol* 2019; 10: 2114. https://doi.org/10.3389/fimmu.2019.02114
10. Wright, A.E. (1903). An experimental investigation on the role of the blood fluids in connection with phagocytosis. *Proc R Soc Lond* 72: 357–370.
11. Porter, R.R. (1959). The hydrolysis of rabbit y-globulin and antibodies with crystalline papain. *Biochem J* 73 (1): 119–126. https://doi.org/10.1042/bj0730119.

12. Edelman, G.M. and Poulik, M.D. (1961). Studies on structural units of the gamma-globulins. *J Exp Med* 113 (5): 861–884. https://doi.org/10.1084/jem.113.5.861.
13. Hozumi, N. and Tonegawa, S. (1976). Evidence for somatic rearrangement of immunoglobulin genes coding for variable and constant regions. *Proc Natl Acad Sci USA* 73 (10): 3628–3632. https://doi.org/10.1073/pnas.73.10.3628.
14. Sabin FR. Cellular reactions to a dye-protein with a concept of the mechanism of antibody formation. *J Exp Med* 1939; 70(1): 67–82. https://doi.org/10.1084/jem.70.1.67.
15. Fagraeus A Plasma cellular reaction and its relation to the formation of antibodies in vitro. *Nature* 1947; 159(4041): 499. https://doi.org/10.1038/159499a0.
16. Van Leeuwenhoek, M. (1674). Microscopical observations from Mr Leeuwenhoek, concerning blood, milk, bones, the brain, spitle, cuticula, sweat, fat, teares; communicated by the said observer to the Publisher in a letter, dated June 1 1674. *Philos Trans R Soc Lond* 9: 121–131. https://doi.org/10.1098/rstl.1674.0030.
17. Lieutaud, J. (1749). *Elementa Physiologiae*. Amsterdam: Fratrum Detournes.
18. Senac, J.B. (1749). *Traité de la structure du cœur, de son action, et de ses maladies*. Paris: Jacques Vincent.
19. Addison, W. (1845). *The Actual Process of Nutrition and in Inflammation in the Living Structure Demonstrated by the Microscope* (ed. J. Chruchill) (London).
20. Schultze, J.S. (1865). Ein heizbarer Objecttisch und seine Verwendung bei Untersuchungen des Blutes. *Arch Mikrosc Anat* 1: 1–42.
21. Ehrlich, P. (1879). Beiträge zur Kenntniss der granulirten Bindegewebszellen und der eosinophilen Leukocythen. *Arch Anat Physiol (Leipzig)* 3: 166–169.
22. Erlich, P. (1877). Beiträge zur Kenntniss der Anilinfärbungen und ihrer Verwendung in der mikroskopischen Technik. *Arch Mikr Anat* 13: 263–277.
23. Cavaillon JM, Legout S. Centenary of the death of Elie Metchnikoff: a visionary and an outstanding team leader. *Microbes Infect* 2016; 18(10): 577–594. https://doi.org/10.1016/j.micinf.2016.05.008.
24. Metchnikoff, E. (1883). Unterchungen über die mesodermalen phagocyten einiger wirbeltiere. *Biol Centralbl* 3 (18): 560–565.
25. Metchnikoff, E. (1884). Untersuchungen über die intracellular verdauung bei wirbellosen thieren. *Arb Zool Inst Univ Wien* 5: 141–168.
26. Gordon S, Plüddemann A. Tissue macrophages: heterogeneity and functions. *BMC Biol* 2017; 15(1): 53. https://doi.org/10.1186/s12915-017-0392-4.
27. Cooper MD, Peterson RD, Good RA. Delineation of the thymic and bursal lymphoid systems in the chicken. *Nature*. 1965; 205: 143–146. https://doi.org/10.1038/205143a0 .
28. Miller JF, Mitchell GF. Cell to cell interaction in the immune response. I. Hemolysin-forming cells in neonatally thymectomized mice reconstituted with thymus or thoracic duct lymphocytes. *J Exp Med* 1968; 128(4): 801–820. https://doi.org/10.1084/jem.128.4.801.
29. Cerottini JC, Nordin AA, Brunner KT. Specific in vitro cytotoxicity of thymus-derived lymphocytes sensitized to alloantigens. *Nature* 1970; 228(5278): 1308–1309. https://doi.org/10.1038/2281308a0.
30. Mosmann, T.R., Cherwinski, H., Bond, M.W. et al. (1986). Two types of murine helper T cell clone. I. Definition according to profiles of lymphokine activities and secreted proteins. *J Immunol* 136 (7): 2348–2357.
31. Steinman RM, Cohn ZA. Identification of a novel cell type in peripheral lymphoid organs of mice. I. Morphology, quantitation, tissue distribution. *J Exp Med* 1973; 137(5): 1142–1162. https://doi.org/10.1084/jem.137.5.1142.
32. Kiessling R, Klein E, Wigzell H. "Natural" killer cells in the mouse. I. Cytotoxic cells with specificity for mouse Moloney leukemia cells. Specificity and distribution according to genotype. *Eur J Immunol* 1975; 5(2): 112–117. https://doi.org/10.1002/eji.1830050208.
33. Vivier E, van de Pavert SA, Cooper MD, Belz GT. The evolution of innate lymphoid cells. *Nat Immunol* 2016; 17(7): 790–794. https://doi.org/10.1038/ni.3459.

34. Cavaillon JM, Legout S. Louis Pasteur: between myth and reality. *Biomolecules* 2022; 12(4): 596. https://doi.org/10.3390/biom12040596.
35. Fan, T., Zhang, M., Yang, J. et al. (2023). Therapeutic cancer vaccines: advancements, challenges and prospects. *Signal Transduct Target Ther* 8: 450. https://doi.org/10.1038/s41392-023-01674-3.
36. Dunning, R. (1800). Some observations on vaccination or the inoculated cow-pox. London. March and Teape, Tower-Hill
37. von Leyden, E. and Blumenthal, F. (1902). Vorlacufige mittheilungen ueber einige ergebnisse der kerbsforschung auf der 1. Medizinischen Klinik. *Deut Med Wschr* 28: 637–638.
38. Graham, J.B. and Graham, R.M. (1959). The effect of vaccine on cancer patients. *Surg Gynecol Obstet* 109 (2): 131–138.
39. Gold, P. and Freedman, S.O. (1965). Demonstration of tumor-specific antigens in human colonic carcinomata by immunological tolerance and absorption techniques. *J Exp Med* 121: 439–462. https://doi.org/10.1084/jem.121.3.439.
40. Hu, S.L. and Plowman, G.D. (1988). Characterization of a recombinant vaccinia virus expressing human melanoma-associated antigen p97. *J Virol* 62: 176–180. https://doi.org/10.1128/jvi.62.1.176-180.198.
41. Otsuji, E., Park, Y., Tashiro, K. et al. (1995). Inhibition of b16 melanoma metastasis by administration of g(m3)- or gg3- liposomes – blocking adhesion of melanoma-cells to endothelial-cells (antiadhesion therapy) via inhibition of g(m3)-gg3cer or g(m3)-laccer interaction. *Int J Oncol* 6 (2): 319–327. https://doi.org/10.3892/ijo.6.2.319.
42. Kashmiri SV, Shu L, Padlan EA, et al. Generation, characterization, and in vivo studies of humanized anticarcinoma antibody CC49. *Hybridoma* 1995 ;14(5):461–473. https://doi.org/10.1089/hyb.1995.14.461.
43. Flores JE, Thompson AJ. The global impact of hepatitis B vaccination on hepatocellular carcinoma. *Vaccines (Basel)* 2022; 10(5): 793. https://doi.org/10.3390/vaccines10050793.
44. Frazer, I.H. (2019). The HPV vaccine story. *ACS Pharmacol Transl Sci* 2: 210–212. https://doi.org/10.1021/acsptsci.9b00032.
45. Behring, E. and Kitasato, S. (1890). Ueber das Zustandekommen der Diphtherie-Immunitat and der Tetanus-Immunität bei Thieren. *Dtsch Med Wochenschr* 16: 1113–1114.
46. Baginsky, A. (1895). *Die Serumtherapie Der Diphtherie Nach Den Beobachtungen Im Kaiser und Kaiserin Friedrich Kinderkrankenhause in Berlin*. Berlin, Germany: Kessinger Publishing, LLC.
47. Roux, E., Martin, L., and Chaillou, A. (1894). Trois cents cas de diphtérie traités par le sérum anti-diphtériques. *Ann Inst Pasteur* 8: 640–661.
48. Yersin, A. (1894). peste bubonique à Hong Kong. *Ann Inst Pasteur* 8: 662–667.
49. Yersin, A., Calmette, A., and Borrel, A. (1895). La peste bubonique: Deuxième note. *Ann Inst Pasteur* 9: 589–592.
50. Yersin, A. (1896). Historique du premier cas de peste traité et guéri par l'emploi du sérum antipesteux. *Bull Acad Méd* XXXVI: 195–196.
51. Simond P-L (1898). Rapport sur les cas de peste traités dans l'Inde anglaise au moyen du sérum antipesteux préparé à l'Institut Pasteur de Paris par M. le Dr Roux. *AHMC* 1: 349–361.
52. Zemmers, N. (1893). Rinderpest infektion und immunisierung und schutzimpfung gegen rinderpest. *Berl Tierärztl Wochenschr* 23: 590–591.
53. Busch, W. (1868). Aus der Sitzung der medicinischen Section vom 13 November 1867. *Berl Klin Wochenschr* 5: 137.
54. Fehleisen, F. (1882). Ueber die züchtung der erysipelkokken auf künstlichem nährboden und ihre übertragbarkeit auf den menschen. *Dtsch Med Wochenschr* 8: 553–554.
55. Coley, W.B. (1893). The treatment of malignant tumors by repeated inoculations of erysipelas: with a report of ten original cases. *Am J Med Sci* 105: 487–510.

56. Decker WK, da Silva RF, Sanabria MH, et al. Cancer immunotherapy: historical perspective of a clinical revolution and emerging preclinical animal models. *Front Immunol* 2017;8: 829. https://doi.org/10.3389/fimmu.2017.00829.
57. Coley, W.B. (1898). The treatment of inoperable sarcoma with the mixed toxins of erysipelas and bacillus prodigiosus. Immediate and final results in one hundred and forty cases. *J Am Med Ass* 31: 456–465.
58. Ehrlich, P. (1909). Über den jetzigen stand der karzinomforschung. *Ned Tijdschr Geneeskd* 5: 273–290.
59. Burnet FM. Cancer—a biological approach. *Br Med J* 1957;1:841–847. https://doi.org/10.1136/bmj.1.5023.841.
60. Hartwell, J.L., Shear, M.J., Adams, J.R., and Perrault, A. (1943). Chemical treatment of tumors. VII nature of hemorrhage-producing fraction from *Serratia marcescens* (*Bacillus prodigiosis*) culture filtrates. *J. Natl Cancer Inst* 4: 107–122.
61. Hedlund, G., Dohlsten, M., Petersson, C., and Kalland, T. (1993). Superantigen-based tumor therapy: in vivo activation of cytotoxic T cells. *Cancer Immunol Immunother* 36: 89–93.
62. Pearl, R. (1928). On the pathological relations between cancer and tuberculosis. *Exp Biol Med* 26 (1): 73–75.
63. Holmgren, I. (1936). Employment of BCG, especially in intravenous injection. *Acta Med Scand* 90 (Suppl): 350–361.
64. Villasor, R.P., Fetalino, M.S., and Ramirez, A.T. (1963). The clinical use of BCG vaccine in stimulating host resistance to cancer. *Philippines J Surg Surg Spec* 18: 85–93.
65. Mathé, G., Amiel, J.L., Schwarzenberg, L. et al. (1969). Active immunotherapy for acute lymphoblastic leukaemia. *Lancet* 1 (7597): 697–699. https://doi.org/10.1016/s0140-6736(69)92648-8.
66. Morales, A., Eidinger, D., and Bruce, A.W. (1976). Intracavitary *Bacillus Calmette-Guerin* in the treatment of superficial bladder tumors. *J Urol* 116 (2): 180–183. https://doi.org/10.1016/s0022-5347(17)58737-6.
67. Moolten F, Zajdel S, Cooperband S. Immunotherapy of experimental animal tumors with antitumor antibodies conjugated to diphtheria toxin or ricin. *Ann N Y Acad Sci* 1976;277(00):690–699. https://doi.org/10.1111/j.1749-6632.1976.tb41740.x.
68. Blythman HE, Casellas P, Gros O, et al. Immunotoxins: hybrid molecules of monoclonal antibodies and a toxin subunit specifically kill tumour cells. *Nature.* 1981 290; (5802):145–146. https://doi.org/10.1038/290145a0.
69. Williams DP, Parker K, Bacha P, et al. Diphtheria toxin receptor binding domain substitution with interleukin-2: genetic construction and properties of a diphtheria toxin-related interleukin-2 fusion protein. *Protein Eng* 1987 ;1(6):493–498. https://doi.org/10.1093/protein/1.6.493.
70. Calmette, A., Saenz, A., and Costil, L. (1933). Effects du venin de cobra sur les greffes cancereuses et sur le cancer spontané (adeno-carcinome) de la souris. *CR Acad Sci* 197: 205–210.
71. Dock, G. (1904). The influence of complicating diseases upon leukaemia. *Am J Med Sci* 127: 561–592.
72. Moore AE. Enhancement of oncolytic effect of Russian encephalitis virus. *Proc Soc Exp Biol Med* 1951 Apr;76(4):749–754. https://doi.org/10.3181/00379727-76-18619.
73. Higgins, G.K. and Pack, G.T. (1951). Virus therapy in the treatment of tumors. *Bull Hosp Joint Dis* 12: 379–382.
74. Southam, C.M. and Moore, A.E. (1952). Clinical studies of viruses as antineoplastic agents with particular reference to Egypt 101 virus. *Cancer* 5: 1025–1034.
75. Bierman, H.I., Crile, D.M., Dod, K.S. et al. (1953). Remissions in leukemia of childhood following acute infectious disease. *Cancer* 6 (3): 591–605. https://doi.org/10.1002/1097-0142(195305)6:3<591::aid-cncr2820060317>3.0.co;2-m.

76. Smith, R.R., Huebner, R.J., Rowe, W.P. et al. (1956). Studies on the use of viruses in the treatment of carcinoma of the cervix. *Cancer* 9: 1211–1218. https://doi.org/10.1002/1097-0142(195611/12)9:6<1211::aid-cncr2820090624>3.0.co;2-7.
77. Pack, G.T. (1950). Note of the experimental use of rabies vaccine for melanomatosis. *Arch Dermatol* 62: 694–695.
78. Kelly E, Russell SJ. History of oncolytic viruses: genesis to genetic engineering. *Mol Ther* 2007 Apr;15(4):651–659. https://doi.org/10.1038/sj.mt.6300108.
79. Cohn, E.J., Oncley, J.L., Strong, L.E. et al. (1944). Chemical, clinical, and immunological studies on the products of human plasma fractionation. I. The characterization of the protein fractions of human plasma. *J Clin Invest* 23 (4): 417–432. https://doi.org/10.1172/JCI101508.
80. Stokes, J., Maris, E.P., and Gellis, S.S. (1944). Chemical, clinical, and immunological studies on the products of human plasma fractionation. XI. The use of concentrated normal human serum gamma globulin (human immune serum globulin) in the prophylaxis and treatment of measles. *J Clin Invest* 23 (4): 531–540. https://doi.org/10.1172/JCI101518.
81. Bruton, O.C. (1952). Agammaglobulinemia. *Pediatrics* 9: 722–728.
82. Schultze, H.E. and Schwick, G. (1962). Über neue Möglichkeiten intravenöser Gammaglobulin-Applikation. *Deuthsche Med Wchnschr* 87 (34): 1643–1650. https://doi.org/10.1055/s-0028-1113997.
83. Pan B, Sun P, Pei R, et al. Efficacy of IVIG therapy for patients with sepsis: a systematic review and meta-analysis. *J Transl Med* 2023;21(1):765. https://doi.org/10.1186/s12967-023-04592-8.
84. Alwakeel M, Abi Fadel F, Nanah A, et al. Efficacy of COVID-19 treatments in intensive care unit: a systematic review and meta-analysis of randomized controlled trials. *Crit Care Res Pract* 2024;2024:2973795. https://doi.org/10.1155/ccrp/2973795.
85. Hooper, J.A. (2015). The history and evolution of immunoglobulin products and their clinical indications. *LymphoSign J* 2: 181–194. https://doi.org/10.14785/lpsn-2014-0025.
86. Köhler G, Milstein C. Continuous cultures of fused cells secreting antibody of predefined specificity. *Nature.* 1975 ;256(5517):495–497. https://doi.org/10.1038/256495a0.
87. Milstein C. The hybridoma revolution: an offshoot of basic research. *Bioessays* 1999 ;21(11):966–973. https://doi.org/10.1002/(SICI)1521-1878(199911)21:11<966::AID-BIES9>3.0.CO;2-Z.
88. Hulett, H.R., Bonner, W.A. et al. (1969). Cell sorting: automated separation of mammalian cells as a function of intracellular fluorescence. *Science* 166 (3906): 747–749. https://doi.org/10.1126/science.166.3906.747.
89. Fulwyler MJ. Electronic separation of biological cells by volume. *Science* 1965; 150(3698):910–911. https://doi.org/10.1126/science.150.3698.910.
90. Green LL, Hardy MC, Maynard-Currie CE, et al. Antigen-specific human monoclonal antibodies from mice engineered with human Ig heavy and light chain YACs. *Nat Genet* 1994;7:13–21. https://doi.org/10.1038/ng0594-13.
91. Lonberg N, Taylor LD, Harding FA, et al. Antigen-specific human antibodies from mice comprising four distinct genetic modifications. *Nature* 1994;368:856–859. https://doi.org/10.1038/368856a0.
92. Clackson T, Hoogenboom HR, Griffiths AD, Winter G. Making antibody fragments using phage display libraries. *Nature* 1991 6336;352:624–628. https://doi.org/10.1038/352624a0.
93. Steinitz, M. (2009). Three decades of human monoclonal antibodies: past, present and future developments. *Human Antibodies* 18: 1–10. https://doi.org/10.3233/HAB-2009-0196.
94. Cosimi, A.B., Colvin, R.B., Burton, R.C. et al. (1981). Use of monoclonal antibodies to T-cell subsets for immunologic monitoring and treatment in recipients of renal allografts. *N Engl J Med* 305: 308–314.
95. Press, O.W., Appelbaum, F., Ledbetter, J.A. et al. (1987). Monoclonal antibody 1F5 (anti-CD20) serotherapy of human B cell lymphomas. *Blood* 69 (2): 584–591.

96. Mössner E, Brünker P, Moser S, et al. Increasing the efficacy of CD20 antibody therapy through the engineering of a new type II anti-CD20 antibody with enhanced direct and immune effector cell-mediated B-cell cytotoxicity. *Blood* 2010;115:4393–4402. https://doi.org/10.1182/blood-2009-06-225979.
97. Marcus R, Davies A, Ando K, et al. Obinutuzumab for the first-line treatment of follicular lymphoma. *N Engl J Med* 2017377;(14):1331–1344. https://doi.org/10.1056/NEJMoa1614598.
98. Soulillou, J.P., Le Mauff, B. et al. (1988). Anti-IL-2-R monoclonal antibody in allograft recipients. *J Autoimmun* 1: 655–661.
99. Soulillou JP, Cantarovich D, le Mauff B, et al. Randomized controlled trial of a monoclonal antibody against the interleukin-2 receptor (33B3.1) as compared with rabbit antithymocyte globulin for prophylaxis against rejection of renal allografts. *N Engl J Med* 1990;322(17):1175–1782. https://doi.org/10.1056/NEJM199004263221702.
100. Waterhouse P, Penninger JM, Timms E, et al. Lymphoproliferative disorders with early lethality in mice deficient in CTLA-4. *Science* 1995; 270 (5238): 985–988. https://doi.org/10.1126/science.270.5238.985.
101. Tivol EA, Borriello F, Schweitzer AN, et al. Loss of CTLA-4 leads to massive lymphoproliferation and fatal multiorgan tissue destruction, revealing a critical negative regulatory role of CTLA-4. *Immunity* 1995; 3(5): 541–547. https://doi.org/10.1016/1074-7613(95)90125-6.
102. Ishida Y, Agata Y, Shibahara K, Honjo T Induced expression of PD-1, a novel member of the immunoglobulin gene superfamily, upon programmed cell death. *EMBO J* 1992; 11(11): 3887–3895. https://doi.org/10.1002/j.1460-2075.1992.tb05481.x.
103. Hodi, F.S., O'Day, S.J., McDermott, D.F. et al. (2010). Improved survival with ipilimumab in patients with metastatic melanoma. *N Engl J Med* 363: 711–723. https://doi.org/10.1056/NEJMoa1003466.
104. Topalian SL, Hodi FS, Brahmer JR, et al. Safety, activity, and immune correlates of anti-PD-1 antibody in cancer. *N Engl J Med* 2012; 366(26): 2443–2454. https://doi.org/10.1056/NEJMoa1200690.
105. Isaacs, A. and Lindenmann, J. (1957). Virus interference. I. The interferon. *Proc R Soc London B Biol Sci* 147: 258–267.
106. Nagano, Y. and Kojima, Y. (1954). Immunizing property of vaccinia virus inactivated by ultraviolets rays. *C R Séances Soc Biol Fil* 148: 1700–1702.
107. Masucci MG, Szigeti R, Klein E, et al. Effect of interferon-alpha 1 from *E. coli* on some cell functions. *Science* 1980;209(4463):1431–1435. https://doi.org/10.1126/science.6158096.
108. Horning, S.J., Levine, J.F., Miller, R.A. et al. (1982). Clinical and immunologic effects of recombinant leukocyte A interferon in eight patients with advanced cancer. *JAMA* 247 (247): 1718–1722.
109. Sherwin, S.A., Knost, J.A., Fein, S. et al. (1982). A multiple-dose phase I trial of recombinant leukocyte A interferon in cancer patients. *JAMA* 248: 2461–2466.
110. Bloom BR, Bennett B. Mechanism of a reaction in vitro associated with delayed-type hypersensitivity. *Science* 1966;153(3731):80–82. https://doi.org/10.1126/science.153.3731.80.
111. Cohen, S., Bigazzi, P.E., and Yoshida, T. (1974). Similarities of T cell function in cell-mediated immunity and antibody production. *Cell Immunol* 12: 150–159. https://doi.org/10.1016/0008-8749(74)90066-5.
112. Menkin, V. (1944). Chemical basis of fever. *Science* 100: 337–338. https://doi.org/10.1126/science.100.2598.337.
113. Wood, B. (1958). The role of endogenous pyrogen in the genesis of fever. *The Lancet* 2: 53–57. https://doi.org/10.1016/s0140-6736(58)91237-6.
114. Bennett, I.L. Jr. and Beeson, P.B. (1953). Studies on the pathogenesis of fever. II. Characterization of fever-producing substances from polymorphonuclear leukocytes and from the fluid of sterile exudates. *J Exp Med* 98 (5): 493–508. https://doi.org/10.1084/jem.98.5.493.

115. Atkins, E. and Wood, W.B. Jr. (1955). Studies on the pathogenesis of fever. I. The presence of transferable pyrogen in the blood stream following the injection of typhoid vaccine. *J Exp Med* 101 (5): 519–528. https://doi.org/10.1084/jem.101.5.519.
116. Auron P E, Webb AC, Rosenwasser LJ, et al. (1984). Nucleotide sequence of human monocyte interleukin-1 precursor cDNA. *PNAS* 81 (24): 7907–7911.
117. Lomedico, P.T., Gubler, U., Hellmann, C.P. et al. (1984). Cloning and expression of murine interleukin-1 cDNA in *Escherichia coli*. *Nature* 312: 458–462. https://doi.org/10.1038/312458a0.
118. Morgan, D.A., Ruscetti, F.W., and Gallo, R. (1976). Selective in vitro growth of T lymphocytes from normal human bone marrows (external link). *Science* 193 (4257): 1007–1008.
119. Carswell EA, Old LJ, Kassel RL, et al. An endotoxin-induced serum factor that causes necrosis of tumors. *Proc Natl Acad Sci USA* 1975 ;72(9):3666–3670. https://doi.org/10.1073/pnas.72.9.3666.
120. Beutler, B., Greenwald, D., Hulmes, J.D. et al. (1985). Identity of tumour necrosis factor and the macrophage-secreted factor cachectin. *Nature* 316 (5): 52–54. https://doi.org/10.1038/316552a0.
121. Yoshimura, T., Matsushima, K., Oppenheim, J.J., and Leonard, E.J. (1987). Neutrophil chemotactic factor produced by lipopolysaccharide (LPS)-stimulated human blood mononuclear leukocytes: partial characterization and separation from interleukin 1 (IL 1). *J Immunol* 139 (3): 788–793.
122. Metcalf D. The colony-stimulating factors and cancer. *Nat Rev Cancer* 2010 Jun;10(6):425–434. https://doi.org/10.1038/nrc2843.
123. Cavaillon, J.M. (2001). Pro- versus anti-inflammatory cytokines: myth or reality. *Cell Mol Biol (Noisy-le-grand)* 47 (4): 695–702.
124. Taniguchi T, Matsui H, Fujita T, et al. Structure and expression of a cloned cDNA for human interleukin-2. *Nature* 1983;302(5906):5305–5310. https://doi.org/10.1038/302305a0.
125. Dopfer R, Niethammer D, Peter HH, et al. In vivo effects of interleukin 2 on lymphocyte subpopulations in a patient with a combined immunodeficiency. *Immunobiology* 1984;167(5):452–461. https://doi.org/10.1016/S0171-2985(84)80077-7.
126. Rosenberg, S.A., Mulé, J.J., Spiess, P.J. et al. (1985). Regression of established pulmonary metastases and subcutaneous tumor mediated by the systemic administration of high-dose recombinant interleukin 2. *J Exp Med* 161 (5): 1169–1188. https://doi.org/10.1084/jem.161.5.1169.
127. Hooper WC, Barth RF, Shah NT. Lack of natural killer cell activity in hairy cell leukemia patients and partial restoration with interleukin-2. *Cancer* 1986; 57(5): 988–993. https://doi.org/10.1002/1097-0142(19860301)57:5<988::aid-cncr2820570519>3.0.co;2-2.
128. Lotze, M.T., Custer, M.C., Ettinghausen, S.E. et al. (1987). In vivo administration of purified human interleukin-2 to patients with cancer: development of interleukin-2 receptor positive cells and circulating soluble interleukin-2 receptors following interleukin-2 administration. *Cancer Res* 47: 2188–2195.
129. Gianni AM, Siena S, Bregni M, et al. Granulocyte-macrophage colony-stimulating factor to harvest circulating haemopoietic stem cells for autotransplantation. *Lancet* 1989; 2(8663): 580–585. https://doi.org/10.1016/s0140-6736(89)90711-3.
130. Dührsen, U., Villeval, J.L., Boyd, J. et al. (1988). Effects of recombinant human granulocyte colony-stimulating factor on hematopoietic progenitor cells in cancer patients. *Blood* 72 (6): 2074–2081.
131. Nierhaus A, Montag B, Timmler N, et al. Reversal of immunoparalysis by recombinant human granulocyte-macrophage colony-stimulating factor in patients with severe sepsis. *Intensive Care Med* 2003; 29(4): 646–651. https://doi.org/10.1007/s00134-003-1666-6.
132. Döcke WD, , Randow F, Syrbe U, et al. Monocyte deactivation in septic patients: restoration by IFN-gamma treatment. *Nat Med* 1997; 3(6): 678–681. https://doi.org/10.1038/nm0697-678.

133. Venet F, Foray AP, Villars-Méchin A, et al. IL-7 restores lymphocyte functions in septic patients. *J Immunol* 2012; 189(10): 5073–5081. https://doi.org/10.4049/jimmunol.1202062.
134. Hotchkiss RS, Colston E, Yende S, et al. Immune checkpoint inhibition in sepsis: a phase 1b randomized study to evaluate the safety, tolerability, pharmacokinetics, and pharmacodynamics of nivolumab. *Intensive Care Med* 2019; 45(10): 1360–1371. https://doi.org/10.1007/s00134-019-05704-z.
135. Cavaillon JM, Chousterman BG, Skirecki T. Compartmentalization of the inflammatory response during bacterial sepsis and severe COVID-19. *J Intensive Med* 2024; 4(3): 326–340. https://doi.org/10.1016/j.jointm.2024.01.001.
136. Cavaillon JM, Eisen D, Annane D Is boosting the immune system in sepsis appropriate? *Crit Care* 2014 ; 18(2): 216. https://doi.org/10.1186/cc13787.
137. Roquilly A, Francois B, Huet O, et al. Interferon gamma-1b for the prevention of hospital-acquired pneumonia in critically ill patients: a phase 2, placebo-controlled randomized clinical trial. *Intensive Care Med* 2023; 49(5): 530–544. https://doi.org/10.1007/s00134-023-07065-0.
138. Daix T, Mathonnet A, Brakenridge S, et al. Intravenously administered interleukin-7 to reverse lymphopenia in patients with septic shock: a double-blind, randomized, placebo-controlled trial. *Ann Intensive Care* 2023; 13(1): 17. https://doi.org/10.1186/s13613-023-01109-w.
139. Bonvalot S, Laplanche A, Lejeune F, et al. Limb salvage with isolated perfusion for soft tissue sarcoma: could less TNF-alpha be better? *Ann Oncol* 2005; 16(7): 1061–1068. https://doi.org/10.1093/annonc/mdi229.
140. Levin AM, Bates DL, Ring AM, et al. Exploiting a natural conformational switch to engineer an interleukin-2 'superkine'. *Nature* 2012; 484(7395): 529–533. https://doi.org/10.1038/nature10975.
141. Lopes, J.E., Fisher, J.L., Flick, H.L. et al. (2020). ALKS 4230: a novel engineered IL-2 fusion protein with an improved cellular selectivity profile for cancer immunotherapy. *J Immunother Cancer* 8 (1): e000673. https://doi.org/10.1136/jitc-2020-000673.
142. Stagg, J., Wu, J.H., Bouganim, N., and Galipeau, J. (2004). Granulocyte-macrophage colony-stimulating factor and interleukin-2 fusion cDNA for cancer gene immunotherapy. *Cancer Res* 64: 8795–8799. https://doi.org/10.1158/0008-5472.CAN-04-1776.
143. Acres B, Gantzer M, Remy C, et al. Fusokine interleukin-2/interleukin-18, a novel potent innate and adaptive immune stimulator with decreased toxicity. *Cancer Res* 2005;65(20):9536–9546. https://doi.org/10.1158/0008-5472.CAN-05-0691.
144. Rafei M, Wu JH, Annabi B, et al. A GMCSF and IL-15 fusokine leads to paradoxical immunosuppression in vivo via asymmetrical JAK/STAT signaling through the IL-15 receptor complex. *Blood* 2007 109;(5):2234–2342. https://doi.org/10.1182/blood-2006-07-037473
145. Bhatt S, Parvin S, Zhang Y, et al. Anti-CD20-interleukin-21 fusokine targets malignant B cells via direct apoptosis and NK-cell-dependent cytotoxicity. *Blood* 2017;129(16):2246–2256. https://doi.org/10.1182/blood-2016-09-738211.
146. Cavaillon JM, Singer M, Skirecki T. Sepsis therapies: learning from 30 years of failure of translational research to propose new leads. *EMBO Mol Med* 2020; 12(4): e10128. https://doi.org/10.15252/emmm.201810128.
147. Ospina-Tascón GA, Büchele GL, Vincent JL. Multicenter, randomized, controlled trials evaluating mortality in intensive care: doomed to fail? *Crit Care Med* 2008; 36(4): 1311–1322. https://doi.org/10.1097/CCM.0b013e318168ea3e.
148. Elliott MJ, Maini RN, Feldmann M, et al. Randomised double-blind comparison of chimeric monoclonal antibody to tumour necrosis factor alpha (cA2) versus placebo in rheumatoid arthritis. *Lancet* 1994; 344(8930): 1105–1110. https://doi.org/10.1016/s0140-6736(94)90628-9.
149. Genovese MC, Van den Bosch F, Roberson SA, et al. LY2439821, a humanized anti-interleukin-17 monoclonal antibody, in the treatment of patients with rheumatoid arthritis: a phase I randomized, double-blind, placebo-controlled, proof-of-concept study. *J Arthritis Rheum* 2010; 62(4): 929–939. https://doi.org/10.1002/art.27334.

150. Smolen JS, Beaulieu A, Rubbert-Roth A, et al. Effect of interleukin-6 receptor inhibition with tocilizumab in patients with rheumatoid arthritis (OPTION study): a double-blind, placebo-controlled, randomised trial. *Lancet* 2008 371(9617): 987–997. https://doi.org/10.1016/S0140-6736(08)60453-5.
151. van Dullemen HM, van Deventer SJ, Hommes DW, et al. Treatment of Crohn's disease with anti-tumor necrosis factor chimeric monoclonal antibody (cA2). *J. Gastroenterol* 1995; 109(1): 129–135. https://doi.org/10.1016/0016-5085(95)90277-5.
152. Targan SR, Hanauer SB, Deventer SJ, et al. A short-term study of chimeric monoclonal antibody cA2 to tumor necrosis factor alpha for Crohn's disease. Crohn's Disease cA2 Study Group. *N Engl J Med* 1997 ; 337(15): 1029–1035. https://doi.org/10.1056/NEJM199710093371502.
153. Chaudhari U, Romano P, Mulcahy LD, et al. Efficacy and safety of infliximab monotherapy for plaque-type psoriasis: a randomised trial. *Lancet* 2001; 357(9271): 1842–1847. https://doi.org/10.1016/s0140-6736(00)04954-0.
154. Ghoreschi K, Thomas P, Breit S, et al. Interleukin-4 therapy of psoriasis induces Th2 responses and improves human autoimmune disease. *Nat Med* 2003;9(1):40–46. https://doi.org/10.1038/nm804.
155. Leonardi C, Matheson R Zachariae C, et al. Anti-interleukin-17 monoclonal antibody ixekizumab in chronic plaque psoriasis. *N Engl J Med* 2012;366(13):1190–1199. https://doi.org/10.1056/NEJMoa1109997.
156. Papp, K.A., Leonardi, C., Menter, A. et al. (2012). Brodalumab, an anti-interleukin-17-receptor antibody for psoriasis. *N Engl J Med* 366 (13): 1181–1189. https://doi.org/10.1056/NEJMoa1109017.
157. Papp KA, Langley RG, Lebwohl M, et al Efficacy and safety of ustekinumab, a human interleukin-12/23 monoclonal antibody, in patients with psoriasis: 52-week results from a randomised, double-blind, placebo-controlled trial (PHOENIX 2). *Lancet* 2008;371(9625):1675–1684. https://doi.org/10.1016/S0140-6736(08)60726-6.
158. Poeta V, Massara M, Capucetti A, Bonecchi R Chemokines and chemokine receptors: new targets for cancer immunotherapy. *Front Immunol* 2019;10: 379. https://doi.org/10.3389/fimmu.2019.00379.
159. Coleman RL, Duska LR, Ramirez PT, et al. Phase 1-2 study of docetaxel plus aflibercept in patients with recurrent ovarian, primary peritoneal, or fallopian tube cancer. *Lancet Oncol* 2011;12(12):1109–1117. https://doi.org/10.1016/S1470-2045(11)70244-3.
160. Fulciniti M, Hideshima T, Vermot-Desroches C, et al. A high-affinity fully human anti-IL-6 mAb, 1339, for the treatment of multiple myeloma. *Clin Cancer Res* 2009;15(23):7144–7052. https://doi.org/10.1158/1078-0432.CCR-09-1483.
161. Nair P, Pizzichini MM, Kjarsgaard M, et al. Mepolizumab for prednisone-dependent asthma with sputum eosinophilia. *N Engl J Med* 2009;360(10):985–993. https://doi.org/10.1056/NEJMoa0805435.
162. Corren J, Lemanske RF, Hanania NA, et al. Lebrikizumab treatment in adults with asthma. *N Engl J Med* 2011 365;(12):1088–1098. https://doi.org/10.1056/NEJMoa1106469.
163. Beck LA, Thaçi D, Hamilton JD, et al. Dupilumab treatment in adults with moderate-to-severe atopic dermatitis. *N Engl J Med* 2014 ;371(2):130–139. https://doi.org/10.1056/NEJMoa1314768.
164. Soulillou, J.P., Cantarovich, D., le Mauff, B. et al. (1990). Randomized controlled trial of a monoclonal antibody against the interleukin-r Receptor (33B3.1) as compared with rabbit antithymocyte globulin for prophylaxis against rejection of renal allografts. *N Engl J Med* 322: 1175–1182. https://doi.org/10.1056/NEJM199004263221702.
165. Wynn D, Kaufman M, Montalban X, et al. Daclizumab in active relapsing multiple sclerosis (CHOICE study): a phase 2, randomised, double-blind, placebo-controlled, add-on trial with interferon beta. *Lancet Neurol* 2010;9(4):381–390. https://doi.org/10.1016/S1474-4422(10)70033-8.

166. Merrill JT, Wallace DJ, Petri M, et al. Safety profile and clinical activity of sifalimumab, a fully human anti-interferon α monoclonal antibody, in systemic lupus erythematosus: a phase I, multicentre, double-blind randomised study. *Ann Rheum Dis* 2011;70(11):1905–1913. https://doi.org/10.1136/ard.2010.144485.
167. Cummings SR, San Martin J, McClung MR, et al. Denosumab for prevention of fractures in postmenopausal women with osteoporosis. *N Engl J Med* 2009361; (8):756–765. https://doi.org/10.1056/NEJMoa0809493.
168. Hench PS, Kendall EC, Slocumb CH, Polley HF The effect of a hormone of the adrenal cortex (17-hydroxy-11-dehydrocorticosterone: compound E) and of pituitary adrenocortical hormone in arthritis: preliminary report. *Ann Rheum Dis* 1949;8(2):97–104. https://doi.org/10.1136/ard.8.2.97.
169. Lannan, E.A., Galliher-Beckley, A.J., Scoltock, A.B., and Cidlowski, J.A. (2012). Proinflammatory actions of glucocorticoids: glucocorticoids and TNFα coregulate gene expression *in vitro* and *in vivo*. *Endocrinology* 153 (8): 3701–3712. https://doi.org/10.1210/en.2012-1020.
170. Staruch, M.J. and Wood, D.D. (1985). Reduction of serum Interleukin-1-like activity after treatment with dexamethasone. *J Leukoc Biol* 37 (2): 193–207. https://doi.org/10.1002/jlb.37.2.193.
171. Arya, S.K., Wong-Staal, F., and Gallo, R.C. (1984 Jul). Dexamethasone-mediated inhibition of human T cell growth factor and gamma-interferon messenger RNA. *J Immunol* 133 (1): 273–276.
172. Culpepper, J.A. and Lee, F. (1985). Regulation of IL 3 expression by glucocorticoids in cloned murine T lymphocytes. *J Immunol* 135 (5): 3191–3197.
173. Kelso, A. and Munck, A. (1984). Glucocorticoid inhibition of lymphokine secretion by alloreactive T lymphocyte clones. *J Immunol* 133 (2): 784–791.
174. Waage, A. and Bakke, O. (1988). Glucocorticoids suppress the production of tumour necrosis factor by lipopolysaccharide-stimulated human monocytes. *Immunology* 63 (2): 299–302.
175. Calandra T, Bernhagen J, Metz CN, et al. MIF as a glucocorticoid-induced modulator of cytokine production. *Nature* 1995; 377(6544): 68–71. https://doi.org/10.1038/377068a0.
176. Tabardel Y, Duchateau J, Schmartz D, et al. Corticosteroids increase blood interleukin-10 levels during cardiopulmonary bypass in men. *Surgery* 1996; 119(1): 76–80. https://doi.org/10.1016/s0039-6060(96)80217-0.
177. Fantuzzi G, Ghezzi P. Glucocorticoids as cytokine inhibitors: role in neuroendocrine control and therapy of inflammatory diseases. *Mediators Inflamm* 1993;2(4):263–270. https://doi.org/10.1155/S0962935193000365.
178. Opal SM, Fisher CJ Jr, Dhainaut JF, et al. Confirmatory interleukin-1 receptor antagonist trial in severe sepsis: a phase III, randomized, double-blind, placebo-controlled, multicenter trial. The Interleukin-1 Receptor Antagonist Sepsis Investigator Group. *Crit Care Med* 1997;25(7):1115–1124. https://doi.org/10.1097/00003246-199707000-00010.
179. Shakoory, B., Carcillo, J.A., Chatham, W.W. et al. (2016). Interleukin-1 receptor blockade is associated with reduced mortality in sepsis patients with features of macrophage activation syndrome: reanalysis of a prior phase III trial. *Crit Care Med* 44 (2): 275–281. https://doi.org/10.1097/CCM.0000000000001402.
180. Dimopoulos G, de Mast Q, Markou N, et al. Favorable Anakinra responses in severe Covid-19 patients with secondary hemophagocytic lymphohistiocytosis. *Cell Host Microbe* 2020 28;(1):117–123.e1. https://doi.org/10.1016/j.chom.2020.05.007.
181. Larsen CM, Faulenbach M, Vaag A, et al. Interleukin-1-receptor antagonist in type 2 diabetes mellitus. *N Engl J Med* 2007 ;356(15):1517–1526. https://doi.org/10.1056/NEJMoa065213.
182. So A, De Smedt T, Revaz S, Tschopp J A pilot study of IL-1 inhibition by anakinra in acute gout. *Arthritis Res Ther* 2007;9(2):R28. https://doi.org/10.1186/ar2143.

183. Botsios C, Sfriso P, Furlan A, et al. Resistant Behçet disease responsive to anakinra. *Ann Intern Med* 2008;149(4):284–286. https://doi.org/10.7326/0003-4819-149-4-200808190-00018.
184. Abbate A Kontos MC, Grizzard JD, et al. Interleukin-1 blockade with anakinra to prevent adverse cardiac remodeling after acute myocardial infarction (Virginia Commonwealth University Anakinra Remodeling Trial [VCU-ART] pilot study). *Am J Cardiol* 2010 ;105(10):1371–1377.e1. https://doi.org/10.1016/j.amjcard.2009.12.059.
185. Aksentijevich I, Masters SL, Ferguson PJ, et al. An autoinflammatory disease with deficiency of the interleukin-1-receptor antagonist. *N Engl J Med* 2009;360(23):2426–2437. https://doi.org/10.1056/NEJMoa0807865.
186. Lachmann HJ, Kone-Paut I, Kuemmerle-Deschner JB, et al. Use of canakinumab in the cryopyrin-associated periodic syndrome. *N Engl J Med* 2009 ;36023:2416–2425. https://doi.org/10.1056/NEJMoa0810787.
187. Bovet, D. and Staub, A.M. (1937). Action de la thymoxyéthyldiéthylamine (929 F) et des éthers phénoliques sur le choc anaphylactique du cobaye. *C R Soc Biol* 125: 818–823.
188. Kan, N., Ohgaki, K., Yamasaki, N. et al. (1983). Cancer immunotherapy by local transfer of autologous T lymphocytes cultured with T cell growth factor and autologous tumor extract: a clinical trial. *Arch Jpn Chir* 52 (6): 841–853.
189. Mazumder, A. and Rosenberg, S.A. (1984). Successful immunotherapy of natural killer-resistant established pulmonary melanoma metastases by the intravenous adoptive transfer of syngeneic lymphocytes activated in vitro by interleukin 2. *J Exp Med* 159 (2): 495–507. https://doi.org/10.1084/jem.159.2.495.
190. Mulé, J.J., Shu, S., Schwarz, S.L., and Rosenberg, S.A. (1984). Adoptive immunotherapy of established pulmonary metastases with LAK cells and recombinant interleukin-2. *Science* 225 (4669): 1487–1489. https://doi.org/10.1126/science.6332379.
191. Rosenberg, S.A., Spiess, P., and Lafreniere, R. (1986). A new approach to the adoptive immunotherapy of cancer with tumor-infiltrating lymphocytes. *Science* 233 (4770): 1318–1321. https://doi.org/10.1126/science.3489291.
192. Miescher, S., Whiteside, T.L., Carrel, S., and von Fliedner, V. (1986). Functional properties of tumor-infiltrating and blood lymphocytes in patients with solid tumors: effects of tumor cells and their supernatants on proliferative responses of lymphocytes. *J Immunol.* 136 (5): 1899–1907.
193. Rosenberg, S.A., Packard, B.S., Aebersold, P.M. et al. (1988). Use of tumor-infiltrating lymphocytes and interleukin-2 in the immunotherapy of patients with metastatic melanoma. A preliminary report. *N Engl J Med* 319 (25): 1676–1680. https://doi.org/10.1056/NEJM198812223192527.
194. Kuwana, Y., Asakura, Y., Utsunomiya, N. et al. (1987). Expression of chimeric receptor composed of immunoglobulin-derived V regions and T-cell receptor-derived c regions. *Biochem Biophys Res Commun* 149: 960–968. https://doi.org/10.1016/0006-291X(87)90502-X.
195. Hwu, P., Shafer, G.E., Treisman, J. et al. (1993). Lysis of ovarian cancer cells by human lymphocytes redirected with a chimeric gene composed of an antibody variable region and the fc receptor gamma chain. *J Exp Med* 178: 361–366. https://doi.org/10.1084/jem.178.1.361.
196. Hwu, P., Yang, J.C., Cowherd, R. et al. (1995). In vivo antitumor activity of T cells redirected with chimeric antibody/T-cell receptor genes. *Cancer Res* 55 (15): 3369–3373.
197. Neelapu, S.S., Locke, F.L., Bartlett, N.L. et al. (2017). Axicabtagene ciloleucel CAR T-cell therapy in refractory large B-cell lymphoma. *N Engl J Med* 377 (26): 2531–2544. https://doi.org/10.1056/NEJMoa1707447.
198. Teachey, D.T., Lacey, S.F., Shaw, P.A. et al. (2016). Identification of predictive biomarkers for cytokine release syndrome after chimeric antigen receptor T-cell therapy for acute lymphoblastic leukemia. *Cancer Discov* 6 (6): 664–679. https://doi.org/10.1158/2159-8290.CD-16-0040.

199. Liu, E., Marin, D., Banerjee, P. et al. (2020). Use of CAR-Transduced natural killer cells in CD19-positive lymphoid tumors. *N Engl J Med* 382: 545–553. https://doi.org/10.1056/NEJMoa1910607.
200. Inaba, K., Metlay, J.P., Crowley, M.T., and Steinman, R.M. (1990). Dendritic cells pulsed with protein antigens in vitro can prime antigen-specific, MHC-restricted T cells in situ. *J Exp Med* 172 (2): 631–640. https://doi.org/10.1084/jem.172.2.631.
201. Hsu FJ, Benike C, Fagnoni F, et al. Vaccination of patients with B-cell lymphoma using autologous antigen-pulsed dendritic cells. *Nat Med* 1996 ;2(1):52–58. https://doi.org/10.1038/nm0196-52.
202. Selye, H. (1936). A syndrome produced by diverse nocuous agents. *Nature* 138: 32.
203. Tracey KJ. Physiology and immunology of the cholinergic antiinflammatory pathway. *J Clin Invest* 2007 ; 117(2): 289–296. https://doi.org/10.1172/JCI30555.
204. Koopman FA, Chavan SS, Miljko S, et al. Vagus nerve stimulation inhibits cytokine production and attenuates disease severity in rheumatoid arthritis. *Proc Natl Acad Sci USA* 2016; 113(29): 8284–8289. https://doi.org/10.1073/pnas.1605635113.
205. Bonaz B, Sinniger V, Hoffmann D, et al. Chronic vagus nerve stimulation in Crohn's disease: a 6-month follow-up pilot study. *Neurogastroenterol Motil* 2016; 28(6): 948–953. https://doi.org/10.1111/nmo.12792.
206. Kohoutova M, Horak J, Jarkovska D et al. Vagus nerve stimulation attenuates multiple organ dysfunction in resuscitated porcine progressive sepsis. *Crit Care Med* 2019;47(6):e461–e469. https://doi.org/10.1097/CCM.0000000000003714.
207. Wu Z, Zhang X, Cai T, et al. Transcutaneous auricular vagus nerve stimulation reduces cytokine production in sepsis: an open double-blind, sham-controlled, pilot study. *Brain Stimul* 2023;16(2):507–514. https://doi.org/10.1016/j.brs.2023.02.008.
208. Osuchowski, M. and Cavaillon, J.M. (2025). Obituary Tomasz Skirecki (May 22nd, 1987–January 21st, 2025). *Microb Infect* 27 (3): 105525. https://doi.org/10.1016/j.micinf.2025.105482.

2

Introduction to Immunology and Immune Modulation

JANIN CHANDRA, LAKSHITA PATIL, AND GRAHAM LEGGATT
Frazer Institute, Faculty of Health, Medicine and Behavioural Sciences, The University of Queensland, Brisbane, Queensland, Australia

LEARNING OBJECTIVES

- Overview of immune cells and their functions
- Understand how immunity to pathogens is activated
- Recognise key differences between innate and adaptive immune mechanisms
- Know key aspects of immune regulation and how they relate to immune-driven diseases

2.1 THE FRONTLINES OF IMMUNE DEFENCE

The body is protected from the outside world through the skin and the mucosal epithelium [1]. The skin contains a densely packed layer of keratinocytes called the epidermis. The outermost layer of the epidermis, the stratum corneum, consists of dead keratinised cells and is waterproof, thereby resisting pathogen entry. In addition, the epidermis continuously renews, and surface-attached pathogens are expelled together with dead keratinocytes. The skin further produces sweat and sebum, which contain antimicrobial molecules like lysozymes, defensins, and cathelicidins. On inner surfaces, the mucosal epithelium is a key barrier to infection, assisted by the production of an overlying mucous layer. Mucus serves both as a physical and a chemical barrier to stop pathogen invasion [2]. Physically, it traps pathogens, and chemically, it contains antimicrobial substances including lysozymes, defensins, and lactoferrin. This mucus also has an 'outward' flow direction, facilitating expulsion of pathogens, for example, upwards from the lungs into the mouth and nose, and downwards and out from the intestinal and female reproductive system. The eye has developed a special biochemical barrier called tears [3]. Tears consist of mucus, water, oil, and soluble immunoglobulin (Ig)A antibodies, contain antimicrobial properties, and are designed to wash out dust and neutralise pathogens while preserving ocular surface integrity.

If pathogens manage to overcome these first physical and biochemical barriers, they will then have to breach the epithelial cell layers to enter the body. Epithelial cells are therefore firmly connected with tight junctions, including Claudins, Occludins, Zona Occludens proteins and junctional adhesion molecules [1].

The skin and mucosal epithelia of the body are further heavily populated with cells of the innate and adaptive immune system. In fact, the skin contains twice the number of immune cells than present in the blood [4]. While the epithelial cells are static, the immune cells are mobile and can move towards biochemical signals that suggest danger or invasion, and enter or exit the epithelium.

2.2 PAMPS AND DAMPS

The immune system has developed a range of molecular detectors of so-called pathogen- or damage-associated molecular patterns (PAMPs or DAMPs). These detectors, called pattern recognition receptors (PRRs), can recognise components of bacteria, viruses, fungi, and parasites, or cellular damage related to injury, mechanical stress, and cell death [5]. Common PAMPs are bacterial cell wall components including lipopolysaccharides (Gram-negative bacteria), peptidoglycans (Gram-positive bacteria), and flagellin (motile bacteria), as well as unmethylated bacterial and viral CpG DNA, double- and single-stranded viral RNA, and fungal components such as zymosan, mannan, and glucans. DAMPs often represent molecules intrinsic to the host (referred to as 'self'), such as high levels of ATP, DNA or histones in the cytoplasm of dying cells, heat shock and S100 proteins, calreticulin as an indicator of endoplasmic reticulum (ER) stress and apoptosis, or oxidised phospholipids as a sign of damaged membranes. PRRs are groups of receptors, including the Toll-like receptors (TLRs), NOD-like receptors (NLRs), RIG-I-like receptors (RLRs), and C-type lectin receptors (CLRs). The recognition of PAMPs and DAMPs is often the first step of immune detection. While all immune cells express some PRRs, specialised tissue-resident and patrolling immune cells called macrophages and dendritic cells detect the broadest range of PAMPs and DAMPs, positioning them as central coordinators of immune surveillance and early alarm signalling.

2.3 COMPLEMENT SYSTEM

The complement system is a truly ancient part of the innate immune system, which first evolved more than 1,000 million years ago in protostomes, and continues to play a fundamental role in the immune defence in higher vertebrates, including humans [6]. It consists of over 30 proteins, providing an immediate soluble barrier to defend against pathogens, clear dead cells, and amplify inflammation. It is activated either by specific PAMPs such as microbial carbohydrates or by immune complexes including antibodies. Complement proteins coat pathogens, a process termed opsonisation, thereby facilitating phagocytosis by specialised innate immune cells. It further generates potent inflammatory mediators, leading to the recruitment of immune cells. Specific complement proteins can also directly induce the death of Gram-negative bacteria by forming membrane-attack complexes.

2.4 INNATE IMMUNE CELLS

The first line of an immune response in the epithelium often involves the release of DAMPs and immune signalling molecules called **alarmins** by epithelial cells in response to infection, injury, or cellular stress (Figure 2.1a). These

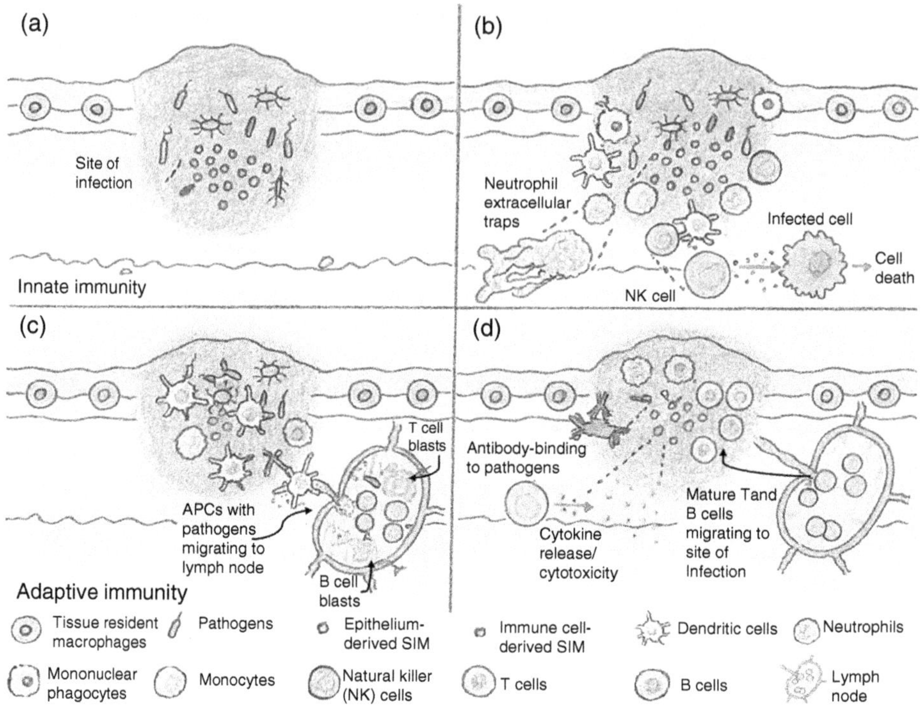

FIGURE 2.1 **A basic overview of an immune response to infection.** (a) A viral or bacterial infection to the epithelium leads to local inflammation by the release of alarmins and cytokines by epithelial cells and tissue-resident innate immune cells. (b) This inflammation leads to the recruitment of other innate immune cells, including neutrophils, monocytes, dendritic cells, and NK cells. Neutrophils and NK cells will contain the infection by the release of cytotoxic cytokines and NETs. Dendritic cells and macrophages will phagocytose pathogens and migrate to the draining lymph node. (c) In the lymph node, dendritic cells and macrophages will present antigen and activate T cells and B cells, leading to T cell and B cell expansion. (d) Adaptive T cells and B cells will then migrate to the site of inflammation using chemokine gradients and destroy the infected cells and pathogens using antibodies and cytotoxic effector molecules. Soluble immune mediators (SIM): alarmins, chemokines, cytokines, cytotoxic molecules. Created by the authors. Original figure; copyright held by the chapter contributors.

epithelial-cell-derived molecules, together with **cytokines** secreted by surveilling **tissue-resident macrophages** in response to PAMPs and DAMPs, trigger the activation of endothelial cells, leading to the recruitment of other circulating immune cells from the blood. Endothelial cells exposed to alarmins and an inflammatory cytokine milieu will upregulate adhesion molecules, including E- and P-selectins, as well as ICAM-1 and VCAM-1, to increase vascular permeability and allow immune cells to enter the site of harm. Innate immune cells in circulation, such as neutrophils, monocytes, and dendritic cells (DCs), will roll along the activated endothelium and eventually migrate through the endothelium by connecting firmly with endothelial cells and following a gradient of **chemokines**. Chemokines are small proteins that induce the activation and migration of cells bearing the corresponding chemokine receptor. Once in the tissue, these innate immune cells will destroy, trap or phagocytose pathogens, release additional cytokines, and amplify the immune response (Figure 2.1b).

Neutrophils are the first innate immune cells to be recruited to the site of inflammation from the bloodstream. They can contain pathogens through mechanisms of phagocytosis, the release of cytotoxic granules, cytokine communication to other immune cells, and the expel of so-called neutrophil extracellular traps (NETs) [7]. NETs are a web of neutrophil DNA containing cytotoxic granule proteins that help to trap and degrade pathogens, and their expulsion is often associated with neutrophil cell death termed NETosis. With NETosis leading to cell rupture, this process often contributes to the inflammatory process by triggering a DAMP response in addition to the recognition of PAMPs. **Mast cells**, **basophils** and **eosinophils** are also recruited through chemokine gradients and play roles in tissue repair and wound healing, in the defence against parasites through the release of inflammatory mediators, and in the allergy response.

A cytotoxic innate immune cell called the **natural killer (NK) cell** is recruited through proinflammatory cytokines, interleukin (IL)-12, IL-15, and IL-18, typically released by neutrophils and tissue-resident macrophages. The activation of NK cells is controlled by the balance of signals from activating and inhibitory receptors on the NK cell surface. NK cells respond to the downregulation of inhibitory ligands such as major histocompatibility complex class I (MHCI), a molecule normally expressed by all nucleated cells and involved in antigen presentation. They also detect activating stress signals on infected cells, including the MHCI-related molecules MICA and MICB, enabling NK cell engagement even in the absence of pathogen-specific antigen recognition. [8]. Due to their cytotoxic potential, NK cells are able to provide a fast response by directly killing infected cells through the release of the cytotoxic effector molecules perforin and granzymes (Figure 2.1b). Through these mechanisms, NK cells also contribute to the killing of tumour cells.

While these innate immune effector cells work to contain the spread of infection, other innate immune cells with the ability to activate the adaptive immune arm come into play. **Macrophages** and **DCs** belong to the mononuclear phagocyte system, due to their specialised function in phagocytosis (Figure 2.1c) [9]. Macrophages and DCs are highly abundant throughout all epithelia [10] and are further recruited from the blood during inflammation. Both act as professional **antigen-presenting cells (APCs)** and play a pivotal role in the first sensing of damage and pathogens. APCs are classified as innate immune cells due to their capability of PAMP and DAMP sensing through PRRs, phagocytosis, and cytokine release capabilities, but are further essential in bridging the innate and adaptive immune functions through the process of antigen presentation. Macrophages play a primary role in tissue in phagocytosis, the clearance of debris, wound healing, and local cytokine signalling. DCs are more specialised to migrate via lymphatics to the draining lymph node and present processed antigens to naïve T cells. The macrophage ontogeny depends on the sensing of macrophage colony-stimulating factor (M-CSF) through CSF1 receptor, and macrophages therefore represent one immune lineage. DCs can be further categorised into multiple lineages. These include **plasmacytoid DCs (pDC)** and **conventional DCs (cDC)**. The classification of pDCs as DCs is currently controversial as these cells play important roles in innate immunity through their rapid and strong release of type I interferons upon PAMP and DAMP sensing, while they have limited antigen presentation capability [11]. In contrast, cDC are characterised by a high capability of antigen presentation and T cell activation; however, further lineage distinction is important for ontogeny and function. Type 1 cDC (**cDC1**) are specialised in cross-presentation of antigens, a process that will be further explained below, and is important for the initiation of cytotoxic T cell responses. cDC1 therewith play a major role in viral responses and in tumour immunity. The **cDC2** immune lineage has recently been delineated into further subsets, where their nomenclature and lineage identity are still being established [12]. They play an important role in the initiation of helper T cell responses. Other DC subtypes have recently been described, including DC3, but their lineage identity and function have not been fully resolved yet [12].

2.5 ANTIGEN PRESENTATION

Antigen presentation describes the processing and presentation of protein antigens that lymphocytes of the adaptive immune arm can recognise through specialised receptors [13]. Peptide fragments, derived from protein antigens, are presented to T cells through molecules called **MHC**. MHC exists as class I and class II molecules. While MHCI is expressed by all nucleated cells in the body, MHCII is primarily expressed by APCs of the mononuclear phagocyte system.

MHC molecules are always loaded with peptide antigens. These peptides are either self-antigens or foreign antigens derived from pathogens. APCs capture foreign antigens either through phagocytosis of pathogens or pathogen-infected cells or through direct infection by viruses or bacteria. Self-antigen presented in the absence of danger signals will induce tolerance. The induction of adaptive immunity to foreign antigens depends on a combination of signals from APCs to T cells . When APCs sense danger through PRRs, they upregulate co-stimulatory molecules and express proinflammatory cytokines. A T cell which recognises the MHC-presented peptide through their T cell receptor (TCR) is then activated and will proliferate and develop a functional programme which depends on the specific additional signals the APC provides as co-simulation and cytokines. The corresponding T cell outcomes can be highly varied and are orchestrated to suit the specific need.

Antigen presentation plays a major role in the regulation of anti-tumour immunity. APCs must acquire tumour cell-derived antigen to induce tumour-directed T cell responses. This is complicated when the tumour antigen is also a self-antigen and will not trigger conventional PRRs, often leading to tolerance induction and immune escape (see Chapter 3).

2.6 ADAPTIVE IMMUNITY

The adaptive immune system is composed of **T cells** and **B cells**, with each individual cell being defined by the expression of a unique TCR or B cell receptor (BCR) [14]. These receptors are composed of two protein chains each constructed to contain a variable region, responsible for ligand binding and encoded by random recombination of a highly diverse set of genes, fused with a constant region encoded by a smaller set of conserved genes. The two protein chains in conventional T cells are the TCR alpha and beta chain which combine to form a heterodimeric receptor that functions at the cell surface to recognise the peptide/MHC complex. In contrast,

B cells express heavy and light chain proteins, each composed of a variable and constant region, that fold together to produce the surface-bound BCR or a secreted receptor known as antibody. BCRs bind to a variety of soluble or cell-bound ligands, also referred to as antigens, via the variable regions of the heavy and light chains. In more recent times, the term 'antigen' has been more broadly used for any ligands recognised by TCR or BCR. The B cell heavy chain protein has a selection of five different constant region genes (IgM, IgD, IgG, IgE, IgA), each of which conveys different functional properties to the secreted antibodies. It is estimated that random recombination within the TCR/BCR variable regions of each protein chain can generate $>10^{10}$ different sequences, with each individual T or B cell inheriting just one receptor sequence. T and B cells that encounter the matching ligand for their TCR/BCR undergo clonal expansion and gain effector function during the course of an immune response. The adaptive immune cells also display **memory** for previously encountered ligands, whereby some activated/effector T and B cells will enter a resting state until further challenge with the same ligand, a feature which is central to the success of prophylactic vaccines.

2.6.1 Development of T and B Cells

Most cells that constitute the immune system are generated from haematopoietic stem cells arising in the bone marrow after birth. Both surface interactions and soluble molecules released within the bone marrow microenvironment direct stem cells into a lymphoid lineage – giving rise to T and B cells, or a myeloid lineage – giving rise to many of the innate immune cells. While B cell development from the lymphoid lineage occurs in the bone marrow, precursors for T cells migrate under the influence of chemokines to the thymus for further development [15]. In both the bone marrow and the thymus, TCRs and BCRs are generated through gene rearrangements, thus committing the lymphoid precursors to a T cell or B cell lineage. Conventional T cells express a heterodimeric TCR composed of an alpha and beta chain, while the alternate combination of a gamma and delta TCR chain leads to the formation of gamma delta T cells, a cell type that recognises a diverse array of common pathogen-derived metabolites and is generally involved in innate immune function. Among T cells with an alpha beta TCR, there are **unconventional T cells**, such as **natural killer T (NKT) cells** and **mucosal-associated invariant T (MAIT) cells**, which can express a conserved alpha chain and a more limited range of beta chains. These T cell subsets have TCRs that can recognise non-peptide components of pathogens such as glycolipids and Vitamin B metabolites. In the late stages of thymic development, **conventional T cells** express either a CD4 or CD8 co-receptor, which assists the signal transmitted through the TCR. B cells in the bone marrow will initially express a membrane-bound form of IgM, which acts as the BCR. Given the large array of random BCR and TCR sequences generated during development, receptors may be generated that are reactive to molecules/antigens within the body that it is aiming to protect. These molecules are commonly referred to as **self**. Both B and T cells are tested for reactivity to self-antigens during selection processes in the bone marrow or thymus. High-affinity TCR/BCR binding to self-antigen leads to apoptosis of the cell, thus reducing the chance of autoimmune diseases once the B or T cells are released into the blood. This process in the thymus is referred to as **central tolerance**. At the conclusion of selection events, the cells are released into the bloodstream, where they are now referred to as naïve T and B cells. Due to their unique pattern of adhesion molecules and chemokine receptors, the majority of naïve B and T cells circulate between the blood and lymphatics, where they will encounter secondary lymphoid organs such as the lymph nodes and spleen. In these secondary lymphoid organs, both B and T cells have the opportunity to transition from a naïve cell into an activated, effector cell phenotype.

2.6.2 Naïve T Cell Activation

L-selectin and CCR7 are two key surface molecules that allow migration of T cells from the high endothelial venules of the blood into the lymph node. There are a large number of lymph nodes throughout the body to capture draining fluids and cells that have been transported through lymphatic vessels from local tissue sites. The spleen acts as a similar filter for antigens circulating in the blood. Importantly, DCs capture antigens from the tissue sites, degrade protein into peptides, and move to the draining lymph node to present these peptides in association with MHC molecules to naïve T cells (Figure 2.2). This process of engaging naïve T cells with antigen-bearing DCs in the lymph node (or spleen) is called T activation. T cell activation and differentiation require three signals within the lymph node microenvironment.

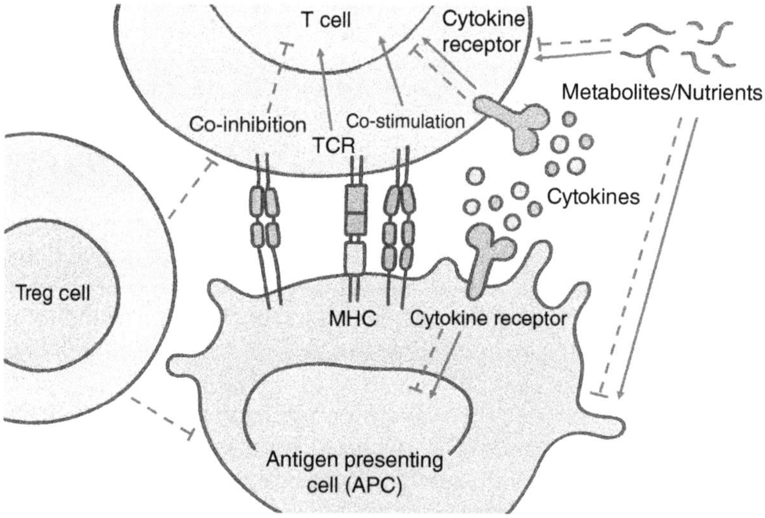

FIGURE 2.2 T cell activation and modulation by co-stimulation, co-inhibition, and Tregs. T cell activation occurs when antigen-presenting cells (APCs) present peptide/MHC to the T cell receptor (TCR) on naïve T cells. However, this initial signal alone is insufficient for full activation. A secondary signal, either co-stimulatory or co-inhibitory, is required to determine whether T cell activation is successful. Co-stimulatory signals, delivered through interactions such as CD28 on T cells and CD80/86 on APCs, promote activation, while co-inhibitory signals, such as CTLA-4 binding, inhibit T cell activation. Tregs also play a critical role in modulating both APC and T cell responses, providing an indirect regulatory effect on the immune activation process. Additionally, cytokines released during infection bind to cytokine receptors on both APCs and T cells, further influencing their activation or inhibition. Nutrients and metabolites also impact antigen presentation by APCs and the activation of T cells, contributing to the overall immune response. Created by the authors. Original figure; copyright held by the chapter contributors.

Firstly, the correct peptide/MHC complex has to be presented on the DC surface to the TCR, and this represents **signal 1.** The interaction between CD28 on the T cell and CD80/86 provides **signal 2,** which is critical to activation, while a number of different cytokines or cell surface interactions give **signal 3**, which differentiates the naïve T cell into one of many different functional T cell subsets. The process of activation can be enhanced by other co-stimulatory molecules, such as CD137, or suppressed by inhibitory receptors on the T cell surface such as cytotoxic T-lymphocyte-associated protein-4 (CTLA-4) and programmed cell death protein 1 (PD-1) [16]. Following the delivery of the three signals, the individual T cell will undergo clonal expansion (facilitated by growth factors such as IL-2) and finally gain function and differentiate into an activated, effector T cell. Effector T cells have several key differences with naïve T cells, including a change in adhesion molecules allowing for exit from the lymph node and passage into inflamed tissue sites, upregulation of chemokine receptors that help direct the T cell from the bloodstream towards sources of tissue inflammation, and the gain of effector molecules, which may be held in secretory granules within the cell.

2.6.3 Naïve B Cell Activation

Naïve B cells enter secondary lymphoid organs in a similar manner to naïve T cells. Within the lymphoid organ, the B cells accumulate within B cell follicles and can form **germinal centres** [17]. Antigens that activate B cells enter secondary lymphoid organs from the blood or lymphatics either as soluble molecules or bound to the surface of DCs. Critical to the activation of most naïve B cells are signals derived from CD4 T cells. Naïve B cells that bind to foreign antigens via their BCR will internalise the antigen and peptides derived from the enzymatic digestion of proteins and the antigen will be displayed on MHC II molecules at the B cell surface. Effector CD4 T cells, which recognise these peptide/MHC II complexes, will then provide activation signals through secreted cytokines (e.g. IL-5) or cell surface receptor interactions (e.g. CD40–CD40L). The activation process for B cells has parallels with T cell activation, where BCR interaction with antigen is signal 1, and CD4 T cell interactions provide the second and third signals. Although most naïve B cell activation requires T cell help, there are naïve B cells which can be activated by certain pathogen-derived structures (e.g. lipopolysaccharide, LPS, and bacterial lectins) such that the need for T cell help is bypassed (T-independent antibody responses). Once activated, B cells can uniquely make changes to their BCR through the introduction of random mutations and subsequent receptor selection such that the affinity of the BCR for antigen is increased. Cytokines/surface interactions in the lymph node can also result in **isotype switching**, whereby the initial IgM heavy chain is replaced by other heavy chains (e.g. IgG). Following activation, B cells can cease to produce a surface BCR and instead become a **plasma cell**, which now secretes the BCR into the bodily fluids as a soluble molecule called immunoglobulin or antibody.

2.6.4 Effector T Cells

The two key conventional effector T cells are CD4 and CD8 T cells. CD8 T cells are commonly referred to as **cytotoxic T cells,** as they are capable of secreting molecules that enter the target cell and induce apoptosis. During differentiation, CD8 T cells acquire cytotoxic granules, which contain proteins such as perforin and granzymes that can be released from the T cell across the cellular synapse towards the engaged target cell, resulting in internalisation and granzyme-mediated activation of target cell apoptosis. To trigger release of cytotoxic granules, it is required that the effector T cells engage their TCR with the same peptide/MHC complex that caused T cell activation in the lymph node. The second and third signals are not a requirement for the effector function of activated T cells. Signalling from the CD8 T cell TCR can also result in the secretion of cytokines (e.g. IFN-γ) or upregulation of cell surface molecules (e.g. FasL) that assist with target cell clearance. Effector T cell function routinely occurs in the inflamed/infected tissues of the body. CD4 T cells are also known as **helper T cells (Th)** due to their secretion of cytokines or expression of surface ligands, which assist with the function of other immune cells. Early research separated CD4 T cells into two subsets, Th1 and Th2, based on the T cell production of the cytokines IFN-γ and IL-4, respectively. IFN-γ was important in assisting macrophages with phagocytosis and the killing of intracellular bacteria, while IL-4 promoted immunity against helminth worms and assisted with antibody production. Further characterisation of CD4 T cells led to the identification of other prominent helper T cell subsets such as Th17 and T follicular helper T (Tfh) cells. Th17 cells are involved in promoting inflammation through secretion of IL-17, which primarily acts on non-immune cells to induce chemokines which attract neutrophils. Tfh cells take up specialised niches within the lymph node follicles and assist with antibody production through cytokines such as IL-21. During differentiation and in the presence of cytokines such as transforming growth factor-beta (TGF-β), or weak co-stimulation and strong co-inhibition by APCs, some peripheral CD4 T cells can differentiate into **peripherally-derived regulatory T cells (pTreg)** [18]. Treg can also be generated in the thymus during T cell development based on an intermediate level of TCR signalling when presented with self-antigen, and are referred to as **thymus-derived regulatory T cells (tTreg)**. Both types of Treg are involved in **immune tolerance** by suppressing immune responses against infection or cancer and preventing autoimmune responses. The secretion of IL-10/TGF-β and surface interactions involving CTLA-4 are two key mechanisms by which Treg achieve their suppressive role in the immune system.

2.6.5 Effector B Cells and Antibody

A key role of effector B cells is to differentiate into plasma cells which no longer express a surface BCR and instead secrete large quantities of that same receptor as soluble antibody into the bloodstream. The first release is characterised by a predominance of IgM isotype antibodies, which then switch to IgG, IgA, and IgE, dependent on the cytokine microenvironment and signals provided by the CD4 helper T cells. Each isotype of antibody has a preferred different location within the body or performs a particular function. IgM forms pentameric structures, which are largely restricted to the bloodstream and will interact with complement proteins effectively. IgG is the most frequent antibody in the blood and has the ability to pass across the placenta to provide maternal antibody protection to the developing foetus. IgG antibodies can also attach to antigens on the surface of cells, resulting in binding of NK cells to the constant region of the IgG and the induction of **antibody-dependent cellular cytotoxicity (ADCC)**, resulting in apoptosis of the cell. Mucosal surfaces and fluids are largely dominated by dimeric IgA antibodies which are capable of being transcytosed through epithelial cells and into the luminal mucous secretions. This is particularly important as breast milk will transfer maternal IgA to the newborn gut to assist in protection against colonisation with pathogenic gut organisms. IgE antibodies are commonly found on the surface of mast cells expressing a surface receptor which binds to the constant region of the IgE molecule. On the mast cells, the IgE antibody can attach to allergens (e.g. bee venom, grass pollens), resulting in the formation of allergic disease, or attach to parasites, resulting in mast cell degranulation and destruction of large parasites.

2.6.6 Immunological Memory

Both T and B cells that have undergone activation in response to antigen have the capability to form long-lived immune cells referred to as **memory T and B cells** [19]. Memory cells can reside in the secondary lymphoid organs (spleen, lymph nodes) or bone marrow, or establish within previously infected tissues as **resident memory cells**. Memory B and T cells have also undergone epigenetic changes and membrane rearrangement of antigen receptors such that they are capable of responding much more rapidly to a second antigen challenge. Vaccination leverages this principle by generating these long-lived memory T and B cells in advance of infection, enabling a rapid and highly effective response upon real pathogen exposure by markedly shortening the lag time to effector response and thereby reducing the severity of symptoms.

2.6.7 Modulation of the Adaptive Immune Response

To avoid the development of autoimmune reactions or to reduce immune function following clearance of a pathogen, the immune system counterbalances immune activation with suppressive and inhibitory mechanisms (Figure 2.2). Non-responsiveness of lymphocytes to antigens present outside the thymus is referred to as **peripheral tolerance**.

Immune checkpoint inhibitors represent a class of surface proteins that transmit suppressive intracellular signals when engaged with ligand or compete with activating receptors to successfully shut down adaptive immune cell function. Upregulation of these inhibitory proteins on T cells is often associated with chronic antigen engagement, thus giving rise to the term '**exhausted T cells**' [20]. While these counterbalances have an important role in dampening the immune response after pathogen clearance, these same mechanisms can be hijacked by tumours to minimise the anti-tumour immune response, as has been observed with immunoinhibitory receptors such as PD-1 and LAG-3. Secreted cytokines such as TGF-β and IL-10 also produce immunosuppressive signals when engaged with their respective cytokine receptors on T and B cells. Cytokine-mediated suppression represents one of the key mechanisms used by Treg, an inhibitory subset of CD4 T cells, to dampen immune responses. Another key mechanism that limits immune cell activation and function is the availability of nutrients. Nutrients critical to T cell and B cell survival and function may be depleted within the local microenvironment by non-immune cells, leading to T cell and B cell **anergy** or apoptosis. An example of the evolutionary purpose of anergy is the production of the IDO enzyme within the placenta, which depletes tryptophan thus limiting the function of maternal T cells recognising paternal antigens bound to MHC expressed by the embryo, thus protecting the developing embryo from its mothers immune system [21]. Adaptive immune cell function may also be limited by physical access to the tissue in areas such as the brain, retina, or developing embryo under homeostatic conditions. Finally, a downregulation of immune-activating signals can also result in a modulation of adaptive immune cell function at the conclusion of an immune response.

2.7 TRAINED IMMUNITY – A DIFFERENT KIND OF IMMUNE MEMORY

The term immune memory is conventionally reserved for the recall response capabilities of T and B cells. However, more recent advances have identified mechanisms in **innate immune memory** (also termed **trained immunity**), leading to enhanced responsiveness to repeated challenges [22]. Examples of this are the 30% decrease in all-cause mortality in children vaccinated against measles, or the reduction of overall mortality in children from countries with high infectious burden after inoculation with the live vaccine bacillus Calmette–Guérin (BCG). Innate immune memory is mediated by **epigenetic and metabolic reprogramming** of innate immune cells after stimulation with PAMPs and DAMPs. Epigenetic changes are mediated through long-term histone modifications, influencing gene accessibility and transcription. Metabolic reprogramming is achieved by switching from oxidative phosphorylation to glycolysis or glutaminolysis for faster energy production and the Krebs cycle for lipid synthesis. As a result, these reprogrammed innate immune cells display enhanced functional responses upon subsequent stimulations, including increased cytokine release and antigen processing and presentation. Curiously, this trained immunity can also occur in non-immune cells, including in endothelial cells, epithelial cells, and fibroblasts, which also participate in immune initiation and regulation.

Because innate immune cells often have a short half-life, the proposition of a trained innate memory poses the question of whether systemic inflammation leads to reprogramming of haematopoietic progenitors and stem cells. Indeed, recent studies have identified long-lasting changes in circulating monocytes and neutrophils after BCG vaccination, and murine studies demonstrated epigenetic changes in multi-potent hematopoeitic stem cells in the bone marrow. These findings suggest that long-term innate immune 'memory' may be possible.

The advantage of trained immunity is its broad non-specific protection against pathogens, contributing to the overall buildup of immunity in young individuals. It can, however, also contribute to the development of chronic inflammation and its associated disorders, and more research is required to understand the delicate balance between these states of existence. This emerging field of research also opens up opportunities for the development of applications that specifically target trained innate immunity.

2.8 EXAMPLES OF FAILING IMMUNE REGULATION

The immune system has developed a range of immunoregulatory mechanisms that allow it to escalate and retract as needed. The balance between immune escalation and retraction is critical to allow the body to eliminate or control microbial invasion while limiting tissue damage. Life-threatening diseases can emerge when appropriate immune regulation is failing. These diseases include cancer, immunopathology after infections, and autoimmune diseases. Clinical approaches of immunotherapy aim to target these immunoregulatory mechanisms with the goal of restoring immune homeostasis and immune function. Below are examples of diseases triggered by a failure to regulate immune responses.

2.8.1 Cancer

Immune surveillance is the process by which the immune system continuously monitors the body for abnormal cells, such as infected, stressed, or transformed (cancerous) cells, and eliminates them to maintain tissue integrity and prevent disease. Therefore, the immune system has the ability to detect **tumour neoantigens**, antigens that are different from normal cells through the accumulation of mutations, initiating a cytotoxic T cell response. Stress-induced signals such as MICA/MICB and downregulation of MHC I molecules can be detected by NK cells to identify abnormal cells, and will trigger a cytotoxic killing response. When these immune surveillance mechanisms fail, abnormal cell growth can lead to tumour formation and invasive cancer. Tumours have developed a range of mechanisms to actively evade the immune system, a process that is explained in more detail in Chapter 3 and their immunotherapeutic opportunities in Part II (Chapters 4–7) of this book.

2.8.2 Immunopathology After Infection

Infection is one mechanism that can trigger **immunopathology** due to immune dysregulation. For example, excessive activation of innate and adaptive immune cells can lead to uncontrolled release of proinflammatory cytokines, leading to an acute cytokine storm. A systemic cytokine storm can lead to vascular leakage, coagulopathy, and multi-organ failure. Examples of these are vascular collapse after Ebola virus infection, due to massive cytokine release, and vascular leakage after Dengue virus infection. Sepsis due to bacterial blood infection can lead to thrombosis and organ failure. In contrast to this acute immune dysregulation, a chronic inflammation mediated by prolonged immune cell activity can lead to fibrosis. Post-virus lung fibrosis has been described after COVID-19 infection, and hepatitis B and C infection can lead to liver fibrosis and cirrhosis. Chronic tuberculosis can lead to the formation of granulomas, causing lung cavitation. Persistent viral infections such as with human immunodeficiency virus (HIV) or hepatitis B and C virus can lead T cells to become exhausted after chronic antigen exposure, enabling persistent inflammation and failure to clear infection. These are key examples where immunotherapeutic approaches are needed to overcome immunopathology after infection and chronic inflammation, and these will be specifically discussed in Part III (Chapters 8–10) of this book.

2.8.3 Chronic Inflammatory Diseases

While inflammation is critical to facilitate wound healing and the response to pathogens, if not resolved, chronic inflammatory conditions can develop. Examples of these are ulcerative colitis (gut inflammation), atopic dermatitis and hidradenitis suppurativa (skin inflammation), or atherosclerosis (arterial wall inflammation). The cytokine tumour necrosis factor alpha (TNF-α) is a key mediator of inflammation and is primarily produced by macrophages and monocytes at acute stages, while T and NK cells contribute to TNF-α production under chronic inflammatory conditions. TNF-α leads to a cascade in cytokine production, including proinflammatory cytokines IL-1 and IL-6, as well as nuclear factor-kappa B (NF-κB) activation in immune cells. It further activates endothelial cells and increases vascular permeability, resulting in swelling and the infiltration of immune cells. If persistent, TNF-α signalling can lead to tissue damage, fibrosis, and cachexia. Therefore, drugs neutralising TNF-α, IL-1, or IL-6 are widely used immunotherapies for treating chronic inflammation.

2.8.4 Autoimmune Diseases

The immune system has evolved safeguard mechanisms that allow it to distinguish 'foreign' (invader) from 'self', through the tightly regulated processes of central and peripheral tolerance. However, an estimated 5–8%, or over 400 million people globally, experience autoimmune diseases, conditions where the immune system attacks its own tissues. For most autoimmune diseases, the exact cause of tolerance breakdown is not yet known. Yet, multiple mechanisms are likely to occur. For example, T cells reactive to a self-antigen fail to be eliminated during thymic development, representing a failure of central tolerance. Another mechanism is through the dysregulation of Treg. Treg play a pivotal role in suppressing effector T cell responses, and a failure in their function can lead to overactivity of self-reactive effector T cells and tissue pathology. A process by which such auto-reactive T and B cells may become activated is **molecular mimicry**, where pathogen antigens closely resemble self-antigens, leading to cross-reactive immune responses. One such example is the development of rheumatic fever after *Streptococcus pyogenes* infection, where antibodies against the bacterial M protein also cross-react with heart tissue, and can lead to chronic valve damage, heart failure, arrhythmias, and stroke. Global investigations in the treatment of type 1 diabetes, Crohn's disease, systemic lupus, rheumatoid arthritis, and multiple sclerosis are actively pursuing new therapeutic opportunities to restore immune tolerance, some of which are discussed in further detail in Part IV (Chapters 11–13) of this book.

2.9 CASE STUDY – IMMUNE MODULATION GONE WRONG

In 2006, a first-in-human Phase 1 clinical trial was conducted using a superagonistic anti-CD28 antibody (theralizumab, TGN1412) to establish safety in a cohort of six healthy male participants [23]. This antibody was designed to activate T cells independent of TCR-antigen recognition, intended as a therapeutic for the treatment of B cell chronic lymphocytic leukaemia. All healthy participants received the infusion of the antibody intravenously and 10 minutes apart, and developed life-threatening cytokine release syndrome (CRS), also known as cytokine storm, within 90 minutes to hours. Blood analysis indicated strong release of TNF-α within 1 hour of infusion. The participants developed high fevers, severe pain, delirium, vomiting, diarrhoea, multi-organ failure, and severe tissue swelling. One's man head swelled so severely that he was named the 'Elephant Man' in the media, and one participant required amputation of fingertips, toes, and part of his foot. All participants were admitted to the intensive care unit, and while all patients survived, long-term effects persisted [24].

In the aftermath of this incident, investigations determined that the antibody had been thoroughly tested in preclinical *in vivo* studies, including in non-human primate models, with no indication of serious side effects [25]. However, further studies identified that amino acid sequence differences of up to 4% in the CD28 molecule exist between humans and non-human primates used for preclinical evaluation, and may explain the difference in response. This is an example that preclinical *in vivo* testing in other species, including in non-human primates, is not always predictive of serious side effects in humans, and any first-in-human clinical trial must expect the unexpected. Therefore, the largest error in the conduct of this clinical trial was that all six participants received treatment at the same time, without allowing time to monitor for acute side effects before treating the next participant.

KEY TERMS & DEFINITIONS SIDEBAR

The innate immune system is the body's first, fast, and non specific line of defence. It recognises common danger signals and responds immediately to infection or tissue damage. It includes physical barriers (skin, epithelium), soluble factors (complement, cytokines), and sentinel cells such as macrophages, dendritic cells, neutrophils, and NK cells.

The adaptive immune system is the body's slower but highly specific and memory forming defence. It relies on antigen specific receptors on B cells and T cells, enabling precise pathogen targeting and long lasting immunity.

Phagocytosis is the process by which specialised immune cells engulf, internalise, and degrade microbes, debris, or dying cells to eliminate them from tissues.

Alarmins are host derived danger molecules released during tissue stress or damage that rapidly activate innate immunity and initiate inflammation.

Cytokines are small, secreted signalling proteins that allow immune and non immune cells to communicate, coordinating inflammation, defence, and tissue repair.

Chemokines are small signalling proteins that direct the movement of immune cells by creating localised chemical gradients that guide cell migration.

Immunological memory is the long lasting ability of the immune system to respond faster and more effectively to a previously encountered antigen after the initial response has resolved.

Trained immunity is the process by which innate immune cells undergo lasting epigenetic and metabolic reprogramming after a primary stimulus, enabling them to mount a more robust response to subsequent challenges.

Immune tolerance is the state in which the immune system actively avoids attacking the body's own cells and harmless antigens, maintaining self nonreactivity and preventing unnecessary inflammation.

Anergy is a durable hyporesponsive state in which a lymphocyte remains alive but fails to activate or proliferate upon antigen encounter, typically because it received antigen recognition without the necessary co stimulatory or cytokine signals.

Immune homeostasis is the balanced state in which the immune system maintains effective defence while actively preventing excessive or inappropriate inflammation, preserving tissue integrity and normal physiological function.

Immunopathology is tissue damage or disease that arises from an inappropriate, excessive, or dysregulated immune response rather than from the pathogen or insult itself.

A cytokine storm is an uncontrolled, self amplifying surge of pro inflammatory cytokines that overwhelms normal regulatory mechanisms, leading to widespread tissue damage, vascular leakage, and systemic pathology.

An antibody is a Y shaped protein produced by B cells that specifically recognises and binds to an antigen, marking it for neutralisation or elimination by the immune system.

An antigen is any molecule that can be specifically recognised by antibodies or T cell receptors, triggering an adaptive immune response.

Molecular mimicry is the phenomenon in which structural similarity between pathogen derived molecules and host self antigens causes immune responses against the pathogen to inadvertently cross react with and damage host tissues.

LIST OF ABBREVIATIONS

ADCC	antibody-dependent cellular cytotoxicity
APC	antigen-presenting cell
BCR	B cell receptor
BCG	bacillus Calmette–Guérin (tuberculosis vaccine)
cDC	conventional dendritic cell
CLR	C-type lectin receptor
CRS	cytokine release syndrome
DAMP	damage-associated molecular pattern
DC	dendritic cell
IL	interleukin
MAIT	mucosal-associated invariant T cell
NET	neutrophil extracellular trap
NK	natural killer (cell)
NLR	NOD-like receptor
pTreg	peripherally-derived regulatory T cell
PAMP	pathogen-associated molecular pattern
pDC	plasmacytoid dendritic cell
RLR	RIG-I-like receptor
TCR	T cell receptor
Th	T helper (cell)
TLR	Toll-like receptor
Treg	regulatory T cells
tTreg	thymus-derived regulatory T cell

REVIEW QUESTIONS

1. Compare and contrast the key properties of macrophages and neutrophils in the innate immune system.
2. How do T cells and B cells differ in their function during an immune response?
3. Outline the role of DCs in activating naïve CD4 and CD8 T cells.
4. What are the key mechanisms that limit activation of lymphocytes or prevent autoimmune disease in the tissues?

REFERENCES

1. Zhang, C., Merana, G.R., Harris-Tryon, T., and Scharschmidt, T.C. (2022). Skin immunity: dissecting the complex biology of our body's outer barrier. *Mucosal Immunol* 15 (4): 551–561.
2. Vancamelbeke, M. and Vermeire, S. (2017). The intestinal barrier: a fundamental role in health and disease. *Expert Rev Gastroenterol Hepatol* 11 (9): 821–834.
3. de Paiva, C.S., St Leger, A.J., and Caspi, R.R. (2022). Mucosal immunology of the ocular surface. *Mucosal Immunol* 15 (6): 1143–1157.
4. Sender, R., Weiss, Y., Navon, Y. et al. (2023). The total mass, number, and distribution of immune cells in the human body. *Proc Natl Acad Sci USA* 120 (44): e2308511120.
5. Takeuchi, O. and Akira, S. (2010). Pattern recognition receptors and inflammation. *Cell* 140 (6): 805–820.
6. Revel M, Zarantonello A, Roumenina LT. The complement system. *Adv Exp Med Biol* 2025;1476:147–198.
7. Borregaard, N. (2010). Neutrophils, from marrow to microbes. *Immunity* 33 (5): 657–670.
8. Björkström, N.K., Strunz, B., and Ljunggren, H.-G. (2022). Natural killer cells in antiviral immunity. *Nat Rev Immunol* 22 (2): 112–123.
9. Geissmann, F., Manz, M.G., Jung, S. et al. (2010). Development of monocytes, macrophages, and dendritic cells. *Science* 327 (5966): 656–661.
10. Hume, D.A., Irvine, K.M., and Pridans, C. (2019). The mononuclear phagocyte system: the relationship between monocytes and macrophages. *Trends Immunol* 40 (2): 98–112.
11. Arroyo Hornero, R. and Idoyaga, J. (2023). Plasmacytoid dendritic cells: a dendritic cell in disguise. *Mol Immunol* 159: 38–45.
12. Heras-Murillo, I., Adán-Barrientos, I., Galán, M. et al. (2024). Dendritic cells as orchestrators of anticancer immunity and immunotherapy. *Nat Rev Clin Oncol* 21 (4): 257–277.
13. Kotsias, F., Cebrian, I., Alloatti, A. et al. (2019). Antigen processing and presentation. In: *Int Rev Cell Mol Biol*, vol. 348, 69–121.
14. Murphy, K.M. and Weaver, C. (2022). *Janeway's Immunobiology: Tenth International Student Edition with Registration Card*. W.W. Norton.
15. Ashby, K.M. and Hogquist, K.A. (2024). A guide to thymic selection of T cells. *Nat Rev Immunol* 24 (2): 103–117.
16. Chen, L. and Flies, D.B. (2013). Molecular mechanisms of T cell co-stimulation and co-inhibition. *Nat Rev Immunol* 13 (4): 227–242.
17. Cyster, J.G. and Allen, C.D.C. (2019). B cell responses: cell interaction dynamics and decisions. *Cell* 177 (3): 524–540.
18. Masopust, D., Awasthi, A., Bosselut, R. et al. (2026). Guidelines for T cell nomenclature. *Nat Rev Immunol* 26: 298–313. https://doi.org/10.1038/s41577-025-01238-2.

19. Lam, N., Lee, Y., and Farber, D.L. (2024). A guide to adaptive immune memory. *Nat Rev Immunol* 24 (11): 810–829.
20. Baessler, A. and Vignali, D.A.A. (2024). T cell exhaustion. *Annu Rev Immunol* 42 (1): 179–206.
21. Sedlmayr, P., Blaschitz, A., and Stocker, R. (2014). The role of placental tryptophan catabolism. *Front Immunol* 5: 230.
22. Domínguez-Andrés, J., dos Santos, J.C., Bekkering, S. et al. (2023). Trained immunity: adaptation within innate immune mechanisms. *Physiol Rev* 103 (1): 313–346.
23. Suntharalingam, G., Perry, M.R., Ward, S. et al. (2006). Cytokine storm in a phase 1 trial of the anti-CD28 monoclonal antibody TGN1412. *N Engl J Med* 355 (10): 1018–1028.
24. Panoskaltsis, N., McCarthy, N.E., Stagg, A.J. et al. (2021). Immune reconstitution and clinical recovery following anti-CD28 antibody (TGN1412)-induced cytokine storm. *Cancer Immunol Immunother* 70 (4): 1127–1142.
25. Attarwala, H. (2010). TGN1412: from discovery to disaster. *J Young Pharm* 2 (3): 332–336.

CHAPTER 3

Mechanisms of Immune Evasion and Immune Surveillance: Cellular Barriers to Immunotherapy

MARION F. BARROS, LIWANG ZHANG, JASON J. LEE, JENNA S. THERON, LIXUE LI, SHANNON R. JOSEPH, AND FIONA SIMPSON

Frazer Institute, The University of Queensland, Brisbane, Queensland, Australia

LEARNING OBJECTIVES

- Understand tumour-inherent mechanisms such as antigen loss that can lead to immune escape.
- Describe key characteristics of the tumour microenvironment that contribute to immunosuppression.
- Understand how tumours can exploit immune cell-specific regulatory functions to evade immunosurveillance.
- Understand the mechanistic similarities between immune evasion in tumours, and commonality with components of microbial pathogenesis and autoimmunity.

3.1 INTRODUCTION

Avoiding immune destruction is one of the 'emerging hallmarks' introduced in the 2011 *Hallmarks of Cancer: the next generation* [1]. Tumours can evolve their immunogenicity to become immune-resistant, a process termed immunoediting. This model was proposed in 2002 to describe the dynamic interactions between tumour cells and the immune system [2]. Immunoediting takes place as a tumour develops and immunosurveillance occurs. There are three phases of immunoediting: elimination, equilibrium, and escape.

The **Elimination** phase is an immunosurveillance phase where tumour cells are killed by immune mechanisms involving both the innate and adaptive immune system. Briefly, innate immune cells recognise stromal damage inflicted by the growing tumour, and inflammatory signals induce innate immune cell infiltration. This leads to a cascade of immune cell activation, culminating in the homing of $CD4^+$ and $CD8^+$ T cells to the tumour site.

The **Equilibrium** phase is the period in which tumour cells that have escaped or avoided elimination are selected for growth. Both lymphocytes and interferon (IFN)-γ exert selection pressure on rapidly mutating, genetically unstable tumour cells.

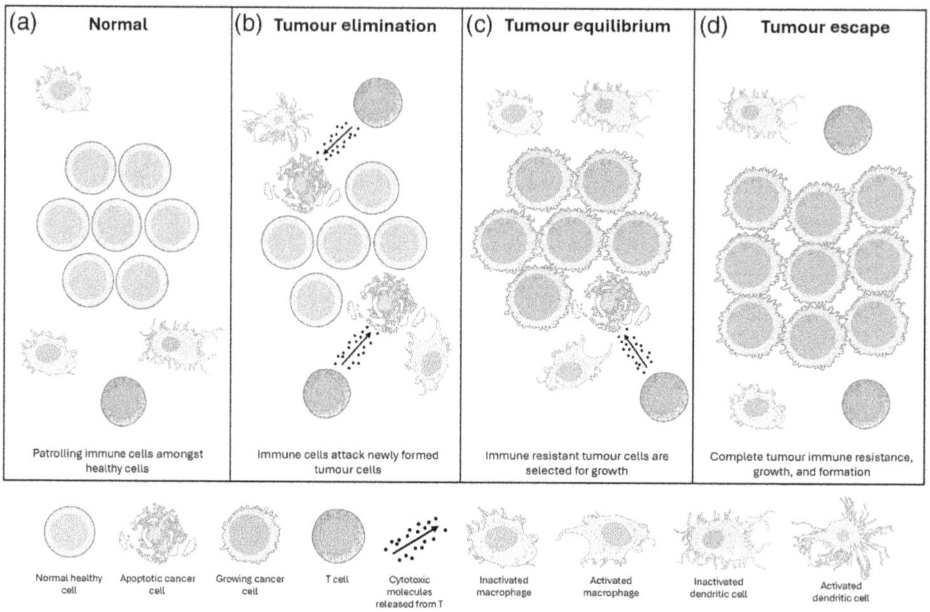

FIGURE 3.1 The (a) normal physiology where healthy cells do not interact with immunosurveillance immune cells, (b) tumour elimination where tumour cells are recognised and eliminated by immune response, (c) tumour equilibrium where tumour cells are killed by the immune cells, but as some tumour cells divide they evolve and evade killing, leading to tumour equilibrium, and (d) tumour cells divide and have evolved immune escape mechanisms and immune cells are no longer activated to kill the tumour cell, thereby enabling tumour escape. Created by the authors, Adapted from NIAID BioArt (NIH).

New tumour cell variants arise, which are even more resistant to immune cell attack. This process can take years, leading to the clinical outcome of tumour recurrence.

The **Escape** phase is the period where tumour cell variants which survived the *equilibrium phase* by evading the host immune defences grow and develop unchecked, with changes conferring further immune resistance (Figure 3.1).

Chapter scope: This chapter focuses on mechanisms by which tumour cells escape the innate and adaptive immune surveillance systems. This is not the same as mechanisms induced by drug therapies (discussed in later chapters), but instead we focus on inherent cellular mechanisms which allow escape from the immune system allowing tumours to form in the host.

3.2 TUMOUR-INTRINSIC EVASION MECHANISMS

3.2.1 Major Histocompatibility Complex Class I Downregulation and Antigen Presentation Loss

Tumour cells divide frequently. As a result, genetic editing is inefficient and allows tumour-specific antigens to be produced. These may be presented by the major histocompatibility complex class I (MHC-I) receptor (human leukocyte antigen (HLA)-I in humans). Tumours can downregulate MHC-I as a key oncogenic feature, bypassing recognition and killing by effector immune cells such as $CD8^+$ T cells. MHC-I downregulation occurs in up to 90% of human tumours [3]. Decreased surface expression of MHC-I allows evasion from T-cell-mediated anti-tumour immunity. T cells are primed by macrophages and dendritic cells (DCs) to specifically recognise these tumour antigens and therefore cannot become activated when these antigens are hidden by decreased MHC-I expression and presentation. Conversely, low MHC-I expression increases cell susceptibility to natural killer (NK) cell-mediated cytotoxicity. MHC-I binds to inhibitory receptors, such as killer cell immunoglobulin-like receptors (KIRs), reducing NK-cell activation. Downregulation of MHC-I causes these inhibitory signals to be absent, allowing enhanced NK-cell activation and cytotoxicity [4]. However, cancer cells are de-differentiated and exhibit plasticity generating physiological alterations which allow evasion of NK- and T-cell-mediated cytotoxicity. As a clinical example, colorectal cancer patients with reversible MHC-I downregulation were compared to patients with irreversible MHC-I downregulation, with the irreversible downregulation showing a better prognosis [5].

Several molecular pathways control MHC-I production and stability, and molecules involved in these pathways have been explored as potential therapeutic targets. Nuclear factor-kappa B (NF-κB) is a central controller of MHC-I expression and is stimulated by tumour necrosis factor alpha (TNF-α), but manipulation of these pathways causes toxicity. It has been reported that upregulation of proteosome subunits increases the half-life of MHC-I [6]. In the context of therapy, several topoisomerase inhibitors, microtubule stabilisers, cisplatin, and radiation therapy increase MHC-I surface expression via NF-κB stabilisation and IFNβ secretion, which may help to decrease tumour immune escape [7, 8].

Tumours bypass MHC-I antigen presentation through several mechanisms, notably through alteration of the transporter associated with antigen processing (TAP) protein complex. In order for peptides to be bound and presented by MHC-I they must be delivered into the endoplasmic reticulum from the cytosol, a function executed by the TAP complex [9]. TAP is an ABC transporter composed of two subunits, TAP1 and TAP2. Upregulation of TAP1 and TAP2 subunits, through the activity of IFNβ and TNF-α cytokines, can enhance MHC-I surface molecule expression above levels constitutively expressed by most cell types. Conversely, tumour cells can secrete interleukin (IL)-10 which is associated with downregulation of both transcription and translation of TAP. This causes reduced cell surface expression of MHC-I antigens and reduced T-cell-specific lysis. Murine IL-10-transduced cells with increased IL-10 production decrease TAP expression, inducing low MHC-I surface expression and reduced T-cell-specific lysis, but enhanced NK-cell-mediated cytotoxicity [10].

Tumours can additionally reduce MHC-I presentation through their loss of β2 microglobulin (B2M). B2M is a component of MHC-I molecules which lies beside the α3 chain of MHC-I on the cell surface and can bind other class I-like molecules such as CD1 and the neonatal Fc receptor. Mouse models deficient for the *B2M* gene have been engineered, demonstrating that B2M is necessary for cell surface expression of MHC-I and stability of its peptide-binding groove. In the absence of B2M, very limited expression of MHC-I molecules can be detected on the surface. In vitro studies show that the *B2M* knockout cell line does not express HLA-I molecules on the cell surface [11]. At the endoplasmic reticulum (ER), B2M forms the peptide loading complex together with tapasin, Erp57, HLA-I, and calreticulin to facilitate the folding of the MHC-I α subunit and load tumour peptide antigens to the peptide-binding groove. B2M expression is regulated by genetic and epigenetic mechanisms. Genetic mutations including nonsense, point, frameshift, and splice site mutations as well as loss of heterozygosity in tumour cells can alter B2M expression, leading to loss of MHC-I presentation. The MHC-I heavy (α) chain accumulates in the ER and is degraded in the cytosol. This is observed in melanoma where distinct mutations in the B2M gene causes loss of the HLA-I antigen, and reintroduction of wild-type B2M in these cells restores cytotoxic T-cell killing. B2M mutations in melanoma cells may be an early event in tumorigenesis [12].

An example of transcriptional changes leading to MHC-I downregulation is observed where the gene *Npm1* is deleted. Nucleophosmin (NPM1) protein associates with the transcription factor interferon regulatory factor (IRF)1, sequestering it from binding to the promotors of genes *Nlrc5* and *Ciita* and thus suppressing expression of both MHC-I and MHC-II molecules in tumours [13]. Cancer cell-intrinsic signalling such as impaired IFN responsiveness, Kirsten rat sarcoma viral oncogene homolog (KRAS) mutations, and myelocytomatosis oncogene cellular homolog (MYC) amplifications can cause reduced or loss of expression of MHC-I [14–16].

As noted, a myriad of alterations in the tumour cells can lead to loss of appropriate tumour cell antigen presentation by MHC-I, thus leading to tumour immune evasion (Figure 3.2).

3.2.2 Other Tumour-Intrinsic Evasion Mechanisms

As tumour cells under selective pressure from immune cells grow, the tumour microenvironment (TME) evolves towards an immunosuppressive environment. These environmental changes can inhibit anti-tumour T cells, reducing their ability to destroy cancer cells. One of these mechanisms is the expression of immune-regulatory molecules, such as programmed death ligand 1 (PD-L1) or non-classical HLA molecules that inhibit T cells within the TME. These 'checkpoint' molecules and their successful therapies are discussed in Chapters 4 and 5. It is of note that such inhibitory receptors are expressed throughout the TME, on cancer-associated fibroblasts (CAFs), macrophages, and other cells inducing immunosuppression. This change in cell surface expression of proteins is a consistent theme in tumour immune evasion. The loss of expression of CD95 receptor can allow evasion from CD95-mediated killing. Alternately, it has been shown that gain of CD95 ligand expression by hepatocellular carcinomas can allow the tumour cells to kill $CD95^+$ immune cells such as lymphocytes by inducing apoptosis in the immune cells [17].

3.2.3 Antigen Loss Under Immune Pressure

Endocytosis is the process by which cell surface proteins, lipids, and fluid from the extracellular environment are packaged, sorted, and internalised into cells. Endocytosis is also a mechanism of drug internalisation into cells [18]. Cancer cells display heterogeneous changes in endocytic activity [19], and this in turn alters display

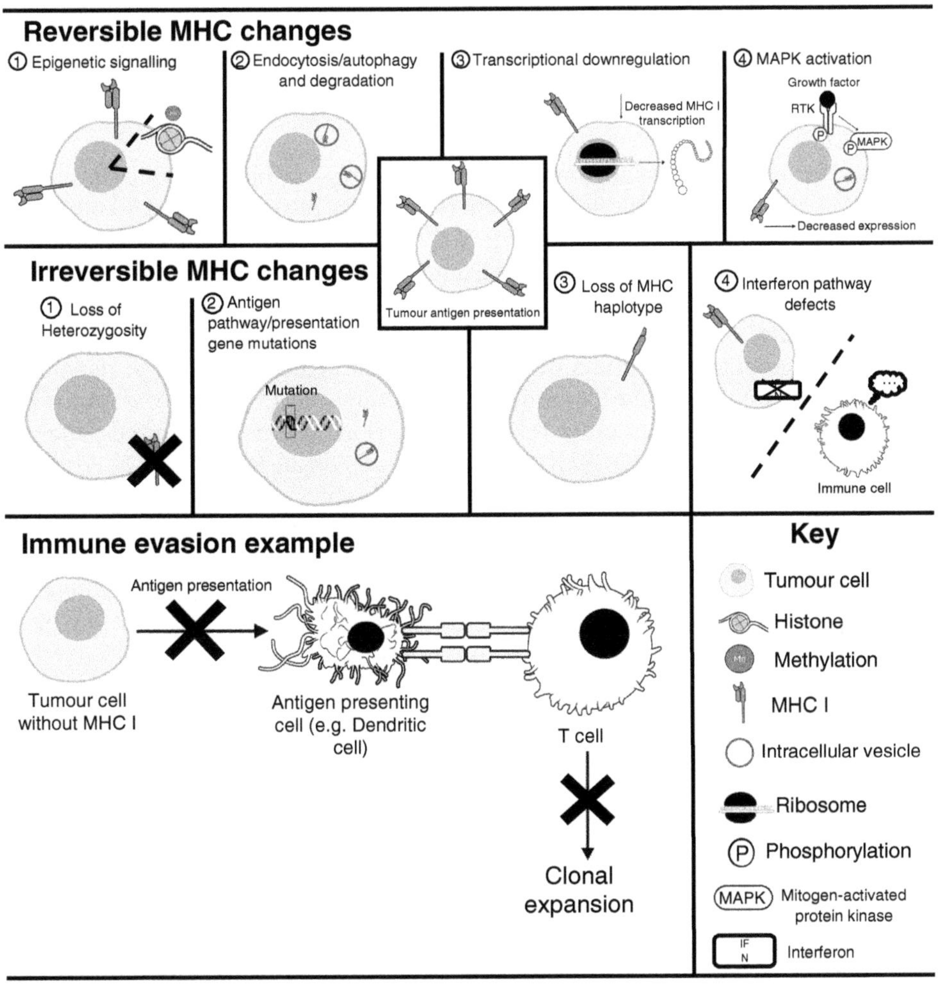

FIGURE 3.2 Some of the reversible and irreversible changes that can affect major histocompatibility complex class I (MHC-I) presentation including: Reversible: changes in epigenetic signalling, changes in endocytic and exocytic pathways, transcriptional downregulation, and activation of the MAPK signalling pathway; Irreversible: loss of heterozygosity, antigen presentation pathway gene mutations, loss of MHC haplotype, and defects in interferon signalling pathways. Created by the authors, Adapted from NIAID BioArt (NIH).

of receptors on the plasma membrane, such as CD44 and CD59. While changes in molecular trafficking lead to several oncogenic changes, these altered mechanisms also facilitate immune evasion and therapy evasion. Anti-programmed death 1 (PD-1) induces 50–60% surface PD-1 internalisation from human and mouse cells, leaving low levels of resistant receptors. The ligand/receptor complexes are retained within the endo-lysosomal system or degraded. $CD4^+$ and $CD8^+$ T cells are additionally induced to increase their expression of cytotoxic molecules, such as perforin and granzyme B, and infiltrate tumours to a greater extent [20].

Case Study: CAR-T Escape: Tumour Evolution Under Therapeutic Pressure

Various forms of successful immunotherapies target tumour-specific antigens. Of significant note and success is chimeric antigen receptor (CAR)-T-cell therapy. This involves genetic engineering of CARs on T cells to recognise tumour-specific antigens. Tumours develop resistance to this pressure by downregulating antigens, a major cause for relapse after CAR-T-cell treatment. This can occur through several mechanisms including genetic mutation of the tumour antigen, epigenetic modifications, and antigen redistribution [21]. The CD19 antigen is a target for therapy in acute lymphoblastic leukaemia (ALL). However, approximately 10–20% of patients suffer relapse. Braig et al. examined relapsed patients after treatment with the CD19/CD3 bispecific T-cell engager (BiTE) [22]. All four of the cases studied showed that the patients' ALL had not changed, except that cancer cells were now CD19 negative. Further study revealed that CD19 in these cells of relapsed patients had disrupted exocytosis from the Golgi and trans-Golgi networks. In this example, the target receptor was not affected by alterations in endocytosis, but by alterations in exocytosis of the newly synthesised receptor. See Chapter 6 for detailed CAR-T and NK-cell discussion.

3.3 TUMOUR-EXTRINSIC EVASION MECHANISMS

In addition to the tumour-intrinsic features of immune evasion, the surrounding stromal cells, pro-tumour immune cells, blood vessels, cytokines, chemokines, and their interactions with one another and tumour cells can promote immune evasion and immunosuppression. These components are referred to as the TME, which contribute to cancer immunoevasion.

3.3.1 Hypoxia and HIF-1α

Hypoxia is a key immunosuppressive feature of the TME, being present in 90% of solid tumours, and a hallmark of cancer [23]. Hypoxia, characterised by tissue oxygen levels dropping below 1% (below 10 mmHg when compared to 40–60 mmHg in most normal tissues), occurs because of increased oxygen consumption relative to delivery and abnormal vascular networks within the TME [24]. These are effects of the proliferative rate of tumour cells and their increasing distance from vessels within the tumour area (Figure 3.3). Hypoxia drives immunosuppression by stabilising and activating the hypoxia-induced factor (HIF) in tumour cells, which mediates several immune-evasive mechanisms. HIF-1α structural stabilisation under hypoxia facilitates binding to HIF-1β, allowing full transcriptional activation. This promotes PD-L1 expression on cancer cells, suppressing immune responses [25]. The HIF-1 complex additionally influences innate and adaptive immune cell activity [26]. HIF-1 inhibits IFN-γ, TNF-α, and granzyme B expression

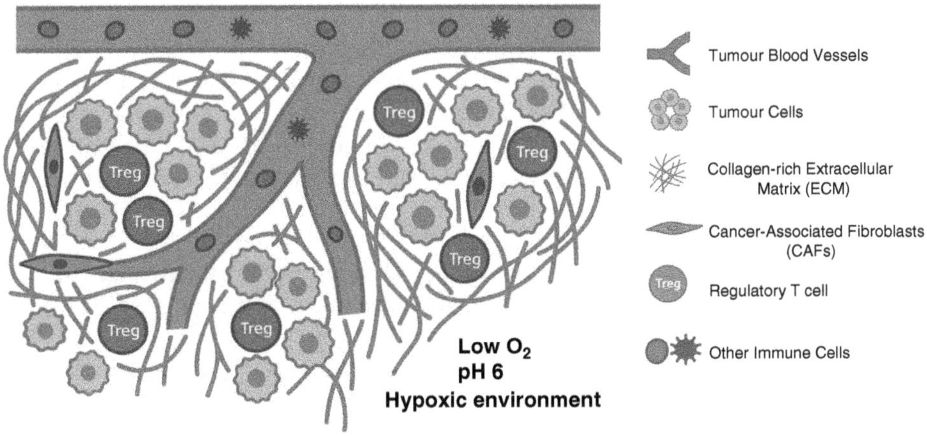

FIGURE 3.3 The tumour microenvironment has many barriers to immune cell activation against tumour cells. As illustrated, lack of blood or lymph vessel infiltration to the tumour area, low pH or hypoxic environment, and increased collagen and extracellular matrix components are physical barriers to immunity. Within the tumour microenvironment are also cellular and molecular barriers such as cancer-associated fibroblasts and T regulatory cells that secrete cytokines which can de-activate anti-tumour immunity. Created by the authors, Adapted from NIAID BioArt (NIH).

in $CD8^+$, $CD4^+$ T, and NK cells. Cumulatively, these changes suppress T-cell toxicity and induce resistance to PD-1/PD-L1 blockade [27]. HIF activation drives the production of the CXCL16 chemokine which recruits myeloid-derived suppressor cells (MDSCs) to the TME [28]. MDSCs subsequently facilitate immunosuppression through their expression of PD-L1, their production of anti-inflammatory cytokines such as IL-10 and TGF-β, and their cell–cell contact with and subsequent suppression of NK cell activation.

An additional target of HIF transcriptional activity is the vascular endothelial growth factor (*VEGF*) gene. VEGF upregulation drives immune evasion by interacting with VEGF receptor on tumours and endothelial cells in the TME. This promotes angiogenesis, the growth of new blood vessels. Through VEGF, these new vessels lack adhesion factors, such as ICAM-1 and VCAM-1, which are essential for anti-tumour immune cell infiltration to the TME [29].

3.3.2 Extracellular Vesicles

Extracellular vesicles (EVs) drive immunosuppression in the TME. EVs are lipid bilayer structures released from all cells. They contain DNA, messenger RNA, micro RNA, protein, surface receptors, and signalling molecules characteristic of the cell from which they are derived [30]. EVs released from tumour cells and CAFs within the TME facilitate immunosuppression and evasion through their contents, namely by altering immune cell phenotypes and induce immune cell apoptosis. In nasopharyngeal carcinoma patients, EVs in the TME were found to contain Galectin-9, which acts as a ligand for Tim-3 receptor on cytotoxic

T cells to induce their apoptosis [31]. EVs additionally induce immunosuppression by infiltrating and manipulating immune interactions within the lymphatic system. Melanoma-derived EVs were found to infiltrate lymph nodes and interact with lymph node endothelial cells to induce apoptosis of tumour antigen-specific $CD8^+$ T cells [32]. EVs were found to deliver the phosphatase and tensin homolog (PTEN) signalling molecule from tumour cells to immune cells in the TME. This PTEN retained its functionality in the recipient cells to induce their apoptosis by driving signalling pathways that upregulated proapoptotic proteins and downregulated anti-apoptotic proteins [33]. EVs can suppress NK-cell function in numerous ways, including NKG2D downregulation and increased SMAD2/3 phosphorylation [34].

In addition to reducing effector immune cells in these ways, EVs actively upregulate immunosuppressive immune cell types. Via their secretion of IL-10 and TGF-β, EVs promote the expansion and activation of T regulatory cells (Tregs) in the TME to suppress cytotoxic cell function [35]. EV-derived TGF-β in conjunction with the prostaglandin E2 (PGE2) molecule additionally drives differentiation and expansion of MDSCs [33]. MDSCs facilitate cytotoxic immune cell apoptosis and inhibition of effector function, as well as expansion of Tregs to create an immunosuppressive TME.

3.3.3 Extracellular Matrix Exclusion

Anti-tumour immune cells are excluded from entering the TME through physical barriers imposed by the extracellular matrix (ECM) [36]. The ECM comprises non-cellular structural carbohydrates, proteoglycans, and fibrous proteins that uphold tissue structure, cell–cell interactions, and biochemical and biomechanical support. Each tissue type has an ECM composition specific to the types of cells present and their function. Tumours manipulate and increase the density of the ECM to shield cancer cells from infiltrating immune cells and promote immune evasion in the TME. This occurs as tumour ECMs have upregulated fibrous proteins such as collagen. Increased TGF-β signalling in the TME acts on CAFs to increase collagen production and cross-linking to form this barrier and inhibit enzymes that degrade excess collagen (Figure 3.3). The increased collagen also engages with immune checkpoint receptors on immune cells to dampen their effector function [37].

3.3.4 Metabolic Regulation

MDSCs which infiltrate tumours can also lead to metabolic changes which suppress the immune cells [38]. These changes are complex and discussed briefly here. The alteration of the tumour environment to hypoxia and increased glycolysis affects key metabolic enzymes such as pyruvate kinase M2, lactate dehydrogenase A, HIF-1α, mammalian target of rapamycin (mTOR), STAT-3, the glucose transporters GLUT-1 and GLUT-3, and lactate dehydrogenase. Increased glycolysis and alteration of fatty acid synthesis and use by the MDSCs leads to depletion of nutrients (such as tryptophan and arginine) as well as increased levels of reactive oxygen species (ROS) and nitric oxide. This metabolic alteration also leads to immunosuppressive cytokines like TGF-β and IL-10. The overall effect of these changes is to suppress the function of anti-tumour immune cells, such as $CD8^+$ T cells.

3.3.5 Interferon Resistance

Interferon was the first cytokine used to treat tumours in patients. However, tumour cells can become entirely resistant to interferon. Impaired IFN signalling or lack of response to IFN treatment is found in different tumour types [39]. There are also several humans who are born with errors in interferon signalling, including complete IFN-γ deficiency [40]. While cytokines are discussed in other chapters, changes in the JAK/STAT pathways via tumour mutation as well as downregulation of MHC-I in tumour cells can lead to interferon resistance [41].

3.4 PARALLELS IN PATHOGENS AND AUTOIMMUNITY

While later chapters describe immunotherapy for viral and microbial infections, correlations exist between pathogen immune evasion and tumour cell immune evasion. Pathogens are evolving entities and respond to the selection pressures exerted by the immune system to survive. These mechanisms are evolutionary, and cancer immune evasion mechanisms are related and adapted from these more archaic systems and thus share commonalities. Some brief examples are described:

3.4.1 Antigenic Variation, Latency, Subversion of MHC Processing

Viruses can avoid $CD8^+$ T-cell recognition when mutations occur in proteins which block antigen processing or MHC-I binding. However, humans express up to six different class I alleles (three class I loci per HLA). For each locus, hundreds of alleles exist at reasonable frequencies in the population. The class I polymorphism means the evolutionary advantage to viruses in altering antigens is limited. Hence viruses have evolved more generalised blockades to antigen processing or presentation [42]. Here the similarities to tumour-intrinsic evasion mechanisms can be seen to have correlations.

Antigen variation: An infectious agent can alter its antigens to avoid recognition. This can be achieved by (a) having a wide variety of antigenic types (b) by antigenic drift and (c) by antigenic variation. An example of antigenic types can be observed in *Streptococcus pneumoniae* which has 84 known types, each of which varies in the polysaccharide capsule structure [43].

Antigenic drift: This has been studied in viruses such as Type A influenza and more recently in COVID-19 infection. Every 2–3 years the influenza virus can gain point mutation changes in the viral surface protein haemagglutinin and its surface protein neuraminidase [44]. This allows it to escape antibody binding. Other mutations allow escape from $CD8^+$ T-cell recognition, so that infected cells are not destroyed [45]. Mutations in viral strains of COVID-19, most concentrated in the Spike protein, affect binding between these mutant peptides and HLA molecules, allowing immune evasion [46, 47].

Antigen swapping: This involved programmed rearrangements of DNA by the pathogen. Trypanosomes, which are parasitic protozoa, are coated with variant-specific glycoprotein (VSG) for which its genome contains nearly 1,000 genes. Each gene encodes a VSG with different antigenic properties, and gene rearrangement mechanisms allow any of these genes being expressed to be replaced [48]. In trypanosomes this is so efficient that they can alter this expression within a host after immune attack, leading to disease 'flare up' or recurrence. The host makes new antibodies against the new VSG. However, this cycle leads to immune exhaustion (i.e. the inability of immune cells to function after prolonged exposure to infection), immune complex damage, neurological damage, and eventually coma [49].

Alteration to MHC-I presentation: Large RNA viruses have developed numerous processes that interrupt the MHC class I antigen presentation pathway. This can occur through multiple mechanisms, a major one being the downregulation of MHC-I transcription. The SARS-CoV-2 virus, for example, produces the ORF6 protein which inhibits the NLRC5 protein of the host cell. NLRC5 is a transcription factor for MHC-I proteins, whose expression is therefore downregulated upon SARS-CoV-2 infection [50].

3.5 EVASION OF THE INNATE IMMUNE SYSTEM

Innate immunity, being the first line of attack and means of immunosurveillance, is the first to fall during tumour progression. Understanding the tumour mechanisms specifically of innate evasion is therefore of key therapeutic interest. Key innate immune populations evaded include NK cells, DCs, and macrophages.

3.5.1 NK-Cell Evasion

NK cells are 'first responders' to oncogenesis, targeting cells that lack surface markers such as MHC-I. NK cells detect tumour-specific antigens, release inflammatory cytokines, and induce apoptosis in target cells via release of perforin and granzyme B from cytotoxic granules. Tumour cells only advance if they avoid this elimination and reach the equilibrium stage as described above. The NK-cell receptors and signalling provide a kill/don't kill balance where NK-cell engagement with another cell either leads to self-tolerance or a cytotoxic response. Tumour cells evade NK-cell cytotoxicity by firstly altering NK-cell plasma membrane content. Specifically, dysregulated serine metabolism in tumour cells contributes to altered sphingomyelin content in NK-cell membranes [51]. This inhibits NK-cell ability to form immunological synapses and secrete cytotoxic granule components onto tumour cells. NK cells in immunosuppressive TMEs additionally have decreased expressions of activating receptors, whose engagement initiates NK-cell binding to tumour targets, immune synapse formation, and killing. The CD226 activating receptor was found downregulated on NK cells in acute myeloid leukaemia patients, disrupting recognition of the CD112 and CD155 ligands expressed on tumour cells [52].

3.5.2 Dendritic Cell Evasion

DCs are the immune system's key surveillance mediators, sampling antigens from the microenvironment and presenting these to T cells to activate the adaptive immune system. DCs comprise the first response to tumour formation, which is bypassed as a tumour progresses through the equilibrium and escape phases. Tumours and the

TME facilitate tolerance to DC function through several soluble mediators such as the CCL2 chemokine. CCL2 induces a tolerogenic DC phenotype by increasing its expression of PD-L1 and reducing its HLA-DR expression [53, 54]. The immunosuppressive TME produces increased levels of IL-10 and TGF-β which inhibit DC maturation and thus antigen presentation. These signalling molecules induce upregulated expression of Inhibitor of Differentiation 1 (Id1) in DCs, causing their switch to an MDSC-like phenotype with immunosuppressive properties [55].

3.5.3 Macrophage Evasion and Phenotypic Change

Macrophages, specifically those of the type I phenotype (M1), have potent antitumorigenic roles in the TME through their phagocytosis of necrotic tumour cells, expression of proinflammatory and cytotoxic mediators including TNF-α, inducible nitric oxide synthase (iNOS), and reactive oxygen species, and MHC-II antigen presentation to enhance Th1 anti-tumour responses [56]. However, macrophages can be polarised to an M2 phenotype by the TME to express arginase 1, IL-10, CD163, and CD206 which promote tumour cell growth, angiogenesis, and metastasis. IL-10 secreted by these macrophages suppresses DCs, further promoting tumour immune escape [57].

KEY TERMS & DEFINITIONS SIDEBAR

Antigen Any molecule or substance that is recognised by the immune system as foreign.

Cytokines Signalling proteins secreted by numerous cell types which contribute to immune activity in both health and disease.

Immunoediting A three-phase process whereby tumours undergo cellular modifications by interacting with the immune system which ultimately result in tumour progression.

Immunosurveillance The continuous surveying and removal of foreign entities and abnormal self-cells by the immune system before they can cause disease.

Inflammation The physiological response to infection, cellular malignancy, or tissue damage which involves the recruitment and activation of both immune and non-immune cells.

Major histocompatibility complex (MHC) A group of genes responsible for coding cell membrane proteins involved in adaptive immunity, tolerance, and foreign particle recognition.

Molecular mimicry Similarities between host protein structures or peptide sequences and pathogens which can lead to immune evasion and/or autoimmunity.

Natural killer (NK) cell A type of cytotoxic innate immune cell capable of eliminating virus-infected and tumour cells.

Tumour microenvironment (TME) The multi-faceted network of cancerous cells, non-cancerous cells, blood vessels, and other extracellular components that interact to promote tumour growth and survival.

LIST OF ABBREVIATIONS

ABC transporter	ATP binding cassette transporter
ADAM10	a disintegrin and metalloproteinase 10
ALL	acute lymphoblastic leukaemia

B2M	β2 microglobulin
BiTE	bispecific T-cell engager
CAF	cancer-associated fibroblast
CAR	chimeric antigen receptor
CCL	chemokine (C–C motif) ligand
CD4	cluster of differentiation 4
CD8	cluster of differentiation 8
COX	cyclooxygenase
CSF1	colony-stimulating factor 1
CXCL	CXC chemokine ligand
DAF	decay accelerating factor
DC	dendritic cell
DNA	deoxyribonucleic acid
ECM	extracellular matrix
EMT	epithelial–mesenchymal transition
ER	endoplasmic reticulum
EV	extracellular vesicle
Fc receptor	fragment crystallisable receptor
GM-CSF	granulocyte-macrophage colony-stimulating factor
HIF	hypoxia-induced family
HIV	human immunodeficiency virus
HLA-1	human leukocyte antigen 1
HTLV-1	human T cell lymphotropic virus type 1
IFN	interferon
Ig	immunoglobulin
IL	interleukin
iNOS	inducible nitric oxide synthase
IRF	interferon regulatory factor
KIR	killer cell immunoglobulin-like receptor
KRAS	Kirsten rat sarcoma viral oncogene homolog
LFA-1	leukocyte function associated 1
MAPK	mitogen-activated protein kinase
MCP	monocyte chemoattractant protein
MDSC	myeloid-derived suppressor cell
MHC-I	major histocompatibility complex class 1
MIC	MHC class I polypeptide-related sequence
MYC	myelocytomatosis oncogene cellular homolog
NCR	natural cytotoxic receptor
NET	neutrophil extracellular trap
NF-κB	nuclear factor kappa B
NK cell	natural killer cell

NO	nitric oxide
NPM1	nucleophosmin 1
PAMP	pathogen-associated molecular pattern
PD-1	programmed death 1
PD-L1	programmed death ligand 1
RNA	ribonucleic acid
ROS	reactive oxygen species
SARS-CoV-2	severe acute respiratory syndrome coronavirus 2
SM	sphingomyelin
STAT3	signal transducer and activator of transcription 3
TAM	tumour-associated macrophage
TAN	tumour-associated neutrophil
TAP	transporter associated with antigen processing
TGF-β	transforming growth factor beta
Th1	T helper 1
TLR	toll like receptor
TME	tumour microenvironment
TNF-α	tumour necrosis factor alpha
Treg	T regulatory cell
VEGF	vascular endothelial growth factor
VSG	variant-specific glycoprotein

REVIEW QUESTIONS

1. Describe two mechanisms used by tumours to downregulate MHC-I expression.
2. Explain hypoxia in tumours and how this phenomenon contributes to tumorigenesis and immunosuppression.
3. What is one mechanism by which tumour cells evade NK cell cytotoxicity?

REFERENCES

1. Hanahan, D. and Weinberg, R.A. (2011). Hallmarks of cancer: the next generation. *Cell* 144 (5): 646–674.
2. Dunn, G.P., Bruce, A.T., Ikeda, H. et al. (2002). Cancer immunoediting: from immunosurveillance to tumor escape. *Nat Immunol* 3 (11): 991–998.
3. Cornel, A.M., Mimpen, I.L., and Nierkens, S. (2020). MHC class I downregulation in cancer: underlying mechanisms and potential targets for cancer immunotherapy. *Cancers* 12 (7): 1760.
4. Anfossi, N., André, P., Guia, S. et al. (2006). Human NK cell education by inhibitory receptors for MHC class I. *Immunity* 25 (2): 331–342.
5. Watson, N.F.S., Ramage, J.M., Madjd, Z. et al. (2006). Immunosurveillance is active in colorectal cancer as downregulation but not complete loss of MHC class I expression correlates with a poor prognosis. *Int J Cancer* 118 (1): 6–10.

6. Vertuani, S., De Geer, A., Levitsky, V. et al. (2003). Retinoids act as multistep modulators of the major histocompatibility class I presentation pathway and sensitize neuroblastomas to cytotoxic lymphocytes. *Cancer Res* 63 (22): 8006–8013.
7. Wan, S., Pestka, S., Jubin, R.G. et al. (2012). Chemotherapeutics and radiation stimulate MHC class I expression through elevated interferon-beta signaling in breast cancer cells. *PLoS One* 7 (3): e32542.
8. Alagkiozidis, I., Facciabene, A., Tsiatas, M. et al. (2011). Time-dependent cytotoxic drugs selectively cooperate with IL-18 for cancer chemo-immunotherapy. *J Transl Med* 9 (1): 77.
9. Suh, W.-K., Cohen-Doyle, M.F., Fruh, K. et al. (1994). Interaction of MHC class I molecules with the transporter associated with antigen processing. *Science* 264 (5163): 1322–1326.
10. Petersson, M., Charo, J., Salazar-Onfray, F. et al. (1998). Constitutive IL-10 production accounts for the high NK sensitivity, low MHC class I expression, and poor transporter associated with antigen processing (TAP)-1/2 function in the prototype NK target YAC-11. *J Immunol* 161 (5): 2099–2105.
11. Lee, O.-H., Lee, S., Park, M. et al. (2022). Generation of a B2M homozygous knockout human somatic cell nuclear transfer-derived embryonic stem cell line using the CRISPR/Cas9 system. *Stem Cell Res* 59: 102643.
12. Hicklin, D.J., Wang, Z., Arienti, F. et al. (1998). Beta2-microglobulin mutations, HLA class I antigen loss, and tumor progression in melanoma. *J Clin Invest* 101 (12): 2720–2729.
13. Wang, X., Chai, Y., Quan, Y. et al. (2024). *NPM1* inhibits tumoral antigen presentation to promote immune evasion and tumor progression. *J Hematol Oncol* 17 (1): 97.
14. Taylor, B.C. and Balko, J.M. (2022). Mechanisms of MHC-I downregulation and role in immunotherapy response. *Front Immunol* 13: 844866.
15. Dhatchinamoorthy, K., Colbert, J.D., and Rock, K.L. (2021). Cancer immune evasion through loss of MHC class I antigen presentation. *Front Immunol* 12: 636568.
16. Ghorani, E., Swanton, C., and Quezada, S.A. (2023). Cancer cell-intrinsic mechanisms driving acquired immune tolerance. *Immunity* 56 (10): 2270–2295.
17. Strand, S., Hofmann, W.J., Hug, H. et al. (1996). Lymphocyte apoptosis induced by CD95 (APO-1/Fas) ligand-expressing tumor cells—a mechanism of immune evasion? *Nat Med* 2 (12): 1361–1366.
18. Banushi, B., Joseph, S.R., Lum, B. et al. (2023). Endocytosis in cancer and cancer therapy. *Nat Rev Cancer* 23 (7): 450–473.
19. Elkin, S.R., Bendris, N., Reis, C.R. et al. (2015). A systematic analysis reveals heterogeneous changes in the endocytic activities of cancer cells. *Cancer Res* 75 (21): 4640–4650.
20. Ben Saad, E., Oroya, A., Anto, N.P. et al. (2024). PD-1 endocytosis unleashes the cytolytic potential of checkpoint blockade in tumor immunity. *Cell Rep* 43 (11): 114907.
21. Lin, H., Yang, X., Ye, S. et al. (2024). Antigen escape in CAR-T cell therapy: mechanisms and overcoming strategies. *Biomed Pharmacother* 178: 117252.
22. Braig, F., Brandt, A., Goebeler, M. et al. (2017). Resistance to anti-CD19/CD3 BiTE in acute lymphoblastic leukemia may be mediated by disrupted CD19 membrane trafficking. *Blood* 129 (1): 100–104.
23. Ye, Y., Hu, Q., Chen, H. et al. (2019). Characterization of hypoxia-associated molecular features to aid hypoxia-targeted therapy. *Nat Metab* 1 (4): 431–444.
24. Brown, J.M. and Wilson, W.R. (2004). Exploiting tumour hypoxia in cancer treatment. *Nat Rev Cancer* 4 (6): 437–447.
25. Ding, X.-C., Wang, L.-L., Zhang, X.-D. et al. (2021). The relationship between expression of PD-L1 and HIF-1α in glioma cells under hypoxia. *J Hematol Oncol* 14 (1): 92.
26. Chen, Z., Han, F., Du, Y. et al. (2023). Hypoxic microenvironment in cancer: molecular mechanisms and therapeutic interventions. *Signal Transduct Target Ther* 8 (1): 70.
27. Ma, S., Zhao, Y., Lee, W.C. et al. (2022). Hypoxia induces HIF1α-dependent epigenetic vulnerability in triple negative breast cancer to confer immune effector dysfunction and resistance to anti-PD-1 immunotherapy. *Nat Commun* 13 (1): 4118.

28. Chaturvedi, P., Gilkes, D.M., Takano, N., and Semenza, G.L. (2014). Hypoxia-inducible factor-dependent signaling between triple-negative breast cancer cells and mesenchymal stem cells promotes macrophage recruitment. *Proc Natl Acad Sci USA* 111 (20): E2120–E2129.
29. Zhang, Y. and Brekken, R.A. (2022). Direct and indirect regulation of the tumor immune microenvironment by VEGF. *J Leukoc Biol* 111 (6): 1269–1286.
30. Kuang, L., Wu, L., and Li, Y. (2025). Extracellular vesicles in tumor immunity: mechanisms and novel insights. *Mol Cancer* 24 (1): 45.
31. Klibi, J., Niki, T., Riedel, A. et al. (2009). Blood diffusion and Th1-suppressive effects of galectin-9–containing exosomes released by Epstein-Barr virus–infected nasopharyngeal carcinoma cells. *Blood* 113 (9): 1957–1966.
32. Leary, N., Walser, S., He, Y. et al. (2022). Melanoma-derived extracellular vesicles mediate lymphatic remodelling and impair tumour immunity in draining lymph nodes. *J Extracell Vesicles* 11 (2): e12197.
33. Sheta, M., Taha, E.A., Lu, Y., and Eguchi, T. (2023). Extracellular vesicles: New classification and tumor immunosuppression. *Biology (Basel)* 12 (1): 110.
34. Coleborn, E., Ghebosu, R., Wolfram, J. et al. (2025). Cancer-derived extracellular vesicles in natural killer cell immune evasion: molecular mechanisms and therapeutic insights. *Mol Ther* 33 (9): 4113–4129.
35. Wang, L., Li, L., and Zhu, G. (2021). Role of extracellular vesicles on cancer lymphangiogenesis and lymph node metastasis. *Front Oncol* 11: 721785.
36. Closset, L., Gultekin, O., Salehi, S. et al. (2023). The extracellular matrix – immune microenvironment crosstalk in cancer therapy: challenges and opportunities. *Matrix Biol* 121: 217–228.
37. Bruni, S., Mercogliano, M.F., Mauro, F.L. et al. (2023). Cancer immune exclusion: breaking the barricade for a successful immunotherapy. *Front Oncol* 13: 1135456.
38. Wang, H., Zhou, F., Qin, W. et al. (2025). Metabolic regulation of myeloid-derived suppressor cells in tumor immune microenvironment: targets and therapeutic strategies. *Theranostics* 15 (6): 2159–2184.
39. Kaplan, D.H., Shankaran, V., Dighe, A.S. et al. (1998). Demonstration of an interferon γ-dependent tumor surveillance system in immunocompetent mice. *Proc Natl Acad Sci USA* 95 (13): 7556–7561.
40. Bustamante, J. (2020). Mendelian susceptibility to mycobacterial disease: recent discoveries. *Hum Genet* 139 (6–7): 993–1000.
41. Kang, Y.H., Biswas, A., Field, M., and Snapper, S.B. (2019). STAT1 signaling shields T cells from NK cell-mediated cytotoxicity. *Nat Commun* 10 (1): 912.
42. Yewdell, J.W. and Bennink, J.R. (1999). Mechanisms of viral interference with MHC class I antigen processing and presentation1. *Annu Rev Cell Dev Biol* 15: 579–606.
43. Ganaie, F.A., Beall, B.W., Yu, J. et al. (2025). Update on the evolving landscape of pneumococcal capsule types: new discoveries and way forward. *Clin Microbiol Rev* 38 (1): e0017524.
44. Han, A.X., de Jong, S.P.J., and Russell, C.A. (2023). Co-evolution of immunity and seasonal influenza viruses. *Nat Rev Microbiol* 21 (12): 805–817.
45. Agerer, B., Koblischke, M., Gudipati, V. et al. (2021). SARS-CoV-2 mutations in MHC-I-restricted epitopes evade $CD8^+$ T cell responses. *Sci Immunol* 6 (57): eabg6461.
46. Wu, D., Kolesnikov, A., Yin, R. et al. (2022). Structural assessment of HLA-A2-restricted SARS-CoV-2 spike epitopes recognized by public and private T-cell receptors. *Nat Commun* 13 (1): 19.
47. Mengist, H.M., Kombe, A.J., Mekonnen, D. et al. (2021). Mutations of SARS-CoV-2 spike protein: implications on immune evasion and vaccine-induced immunity. *Semin Immunol* 55: 101533.
48. Murphy, W.J., Brentano, S.T., Rice-Ficht, A.C. et al. (1984). DNA rearrangements of the variable surface antigen genes of the trypanosomes. *J Protozool* 31 (1): 65–73.

49. Pays, E., Radwanska, M., and Magez, S. (2023). The pathogenesis of African trypanosomiasis. *Annu Rev Pathol: Mech Disease* 18: 19–45.
50. Yoo, J.-S., Sasaki, M., Cho, S.X. et al. (2021). SARS-CoV-2 inhibits induction of the MHC class I pathway by targeting the STAT1-IRF1-NLRC5 axis. *Nat Commun* 12 (1): 6602.
51. Peng, J.-M., Chiu, C.-F., Cheng, J.-H. et al. (2022). Evasion of NK cell immune surveillance via the vimentin-mediated cytoskeleton remodeling. *Front Immunol* 13: 883178.
52. Melo Garcia, L., Gangadharan, A., Banerjee, P. et al. (2025). Overcoming CD226-related immune evasion in acute myeloid leukemia with CD38 CAR-engineered NK cells. *Cell Rep* 44 (1): 115122.
53. Mestrallet, G., Sone, K., and Bhardwaj, N. (2022). Strategies to overcome DC dysregulation in the tumor microenvironment. *Front Immunol* 13: 980709.
54. Jürgens, B., Hainz, U., Fuchs, D. et al. (2009). Interferon-gamma-triggered indoleamine 2,3-dioxygenase competence in human monocyte-derived dendritic cells induces regulatory activity in allogeneic T cells. *Blood* 114 (15): 3235–3243.
55. Papaspyridonos, M., Matei, I., Huang, Y. et al. (2015). Id1 suppresses anti-tumour immune responses and promotes tumour progression by impairing myeloid cell maturation. *Nat Commun* 6: 6840.
56. Cendrowicz, E., Sas, Z., Bremer, E., and Rygiel, T.P. (2021). The role of macrophages in cancer development and therapy. *Cancers (Basel)* 13 (8): 1946.
57. Ruffell, B., Chang-Strachan, D., Chan, V. et al. (2014). Macrophage IL-10 blocks $CD8^+$ T cell-dependent responses to chemotherapy by suppressing IL-12 expression in intratumoral dendritic cells. *Cancer Cell* 26 (5): 623–637.

PART

II

Immunotherapy in Cancer

4

Cancer Immunotherapy: Key Concepts and Techniques

DENISE GOH[1], NG KAI SOON[1], ZHU ZHU[1,2], RACHEL ELIZABETH ANN FINCHAM[3], AND JOE YEONG[1,3,4,5]

[1] Institute of Molecular and Cell Biology (IMCB), Agency for Science, Technology and Research (A*STAR), Singapore, Singapore

[2] Department of Biobank, The First Affiliated Hospital of Zhengzhou University, Zhengzhou, China

[3] Department of Anatomical Pathology, Singapore General Hospital, Singapore, Singapore

[4] Department of Microbiology, Singapore General Hospital, Singapore, Singapore

[5] Duke-NUS Medical School, Singapore, Singapore

LEARNING OBJECTIVES

- Identify the different approaches to immunotherapy.
- Understand how the tumour microenvironment (TME) can influence treatment response.
- Evaluate the applicability of each technique for biomarker discovery and therapeutic assessment.
- Describe how the clinical techniques are used to guide immunotherapy decisions.

4.1 INTRODUCTION

Over the past 10–15 years, immunotherapy has progressed notably, with some of the most promising approaches – including immune checkpoint inhibitors (ICIs), therapeutic cancer vaccines, bi-specific T cell engagers (BiTEs), and adoptive cell therapies (ACT) – sharing a common mechanism of T cell reactivation [1]. However, challenges such as patient response variability remain a major challenge. Given the heterogeneous nature of the disease, the success rate of immunotherapy varies between and within cancer types; some are more sensitive than others. This variability is largely due to differences in the tumour microenvironment (TME) with different immune statuses and biomarker expressions. As such, emerging strategies are now being developed to engage various immune components, including natural killer cells and dendritic cells, that may contribute to therapeutic efficacy. With an expanding landscape of immunotherapy, several laboratory techniques and assays have therefore become essential to reliably characterise immune responses and dissect therapeutic response mechanisms, both in the preclinical and clinical setting.

Previous chapters have covered basic immunology and immune evasion mechanisms. In this chapter, we will describe key concepts that influence treatment response and techniques that have been used in preclinical and clinical settings to assess immune activity.

4.2 APPROACHES IN CANCER IMMUNOTHERAPY

There are four main classes of cancer immunotherapy, differing based on how it modulates the immune system to achieve anti-tumour effects. **ICIs** represent a major class and have significantly improved the prognosis of several cancer types. By blocking the signalling pathways of immune checkpoint molecules, ICIs aim to restore effector T cell activity and achieve durable tumour control. Much evidence, along with long-term study results, has accumulated over the years; a comprehensive overview of ICI mechanisms and their clinical applications will be discussed in-depth in Chapter 5.

Cancer vaccines aim to elicit or amplify tumour-specific immune responses through precisely selected antigens. Advances in next-generation sequencing technologies and neoantigen prediction have accelerated the shift of vaccine strategies from shared-antigen vaccines to personalised, multi-epitope neoantigen formulations. Progress across multiple vaccine platforms – including peptide vaccines, dendritic cell vaccines, DNA/RNA vaccines, and mRNA vaccines – has accelerated clinical translation [2, 3]. Despite challenges such as tumour heterogeneity and immune tolerance, continuous optimisation of antigen prioritisation and delivery systems is expanding the applicability of personalised vaccines across various tumour types (see Chapter 7).

BiTEs induce potent, MHC-independent cytotoxic responses by simultaneously binding CD3-positive T cells and tumour-associated antigens (TAAs), forcing them into close proximity. This approach has achieved notable clinical success in haematologic malignancies but remains challenging in solid tumours due to antigen heterogeneity and the immunosuppressive TME. Ongoing innovations – including half-life extension structures, dual-epitope constructs, and conditionally activated molecules – are progressively improving the efficacy and safety of BiTEs [4, 5], enabling novel BiTE structures and TME-responsive designs for the expansion of this approach into selected solid tumour contexts. Detailed description is given in Chapter 18.

ACTs are personalised immunotherapies that involve collecting a patient's own immune cells to be expanded and functionally enhanced before being reinfused to boost anti-tumour immunity. As one of the fastest-growing areas in immunotherapy, established modalities include chimeric antigen receptor (CAR)-T cell therapy, tumour-infiltrating lymphocyte (TIL) therapy, and genetically engineered T cell receptor (TCR) therapy. FDA-approved CAR-T products, like Yescarta and Kymriah, showed remarkable efficacy in haematologic malignancies, and ongoing efforts are extending these approaches to solid tumours. TIL therapy enriches lymphocyte count with highly active TILs, while TCR-engineered therapy enhances recognition of MHC-presented intracellular antigens. Collectively, ACTs are designed to elicit stronger and more robust anti-tumoural responses. These strategies continue to evolve through advances in cellular engineering and antigen selection, with further developments discussed in later chapters.

4.3 KEY CONCEPTS IN IMMUNOTHERAPY

Immune evasion is now considered a core hallmark (initially included within the 'emerging hallmarks') of cancer. While various escape mechanisms of tumour cells in avoiding immune destruction have been described in the previous chapter, we detail other key concepts that influence immunotherapy response.

4.3.1 Cancer Immunity Cycle

The key, iterative steps which are necessary to generate an effective anti-cancer immune response are neatly summarised in the cancer-immunity cycle framework [6, 7]. Briefly, neoantigens released by cancer cells are captured by dendritic cells and presented to T cells on MHC class I and II molecules. T cells become primed and activated in response to the tumour neoantigens and traffic to the tumour site, infiltrating the tumour bed. T cells recognise cancer cells and bind to the target cell via the TCR. Tumour cells are subsequently eliminated, and tumour-associated neoantigens are released, restarting the cycle [6]. This classic version of the cancer-immunity cycle succinctly outlines the anti-tumour-immune response; however, increasing evidence demonstrating the complex, immunomodulatory nature of the TME has further necessitated the addition of a cancer-immunity sub-cycle [7].

T cell interaction with stromal elements has been demonstrated to have a significant impact on functionality and phenotype, often leading to cellular dysfunction and exhaustion [8]. Thus, previously primed T cells may no longer be able to effectively eliminate cancer cells. Alternatively, T cells may interact with tertiary lymphoid structures (TLS) within the TME, leading to further potentiation of anti-tumoural activity [9]. Specifically, dendritic cells associated with TLS may present additional tumour neoantigens to the T cells, further priming these cytotoxic lymphocytes for direct tumour cell killing. Thus, a subset of T cells may maintain their functional effector state, leading to T-cell-mediated destruction of tumoural cells [7] (Figure 4.1). These additional complexities provide valuable insights into the dynamic interaction between malignant and immune cells and the TME and provide the foundation for further research exploring novel targets for therapeutic interventions.

4.3.2 TME Immunophenotypes

Dynamic relationships between different cell types and cancer cells serve to either promote or suppress tumour growth. The absence, presence and spatial organisation of immune cells within the TME define key immunophenotypes, broadly categorised as 'hot' and 'cold' tumours. Hot tumours are characterised by increased T cell infiltration, PD-L1 expression and tumour mutational burden (TMB), reflecting an inflammatory phenotype generally poised to respond better to ICIs [12]. Their therapeutic strategy focuses on strengthening anti-tumoural immunity by reinvigorating cytotoxic T cell activity. With higher intra-tumoural T cell density, ICIs can more effectively release inhibitory checkpoints, leading to tumour cell lysis [13]. Higher

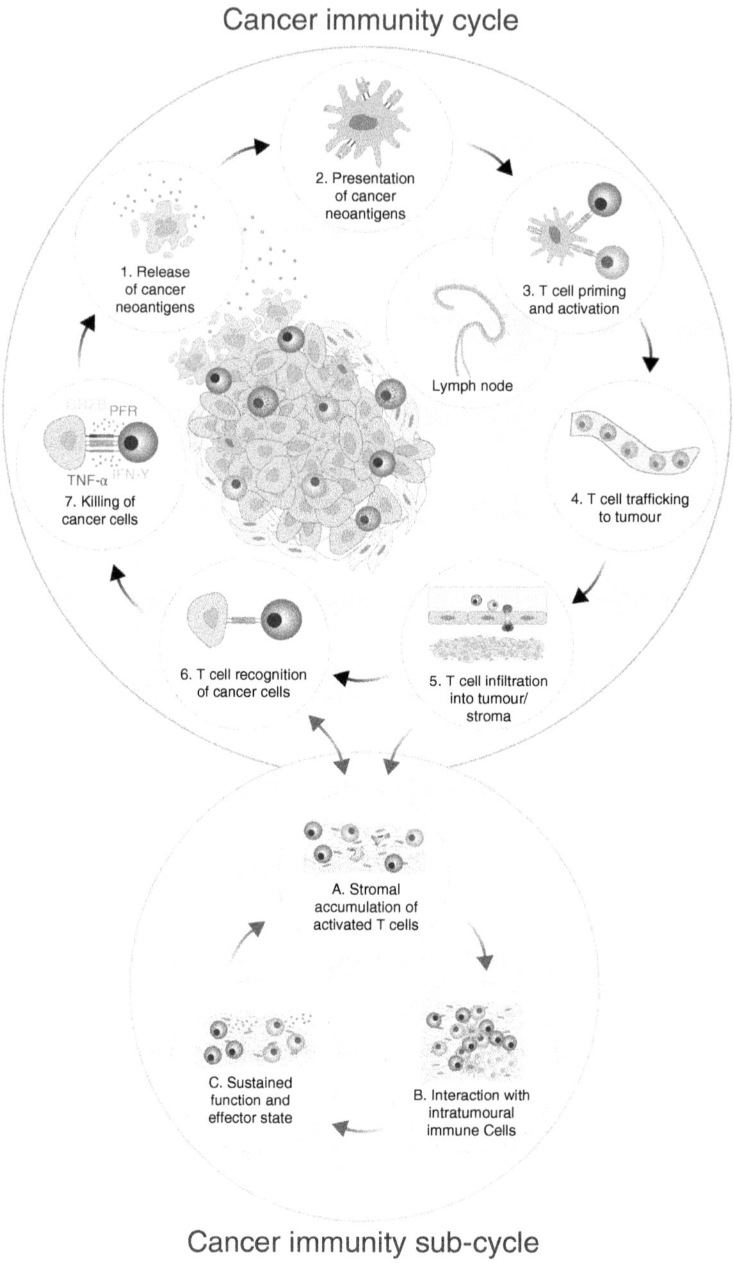

FIGURE 4.1 Summary of the cancer-immunity cycle and cancer-immunity sub-cycle. Neoantigens are released by cancer cells (step 1) and captured by antigen-presenting cells, such as dendritic cells. Dendritic cells then present the neoantigens to T cells via MHC class I and II molecules (step 2), priming and activating the immune cells (step 3). T cells then traffic to the site of malignancy (step 4), where they infiltrate into the tumour/stroma (step 5). Once within the tumour, the primed T cells recognise cancer cells (step 10) and eliminate them (step 11), resulting in the release of cancer-derived neoantigens and restarting the cycle. Concurrently, upon T cell extravasation, the activated T cells may accumulate within the stoma (A). Stromal T cells interact with additional stromal immune cells, such as dendritic cells or tertiary lymphoid structures (B), sustaining T cell function and effector state (C). These T cells may then rejoin the cancer immunity cycle or remain within the stromal sub-cycle. Generated with AI using Inkscape (version 1.3).

TMB also increases the probability of neoantigen expression on cancer cells, which induces neoantigen-specific T cells and amplifies anti-tumoural activity [14]. Typical examples of hot tumours are melanoma, non-small cell lung carcinoma (NSCLC), and renal cancers, with ICI therapy notably transforming lung cancer prognosis over the last two decades [15, 16].

In contrast, cold tumours are characterised by reduced T cell infiltration, low PD-L1 expression and decreased TMB [12, 17]. Their immune-excluded and desert phenotype is often enriched with immunosuppressive cells, such as tumour-associated macrophages, regulatory T cells, and myeloid-derived suppressor cells that drive T cell exhaustion and immune evasion, thereby limiting ICI efficacy [13, 18]. Therefore, therapeutic strategies for cold tumours typically combine ICI with other therapies (i.e. radiotherapy and chemotherapy) to enhance ICI sensitivity by promoting anti-tumoural response. Common examples include liver, pancreatic, and breast cancer. In advanced hepatocellular carcinoma (HCC) not suitable for curative surgery, combination treatment with yttrium-90 radioembolisation and ICI has shown encouraging objective response rate and clinical benefit [19, 20]. Treatment responders exhibited a higher proportion of intra-tumoural $CXCL9^+$/$CXCR3^+$ macrophages, demonstrating that immune activation underlies the sustained clinical response [21, 22].

The dynamic interplay between tumour and immune cells has a profound influence on immunotherapy efficacy. With various techniques, especially computational models, comprehensive TME profiling and analysis can identify unique immune signatures to enhance the effectiveness of immunotherapy.

4.3.3 Cellular Components

Cellular components play an active role in shaping the TME and influencing disease progression [23]. As described in Chapter 2, innate immune cells represent the first line of host defence against damaged cells and cancer cells, while adaptive immune cells serve as the second line of defence. In addition to these immune cell types, non-immune cells, such as cancer-associated fibroblasts (CAFs), endothelial cells, and tumour cells, also actively contribute to shaping the TME (i.e. hot or cold immunophenotype) by modulating immune infiltration, nutrient availability, and local signalling pathways.

CAFs are typically key orchestrators of the cold tumour phenotype, as they secrete extracellular matrix proteins that form dense fibrotic structures, which impede immune cell infiltration, while secreting growth factors and cytokines that promote tumour growth, immune exclusion, and treatment resistance [24, 25]. Similarly, tumour-associated endothelial cells exhibit aberrant cell-adhesion molecules and abnormal angiogenesis, limiting T cell infiltration while supporting tumour progression, intravasation and metastasis [23]. Together, these non-immune stromal components represent promising therapeutic targets to reprogramme cold tumours into hot, immunotherapy-responsive states.

4.3.4 Biomarker Expression

In immunotherapy, biomarker expression offers valuable insights into the patient's tumour and immune landscape. This helps to guide patient selection for treatments, predict therapeutic outcomes, and provide an understanding of the mechanisms of therapy resistance. The most well-characterised biomarkers are **immune checkpoint molecules**, which play a pivotal role in regulating immune activation and suppression. Therapeutic blockade of these molecules has proven transformative and has become a central pillar of modern immunotherapy. The therapeutic mechanisms and clinical treatments involving existing and emerging checkpoint molecules will be covered in greater depth in Chapter 5.

Another class of immune biomarker is the **cytokine** family. These are key mediators of communication and interactions between different cell types within the TME [26]. Their effects are context-dependent, and some are identified as predictive and/or prognostic biomarkers of immunotherapy. As discussed in Chapter 3, cytokines are released as part of an immune response to infection. In cancer immunotherapy, pro-inflammatory IL-2 is the first immunotherapeutic approved by the FDA with notable efficacy in metastatic melanoma and renal carcinoma [27]. NSCLC patients receiving neoadjuvant immunotherapy further showed that higher levels of IL-2 are associated with response [28]. However, IL-2 is also capable of activating regulatory T cells, and high doses can lead to unfavourable side effects such as neurotoxicity [29]. This is an example of a cytokine with dual roles and paradoxical functions in cancer immunity that complicates its usage in immunotherapy. It highlights the importance of considering dual-role implications and focusing on enhancing the antitumour activity while diminishing the pro-tumour effects.

CASE STUDY: IL-2 AS THE FIRST IMMUNOTHERAPY APPROVED FOR CANCER TREATMENT [27]

Alternative names: Aldesleukin, Proleukin®

Approved for: Metastatic melanoma and renal cell carcinoma

In 1984, a patient with metastatic melanoma who had progressed through multiple treatments received a high IL-2 infusion. Within one month posttreatment, her tumours showed extensive shrinkage. Two months posttreatment, all tumours were shrinking. A few months later, there were no signs of cancer. The patient remained disease-free for the next 29 years.

Mechanism of action: Immuno-stimulating; IL-2 is a pro-inflammatory cytokine that activates T cells and other immune cells to attack the cancer.

Limitation: Its broad action also activates immunosuppressive regulatory T cells, resulting in peripheral tolerance and causing significant toxicity.

Tumour biomarkers, including neoantigens and TAAs, are alternative immunotherapeutic targets. **Neoantigens** arise from tumour-specific mutations that are absent in normal tissues, where their presence is associated with high TMB and improved ICI response [30]. This supports their role in the development of personalised vaccines and TCR-engineered T cell therapies. Emerging studies also focused on **'dark proteins'** derived from noncoding RNAs, pseudogenes, untranslated regions, and altered reading frame sources [31]. These unique epitopes are limited in quantity and often degraded through the nonsense-mediated decay pathway; research is ongoing to suppress the pathway, aiming to stabilise these epitopes for MHC-I antigen presentation as potential neoantigens [32].

In contrast, **TAAs** are self-antigens defined by their aberrant expression [33–35]. These TAAs are not tumour-specific but have established relevance in immunotherapy, as they serve as shared targets across diverse tumour types [36]. Interesting examples are CEACAM5 and CEACAM6, which are commonly overexpressed in certain cancers. However, with modification at its N256-glycosylation site, these antigens can become tumour-specific [37]. A clinical trial currently evaluates the use of pembrolizumab (anti-PD-1) with EBC-129, an antibody–drug conjugate targeting this modified epitope, which has received fast-track designation for the treatment of advanced pancreatic ductal adenocarcinoma (PDAC) [38].

The understanding of biomarker expression is crucial in immunotherapy. It helps to guide patient selection and personalised treatment, making sure each patient receives the most suitable therapy. This provides a window for early intervention and the prevention of ineffective therapies. Biomarker expression can also provide greater insight into therapeutic resistance (covered in Chapter 5), allowing for more informed research and facilitating the development of more effective drugs.

4.4 KEY TECHNIQUES FOR IMMUNOTHERAPY ASSESSMENT

Building on the key concepts, we next outline some laboratory techniques used to study and evaluate immune-based therapies in the preclinical and clinical settings.

4.4.1 Preclinical Setting

Within the preclinical setting, several immuno-oncology techniques are routinely used to characterise immune cell subsets, quantify cytokine production, and assess functional immune responses. The main characteristics of each technology are summarised in Table 4.1.

RNA sequencing has revolutionised transcriptome analysis, highlighting not only differential gene expression but also revealing gene fusions, mutations and splicing variants [39]. Bulk RNA sequencing analyses gene expression at the tissue level, averaging global expression. Consequently, it often overlooks tissue and cell heterogeneity, which obscures key driving signals and limits insights into the TME. This led to the development of single-cell RNA sequencing (scRNA-seq), which adds a critical single-cell level resolution to our understanding of the TME, using barcoded labelling of individual cells to reveal individual cellular variation, highlighting tissue heterogeneity within samples [40, 41]. Success stories include the identification of a novel group of immunosuppressive T cells in patients with glioblastoma as a new potential immunotherapy strategy [42] and the identification of deviating differentiation trajectories in a subgroup of cancer cells in metastatic lung cancer, which provides a framework for advancing the discovery of molecular and therapeutic targets [43]. Despite encouraging results, scRNA-seq has limitations, including stress-induced gene expression from cellular dissociation and challenges in clustering, which can obscure accurate identification of cell types and heterogeneity [40, 41]. Thus, a combination with other techniques is often considered for validation. Other advanced methodologies involving RNA sequencing on intact tissues are collectively known as spatial transcriptomics, which will be covered in Chapter 15.

Flow cytometry is a conventional protein profiling technique that enables the detection and quantification of immune proteins that contribute to anti-tumoural response and tumour-immune evasion. It is a high-throughput, single-cell technique

TABLE 4.1 Routine immune-oncology techniques are used in preclinical studies.

Techniques	Detection	Type of analysis	Type of tissue	Typical readouts
RNA sequencing	Transcriptome	Quantitative and qualitative	Dissociated tissue *Intact tissue, see Chapter 15	Gene expression levels, differential gene expression, novel transcripts
Flow cytometry	Surface and intracellular protein expression	Quantitative	Dissociated tissue/ PBMCs/TILs/ Cell lines	Cellular populations and subsets, biomarker expression
ELISA	Soluble proteins	Quantitative	Dissociated tissue PBMCs/TILs	Cytokine concentration
ELISpot	Immune cells secreting antibodies/ cytokines	Quantitative	Dissociated tissue PBMCs/TILs	Antigen-specific immune cells
In vitro functional assays	Functional activity	Quantitative	Dissociated tissue/PBMCs/ Cell lines	Cytotoxicity, proliferation, viability
Immuno histochemistry	Protein expression	Quantitative and qualitative	Intact tissue	Protein localisation, immune infiltration and distribution
In vivo tumour models	Tumour-immune interaction	Quantitative and qualitative	Living organism	Immune infiltration, treatment response, and drug discovery evaluation

that analyses cells in suspension, using lasers as light sources to detect fluorescence signals. Advances in flow cytometry have led to the development of spectral flow cytometry, which detects the complete emission spectrum of fluorochromes rather than just detecting the peak emission as in the case of conventional flow cytometry. This enables the use of fluorochromes with highly overlapping emission spectrums in the same panel [44], thus significantly expanding the panel size to accommodate 25–40 colours. For instance, spectral flow cytometric analysis of surface and intracellular proteins on peripheral blood mononuclear cells (PBMCs) and TILs revealed that >99% of tumour-specific $CD8^+$ T cells expressed CD39 and that increased CD39 expression on $CD8^+$ T cells was found to predict the response to ICB therapy in a small cohort of triple-negative breast cancer (TNBC) patients [45].

Cell culture and functional testing are complementary techniques that provide a detailed evaluation of tumour-immune interaction under controlled conditions. **Cell cultures** can be two-dimensional or three-dimensional, with varying complexity. These models allow precise control over variables, including cytokine concentration, drug dosage, and growth factors, to support mechanistic investigation that would be difficult to evaluate in *in vivo* models. The simplest culture system would be the expansion of primary cells or an established cell line, followed by a co-culture system, which allows the growth of multiple cell types together in the same culture to study their specific interaction and influence on each other. However, these are not a complete representation of the complex TME. Meanwhile, three-dimensional cell cultures can be manipulated to mimic cellular behaviour *in vivo* to provide more accurate data on cell–cell interactions, tumour characteristics, and drug mechanisms. **Functional assays** can be applied to these models to directly measure the biological activity (i.e. cytotoxicity and proliferation) of the cells in response to a stimulus. Specifically, it can help determine the efficacy of immune effector cells and therapeutic agents in modulating anti-tumour immunity.

The **enzyme-linked immunosorbent assay** (ELISA) technique is a biochemical assay that uses antibodies to detect and quantify target proteins in a liquid sample. While it can be differentiated into four types – direct, indirect, sandwich, and competitive – based on how the antibodies are used to detect the antigen, it all follows the same principle: target proteins are captured by antigen- or antibody-coated plates, detected using an enzyme-linked secondary antibody, and quantified via a colourimetric or chemiluminescent readout proportional to protein concentration. This makes ELISA a standard tool for assessing drug effects and monitoring immune responses. As an extension, **enzyme-linked immunospot (ELISpot)** measures the frequency of protein-secreting cells at the single-cell level. It is a highly sensitive functional immunoassay that has a similar workflow to sandwich ELISA, where it involves coating the plate with capture antibody, adding cells, stimulating them, and detecting secreted proteins. Thus, this technique can be used as a fast and simple tool to assess T cell response and vaccine efficacy. With every protein-secreting cell forming a visible spot that allows for quantitative analysis, it is capable of measuring antigen-specific T cell response through cytokine production upon exposure to a specific antigen.

Immunohistochemistry (IHC) is a tissue-based approach that uses antibodies to detect and visualise specific protein expression within intact tissue sections, making it one of the most widely used techniques for protein localisation studies. Preclinical studies have identified numerous proteins as prognostic and/or predictive biomarkers for immunotherapy, yet rigorous validation is still required before they can be reliably translated into clinical practice. **Multiplex IHC** further enables simultaneous detection of multiple proteins on a single tissue section that allows better understanding and elucidation of the spatial relationship of different cell types within the TME. A detailed description of these techniques will be covered alongside emerging new technologies for spatial studies in Chapter 15.

Until now, we have described *ex vivo* (outside their native organism) techniques; however, one important aspect of preclinical studies involves ***in vivo* tumour models** (within the native organism) to enable in-depth evaluation of immunotherapy efficacy and mechanisms in a controlled biological context. Many types of tumour models, predominantly mice (Figure 4.2), have been established to cater to different research needs [46]. Cell-line-derived xenografts are well-characterised models where established human cancer cell lines are grown *in vitro* and then implanted in immunodeficient mice. These are widely used for antitumour drug discovery evaluation and combination immunotherapy assessment. Patient-derived xenografts are somewhat similar, but they are generated by transferring patient tumour tissues directly into the mice to induce cancer. It holds an advantage compared to those derived from cell lines by being able to mimic the original features of the patient's tumour. One example is the orthotopic tumour model, where patient tumour tissue is transferred into the corresponding mouse organ. Genetically engineered mouse models (GEMM) facilitate *de novo* tumourigenesis, without requiring immunodeficient mice. Through genetic manipulations such as knock-out and knock-in genes and inducible systems, GEMM tumours closely resemble their human counterparts and can progress spontaneously, allowing metastatic studies [47]. Syngeneic mouse models are generated by implanting mouse tumour cells into immunocompetent mice of the same genetic background to avoid tumour rejection and to assess the effect of combination immunotherapy and immune response. Immunodeficient humanised mice that recapitulate human immunity are generated by co-engrafting with a human tumour and an immune component. It has been effectively used to assess the treatment efficacy and safety of various cancer immunotherapies, along with the predictive biomarker discovery.

Together, these preclinical techniques provide complementary insights into the TME, with each technique contributing a unique mechanistic understanding. Continued efforts are being made to identify and validate candidate targets for treatment response and clinical outcomes. Therefore, with these techniques thoughtfully integrated, a robust foundation for advancing immunotherapy research can be provided, guiding the translation of these targets towards clinical application.

4.4.2 Clinical Setting

In the clinic, a range of assays are used to characterise patient's immune profiles and guide immunotherapy decision-making. **PBMC immune profiling** and specific immune subset identification provide valuable insights into disease progression and treatment response, reflecting systemic immune responses that may mirror the TME. Compared to traditional biopsies, drawing peripheral blood is minimally invasive and therefore allows for repeated blood draws at multiple timepoints to enable longitudinal immuno-monitoring of patients to assess the trajectory of immune responses across the course of treatment. With spectral flow cytometry, PBMCs can undergo deep immunophenotyping, comprehensive characterisation of activation, exhaustion, and differentiation markers that may correlate with clinical outcome or treatment response, and the discovery of rare cell types that can be missed by conventional flow cytometry [48].

ELISA assays can additionally measure soluble factors with prognostic value in plasma and/or serum samples. For example, carcinoembryonic antigen [49] and CA15-3 [50] are routinely tested via these immunoassays due to their implications in disease metastasis and treatment resistance and prognostic value in breast cancer, respectively. From blood plasma, cell-free DNA (cfDNA) and circulating tumour DNA (ctDNA) are also promising oncological markers that are becoming increasingly measured in clinical settings, termed as 'liquid biopsies'. Quantifiable using

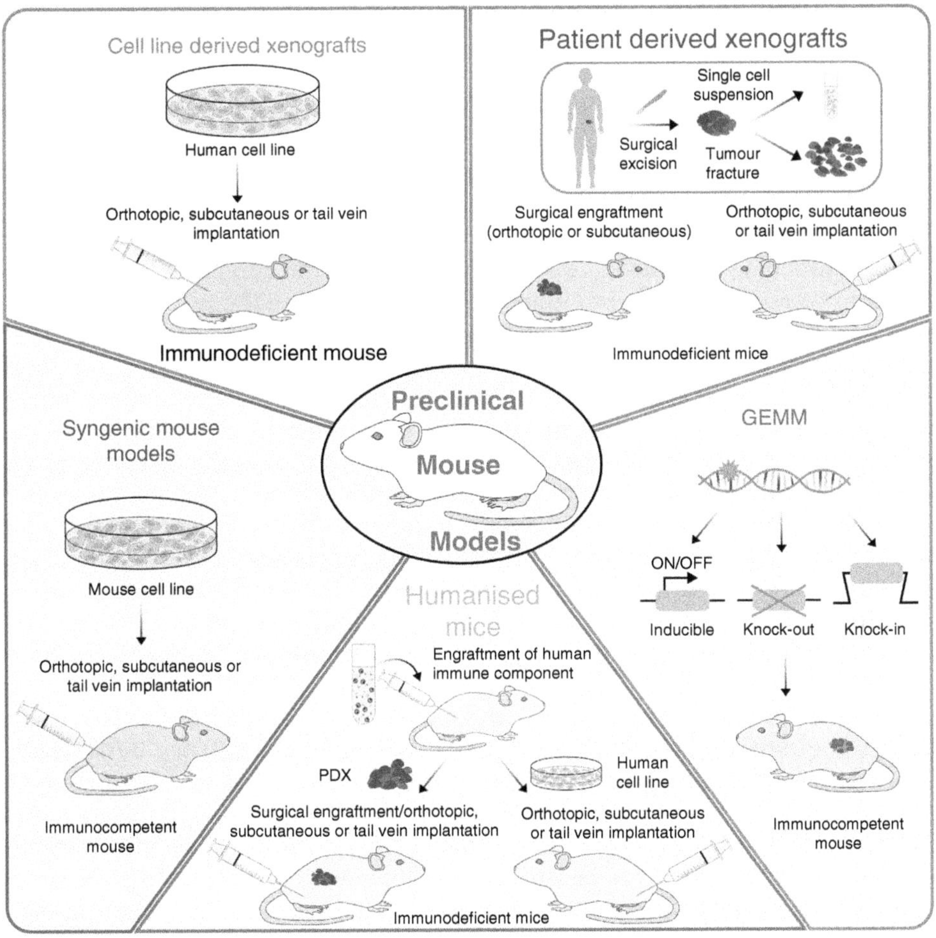

FIGURE 4.2 Summary of preclinical mouse models used in oncology research. Cell line-derived xenograft (CDX) models derive from human cell lines, which are cultured and harvested for implantation into immunodeficient mice. The transfer of cells can be conducted orthotopically (to the same site as the tumour of origin), subcutaneously, or via the tail vein. In patient-derived xenografts (PDX), tumour tissue is surgically excised from cancer patients. This tissue is then either fragmented into small tumour sections, preserving some of the tissue architecture, or processed into a single-cell suspension. The tissue fragments are surgically engrafted, or cell suspensions are implanted, into the immunodeficient mice. Genetically engineered mouse models harness gene editing techniques to facilitate the de novo generation of tumours within immunocompetent mice. Humanized mouse models rely on the engraftment of human immune components into immunodeficient mice. Once established, the immune component of humanized mice mimics their human counterpart. PDX and CDX models can then be established within the model. Finally, syngeneic models harness the implantation of murine cell lines in immuno competent mice. This implantation can be orthotopic, subcutaneous or via the tail vein. Generated with AI using Inkscape (version 1.3).

PCR-based methods such as quantitative PCR or droplet digital PCR, cfDNA and ctDNA levels are often elevated in various cancers compared to healthy individuals, possibly due to attenuated DNase activity and increased necrosis in cancer cells. Elevated levels are correlated with worse prognosis and treatment resistance following immunotherapy [51].

Beyond PBMCs, **TILs** play a crucial role in the TME and are responsible for mounting an anti-tumoural response. High levels of TILs have been linked to better prognosis in various cancer types, including HCC and NSCLC cancer [52]. $CD3^+$ TILs, in particular, are indicative of a more 'inflamed' phenotype and are generally poised to respond better to immunotherapy [53]. While TILs in circulation have been detected sharing TCR clonality and phenotype as those in the tumour, their low frequency warrants the need for histological assessment of tumour sections to evaluate the extent of lymphocyte infiltration within the TME: the most common approach is haematoxylin and eosin staining on formalin-fixed paraffin-embedded tissue slides, which will be subsequently scored by trained pathologists. However, due to high inter-observer variability, there remains a need for standardisation of scoring guidelines, plausibly through computational and deep learning methods. Additionally, with the heterogeneous nature of TILs, it is often necessary to further characterise them into specific immune cell types via methods such as multiplex IHC. To maintain high reproducibility and throughput, a couple of multiplex IHC protocols have already been developed to incorporate the use of diagnostic autostainers [54, 55].

Other analytical techniques used in the clinic also include **PD-L1 IHC assays** and **TMB quantification**. PD-L1 expression is widely tested during initial cancer diagnosis, and its assessment is used to guide treatment decisions by identifying patients who may benefit from immunotherapy (more to be covered in Chapter 5). TMB is defined by the average number of somatic mutations per defined region of a tumour genome [56]. It has become widely accepted that high TMB gives rise to increased neoantigen expression on the surface of tumour cells, making them more detectable by immune cells, which increases immunotherapy sensitivity. In the clinic, these techniques have improved treatment efficacy by facilitating patient triage and guiding decision-making.

Many of these techniques are complementary and may be carried out in conjunction. For instance, as peripheral blood profiling analyses single cells or analytes in suspension, spatial information is lacking to provide accurate mapping and visualisation within the TME. Therefore, in recent years, innovative spatial profiling techniques, along with artificial intelligence (AI) integration, have emerged to perform molecular analyses within the native tissue. More of these advanced techniques will be detailed in Chapter 15.

4.5 FUTURE DIRECTIONS

Cancer immunotherapy has transformed cancer care, offering durable benefits even in cancers once associated with poor prognoses. Despite this progress, major challenges remain – including the persistence of cold tumours with an immunosuppressive TME and the development of therapeutic resistance. While substantial efforts have been made in biomarker discovery and promising results have been observed in preclinical testing, many candidate targets often fail to deliver in early-phase human studies. This underscores the urgent need to identify reliable predictive biomarkers that can better guide therapeutic selection and improve patient outcomes.

The future of immunotherapy points towards a more personalised and multifaceted approach, tailored to the tumour characteristics and immunological profile of each patient to enhance efficacy and overcome resistance. In addition, emerging strategies that harness dark proteins, modulate the gut microbiome to enhance efficacy, and employ oncolytic viruses or nanodelivery platforms to precisely target cancer cells hold great promise. Over the next five years, we may begin to see the efficacy of these emerging therapeutics. Moreover, AI will likely play a crucial role in supporting therapeutic decision-making for immunotherapies, with its unique ability to model and predict treatment response, facilitating truly personalised therapy. Continued innovation and integrative approaches are crucial to overcoming current barriers and further broadening the impact of immunotherapy.

KEY TERMS & DEFINITIONS SIDEBAR

Adoptive cell therapy A form of personalised immunotherapies that involve collecting a patient's own immune cells to be expanded and functionally enhanced before being reinfused to boost anti-tumour immunity.

Biomarker A measurable biological molecule (RNA, DNA, or protein) that can be objectively evaluated as an indicator of normal biological or pathological processes.

Clinical research Studies conducted on human volunteers (patients and healthy subjects) to apply knowledge in a real-world setting.

Immunohistochemistry A laboratory technique that exploits the specific binding between an antibody and antigen (specific protein) in tissue sections to detect and reveal their location and abundance.

Immunophenotype Classification of the tumour microenvironment based on composition and function state of immune cells infiltrating the tumour.

Preclinical research Laboratory and animal studies before first-in-human trials, often used for testing theoretical science.

Tumour microenvironment The complex ecosystem that surrounds a tumour, comprising of cancer cells, immune cells, stromal cells, blood vessels and extracellular matrix.

Tumour mutational burden An indicator that measures the total number of genetic mutations within a cancer cell's genome, reported as the number of mutations per megabase.

Tumour infiltrating lymphocytes A diverse population of immune cells that have migrated from the blood into the tumour to play key roles in anti-tumour immunity.

LIST OF ABBREVIATIONS

CAF cancer-associated fibroblast

HCC hepatocellular carcinoma

ICI immune checkpoint inhibitor

IHC immunohistochemistry

NSCLC non-small cell lung carcinoma

PDAC pancreatic ductal adenocarcinoma
TLS tertiary lymphoid structures
TME tumour microenvironment
TIL tumour-infiltrating lymphocyte
TMB tumour mutational burden
TNBC triple-negative breast cancer

REVIEW QUESTIONS

1. What are the factor(s) that contribute to variable patient responses in immunotherapy?
2. What are the different approaches of immunotherapy, and how do their mechanisms differ?
3. Which technique(s) would you use to assess tumour-immune interactions and quantify specific immune cell subsets within the TME?

REFERENCES

1. Dagher, O.K., Schwab, R.D., Brookens, S.K., and Posey, A.D. Jr. (2023). Advances in cancer immunotherapies. *Cell* 186: 1814–1814.e1.
2. Blass, E. and Ott, P.A. (2021). Advances in the development of personalized neoantigen-based therapeutic cancer vaccines. *Nat Rev Clin Oncol* 18 (4): 215–229.
3. Fan, T., Zhang, M., Yang, J. et al. (2023). Therapeutic cancer vaccines: advancements, challenges, and prospects. *Signal Transduct Target Ther* 8 (1): 450.
4. Goebeler, M.E. and Bargou, R.C. (2020). T cell-engaging therapies – BiTEs and beyond. *Nat Rev Clin Oncol* 17 (7): 418–434.
5. Blanco, B., Dominguez-Alonso, C., and Alvarez-Vallina, L. (2021). Bispecific immunomodulatory antibodies for cancer immunotherapy. *Clin Cancer Res* 27 (20): 5457–5464.
6. Chen D.S., and Mellman, I. (2013). Oncology meets immunology: the cancer-immunity cycle. *Immunity* 39 (1): 1–10.
7. Mellman, I., Chen, D.S., Powles, T., and Turley, S.J. (2023). The cancer-immunity cycle: indication, genotype, and immunotype. *Immunity* 56 (10): 2188–2205.
8. Zhang, Z., Liu, S., Zhang, B. et al. (2020). T cell dysfunction and exhaustion in cancer. *Front Cell Dev Biol* 8: 10.
9. Reste, M., Ajazi, K., Sayi-Yazgan, A. et al. (2024). The role of dendritic cells in tertiary lymphoid structures: implications in cancer and autoimmune diseases. *Front Immunol* 15: 1439413.
10. Neelapu, S.S., Jacobson, C.A., Ghobadi, A. et al. (2023). Five-year follow-up of ZUMA-1 supports the curative potential of axicabtagene ciloleucel in refractory large B-cell lymphoma. *Blood* 141 (19): 2307–2315.
11. Laetsch, T.W., Maude, S.L., Rives, S. et al. (2023). Three-year update of tisagenlecleucel in pediatric and young adult patients with relapsed/refractory acute lymphoblastic leukemia in the ELIANA trial. *J Clin Oncol* 41 (9): 1664–1669.
12. Liu, Y.T. and Sun, Z.J. (2021). Turning cold tumors into hot tumors by improving T-cell infiltration. *Theranostics* 11 (11): 5365–5386.
13. Wu, B., Zhang, B., Li, B. et al. (2024). Cold and hot tumors: from molecular mechanisms to targeted therapy. *Signal Transduct Target Ther* 9 (1): 274.
14. Chan, T.A., Yarchoan, M., Jaffee, E. et al. (2019). Development of tumor mutation burden as an immunotherapy biomarker: utility for the oncology clinic. *Ann Oncol* 30 (1): 44–56.

15. Hapuarachi, B., Danson, S., Wadsley, J., and Muthana, M. (2023). Exercise to transform tumours from cold to hot and improve immunotherapy responsiveness. *Front Immunol* 14: 1335256.
16. Ferreira, M. and Reckamp, K.L. (2022). Editorial: impact of immunotherapy in lung cancer. *Front Oncol* 12: 1083524.
17. Ouyang, P., Wang, L., Wu, J. et al. (2024). Overcoming cold tumors: a combination strategy of immune checkpoint inhibitors. *Front Immunol* 15: 1344272.
18. Chen, Q., Sun, T., and Jiang, C. (2021). Recent advancements in nanomedicine for 'cold' tumor immunotherapy. *Nanomicro Lett* 13: 92.
19. Fenton, S.E., Kircher, S.M., Mulcahy, M.F. et al. (2021). A phase I study of nivolumab (NIVO) in combination with TheraSphere (Yttrium-90) in patients with advanced hepatocellular cancer. *J Clin Oncol* 39 (15_suppl): e16183-e.
20. Tai, D., Loke, K., Gogna, A. et al. (2021). Radioembolisation with Y90-resin microspheres followed by nivolumab for advanced hepatocellular carcinoma (CA 209-678): a single arm, single centre, phase 2 trial. *Lancet Gastroenterol Hepatol* 6 (12): 1025–1035.
21. Chew, V., Lee, Y.H., Pan, L. et al. (2019). Immune activation underlies a sustained clinical response to Yttrium-90 radioembolisation in hepatocellular carcinoma. *Gut* 68 (2): 335–346.
22. Kaya, N.A., Tai, D., Lim, X. et al. (2023). Multimodal molecular landscape of response to Y90-resin microsphere radioembolization followed by nivolumab for advanced hepatocellular carcinoma. *J Immunother Cancer* 11 (8): e007106.
23. Anderson, N.M. and Simon, M.C. (2020). The tumor microenvironment. *Curr Biol* 30 (16): R921–R925.
24. Ozmen, E., Demir, T.D., and Ozcan, G. (2024). Cancer-associated fibroblasts: protagonists of the tumor microenvironment in gastric cancer. *Front Mol Biosci* 11: 1340124.
25. Sarkar, M., Nguyen, T., Gundre, E. et al. (2023). Cancer-associated fibroblasts: the chief architect in the tumor microenvironment. *Front Cell Dev Biol* 11: 1089068.
26. Wang, H., Wang, T., Yan, S. et al. (2024). Crosstalk of pyroptosis and cytokine in the tumor microenvironment: from mechanisms to clinical implication. *Mol Cancer* 23 (1): 268.
27. Rosenberg, S.A. (2014). IL-2: the first effective immunotherapy for human cancer. *J Immunol* 192 (12): 5451–5458.
28. Yi, L., Xu, Z., Ma, T. et al. (2024). T-cell subsets and cytokines are indicative of neoadjuvant chemoimmunotherapy responses in NSCLC. *Cancer Immunol Immunother* 73 (6): 99.
29. Im, S.J., Lee, K., and Ha, S.-J. (2024). Harnessing IL-2 for immunotherapy against cancer and chronic infection: a historical perspective and emerging trends. *Exp Mol Med* 56 (9): 1900–1908.
30. Ott, P.A., Hu, Z., Keskin, D.B. et al. (2017). An immunogenic personal neoantigen vaccine for patients with melanoma. *Nature* 547 (7662): 217–221.
31. Rospo, G., Chila, R., Matafora, V. et al. (2024). Non-canonical antigens are the largest fraction of peptides presented by MHC class I in mismatch repair deficient murine colorectal cancer. *Genome Med* 16 (1): 15.
32. Periasamy, P., Joseph, C., Campos, A. et al. (2024). Regulation of non-canonical proteins from diverse origins through the nonsense-mediated mRNA decay pathway. *Proteomics* 24 (18): e2300361.
33. Baxevanis, C.N., Sotiriadou, N.N., Gritzapis, A.D. et al. (2006). Immunogenic HER-2/neu peptides as tumor vaccines. *Cancer Immunol Immunother* 55 (1): 85–95.
34. Alsalloum, A., Shevchenko, J.A., and Sennikov, S. (2024). NY-ESO-1 antigen: a promising frontier in cancer immunotherapy. *Clin Transl Med* 14 (9): e70020.
35. Schooten, E., Di Maggio, A., van Bergen En Henegouwen, P.M.P. et al. (2018). MAGE-A antigens as targets for cancer immunotherapy. *Cancer Treat Rev* 67: 54–62.
36. Leko, V. and Rosenberg, S.A. (2020). Identifying and targeting human tumor antigens for T cell-based immunotherapy of solid tumors. *Cancer Cell* 38 (4): 454–472.
37. Ng, M.C.H., Yong, W.P., Meric-Bernstam, F. et al. (2024). 653P A phase I dose escalation study of EBC-129, a first-in-class, anti-N-glycosylated CEACAM5 & CEACAM6 antibody-drug conjugate (ADC) in patients with solid tumors. *Ann Oncol* 35: S516.

38. Lentz, R.W., Ng, M.C.H., Yong, W.-P. et al. (2025). Clinical activity of EBC-129, a first-in-class, anti-N256-glycosylated CEACAM5 and CEACAM6 antibody-drug conjugate (ADC), in patients with pancreatic ductal adenocarcinoma (PDAC) in a phase 1 study. *J Clin Oncol* 43 (16_suppl): 4018.
39. Li, X. and Wang, C.-Y. (2021). From bulk, single-cell to spatial RNA sequencing. *Int J Oral Sci* 13 (1): 36.
40. Jovic, D., Liang, X., Zeng, H. et al. (2022). Single-cell RNA sequencing technologies and applications: a brief overview. *Clin Transl Med* 12 (3): e694.
41. Cheng, C., Chen, W., Jin, H., and Chen, X. (2023). A review of single-cell RNA-seq annotation, integration, and cell-cell communication. *Cells* 12 (15): 1970.
42. Long, X., Zhang, Z., Li, Y. et al. (2024). ScRNA-seq reveals novel immune-suppressive T cells and investigates CMV-TCR-T cells cytotoxicity against GBM. *J Immunother Cancer* 12 (4): e008967.
43. Kim, N., Kim, H.K., Lee, K. et al. (2020). Single-cell RNA sequencing demonstrates the molecular and cellular reprogramming of metastatic lung adenocarcinoma. *Nat Commun* 11 (1): 2285.
44. Sahir, F., Mateo, J.M., Steinhoff, M., and Siveen, K.S. (2020). Development of a 43 color panel for the characterization of conventional and unconventional T-cell subsets, B cells, NK cells, monocytes, dendritic cells, and innate lymphoid cells using spectral flow cytometry. *Cytometry A* 105 (5): 404–410.
45. Meng, J., Tan, J.Y.T., Joseph, C.R. et al. (2024). The prognostic value of CD39 as a marker of tumor-specific T cells in triple-negative breast cancer in Asian women. *Lab Investig* 104 (3): 100303.
46. Zhang, C., Sui, Y., Liu, S., and Yang, M. (2024). In vitro and in vivo experimental models for cancer immunotherapy study. *Curr Res Biotechnol* 7: 100210.
47. Kersten, K., de Visser, K.E., van Miltenburg, M.H., and Jonkers, J. (2017). Genetically engineered mouse models in oncology research and cancer medicine. *EMBO Mol Med* 9 (2): 137–153.
48. Spasic, M., Ogayo, E.R., Parsons, A.M. et al. (2024). Spectral flow cytometry methods and pipelines for comprehensive immunoprofiling of human peripheral blood and bone marrow. *Cancer Res Commun* 4 (3): 895–910.
49. Niedzielska, J. and Jastrzębski, T. (2025). Carcinoembryonic antigen (CEA): origin, role in oncology, and concentrations in serum and peritoneal fluid. *J Clin Med* 14 (9): 3189.
50. Ryu, J.M., Kang, D., Cho, J. et al. (2023). Prognostic impact of elevation of cancer antigen 15-3 (CA15-3) in patients with early breast cancer with normal serum CA15-3 level. *J Breast Cancer* 26 (2): 126–135.
51. Sanz-Garcia, E., Zhao, E., Bratman, S.V., and Siu, L.L. (2022). Monitoring and adapting cancer treatment using circulating tumor DNA kinetics: current research, opportunities, and challenges. *Sci Adv* 8 (4): eabi8618.
52. Berele, B.A., Cai, Y., and Yang, G. (2021). Prognostic value of tumor-infiltrating lymphocytes in nasopharyngeal carcinoma patients: meta-analysis. *Technol Cancer Res Treat* 20: 15330338211034265.
53. Presti, D., Dall'Olio, F.G., Besse, B. et al. (2022). Tumor-infiltrating lymphocytes (TILs) as a predictive biomarker of response to checkpoint blockers in solid tumors: a systematic review. *Crit Rev Oncol Hematol* 177: 103773.
54. Sun, Z., Nyberg, R., Wu, Y. et al. (2021). Developing an enhanced 7-color multiplex IHC protocol to dissect immune infiltration in human cancers. *PLoS One* 16 (2): e0247238.
55. Lim, J.C.T., Yeong, J.P.S., Lim, C.J. et al. (2018). An automated staining protocol for seven-colour immunofluorescence of human tissue sections for diagnostic and prognostic use. *Pathology* 50 (3): 333–341.
56. Aggarwal, C., Ben-Shachar, R., Gao, Y. et al. (2023). Assessment of tumor mutational burden and outcomes in patients with diverse advanced cancers treated with immunotherapy. *JAMA Netw Open* 6 (5): e2311181.

CHAPTER 5

Immune Checkpoint Inhibitors in Cancer: Mechanisms, Clinical Use, and Challenges

CAMILLE HANSEN[1,2] AND ARABELLA YOUNG[1,2]
[1] Department of Pathology, University of Utah, Salt Lake City, UT, USA
[2] Huntsman Cancer Institute, University of Utah, Salt Lake City, UT, USA

LEARNING OBJECTIVES

- Understand the mechanism by which immune checkpoint inhibition modifies immune activity against cancer.
- Discuss the clinical applications and limitations of immune checkpoint inhibitor (ICI) use.
- Define predictive biomarkers for ICI response.
- Explain implications for immune-related adverse event (irAE) development and management in the context of ICI treatment.
- Identify emerging immune checkpoints and costimulatory targets, and the challenges in clinical translation.

5.1 INTRODUCTION

Immune checkpoint inhibitors (ICIs) have redefined the treatment landscape for many cancers. The therapeutic activity of ICIs is primarily mediated by blocking inhibitory signals that restrain T cell function, leading to cytotoxic responses against tumour cells that were previously able to evade immune detection. Unlike chemotherapy, radiotherapy or targeted therapies, which act directly on cancer cells, ICIs promote the ability of the immune system to initiate a sustained anti-tumour immune response, which has led to improved survival benefit across multiple cancer types.

Currently in the clinic, ICI treatments encompass a group of monoclonal antibodies directed to four targets: cytotoxic T-lymphocyte-associated protein 4 (CTLA-4), programmed cell death protein 1 (PD-1) or its ligand programmed cell death ligand 1 (PD-L1), and most recently lymphocyte activation gene 3 (LAG-3) (Figure 5.1). These immune checkpoint molecules are normally expressed to maintain immune homeostasis and prevent tissue damage during immune activation, with many initial

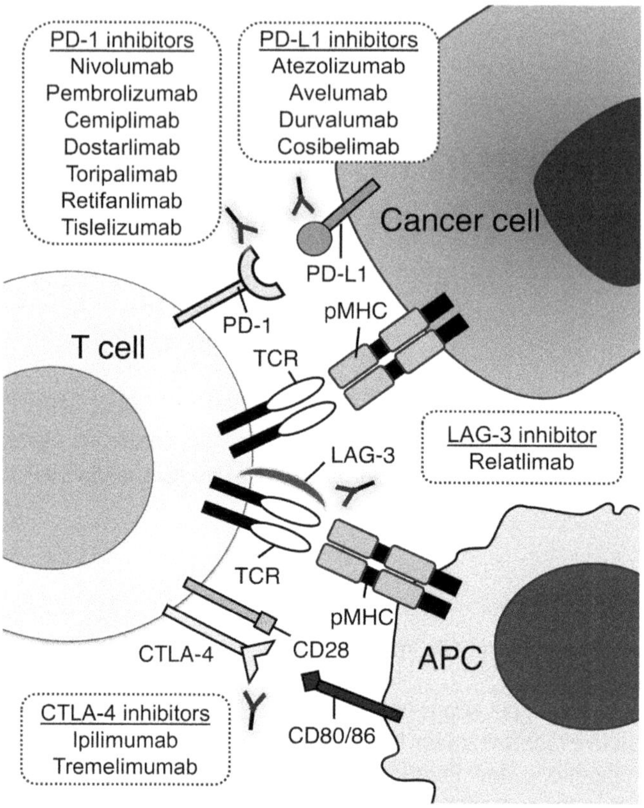

FIGURE 5.1 Mechanism of action for immune checkpoints and their inhibitors. This schematic illustrates the key inhibitory interactions between T cells, APCs, and tumour cells that are disrupted by ICIs. Under normal conditions, T cell activity is regulated through receptor-ligand interactions such as PD-1-PD-L1, CTLA-4-CD80 or CD86, and LAG-3-MHC peptide complex (pMHC), which help to maintain immune tolerance and prevent autoimmunity. Tumours exploit these inhibitory signals to evade immune destruction. Approved ICIs, including monoclonal antibodies against PD-1, PD-L1, CTLA-4, and most recently LAG-3, block engagement of immune checkpoints, improving the ability of T cells to recognise and kill cancer cells. This figure was created by the authors and does not use third-party templates or figure-generation software.

studies defining them as critical for inhibiting immune activity in the context of autoimmunity [1, 2]. However, within the tumour microenvironment (TME), these immunoregulatory molecules are often exploited to disable immune function, leading to suppression of anti-tumour immunity.

Given that the majority of patients with cancer are considered to have an intact immune system, the potential broad applicability of ICI treatments across various cancers has been considered a major clinical advantage for this therapeutic approach. There is a growing number of approvals, with use in solid and haematologic cancers as well as the first-ever cancer-agnostic approval for patients with mismatch repair deficiency (dMMR) cancers [3, 4]. Additionally, ICI treatment continues to be incorporated at different disease stages, including use as a first-line treatment and in the neoadjuvant and adjuvant settings [5, 6]. Yet the widespread application of these therapies has revealed new clinical challenges. Many patients fail to respond to ICIs despite favourable predictive biomarkers, and side effects, termed immune-related adverse events (irAEs), can be unpredictable, long-lasting or permanent, and in some cases life-threatening [7, 8]. As ICIs are increasingly used across more cancer types, including in earlier-stage disease and younger patient populations, understanding and mitigating mechanisms that drive therapeutic resistance and irAEs will be essential in optimising patient outcomes.

This chapter will explore the biological foundations of immune checkpoint regulation, the mechanisms by which ICIs achieve clinical benefit, and limitations for their efficacy and broad utility.

5.2 THE DISCOVERY OF KEY IMMUNE CHECKPOINTS

5.2.1 CTLA-4

CTLA-4 was first identified in 1987, in which it was described as a member of the immunoglobulin superfamily, with expression primarily in activated T cells [9]. Subsequent work demonstrated that CTLA-4 acts as a negative regulator of T cell activation [10]. Following T cell receptor (TCR) signalling, co-stimulation by CD28 in T cells engaging B7 ligands (CD80 or CD86) in antigen-presenting cells (APCs) is critical for T cell activation, survival, and expansion [11]. CTLA-4 is a structural homolog of CD28 with greater affinity for CD80 and CD86. CD28 is constitutively expressed in T cells, whereas CTLA-4 is induced upon TCR signalling, providing a negative feedback signal during T cell activation (Figure 5.1) [12, 13]. CTLA-4 primarily regulates the early phase of T cell responses, acting in secondary lymphoid organs during antigen priming, whereas other checkpoints often maintain tolerance in peripheral organs [13]. Furthermore, *Ctla4*-deficient mice develop a fatal lymphoproliferative disorder characterised by multiorgan autoimmunity, with CTLA-4 haploinsufficiency in humans similarly leading to autoimmunity across multiple organs [1, 14]. Understanding CTLA-4 biology led to a pivotal study that demonstrated that *in vivo* administration of CTLA-4-blocking antibodies could induce tumour regression in preclinical models [15]. This discovery, for which Dr. James Allison received the 2018 Nobel Prize in Physiology or Medicine, provided the initial proof of concept for the therapeutic potential of ICI treatment in patients with cancer.

5.2.2 PD-1/PD-L1

PD-1 was discovered by Dr. Tasuku Honjo in 1992, which led to him also being awarded the 2018 Nobel Prize in Physiology or Medicine, where it was identified as a member of the immunoglobulin superfamily and found on apoptotic immune cells [16]. In contrast to CTLA-4, PD-1 primarily regulates T cell activity in peripheral tissues, including within the TME [17]. PD-1 inhibits T cell activation by interacting with its ligands PD-L1 and programmed cell death ligand 2 (PD-L2), which are often expressed in tumour cells and APCs and can be induced by inflammatory signals, such as interferon (IFN)-γ (Figure 5.1) [18]. Upon binding its ligands, PD-1 recruits phosphatases such as src-homology 2 domain-containing phosphatase 2 (SHP-2), which prevent phosphorylation of downstream signals of the TCR, thereby attenuating T cell-mediated effector functions, such as secretion of IFN-γ and interleukin (IL)-2, T cell proliferation, and survival [17, 19, 20]. Genetic ablation as well as pharmacologic blockade of the PD-1/PD-L1 axis has emphasised its role in maintaining immune tolerance, with mice developing pathologies, such as cardiomyopathy, autoimmune diabetes, and encephalomyelitis, often in a strain-dependent manner [2, 21, 22]. Clinically, multiple antibodies targeting PD-1 or PD-L1 have been approved for the treatment of cancer (Figure 5.1). PD-1 and PD-L1 blockade can target distinct cell types, yet they converge in their ability to reduce suppressive interactions within the TME to primarily promote $CD8^+$ T cell functionality [23]. However, growing evidence indicates that many immune cells, including $CD4^+$ T cells, γδ T cells, and B cells, also respond to these treatments and can contribute to therapeutic efficacy.

5.2.3 LAG-3

Multiple costimulatory and inhibitory receptors have emerged as potential therapeutic targets for cancers in the preclinical setting; however, only antibody blockade against LAG-3 has advanced to clinical use, marking the first regulatory approval of a next-generation ICI. LAG-3 was first described by Frédéric Triebel in 1990, where it was found predominantly on activated lymphocytes [24]. The first ligand discovered for LAG-3 was MHC class II, which binds at a higher affinity than CD4 and is thought to negatively regulate T cell activation by disrupting TCR signalling at the immunological synapse (Figure 5.1). However, LAG-3 has been suggested to have additional binding partners, most notably fibrinogen-like protein 1 (FGL1), which is often enriched in the tumour and periphery of patients with cancer [25]. In autoimmune-prone mice, genetic loss of LAG-3 results in spontaneous immune dysregulation, including an accelerated onset of autoimmune diabetes [26], whereas LAG-3 deficiency in autoimmune-resistant mouse strains does not lead to overt autoimmunity; however, when combined with ablation of PD-1, it can rapidly cause lethal myocarditis [27]. LAG-3 is frequently co-expressed with PD-1 in terminally exhausted T cells in cancer, with dual inhibition leading to complementary functions to overcome dysfunction by bolstering both proliferation and cytotoxicity in a non-redundant manner [28]. Consistent with this, relatlimab (anti-LAG-3) has only been approved for use in combination with nivolumab (anti-PD-1) in patients with metastatic melanoma rather than as a single agent [29].

5.3 APPROVED INDICATIONS AND BIOMARKERS

5.3.1 History of Clinical Approval for ICI Treatment

While ICI treatment is now a cornerstone for multiple cancers, the first clinical trials and approvals occurred in the context of advanced melanoma. Before ICIs, the median survival for patients with stage IV melanoma was less than one year following treatment with chemotherapy, which was largely ineffective. Other immunotherapies, such as cancer vaccines [against glycoprotein (gp) 100, an antigen expressed in both melanocytes and melanoma] and cytokine therapies (such as IL-2 and IFN-α), had been tested and even approved, yet still had minimal impact on survival for patients with melanoma. The phase III trial that led to the approval of ipilimumab (anti-CTLA-4) in metastatic melanoma compared ipilimumab alone, the gp100 cancer vaccine alone, and their combination and demonstrated that treatment arms containing ipilimumab displayed improved overall survival [30]. The use of anti-PD-1 and anti-PD-L1 also rapidly emerged as a viable clinical treatment that could initiate improved therapeutic responses across several cancer types [31, 32]. Given that non-redundant mechanisms of immunosuppression exist in the TME, it was suggested that therapeutic efficacy may be heightened by using ICIs against multiple targets in combination. As of 2024, the ten-year overall survival for patients with melanoma treated with combination nivolumab (anti-PD-1) and ipilimumab (anti-CTLA-4) is 43%, with 37% and 19% for the single agents, respectively [4]. To date, more than 20 cancers have received clinical approval for ICI treatment, highlighting their broad clinical utility.

5.3.2 Approval Based on Tumour Mutation Rate

Approval for ICI use has also been received in a tumour-agnostic manner, based on molecular features rather than cancer type. For instance, dMMR tumours, characterised by a hypermutable genome due to errors in DNA repair machinery that are often microsatellite instability-high (MSI-h), were shown to demonstrate durable responses to ICI treatment, leading to approval of anti-PD-1/PD-L1 use in patients with dMMR cancers in 2020 [33]. The high mutation rate that these tumours harbour is likely to aid in their visibility to the immune system, increasing tumour-infiltrating lymphocytes into the TME. The difference in therapeutic response for dMMR tumours has been particularly evident in colorectal cancer, in which, despite occurring in the same tissue, dMMR tumours demonstrate robust responses to ICI treatment, whereas microsatellite stable (MSS) colorectal cancer receives minimal clinical benefit [3, 34].

The presence of high tumour mutational burden (TMB) in solid tumours, defined as ≥10 mutations per megabase, also received approval for treatment with pembrolizumab (anti-PD-1) in 2020 [35]. High TMB increases the likelihood of neoantigen presentation, which may enhance immune recognition and response to ICIs. High TMB status is frequently observed in tumours arising from chronic exposure to environmental mutagens or carcinogens, such as ultraviolet (UV)-induced melanoma and smoking-associated lung cancer [36]. These molecular indicators demonstrate how biomarkers can help identify patients most likely to benefit from ICI therapy, expanding ICI use beyond traditional histology-based classifications.

5.3.3 Approval Based on PD-L1 Status

Expression of PD-L1 in tumour cells, assessed via immunohistochemistry and known as the tumour proportion score (TPS), is a widely used biomarker to stratify response to anti-PD-1/PD-L1 treatment. In non-small cell lung cancer (NSCLC), high PD-L1 expression (TPS ≥ 50%) is associated with increased therapeutic benefit, whereas tumours with 1–49% or <1% PD-L1 positivity display reduced, but equivalent, survival outcomes [37]. Given this, anti-PD-1 treatment was approved for first-line use in patients with NSCLC that display high PD-L1 expression and has since expanded to other indications. However, PD-L1 shows dynamic expression and intratumour heterogeneity [31, 38]. Moreover, patients with low or absent PD-L1 can still respond to ICI therapy, highlighting the limitations in sensitivity and selectivity when solely relying on PD-L1 expression to determine treatment eligibility.

5.3.4 Early-Stage Use of ICI Treatment

While the majority of ICI administration remains in advanced-stage disease, where systemic therapies are necessary to target both primary and metastatic tumours, their use is expanding into treatment settings that already have curative potential. For instance, neoadjuvant ICI use prior to surgical removal of a tumour has shown promising results in enhancing pathologic complete response rates and survival for patients across multiple cancer types [39–41]. Neoadjuvant treatment is proposed to expand tumour-specific T cells prior to surgical resection, allowing them to be enriched both in the tumour and the periphery [42]. Additionally, adjuvant ICI use, administered after surgery, has been approved for certain early-stage cancers to reduce recurrence risk and prolong cancer-free survival [43], expanding their use in oncologic care.

5.4 CHALLENGES AND CONTROVERSIES

While ICIs have reshaped cancer treatment, their clinical use is impacted by many challenges. A large proportion of patients fail to respond to treatment despite predictive biomarkers (i.e. high TMB and high PD-L1 expression) suggestive of favourable anti-tumour immunity. This emphasises the complexity of immune escape and treatment resistance. Even in responders, ICI use carries the risk of irAEs, which can be unpredictable in onset and variable in severity. Additionally, to overcome ICI resistance, combination therapies are utilised; however, this can further increase the risk of irAEs, highlighting the delicate balance needed for promoting tumour control without immunotoxicity in response to ICI treatment.

5.4.1 ICI Resistance

Resistance to ICI treatment occurs through two main processes: primary or innate resistance, in which patients do not respond to treatment, and secondary or acquired resistance, in which patients display initial therapeutic benefit followed by the evolution of new immunosuppressive mechanisms that lead to tumour progression. Primary resistance is often associated with low TMB, low PD-L1 expression, and an absence or active exclusion of immune cells, particularly $CD8^+$ T cells, from the TME. In contrast, the mechanisms for acquired resistance remain largely unclear and may present unique features for each patient. In some cases, the initial response to ICI treatment has been shown to drive selection of cancer cells that lack recognisable neoantigens, have impaired antigen presentation machinery (such as MHC I loss through beta-2-microglobulin (ß2M) mutations), and that display alterations in IFN-γ signalling [44, 45]. Additionally, the pro-inflammatory TME generated during an initial response to ICI treatment may lead to the recruitment of additional immunosuppressive cells, such as T regulatory cells (Tregs) and myeloid-derived suppressor cells (MDSCs), and the expression of additional immune checkpoints to provide new mechanisms that regulate the immune response. As a result, current clinical strategies to overcome resistance increasingly rely on combination approaches designed to restore anti-tumour immunity.

Over 40% of patients with cancer are eligible to receive ICI treatment in the standard of care setting in the United States; however, less than 15% of patients respond [46]. This highlights the reduced therapeutic benefit observed in the community compared to clinical trials and the urgent need for combination approaches to boost ICI efficacy. For patients who have indicators of primary resistance, they are likely to receive combination treatment, including multiple ICIs or ICIs with conventional therapies, to improve therapeutic benefit through complementary mechanisms [4–6, 29, 47]. Certain forms of chemotherapy and radiotherapy can induce immunogenic cell death (ICD), which releases tumour-associated antigens and inflammatory mediators, such as damage-associated molecular patterns (DAMPs), that can prime anti-tumour immunity and recruit cytotoxic $CD8^+$ T cells. ICD may also upregulate PD-L1 in tumour and stromal cells, creating a more favourable environment for anti-PD-1/PD-L1 treatment. One advantage of localised radiotherapy is that it can promote a distant, or abscopal, response at other tumour sites, which may be further enhanced by ICI treatment. In patients with high-risk cutaneous squamous-cell carcinoma receiving surgical resection followed by localised radiotherapy, the addition of adjuvant cemiplimab (anti-PD-1) provided improved survival benefit across a number of disease-related comparisons, including in the patient group with low PD-L1 expression (TPS $< 1\%$) and presence of metastatic disease [47]. This provides both the rationale and evidence for integrating ICI treatment with conventional therapies, with a need for greater precision in optimising the treatment schedule and dose.

Strategies to reverse acquired resistance remain poorly defined, with patients often transitioning to clinical trials for novel combination approaches. For instance, multiple soluble and metabolic factors with immunosuppressive properties are enriched in the TME, including the accumulation of transforming growth factor-β (TGF-β) and adenosine, as well as other hypoxia-associated pathways. Many of these have been implicated in promoting resistance to ICI treatment, with ongoing clinical trials to assess their combinatorial potential, often with mixed success [48, 49]. Anti-angiogenic therapies, such as vascular endothelial growth factor (VEGF) inhibitors, may also normalise the tumour vasculature and enhance immune infiltration, with combination use alongside ICI treatment approved for multiple solid tumours [50, 51]. However, an incomplete understanding of individualised mechanisms of acquired resistance often hinders the ability to reinvigorate the immune response, highlighting the importance of predictive indicators that extend beyond traditional biomarkers and immune cell types. Moreover, modifiable factors, such as diet, microbiota, concomitant medications, and comorbidities, should be explored for their potential to influence ICI efficacy [52, 53]. Ongoing studies continue to explore approaches involving ICIs and agents targeting metabolic pathways, epigenetic modifiers, oncolytic viruses, cellular therapies, and other immunoregulatory targets, indicative of the breadth of potential therapeutic combinations for use alongside ICI treatment.

5.4.2 irAEs

By enhancing immune activity, ICIs can inadvertently trigger the immune system to attack healthy tissue, resulting in irAEs. These side effects are often unpredictable, with variability in onset ranging from a few weeks to even years after initial ICI exposure, highlighting the need for long-term clinical surveillance [7]. Although irAEs can impact nearly every organ, they most commonly affect the skin, endocrine, and gastrointestinal systems (Figure 5.2). The frequency and severity of irAEs is significantly increased with exposure to combination ICI treatment [4, 29]. Additionally, certain irAEs occur following exposure to specific agents, with anti-CTLA-4 associated with colitis and hypophysitis, while anti-PD-1/PD-L1 exposure is required for autoimmune diabetes [8]. While most irAEs are manageable, some can be chronic, cause permanent organ dysfunction or become life-threatening in severe cases. The mechanisms that govern why some patients develop irAEs remain poorly understood; however, multiple host, tumour, and treatment-related factors are thought to contribute to irAE susceptibility (Figure 5.2).

Several risk factors for irAEs are consistent with those observed in patients developing spontaneous autoimmunity. For instance, human leukocyte antigen (HLA) alleles, which are often strongly linked to autoimmunity, have also been associated with increased susceptibility to ICI-induced autoimmune diabetes, hypothyroidism, and hypophysitis [54, 55]. Genome-wide association studies have also revealed that a variant in *IL7* may contribute to irAE susceptibility, independent of tissue site [56, 57]. In addition, autoantibodies, such as anti-rheumatoid factor (RF), anti-cyclic citrullinated peptide (CCP), anti-thyroid, anti-nuclear, and islet-associated autoantibodies, can be identified in some, but not all, patients and are often significantly less frequent at diagnosis than in patients with spontaneous autoimmunity [55, 58, 59]. This highlights both some similar features between irAEs and spontaneous autoimmunity, as well as the heterogeneity that contributes to the difficulty in predicting ICI-induced irAE development.

New biomarkers for severe and tissue-specific irAEs continue to emerge with an emphasis on understanding changes in the periphery. In patients with melanoma, a higher frequency of activated $CD4^+$ memory T cells and increased peripheral TCR diversity was associated with severe irAEs, even preceding ICI exposure, which may be suggestive of preexisting subclinical autoimmunity [60]. In some cases, irAE development has also been linked to peripheral clonal T cell expansion and cross-reactivity between tumour and self-antigens, such as in the case of vitiligo, where T cells target both healthy melanocytes and melanoma in a non-discriminate manner. Furthermore, several cytokines have been found to be elevated in the blood of patients, both prior to and early during ICI treatment in individuals that develop severe irAEs [61]. These findings demonstrate that host immunity, including preceding ICI exposure, contributes to irAE susceptibility, with further immunoprofiling needed to dissect the underlying heterogeneity for tissue-specific signatures.

Patients that develop irAEs are often afforded improved anti-tumour immunity and overall survival [62]. This positive association is indicative that systemic immune activation, while unfavourable in terms of irAEs, may also contribute to a more robust anti-tumour immune response. As patients now receive ICI treatment in potentially curative settings, the lack of irAE-associated biomarkers represents a

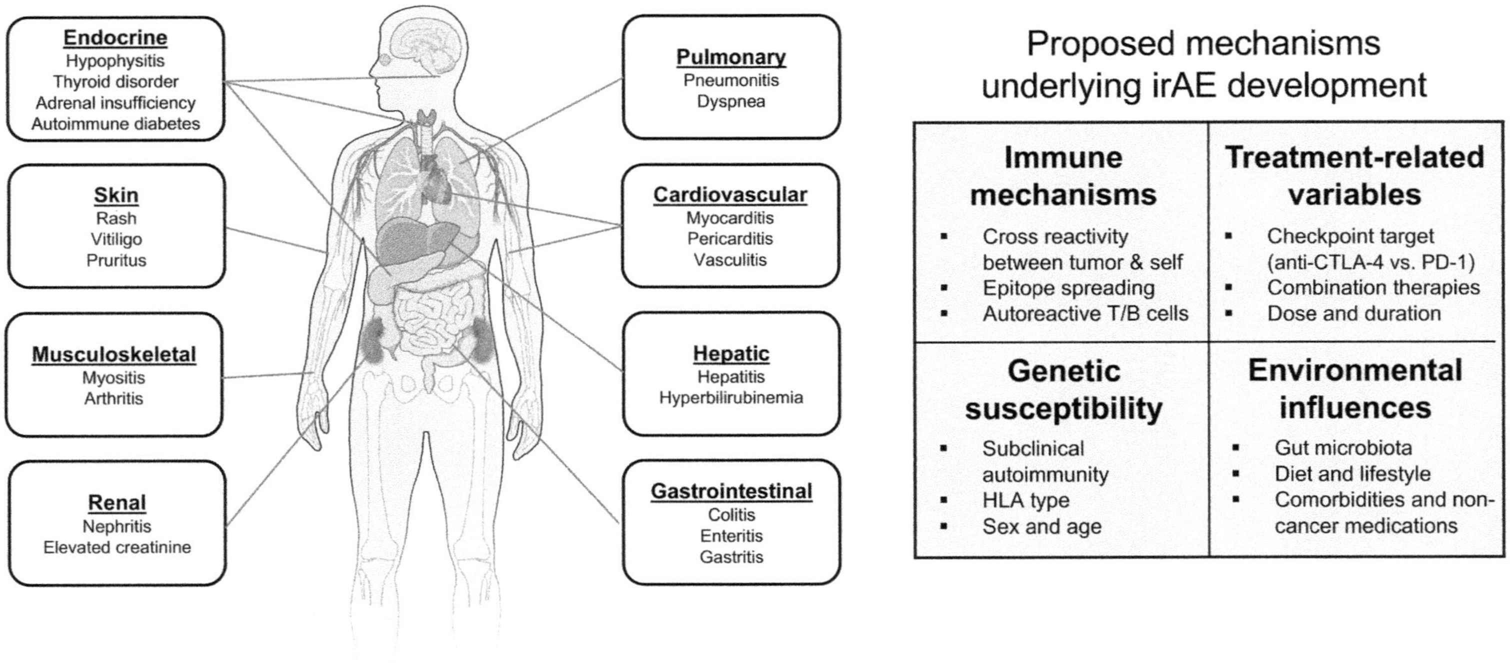

FIGURE 5.2 Clinical and mechanistic overview of irAEs. ICIs can trigger toxicities, termed irAEs, across nearly every organ system, with examples of tissue-specific conditions shown (left panel). The development of irAEs is thought to be due to disruption of tolerance mechanisms that are initiated by multiple underlying causes, including immune mechanisms, treatment regimens, host-intrinsic factors, and environmental influences (right panel). Understanding how these factors interact to drive irAEs remains a critical challenge for balancing both the use and efficacy of ICI treatment. This figure was created by the authors using original artwork and publicly available images adapted from NIH/NIAID BioArt (NIH), and does not use proprietary third-party templates or figure-generation software.

major limitation in performing adequate risk stratification to avoid unnecessary side effects. Additionally, anti-irAE treatments rely largely on immunosuppressive agents, such as systemic corticosteroids, followed by cytokine inhibitors such as anti-tumour necrosis factor (TNF)-α, anti-IL-6R, or anti-IL-17a when steroid-refractory [63]. While often effective in dampening irAE symptoms, these agents may reduce tumour control [62, 64]. This highlights the complexity of this persistent challenge for ICI treatment in balancing anti-tumour immunity and irAE risk.

5.5 CASE STUDIES AND REAL-WORLD EXAMPLES

Several landmark trials illustrate the versatility and challenges across diverse tumour types and clinical settings. The following cases illustrate key themes in ICI therapy, including combination approaches, neoadjuvant strategies, and patient-specific decision-making.

5.5.1 DREAMseq Trial

This trial aimed to test whether patients with BRAF-mutant metastatic melanoma would receive greater clinical benefit with ICIs (anti-CTLA-4 and anti-PD-1) before or after BRAF/MEK inhibitors. Patients treated with BRAF/MEK inhibitors showed better early responses but worse overall survival compared to patients initially receiving ICIs. This study led to the prioritisation of first-line ICI use in patients with BRAF-mutant metastatic melanoma to increase durable responses, even when tumour regression is achievable with targeted therapy [65].

5.5.2 CheckMate 816: Neoadjuvant ICI Use in Early-Stage NSCLC

In CheckMate 816, patients with resectable stage IB-IIIA NSCLC were treated with neoadjuvant nivolumab plus platinum chemotherapy or chemotherapy alone. The ICI regimen significantly improved pathologic complete response rates and overall survival. This was the first trial to address whether immunotherapy could safely be administered before surgery to improve long-term outcomes in early-stage lung cancer [6]. Similar findings have been observed across trials for melanoma and other solid tumours.

5.5.3 Case Report: Neoadjuvant Triplet ICI in Glioblastoma (GBM)

A recent case report described a patient with newly diagnosed isocitrate dehydrogenase (IDH)-wild-type glioblastoma (GBM), an aggressive cancer with low TMB and poor immune infiltrate that often shows minimal response to ICI treatment. The median survival time is 14–15 months for patients with this form of GBM [66]. After a single dose of neoadjuvant triplet ICI (anti-PD-1, anti-CTLA-4, and anti-LAG-3), pathological analysis of the resected tumour revealed dense tumour-infiltrating lymphocytes, suggestive of enhanced immune activation. Remarkably, the patient experienced no disease recurrence after 17 months. This robust therapeutic response has led to the initiation of a clinical trial for neoadjuvant anti-PD-1 and anti-LAG-3 treatment in patients with GBM [67].

5.6 FUTURE DIRECTIONS

The clinical success of ICIs has sparked immense interest in expanding the repertoire of immune-modulating therapies. A new generation of checkpoint molecules, including both inhibitory receptors (TIM-3, TIGIT, VISTA, and BTLA) and costimulatory molecules (4-1BB, CD40, ICOS, and OX40) that have shown preclinical success, are being investigated in early-phase clinical trials (Table 5.1). These agents may broaden therapeutic opportunities, overcome resistance, and extend benefit to a diverse patient population. However, as discussed, biomarkers will be critical for patient selection to ensure that combinatorial strategies enhance therapeutic efficacy over currently approved treatment regimens.

Many inhibitory receptors, such as TIM-3, TIGIT, BTLA, and VISTA, are often co-expressed with PD-1 in T cells, which may represent non-redundant or complementary immunosuppressive mechanisms that are targetable to improve anti-tumour immunity or overcome acquired resistance. To date, clinical trials have often failed to exceed the clinical benefit observed for anti-PD-1/PD-L1 therapies. Most recently, TIGIT, which binds to CD155 and CD112 on tumour cells or APCs and competes with the co-stimulatory receptor CD226, has received much interest for its potential to improve tumour control. While TIGIT blockade has shown promise in preclinical studies, phase III clinical trials have failed to improve outcomes in NSCLC in combination with anti-PD-1 (Table 5.1). Furthermore, a neoadjuvant trial showed that the addition of anti-TIGIT to a bispecific PD-1/LAG-3-targeting antibody resulted in lower response rates compared to the bispecific alone, demonstrating that targeting additional receptors does not necessarily improve patient outcomes [68]. This emphasises the need to improve strategies to stratify patients that are likely to respond to anti-TIGIT or other co-inhibitory receptor therapies, including sub-cohort analyses of the molecular and cellular features that dictate response in early clinical trials.

In contrast, immune agonists targeting costimulatory receptors are being investigated for their ability to promote T cell expansion, survival, and function; yet they have often been associated with concerns relating to increased immunotoxicity. For instance, 4-1BB (CD137) is a member of the TNF receptor superfamily and is expressed in activated T cells and natural killer (NK) cells. 4-1BB engagement promotes survival and cytotoxicity when engaged by its ligand, 4-1BBL. Early trials of 4-1BB agonists were discontinued due to the development of severe irAEs, particularly liver toxicity, though modified and bispecific antibodies are being developed to enhance safety (Table 5.1) [69]. Similarly, agonistic antibodies targeting CD40, a costimulatory molecule expressed on APCs, have shown promise in sensitising preclinical models to ICI treatment by enhancing cross-priming and proinflammatory cytokine production, resulting in increased T cells in poorly immune-infiltrated tumours. Anti-CD40 agonists are under investigation in solid tumours, particularly in pancreatic cancer, which often excludes T cells, frequently in conjunction with chemotherapy or other ICIs [70]. However, CD40 agonists have also shown increased toxicities, including hepatotoxicity and thrombocytopenia, in early clinical trials [71].

Together, this highlights the need for a personalised approach to ICI treatment, guided by tumour- and patient-specific characteristics. As ICIs expand into earlier-stage disease and younger patient populations, optimising safety and tolerability is a

TABLE 5.1 Selected clinical trials targeting emerging immune checkpoints and co-stimulatory molecules.

Target	Agent	Disease	Combination therapy	Stage	Results	NCT identifier
TIM-3	Cobolimab (TSR-022)	Advanced solid tumours	Anti-PD-1, chemotherapy	Phase I	Early-phase data showed only modest response rates in both immunotherapy-naïve and refractory patients.	NCT02817633
	Sabatolimab (MBG453)	Myelodysplastic syndrome	Chemotherapy	Phase II	Phase II evaluation was discontinued due to limited clinical efficacy and a high incidence of ≥ grade 3 toxicities.	NCT04878432
TIGIT	Tiragolumab	NSCLC	Anti-PD-L1	Phase III	A large phase III trial failed to meet primary endpoints for efficacy, representing a late-stage setback for this combinatorial approach.	NCT04294810
	Vibostolimab (MK-7684A)	NSCLC	Anti-PD-1, chemotherapy	Phase III	Early clinical results suggest that combining vibostolimab with PD-1 blockade alone may be insufficient for promoting response, emphasising the need for biomarker-guided patient selection.	NCT05226598
VISTA	SNS-101	Advanced solid tumours	Anti-PD-1	Phase I/II	Early clinical data indicate dose-dependent pharmacodynamic immune activation by this pH-selective antibody.	NCT05864144
4-1BB	Urelumab	Solid tumours/ non-Hodgkin lymphoma	Anti-PD-1	Phase I/II	Early studies showed evidence of immune activation and anti-tumour immune responses, but development was limited by significant hepatotoxicity.	NCT02253992
	Acasunlimab	NSCLC	Anti-PD-1	Phase III	Late-phase clinical trial with this 4-1BBxPD-L1 bispecific antibody, engineered to be Fc-inert to limit treatment-limiting toxicities previously observed.	NCT06635824
ICOS	Vopratelimab	Advanced solid tumours	Anti-PD-1	Phase I/II	Early-phase studies were completed, in which immune activation was demonstrated without consistent objective responses.	NCT02904226
CD40	Mitazalimab	PDAC	Chemotherapy	Phase I/II	Studies have demonstrated manageable safety profiles and encouraging immune activation, supporting advancement into later-stage clinical testing.	NCT04888312

priority to avoid the potential long-term complications and comorbidities that may be associated with unresolved irAEs. Future strategies will need to balance efficacy with quality of life, particularly for patients with curative intent or durable survival benefit following treatment. Clinical trial protocols are restrictive, with patient populations selected on defined criteria that include exclusion due to factors such as age, comorbidities, non-cancer medication exposures, and metastatic sites, which impacts the generalisability of these findings as treatments are used more widely in the community [46]. Such limitations highlight the importance of developing more inclusive trials and expanding real-world data collection when assessing both predictive biomarkers and treatment outcomes, to ensure that patients receive maximal benefit from ICI treatment.

KEY TERMS & DEFINITIONS SIDEBAR

Adjuvant treatment administered after primary therapy, such as surgery, to reduce the risk of tumour recurrence and improve long-term outcomes.

Immune checkpoint inhibitors (ICIs) a class of immunotherapy, specifically monoclonal antibodies that block interactions between immune checkpoints and their ligands, restoring the ability of T cells to kill tumour cells by improving anti-tumour immunity.

Immune-related adverse events (irAEs) autoimmune or autoinflammatory side effects caused by exposure to ICIs, resulting in immune-mediated attacks on noncancerous tissues.

Mismatch repair deficiency (dMMR) a molecular phenotype characterised by an inability to repair DNA, thereby leading to increased mutations and genomic instability. Tumours with dMMR are often microsatellite instability-high (MSI-h).

Neoadjuvant treatment a treatment given to reduce tumour burden prior to the primary therapy, usually surgery, designed to improve therapeutic outcomes.

Overall survival the length of time for which a patient is alive following initiation of cancer treatment. Often used in clinical trials to determine the effect of a new therapeutic modality.

Pathologic complete response the lack of evidence of cancer in samples taken from surgery or biopsy, determined by a pathologist, often associated with a positive prognosis.

Tumour mutational burden (TMB) quantitative measurement of the number of mutations in the DNA across the tumour genome. High TMB is a predictive biomarker of ICI response.

LIST OF ABBREVIATIONS

APC	antigen-presenting cell
ß2M	beta-2-microglobulin
CCP	cyclic citrullinated peptide
CTLA-4	cytotoxic T-lymphocyte-associated protein 4
DAMPs	damage-associated molecular patterns
dMMR	mismatch repair deficiency
FGL1	fibrinogen-like protein 1
GBM	glioblastoma

gp	glycoprotein
HLA	human leukocyte antigen
ICD	immunogenic cell death
ICI	immune checkpoint inhibitor
IFN	interferon
IL	interleukin
irAE	immune-related adverse event
IDH	isocitrate dehydrogenase
LAG-3	lymphocyte activation gene 3
MDSC	myeloid-derived suppressor cell
MHC	major histocompatibility complex
MSI-h	microsatellite instability-high
MSS	microsatellite stable
NIH	National Institutes of Health
NIAID	National Institute of Allergy and Infectious Diseases
NK	natural killer
NSCLC	non-small cell lung cancer
PD-1	programmed cell death protein 1
PD-L1	programmed cell death ligand 1
PD-L2	programmed cell death ligand 2
pMHC	MHC-peptide complex
RF	rheumatoid factor
SHP-2	src-homology 2 domain-containing phosphatase 2
TCR	T cell receptor
TGF-β	transforming growth factor-β
TME	tumour microenvironment
TNF	tumour necrosis factor
TPS	tumour proportion score
Treg	T regulatory cell
UV	ultraviolet
VEGF	vascular endothelial growth factor

REVIEW QUESTIONS

1. What are the differences in targeting CTLA-4 and PD-1 inhibition in terms of mechanism?
2. What are the mechanisms and biomarkers that lead to different forms of ICI resistance?
3. What are irAEs and what factors may predispose certain patients to develop them?
4. What are some of the challenges associated with developing next-generation therapeutic strategies and identifying clinically actionable combination treatments?

ACKNOWLEDGEMENTS

This was supported by the Huntsman Cancer Foundation and National Cancer Institute of the National Institutes of Health under Award Number P30CA042014 (AY), R00CA246061 (AY) and by the National Institute of Allergy and Infectious Diseases of the National Institutes of Health under Award Number T32AI138945 (CH). The content is solely the responsibility of the authors and does not necessarily represent the official views of the National Institutes of Health.

REFERENCES

1. Tivol, E.A., Borriello, F., Schweitzer, A.N. et al. (1995). Loss of CTLA-4 leads to massive lymphoproliferation and fatal multiorgan tissue destruction, revealing a critical negative regulatory role of CTLA-4. *Immunity* 3 (5): 541–547.
2. Nishimura, H., Nose, M., Hiai, H. et al. (1999). Development of lupus-like autoimmune diseases by disruption of the PD-1 gene encoding an ITIM motif-carrying immunoreceptor. *Immunity* 11 (2): 141–151.
3. Le, D.T., Uram, J.N., Wang, H. et al. (2015). PD-1 blockade in tumors with mismatch-repair deficiency. *N Engl J Med* 372 (26): 2509–2520.
4. Wolchok, J.D., Chiarion-Sileni, V., Rutkowski, P. et al. (2025). Final, 10-year outcomes with nivolumab plus ipilimumab in advanced melanoma. *N Engl J Med* 392 (1): 11–22.
5. Cardoso, F., O'Shaughnessy, J., Liu, Z. et al. (2025). Pembrolizumab and chemotherapy in high-risk, early-stage, ER+/HER2− breast cancer: a randomized phase 3 trial. *Nat Med* 31 (2): 442–448.
6. Forde, P.M., Spicer, J., Lu, S. et al. (2022). Neoadjuvant nivolumab plus chemotherapy in resectable lung cancer. *N Engl J Med* 386 (21): 1973–1985.
7. Postow, M.A., Sidlow, R., and Hellmann, M.D. (2018). Immune-related adverse events associated with immune checkpoint blockade. *N Engl J Med* 378 (2): 158–168.
8. Young, A., Quandt, Z., and Bluestone, J.A. (2018). The balancing act between cancer immunity and autoimmunity in response to immunotherapy. *Cancer Immunol Res* 6 (12): 1445–1452.
9. Brunet, J.-F., Denizot, F., Luciani, M.-F. et al. (1987). A new member of the immunoglobulin superfamily—CTLA-4. *Nature* 328 (6127): 267–270.
10. Walunas, T.L., Lenschow, D.J., Bakker, C.Y. et al. (1994). CTLA-4 can function as a negative regulator of T cell activation. *Immunity* 1 (5): 405–413.
11. Thompson, C.B., Lindsten, T., Ledbetter, J.A. et al. (1989). CD28 activation pathway regulates the production of multiple T-cell-derived lymphokines/cytokines. *Proc Natl Acad Sci USA* 86 (4): 1333–1337.
12. Krummel, M.F. and Allison, J.P. (1995). CD28 and CTLA-4 have opposing effects on the response of T cells to stimulation. *J Exp Med* 182 (2): 459–465.
13. Chambers, C.A., Kuhns, M.S., and Allison, J.P. (1999). Cytotoxic T lymphocyte antigen-4 (CTLA-4) regulates primary and secondary peptide-specific CD4(+) T cell responses. *Proc Natl Acad Sci USA* 96 (15): 8603–8608.
14. Schubert, D., Bode, C., Kenefeck, R. et al. (2014). Autosomal dominant immune dysregulation syndrome in humans with CTLA4 mutations. *Nat Med* 20 (12): 1410–1416.
15. Leach, D.R., Krummel, M.F., and Allison, J.P. (1996). Enhancement of antitumor immunity by CTLA-4 blockade. *Science* 271 (5256): 1734–1736.
16. Ishida, Y., Agata, Y., Shibahara, K., and Honjo, T. (1992). Induced expression of PD-1, a novel member of the immunoglobulin gene superfamily, upon programmed cell death. *EMBO J* 11 (11): 3887–3895.

17. Nishimura, H. and Honjo, T. (2001). PD-1: an inhibitory immunoreceptor involved in peripheral tolerance. *Trends Immunol* 22 (5): 265–268.
18. Keir, M.E., Liang, S.C., Guleria, I. et al. (2006). Tissue expression of PD-L1 mediates peripheral T cell tolerance. *J Exp Med* 203 (4): 883–895.
19. Wherry, E.J. (2011). T cell exhaustion. *Nat Immunol* 12 (6): 492–499.
20. Chemnitz, J.M., Parry, R.V., Nichols, K.E. et al. (2004). SHP-1 and SHP-2 associate with the immunoreceptor tyrosine-based switch motif of programmed death 1 upon primary human T cell stimulation, but only receptor ligation prevents T cell activation. *J Immunol* 173 (2): 945–954.
21. Nishimura, H., Okazaki, T., Tanaka, Y. et al. (2001). Autoimmune dilated cardiomyopathy in PD-1 receptor-deficient mice. *Science* 291 (5502): 319–322.
22. Ansari, M.J., Salama, A.D., Chitnis, T. et al. (2003). The programmed death-1 (PD-1) pathway regulates autoimmune diabetes in nonobese diabetic (NOD) mice. *J Exp Med* 198 (1): 63–69.
23. Sun, C., Mezzadra, R., and Schumacher, T.N. (2018). Regulation and function of the PD-L1 checkpoint. *Immunity* 48 (3): 434–452.
24. Triebel, F., Jitsukawa, S., Baixeras, E. et al. (1990). LAG-3, a novel lymphocyte activation gene closely related to CD4. *J Exp Med* 171 (5): 1393–1405.
25. Wang, J., Sanmamed, M.F., Datar, I. et al. (2019). Fibrinogen-like protein 1 is a major immune inhibitory ligand of LAG-3. *Cell* 176 (1–2): 334–347.e12.
26. Bettini, M., Szymczak-Workman, A.L., Forbes, K. et al. (2011). Cutting edge: accelerated autoimmune diabetes in the absence of LAG-3. *J Immunol* 187 (7): 3493–3498.
27. Okazaki, T., Okazaki, I.-m., Wang, J. et al. (2011). PD-1 and LAG-3 inhibitory co-receptors act synergistically to prevent autoimmunity in mice. *J Exp Med* 208 (2): 395–407.
28. Cillo, A.R., Cardello, C., Shan, F. et al. (2024). Blockade of LAG-3 and PD-1 leads to co-expression of cytotoxic and exhaustion gene modules in CD8+ T cells to promote antitumor immunity. *Cell* 187 (16): 4373–4388.e15.
29. Tawbi, H.A., Schadendorf, D., Lipson, E.J. et al. (2022). Relatlimab and nivolumab versus nivolumab in untreated advanced melanoma. *N Engl J Med* 386 (1): 24–34.
30. Hodi, F.S., O'Day, S.J., McDermott, D.F. et al. (2010). Improved survival with ipilimumab in patients with metastatic melanoma. *N Engl J Med* 363 (8): 711–723.
31. Topalian, S.L., Hodi, F.S., Brahmer, J.R. et al. (2012). Safety, activity, and immune correlates of anti-PD-1 antibody in cancer. *N Engl J Med* 366 (26): 2443–2454.
32. Brahmer, J.R., Tykodi, S.S., Chow, L.Q.M. et al. (2012). Safety and activity of anti-PD-L1 antibody in patients with advanced cancer. *N Engl J Med* 366 (26): 2455–2465.
33. Petrelli, F., Ghidini, M., Ghidini, A., and Tomasello, G. (2020). Outcomes following immune checkpoint inhibitor treatment of patients with microsatellite instability-high cancers: a systematic review and meta-analysis. *JAMA Oncol* 6 (7): 1068–1071.
34. André, T., Shiu, K.-K., Kim, T.W. et al. (2020). Pembrolizumab in microsatellite-instability-high advanced colorectal cancer. *N Engl J Med* 383 (23): 2207–2218.
35. Aggarwal, C., Ben-Shachar, R., Gao, Y. et al. (2023). Assessment of tumor mutational burden and outcomes in patients with diverse advanced cancers treated with immunotherapy. *JAMA Network Open* 6 (5): e2311181.
36. Yarchoan, M., Hopkins, A., and Jaffee, E.M. (2017). Tumor mutational burden and response rate to PD-1 inhibition. *N Engl J Med* 377 (25): 2500–2501.
37. Garon, E.B., Rizvi, N.A., Hui, R. et al. (2015). Pembrolizumab for the treatment of non-small-cell lung cancer. *N Engl J Med* 372 (21): 2018–2028.
38. McLaughlin, J., Han, G., Schalper, K.A. et al. (2016). Quantitative assessment of the heterogeneity of PD-L1 expression in non-small-cell lung cancer. *JAMA Oncol* 2 (1): 46–54.
39. Chalabi, M., Verschoor, Y.L., Tan, P.B. et al. (2024). Neoadjuvant immunotherapy in locally advanced mismatch repair-deficient colon cancer. *N Engl J Med* 390 (21): 1949–1958.

40. Forde, P.M., Chaft, J.E., Smith, K.N. et al. (2018). Neoadjuvant PD-1 blockade in resectable lung cancer. *N Engl J Med* 378 (21): 1976–1986.
41. Blank, C.U., Rozeman, E.A., Fanchi, L.F. et al. (2018). Neoadjuvant versus adjuvant ipilimumab plus nivolumab in macroscopic stage III melanoma. *Nat Med* 24 (11): 1655–1661.
42. Luoma, A.M., Suo, S., Wang, Y. et al. (2022). Tissue-resident memory and circulating T cells are early responders to pre-surgical cancer immunotherapy. *Cell* 185 (16): 2918–2935.e29.
43. Luke, J.J., Rutkowski, P., Queirolo, P. et al. (2022). Pembrolizumab versus placebo as adjuvant therapy in completely resected stage IIB or IIC melanoma (KEYNOTE-716): a randomised, double-blind, phase 3 trial. *Lancet* 399 (10336): 1718–1729.
44. Gettinger, S., Choi, J., Hastings, K. et al. (2017). Impaired HLA class I antigen processing and presentation as a mechanism of acquired resistance to immune checkpoint inhibitors in lung cancer. *Cancer Discov* 7 (12): 1420–1435.
45. Zaretsky, J.M., Garcia-Diaz, A., Shin, D.S. et al. (2016). Mutations associated with acquired resistance to PD-1 blockade in melanoma. *N Engl J Med* 375 (9): 819–829.
46. Haslam, A. and Prasad, V. (2019). Estimation of the percentage of US patients with cancer who are eligible for and respond to checkpoint inhibitor immunotherapy drugs. *JAMA Netw Open* 2 (5): e192535.
47. Rischin, D., Porceddu, S., Day, F. et al. (2025). Adjuvant cemiplimab or placebo in high-risk cutaneous squamous-cell carcinoma. *N Engl J Med* 393 (8): 774–785.
48. Metropulos, A.E., Munshi, H.G., and Principe, D.R. (2022). The difficulty in translating the preclinical success of combined TGFbeta and immune checkpoint inhibition to clinical trials. *EBioMedicine* 86: 104380.
49. Vijayan, D., Young, A., Teng, M.W.L., and Smyth, M.J. (2017). Targeting immunosuppressive adenosine in cancer. *Nat Rev Cancer* 17 (12): 709–724.
50. Rini, B.I., Plimack, E.R., Stus, V. et al. (2019). Pembrolizumab plus axitinib versus sunitinib for advanced renal-cell carcinoma. *N Engl J Med* 380 (12): 1116–1127.
51. Finn, R.S., Qin, S., Ikeda, M. et al. (2020). Atezolizumab plus bevacizumab in unresectable hepatocellular carcinoma. *N Engl J Med* 382 (20): 1894–1905.
52. Spencer, C.N., McQuade, J.L., Gopalakrishnan, V. et al. (2021). Dietary fiber and probiotics influence the gut microbiome and melanoma immunotherapy response. *Science* 374 (6575): 1632–1640.
53. Stone, S., McPherson, J.P., Kulkarni, R.P., and Young, A. (2025). The impact of concomitant medications on treatment outcomes in patients with cancer receiving immune checkpoint inhibitors. *Nat Rev Cancer* 26: 137–158.
54. Akturk, H.K., Couts, K.L., Baschal, E.E. et al. (2022). Analysis of human leukocyte antigen DR alleles, immune-related adverse events, and survival associated with immune checkpoint inhibitor use among patients with advanced malignant melanoma. *JAMA Network Open* 5 (12): e2246400.
55. Stamatouli, A.M., Quandt, Z., Perdigoto, A.L. et al. (2018). Collateral damage: insulin-dependent diabetes induced with checkpoint inhibitors. *Diabetes* 67 (8): 1471–1480.
56. Taylor, C.A., Watson, R.A., Tong, O. et al. (2022). IL7 genetic variation and toxicity to immune checkpoint blockade in patients with melanoma. *Nat Med* 28 (12): 2592–2600.
57. Groha, S., Alaiwi, S.A., Xu, W. et al. (2022). Germline variants associated with toxicity to immune checkpoint blockade. *Nat Med* 28 (12): 2584–2591.
58. Borgers, J.S.W., van Wesemael, T.J., Gelderman, K.A. et al. (2024). Autoantibody-positivity before and seroconversion during treatment with anti-PD-1 is associated with immune-related adverse events in patients with melanoma. *J Immunother Cancer* 12 (6): e009215.
59. Osorio, J.C., Ni, A., Chaft, J.E. et al. (2017). Antibody-mediated thyroid dysfunction during T-cell checkpoint blockade in patients with non-small-cell lung cancer. *Ann Oncol* 28 (3): 583–589.

60. Lozano, A.X., Chaudhuri, A.A., Nene, A. et al. (2022). T cell characteristics associated with toxicity to immune checkpoint blockade in patients with melanoma. *Nat Med* 28 (2): 353–562.
61. Lim, S.Y., Lee, J.H., Gide, T.N. et al. (2019). Circulating cytokines predict immune-related toxicity in melanoma patients receiving anti-PD-1-based immunotherapy. *Clin Cancer Res* 25 (5): 1557–1563.
62. Quandt, Z., Lucas, A., Liang, S.I. et al. (2025). Associations between immune checkpoint inhibitor response, immune-related adverse events, and steroid use in RADIOHEAD: a prospective pan-tumor cohort study. *J Immunother Cancer* 13 (5): e011545.
63. Schneider, B.J., Naidoo, J., Santomasso, B.D. et al. (2021). Management of immune-related adverse events in patients treated with immune checkpoint inhibitor therapy: ASCO guideline update. *J Clin Oncol* 39 (36): 4073–4126.
64. Kang, J.H., Bluestone, J.A., and Young, A. (2021). Predicting and preventing immune checkpoint inhibitor toxicity: targeting cytokines. *Trends Immunol* 42 (4): 293–311.
65. Atkins, M.B., Lee, S.J., Chmielowski, B. et al. (2023). Combination dabrafenib and trametinib versus combination Nivolumab and Ipilimumab for patients with advanced BRAF-mutant melanoma: the DREAMseq trial-ECOG-ACRIN EA6134. *J Clin Oncol* 41 (2): 186–197.
66. Stupp, R., Mason, W.P., Bent, M.J.v.d. et al. (2005). Radiotherapy plus concomitant and adjuvant temozolomide for glioblastoma. *N Engl J Med* 352 (10): 987–996.
67. Long, G.V., Shklovskaya, E., Satgunaseelan, L. et al. (2025). Neoadjuvant triplet immune checkpoint blockade in newly diagnosed glioblastoma. *Nat Med* 31 (5): 1557–1566.
68. Long, G.V., Nair, N., Marbach, D. et al. (2025). Neoadjuvant PD-1 and LAG-3-targeting bispecific antibody and other immune checkpoint inhibitor combinations in resectable melanoma: the randomized phase 1b/2 Morpheus-Melanoma trial. *Nat Med* 31 (11): 3700–3712.
69. Segal, N.H., Logan, T.F., Hodi, F.S. et al. (2017). Results from an integrated safety analysis of urelumab, an agonist anti-CD137 monoclonal antibody. *Clin Cancer Res* 23 (8): 1929–1936.
70. Van Laethem, J.-L., Borbath, I., Prenen, H. et al. (2024). Combining CD40 agonist mitazalimab with mFOLFIRINOX in previously untreated metastatic pancreatic ductal adenocarcinoma (OPTIMIZE-1): a single-arm, multicentre phase 1b/2 study. *Lancet Oncol* 25 (7): 853–864.
71. Vonderheide, R.H., Flaherty, K.T., Khalil, M. et al. (2007). Clinical activity and immune modulation in cancer patients treated with CP-870,893, a novel CD40 agonist monoclonal antibody. *J Clin Oncol* 25 (7): 876–883.

6

Advancements in CAR T and CAR NK Cell Therapies

KAREN SLATTERY[1,2], THOMAS J. COLE[1,2], AND PHILLIP K. DARCY[1,2]

[1] Cancer Immunology Program, Peter MacCallum Cancer Centre, Melbourne, Victoria, Australia

[2] Sir Peter MacCallum Department of Oncology, The University of Melbourne, Parkville, Victoria, Australia

LEARNING OBJECTIVES

- Explain key advancements made in CAR T and CAR NK cell therapies to date.
- Understand the advantages and disadvantages of CAR T cell versus CAR NK cell therapies.
- Appreciate and identify future directions for the field of CAR T and NK cell therapy research.

6.1 INTRODUCTION

The concept of CAR T-cell therapies first emerged in the 1980s when two groups developed modified versions of T-cell receptors, that is chimeric antigen receptors (CARs), and demonstrated their enhanced activity against target cells [1]. This led to the development of the first-generation CAR T cells in the 1990s, containing a single-chain variable fragment (scFv) fused to a CD3ζ or FcεRIγ stimulatory domain [2]. Following disappointing clinical trial outcomes, second-generation CAR T cells were developed by incorporating a co-stimulatory domain to provide the essential 'second signal'. Combining CD3ζ and CD28 endodomains dramatically increased the efficacy of CAR T cells [3]. A further key advancement was the integration of the 4-1BB/CD137 signal transduction domain into CAR design, which paved the way for the early success of CAR T cells in the clinic [4]. The first commercial CAR T-cell therapy, tisagenlecleucel (Kymriah), received FDA approval in 2017, and since then, 6 more have entered the clinic, with some achieving remission rates up to 82%. However, all currently approved CAR T-cell therapies target haematological cancers, where relapses are common, and none are approved for solid tumours, which represent 90% of adult and 30% of paediatric cancers. There is therefore an urgent need to improve CAR T-cell therapies so they can function effectively within the tumour microenvironment (TME) and achieve durable clearance of solid tumours.

6.2 ARMOURING CAR T CELLS TO ENHANCE THERAPEUTIC EFFICACY

'Armouring' CAR T cells involves giving them extra tools so they have enhanced efficacy and persistence in tumours. This includes overexpression of key effector molecules such as pro-inflammatory cytokines, chemokines, or co-stimulatory ligands. These modifications aim to boost both the activity of adoptive cell therapy (ACT) and augment endogenous immunity to combat the barrier of tumour antigen heterogeneity.

6.2.1 Armouring with Pro-inflammatory Cytokines

Engineering CAR T cells to secrete pro-inflammatory cytokines has emerged as a powerful strategy to enhance anti-tumour activity and engage endogenous immunity (Figure 6.1a). IL-12-armoured CAR T cells secrete the cytokine locally upon antigen recognition, activating myeloid cells, reducing immunosuppressive MDSCs and

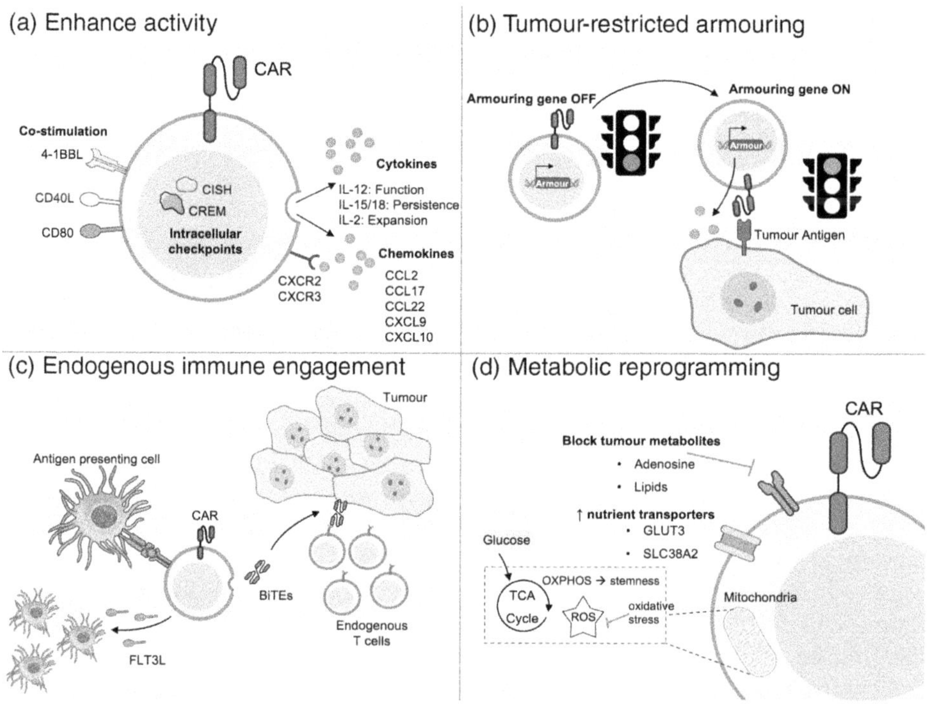

FIGURE 6.1 Next-generation armouring strategies for CAR T- and CAR NK cell therapies. (a) Intrinsic armouring strategies to boost activity include deletion of intracellular checkpoints and overexpression of cytokines and chemokines. (b) Tumour-restricted armouring for payload delivery only to the tumour site. (c) Stimulating engagement with endogenous immunity through FLT3L and BiTE secretion. (d) Optimising metabolism by modulating sensitivity to immunosuppressive metabolites and augmenting nutrient receptor expression. CAR = chimeric antigen receptor, BiTEs = bispecific T-cell engagers, ROS = reactive oxygen species, OXPHOS = oxidative phosphorylation.

TAMs, and promoting pro-inflammatory immune populations [5, 6]. Preclinical studies have demonstrated strong tumour control, and early clinical trials (NCT02498912, NCT01236573) with IL-12-engineered TILs have shown complete responses in some patients, although systemic toxicity remains a concern [7].

Other cytokines offer complementary benefits with potentially improved safety. IL-18-armoured CAR T cells enhance IFN-γ production and recruit host $CD8^+$ T cells, NK cells, NKT cells, dendritic cells, and inflammatory macrophages, while reducing suppressive populations such as Tregs and immunosuppressive macrophages [8]. Early clinical data with IL-18 CAR T cells have shown objective responses with minimal toxicity (NCT04684563) [9]. IL-15 armouring supports CAR T-cell homeostasis, memory stem-like phenotypes, and long-term persistence, enabling robust proliferation and sustained anti-tumour responses even upon tumour rechallenge [10]. Engineered IL-2 variants ('superkines') preferentially expand effector T cells over Tregs, increasing CAR T-cell numbers and enhancing endogenous immune populations, including $CD4^+$ and $CD8^+$ T cells, NK cells, and ILC2s, while reducing MDSCs [11]. Collectively, these strategies highlight how cytokine armouring can simultaneously boost CAR T-cell potency, persistence, and coordination with the host immune system.

6.2.2 Armouring with Co-stimulatory Molecules and Antibody-Like Proteins

CAR T cells can be enhanced through co-stimulatory molecules and antibody-like proteins, which can augment both intrinsic and extrinsic immune responses. CD40L expression on CAR T cells engages CD40 on dendritic cells, promoting DC maturation, IL-12 secretion, and activation of both $CD4^+$ and $CD8^+$ T cells [12]. Constitutive CD40L expression also enhances CAR T cytotoxicity and pro-inflammatory cytokine production while directly increasing tumour immunogenicity by upregulating MHC molecules and Fas ligand on $CD40^+$ tumour cells [13].

Other co-stimulatory strategies further reinforce CAR T activation and persistence. Co-expression of 4-1BB ligand (4-1BBL) and CD80 provides both autocrine survival signals via 4-1BB and trans-costimulation to bystander T cells through CD28, overcoming the lack of immune-stimulatory signals in the TME and enabling eradication of large tumours in preclinical models [14]. Similarly, CAR T cells engineered to secrete anti-PD-1 scFv deliver checkpoint blockade locally, enhancing CAR T proliferation, cytokine secretion, and tumour clearance while minimising systemic toxicity [15]. Together, these approaches show that armouring CAR T cells with co-stimulatory molecules and antibody-like proteins can boost immune functions, recruit host immunity, and counteract tumour-induced immunosuppression.

6.2.3 Armouring with Chemokines

Poor trafficking and retention of CAR T cells within solid tumours remain key limitations to efficacy. Modulation of chemokine signalling has been employed to enhance CAR T-cell migration, persistence, and coordination with other immune subsets in the TME (Figure 6.1b). A key example comes from Adachi et al., who engineered CAR T cells to secrete CCL19 and IL-7, mimicking lymphoid tissue architecture to recruit DCs and naïve T cells while supporting CAR T-cell survival and expansion [16]. This promoted intratumoral immune cell clustering and improved tumour clearance in murine models. Similarly, CXCR2 engineering enhanced CAR T-cell migration towards CXCL1- and CXCL2-expressing tumours, increasing infiltration and tumour control in hepatocellular carcinoma models [17]. Additional strategies have leveraged CCR2b and CCR4 expression to redirect CAR T cells towards chemokines (CCL2, CCL17, CCL22) enriched in neuroblastoma, mesothelioma, and Hodgkin's lymphoma [18, 19]. Notably, this approach may also competitively inhibit recruitment of immunosuppressive Treg and myeloid cells that depend on the same chemokine gradients, thereby indirectly mitigating tumour-induced immunosuppression.

Further advances have focused on restoring tumour expression of chemokines to boost CAR T-cell infiltration. CXCR3 is critical for T-cell trafficking; however, its ligands (CXCL9, CXCL10, and CXCL11) are often epigenetically silenced in solid tumours. Peng et al. showed that combining CAR T therapy with EZH2 and DNA methyltransferase inhibitors reactivated expression of these chemokines, restoring infiltration and anti-tumour function in ovarian cancer models. Collectively, these findings highlight how engineering CAR T cells with tailored chemokine receptors or co-administering agents that modulate tumour chemokine expression can improve CAR T-cell trafficking, persistence, and coordination with endogenous immune cells.

6.3 TUMOUR-RESTRICTED ARMOURING – THE NEXT FRONTIER OF ENHANCED CAR T CELLS

While the armouring of CAR T cells with effector molecules is promising, it raises important safety concerns. For example, peripheral expression of pro-inflammatory cytokines can result in toxicities, for example cytokine release syndrome (CRS) and immune effector cell-associated neurotoxicity syndrome (ICANS). An innovative strategy to overcome this is to restrict the expression of the armouring molecule to the tumour, thus protecting against excessive inflammation in the periphery. This involves putting a target 'armouring' gene under the control of a promoter that is turned on following TCR/CAR activation (Figure 6.1b). This is a rapidly evolving field with key advancements made using the promoters NFAT, NR4A2, and RGS [16].

6.3.1 NFAT-Mediated Tumour-Restricted Payload Delivery

One of the first strategies to restrict gene expression to tumours was by harnessing the promoter of nuclear factor of activated T cells (NFATs). NFATs are a family of transcription factors that are activated in response to TCR signalling. In response to antigen stimulation, NFAT relocates to the nucleus, where it regulates gene expression. Zhang et al. created a vector where IL-12 expression was controlled by the NFAT promoter, and this IL-12 expression was only initiated following TCR activation by tumour antigens [20]. These cells exhibited greater tumour control in a B16 tumour model, and similar results have been observed in a model of hepatocellular carcinoma, where there were no observed toxicities. However, the NFAT promoter can result in 'leaky', extra-tumoral transgene expression, with severe toxicities reported for NFAT-IL-12 CAR T cells in preclinical melanoma models [21].

6.3.2 HDR-Based Engineering for Tumour-Restricted Payload Delivery

While NFAT remains the most widely used strategy for tumour-restricted payload delivery, important toxicity issues remain due to incomplete restriction of transgene expression to the tumour. Indeed, a clinical trial for NFAT-IL-12-armoured T cells was forced to terminate early due to toxicities (NCT01236573) [7]. This demonstrates that the NFAT promoter is not sufficiently tumour-restricted to avoid peripheral inflammation.

To circumvent this, Chen et al. screened for CAR T-cell genes with increased transcription in tumours compared to spleen [22]. They identified the *NR4A2* and *RGS16* as promoters that can drive tumour-restricted expression of cytokine genes. Importantly, they harnessed the CRISPR-based gene editing technique homology-directed repair (HDR) to insert payload genes under the control of these promoters. Using the NR4A2 promoter to express transgenes resulted in better tumour-restricted expression than an NFAT-based promoter. When IL-12 or IL-2 was expressed under the control of the NR4A2 or RGS16 promoter, CAR T cells exhibited potent *in vivo* anti-tumour activity without noticeable toxicity. Thus, by using these endogenous, tumour-activated regulatory elements instead of synthetic promoters, this strategy produced a new generation of armoured CAR T cells with improved safety and efficacy.

Overall, these innovative strategies represent significant advancements in the field of CAR T-cell therapy, aiming to enhance the precision and safety of treatments for solid tumours. By restricting the expression of armouring payloads to the tumour site, these approaches hold promise for improving patient outcomes and broadening the applicability of CAR T-cell therapies.

6.4 ENGAGING CAR T CELLS WITH ENDOGENOUS IMMUNITY

Engaging the host immune system is a promising strategy to enhance tumour clearance in solid cancers by promoting epitope spreading, antigen cross-presentation, and innate immune activation, thereby extending control beyond CAR-specific targets (Figure 6.1c). Bispecific T-cell engagers (BiTEs) use antibodies that link T cells to tumour-associated antigens independently of MHC-TCR interactions. The first-generation BiTEs demonstrated tumour regression in glioma, paving the way for clinical development. Notably, Blinatumomab (CD19×CD3) was the first FDA-approved BiTE, showing efficacy in B-cell acute lymphoblastic leukaemia [23], while Teclistamab (BCMA×CD3), approved in 2022 for multiple myeloma, features an antibody-like IgG4 structure with an improved half-life, allowing intermittent dosing rather than continuous infusion.

6.4.1 CAR T Cells Secreting Bispecific Engagers (CART.BiTEs)

Although the efficacy of bispecific antibodies has been positively demonstrated in patients with haematological malignancies, this triumphant success has not been observed in solid tumours. CART.BiTEs are next-generation constructs in which CAR T cells are engineered to secrete BiTEs targeting additional tumour-associated antigens. This design extends cytotoxicity to **antigen-negative variants** and mobilises **bystander immune cells** against the tumour. In glioblastoma, EGFRvIII-CAR

T cells secreting EGFR-BiTEs broadened antigen recognition and delayed relapse [24]. In hepatocellular carcinoma, GPC3-CAR T cells producing B7-H3-BiTEs resulted in improved tumour killing and activation of endogenous T-cell responses [25]. In ovarian cancer, MUC16-CAR T cells secreting ESK1-BiTEs improved the killing of MUC16-low tumours *in vitro* and *in vivo* [26]. Finally, MesoFAP CAR T cells, targeting mesothelin and fibroblast activation protein, remodelled tumour stroma and enhanced infiltration in pancreatic models. Collectively, these findings suggest that **CART.BiTE platforms** bridge the advantages of monoclonal antibody therapy and adoptive cell transfer, offering a potent and adaptable strategy to overcome intratumoral heterogeneity and immune evasion.

6.4.2 Engaging with Host APCs

The success of immunotherapy has been heavily reliant on the ability of host immune cells to recognise tumour-specific antigens. Hence, it is not surprising that most approaches to enhance ACT have focused on T cells, which are key orchestrators of immunity. However, T cells do not work in solitary. Antigen-presenting cells (APCs) such as DCs play crucial roles in promoting immunity and bridging the link between the adaptive and innate immune responses. Studies have shown that co-treatment with enterotoxin, which links TCRs to MHC-II on APCs, enhances CAR T-cell activation and proliferation, leading to stronger anti-tumour responses and recruitment of host T cells in solid tumour models [27]. Similarly, CLEC9A-targeted approaches have demonstrated potent synergy between DCs and CAR T cells: a tailored nanoemulsion delivering antigen to CLEC9A+. DCs promoted durable tumour regression and immune memory [28], while a bispecific engager linking PD-1 on T cells to CLEC9A on DCs enhanced $CD8^+$ T-cell activation and reduced exhaustion compared to PD-1 blockade alone [29]. Vaccine-based approaches, such as the amphiphilic CAR ligand (Amph-Ligand) vaccine, further enhanced CAR T-cell priming, expansion, and antigen spreading, producing durable tumour control dependent on endogenous T cells [30]. Finally, CAR T cells engineered to secrete FLT3 ligand (FLT3L) expanded intratumoral DC1 populations and activated host $CD8^+$ T cells, thereby overcoming tumour heterogeneity and strengthening anti-tumour efficacy [31]. Collectively, these findings underscore that engaging CAR T cells with APCs, through molecular, bispecific, or vaccine-based strategies, can coordinate adaptive and innate immune responses, sustain antigen spreading, and achieve long-term tumour control.

6.5 ENHANCING CAR T-CELL EFFICACY THROUGH METABOLISM

Metabolism is now widely appreciated to govern all aspects of the T-cell immune response, including differentiation, activation and effector responses [32]. The importance of metabolism for CAR T-cell efficacy was first highlighted by van Bruggen et al. in 2019, with the observation that leukaemia patients who received CAR T cells with superior mitochondrial fitness had better CAR T-cell persistence and responses [33]. Thus, research has begun to explore how metabolism can be harnessed to boost CAR T-cell responses in cancer (Figure 6.1d).

6.5.1 Boosting Bioenergetics by Manipulating Nutrient Receptor Expression

Glucose is a critical nutrient for fuelling metabolism in mammalian cells, including T cells [34]. As glucose can be limiting in the TME [35], overexpression of glucose transporters has emerged as an exciting approach to boost CAR T-cell efficacy [36]. Glut1 is the dominant glucose receptor expressed by T cells, and its overexpression in CAR T cells resulted in enhanced metabolic and cytokine responses and improved in vivo anti-tumour efficacy and long-term persistence [37]. Glut3 is a more context-specific glucose transporter, with a much higher affinity for glucose than Glut1, and therefore may be more suitable for the low glucose environment of tumours. Toledano et al. showed that Glut3-overexpressing CAR T cells had improved in vivo anti-tumour activity in a murine model of melanoma [38]. Increasing expression of the glutamine transporter SLC38A2 in CAR T cells has also demonstrated promising pre-clinical potential [39]. Despite the importance of a range of other nutrients for T-cell responses, the impact of overexpression of other transporters remains unexplored.

As well as being limited in important nutrients such as glucose, the TME is also rich in immunosuppressive metabolites such as lactate, adenosine and certain lipids [40]. Therefore, deletion of receptors for these inhibitory metabolites represents a promising strategy to protect CAR T cells from the hostile TME. CRISPR-mediated deletion of the adenosine A_{2A} receptor ($A_{2A}R$) boosts cytokine responses and *in vivo* therapeutic efficacy in CAR T cells [41], while overexpression of the A_1 receptor, which signals inversely to the A_{2A} receptor, protects CAR T cells against the impact of adenosine [42]. Although not yet explored in CAR T cells, the potential of boosting T-cell responses in cancer by deleting the lipid transporter CD36 and the lactate transporter MCT4 has been demonstrated.

6.5.2 Metabolic Reprogramming During Expansion

The *in vitro* expansion required to generate CAR T cells for the clinic offers opportunities to manipulate metabolism to skew the phenotype and function of the product. This was demonstrated recently by Frisch et al., where modulation of glycolysis using dichloroacetate during *in vitro* expansion drove the development of CAR T cells with enhanced mitochondrial metabolism, histone acetylation and expression of longevity genes [43]. This culminated in increased *in vivo* engraftment and therapeutic efficacy in murine tumour models.

These studies highlight that metabolic modulation represents a powerful avenue to enhance CAR T-cell efficacy. Approaches such as overexpressing nutrient transporters, deleting receptors for immunosuppressive metabolites, and conditioning CAR T cells during in vitro expansion have demonstrated significant preclinical promise by improving persistence, effector function, and anti-tumour activity (Figure 6.1d). Despite these advances, many aspects of T-cell metabolism, such as the targeted manipulation of mitochondrial pathways and metabolic enzymes, remain largely unexplored in CAR T cells. Future work integrating these strategies could provide a comprehensive framework to generate CAR T cells that are not only more resilient within the nutrient-deprived and immunosuppressive TME but also capable of sustaining durable anti-tumour responses.

6.6 ARMOURING CAR NK CELLS FOR INCREASED THERAPEUTIC EFFICACY

NK cells are lymphocytes with an inherent ability to rapidly kill tumour cells. Their potential as a cell therapy was first demonstrated in 1990, when administration of NK cells and IL-2 was tested in renal cell carcinoma patients [44]. Despite this early promise and extensive evidence linking NK cell abundance with improved prognosis in cancer patients [45], research on the importance of NK cells in cancer has historically lagged behind that of T cells, a trend that continues in the field of CAR NK cell therapy.

Nonetheless, NK cells offer several advantages that make them highly attractive for therapeutic development. As sentinels of the innate immune system, they are not reliant on antigen-specific receptors but instead detect tumour cells through a balance of activating and inhibitory receptors that sense stress ligands and MHC-I downregulation. They have a favourable safety profile and are less prone to inducing graft-versus-host disease or CRS compared to CAR T cells [46]. Moreover, research suggests they are particularly important in protection against metastasis [47]. Together, these attributes position NK cells as a potential 'off-the-shelf' allogeneic cell therapy, with multiple biological sources under investigation, including umbilical cord blood (CB), haematopoietic stem cells (HSCs), induced pluripotent stem cells (iPSCs) and immortalised cell lines such as NK-92. This strategy may be particularly advantageous for cancer patients who have undergone intensive chemotherapy and consequently possess reduced or dysfunctional circulating T cells.

Although not as advanced as CAR T cells, research exploring how to armour CAR NK cells with the tools needed to effectively eradicate tumours has grown in recent years. This has been driven and catalysed by the decades of research on optimising and armouring CAR T cells, with efforts focusing on augmenting expression of key effector molecules such as cytokines and chemokines and modulating intracellular molecular switches.

6.6.1 Pro-inflammatory Cytokines

IL-15 is a critical cytokine for many aspects of the NK cell immune response, including survival and activation. CAR NK cells expressing the IL-15 gene are effective in treating B cell malignancies and demonstrate remarkable persistence 1 year post infusion [48]. There were no major toxicities reported in these studies, despite the gene being constitutively expressed. Importantly, IL-15-CAR NK cells have also demonstrated clinical potential in models of solid cancer. Teng et al. showed that treatment with CB-derived IL-15 CAR NK cells increased survival in a murine model of human metastatic pancreatic cancer, with CAR NK cells still detectable 90 days post infusion [49].

IL-21 is a pleiotropic cytokine with the capacity to expand and activate NK cells. NK cells engineered to express IL-21 were safer and more effective at controlling tumours compared to IL-15-NK cells in murine models of glioblastoma [50]. While a wide range of other cytokines are known to promote NK cell responses, including IL-2 and IL-18, the impact of armouring CAR NK cells with these proteins awaits exploration.

6.6.2 Resistance to TGF-β in the TME

TGF-β is a multifunctional cytokine with a wide variety of roles that are dependent on context and timing. TGF-β is often enriched in the TME and circulation of cancer patients and exerts suppressive effects on NK cells in cancer [51]. Engineering CAR NK cells for resistance to TGFβ in the TME has therefore emerged as a powerful approach to enhance efficacy. CRISPR/Cas9-mediated deletion of the TGF-β downstream signalling protein SMAD4 in human CAR NK cells boosted cytotoxicity, *in vivo* tumour infiltration and tumour control in a murine model of breast cancer [52]. Ren *et al.* developed a CAR harbouring the extracellular domains of TGF-β receptor II and transmembrane and intracellular domains of the IL-21 receptor, thus converting the suppressive signal from TGF-β into an activating one. NKG2D-CAR NK cells engineered with this chimeric receptor demonstrated remarkable in vivo tumour control, which was associated with increased NK cell infiltration, activation and persistence in tumours [53]. Moreover, engineering CAR NK cells to release P6 protein, which disrupts TGFβ's inhibitory signalling, increases in vivo anti-tumour activity [54]. Together, these studies highlight the therapeutic potential of reprogramming NK cell responses to overcome TGFβ-mediated immunosuppression, offering a promising avenue to enhance the durability and efficacy of CAR NK cell therapies in solid tumours. Excitingly, a clinical trial is underway examining the safety, tolerability and benefits of TGF-β receptor II KO CB-derived NK cells for treating recurrent glioblastoma (NCT04991870).

6.6.3 Chemokines

Although chemokines are critical for directing NK cell homing to tumours, research modulating chemokine signalling to enhance CAR NK cell efficacy remains in its early stages. Nonetheless, Bonanii et al. demonstrated that blocking CXCR3 in IL-15-activated NK cells promoted bone marrow migration and improved tumour control in multiple myeloma [55], while CXCR1 overexpression in CAR NK cells enhanced tumour homing and increased anti-tumour responses *in vivo* [56]. Although there is broad scope for further research in this area, these findings highlight the potential of manipulating chemokine pathways to improve CAR NK cell trafficking and therapeutic efficacy.

6.6.4 Intracellular Checkpoints

6.6.4.1 Deleting CISH to Unleash IL-15 Signalling

Cytokine-inducible SH2-containing protein (CIS, encoded by *Cish*), a member of the suppressor of cytokine signalling (SOCS) family, negatively modulates cytokine and growth factor signalling. It was first identified as a fundamental regulator of NK cell IL-15 signalling in 2016, where *Cish* knockout drove resistance to tumours in several models, which was dependent on NK cell activity [57]. Subsequent studies have confirmed that *Cish* deletion enhances NK cell therapeutic activity. Bernard et al. showed that *Cish* knockout protected against metastasis in a B16 melanoma model and boosted the functions of NK-92 cells and human primary NK cells [58]. In CB-derived CD19-CAR NK cells, *Cish* knockout boosted functional and metabolic responses, which drove enhanced anti-tumour activity and eradicated tumours in a murine model of lymphoma, without noticeable toxicity. These findings establish CISH as a key intracellular checkpoint in NK cells, and its deletion represents a promising strategy to amplify the potency and persistence of CAR NK cell therapies.

6.6.5 Deleting CREM to Boost NK Cell Responses

Cyclic AMP response element modulator (CREM) is a transcription factor that binds cAMP response element (CRE) to modulate gene expression. Rafei et al. recently showed that CREM is induced by CAR and IL-15 signalling in CAR NK cells and is upregulated in both mouse and human tumours, where it restricts NK cell responses and is associated with exhaustion [59]. *Crem* KO CD70-CAR NK cells had enhanced ability to control tumour growth *in vivo* in models of both lymphoma and metastatic breast cancer, without evidence of severe toxicity. Together, these studies underscore the importance of intracellular checkpoints such as CISH and CREM in regulating NK cell activity (Figure 6.1a), highlighting that their targeted deletion can reinvigorate NK cell function and potentially enhance the efficacy of CAR NK cell therapies against solid and haematologic malignancies.

6.7 BOOSTING CAR NK CELL THERAPEUTIC EFFICACY THROUGH METABOLISM

Oxidative and glycolytic metabolism are essential for driving NK cell functional responses; however, these pathways are frequently disrupted in the TME [60] and even in the circulation of metastatic cancer patients [61], which restricts their anti-tumour activities. This metabolic dysfunction underscores the need to engineer CAR NK cells that can maintain their bioenergetic and biosynthetic capacity in the hostile TME. While strategies to enhance NK cell metabolism in cancer have not yet been widely applied to CAR NK cells, existing work highlights the promising potential of metabolic reprogramming to improve their therapeutic efficacy.

6.7.1 Modulating Metabolism via Cytokine Signalling Pathways

Cytokines are critical regulators of NK cell metabolic responses, and their signalling pathways can be leveraged to modulate metabolism. Daher et al. showed that deletion of *CISH*, which represses IL-15 signalling, increased CB-derived CAR NK cell mTORC1 and cMyc signalling, leading to enhanced glycolysis [62]. These metabolically reprogrammed *CISH* KO CAR NK cells effectively eradicated lymphoma xenografts without inducing toxicity. Similarly, Zhu et al. reported that *CISH* deletion in iPSC-derived NK cells enhanced mTORC1 signalling, promoting both glycolytic and mitochondrial metabolism, which resulted in increased in vivo tumour control and persistence.

The ability to adapt to the hostile TME through metabolic flexibility represents a promising strategy to boost CAR NK cell metabolism in cancer. Poznanski et al. showed that STAT3-mediated expansion of NK cells using feeder cells expressing IL-21 produced NK cells with remarkable substrate flexibility [63], capable of fuelling mitochondrial metabolism with glucose, glutamine and fatty acids. Upon culture in malignant ascites (modelling the TME of ovarian cancer), STAT3-expanded NK cells retained their metabolic and functional responses and had increased cytotoxicity against tumour cells.

While pro-inflammatory cytokines drive NK cell metabolism, TGFβ is a key repressor of NK cell bioenergetics. NK cells from metastatic breast cancer patients have increased intracellular TGFβ signalling, and treating them *ex vivo* with a TGFβ blocking antibody protects their mitochondrial metabolism and enhances their cytotoxicity against tumour cells. Overall, these findings highlight the important role of cytokine signalling in shaping NK cell metabolism.

6.7.2 Protecting Redox Homeostasis

A critical role for certain metabolic pathways is regulating redox homeostasis, including maintaining the balance between reactive oxygen species (ROS) and antioxidant production. NK cells experience high levels of oxidative stress in the TME, which is associated with impaired functional and metabolic responses [61]. Poznanski et al. harnessed the Nrf2 transcription factor, which is a key regulator of the cell response to oxidative stress [63]. Activation of Nrf2 antioxidant activity using the drug RTA-408 enhanced NK cell metabolic and cytotoxic responses in the presence of malignant ascites *in vitro*, while *in vivo* coadministration of RTA-408 and NK cells resulted in remarkable control of tumour growth in an ovarian cancer model.

6.7.3 Targeting Immunosuppressive Metabolites in the TME

Although lipid metabolism supports NK cell homeostasis and responses in certain contexts, excess lipids in the TME can impair NK cell function and metabolism. Kobayashi et al. showed that fatty acids such as palmitic, stearic and oleic acid accumulated in the plasma of lymphoma-bearing mice, which was associated with reduced NK cell anti-tumour activity [64]. Similarly, Slattery et al. showed that malignant ascites from advanced ovarian cancer patients is enriched in polar lipids such as phosphatidylcholines, which the NK cell readily sequesters when exposed to ascites. Importantly, blocking uptake of polar lipids through the transporter SR-B1 protected NK cell cytotoxicity in ascites 60, underscoring the therapeutic potential of targeting lipid uptake pathways to safeguard CAR NK cell immunity in ovarian and other lipid-rich cancers.

Like T cells, excess adenosine in the TME impairs NK cell maturation, function and metabolism [65]. To circumvent this, Young et al. deleted the $A_{2A}R$ in NK cells, which increased NK cell maturation and proliferation and enhanced tumour control in a model of melanoma [65]. In a complementary approach, Chambers et al. engineered human NK cells with a CAR recognising CD73, which is the enzyme responsible for adenosine production by tumour cells. These CD73-CAR NK cells blocked adenosine production by tumour cells and also increased CAR NK cell recognition and killing of CD73+ tumour cells in *in vivo* lung adenocarcinoma tumours, without observable toxicities [66]. Together, these findings highlight the therapeutic potential of engineering CAR NK cells for resistance to the immunosuppressive metabolites of the TME (Figure 6.1d).

6.8 FUTURE DIRECTIONS FOR CAR T AND CAR NK CELL THERAPY

While the advancements made in CAR T and CAR NK cell therapies over the past decade have been remarkable, there remains a wide scope for further optimisation and improvement. One key challenge is the high cost and complexity of manufacturing patient-specific CAR T cells, making off-the-shelf, allogeneic CAR NK cell therapies an attractive and potentially more cost-effective alternative. Developing tumour-restricted payload delivery platforms for CAR NK cells will be crucial to enable localised armouring and minimise toxicity. Additionally, strategies to generate CAR T cells *in vivo*, such as systemic delivery of CAR mRNA using lipid nanoparticles, are being actively explored and may reduce costs while improving accessibility [67].

Achieving robust and durable efficacy in solid tumours remains the greatest and most urgent challenge. Combining the strategies outlined in this chapter with a deeper understanding of CAR T and CAR NK cell dynamics in the TME and periphery will be essential for developing effective, safe, and durable cell therapies for solid cancers.

KEY TERMS & DEFINITIONS SIDEBAR

Antigen spreading expansion of the immune response to secondary targets/antigens.

Bystander T cells T cells that are activated by inflammatory signals during an immune response, although they are not specific to the original stimulus.

Checkpoints a barrier or 'off switch' to the immune response.

Endogenous immunity the natural, preexisting immune system in cell therapy recipients.

Mitochondrial fitness the biological efficiency and general health of mitochondria.

Metabolic flexibility the ability to switch between metabolic pathways and use diverse substrates to fuel metabolism.

Off-the-shelf readily available commercial stocks that can be safely administered to the general population.

Payload the protein product of the gene inserted into CAR T cells.

LIST OF ABBREVIATIONS

ACT	adoptive cell therapy
APC	antigen-presenting cells
CAR	chimeric antigen receptor
CB	cord blood
CIS	cytokine-inducible SH2-containing protein
CRE	cAMP response element
CREM	cyclic AMP response element modulator
CRS	cytokine release syndrome
HSC	haematopoietic stem cells
ICANS	immune effector cell-associated neurotoxicity syndrome

iPSC induced pluripotent stem cell
NFAT nuclear factor of activated T cells
ROS reactive oxygen species
scFv single-chain variable fragment
SOCS suppressor of cytokine signalling
TME tumour microenvironment

REVIEW QUESTIONS

1. Describe key strategies to armour CAR T cells to boost therapeutic efficacy.
2. Explain methods to armour CAR NK cells to enhance therapeutic efficacy.
3. What are the important advantages and disadvantages of using CAR NK cell therapy instead of CAR T-cell therapy?
4. Explain how cellular metabolism can be harnessed to improve the efficacy of CAR T and CAR NK cell therapies.
5. How might cell therapies become more accessible in the clinic?

REFERENCES

1. Kuwana, Y., Asakura, Y., Utsunomiya, N. et al. (1987). Expression of a chimeric receptor composed of immunoglobulin-derived V regions and T-cell receptor-derived C regions. *Biochem Biophys Res Commun* 149 (3): 960–968. https://doi.org/10.1016/0006-291x(87)90502-x.
2. Moritz, D., Wels, W., Mattern, J., and Groner, B. (1994). Cytotoxic T lymphocytes with a grafted recognition specificity for ERBB2-expressing tumor cells. *Proc Natl Acad Sci USA* 91 (10): 4318–4322. https://doi.org/10.1073/pnas.91.10.4318.
3. Savoldo, B., Ramos, C.A., Liu, E. et al. (2011). CD28 costimulation improves expansion and persistence of chimeric antigen receptor-modified T cells in lymphoma patients. *J Clin Invest* 121 (5): 1822–1826. https://doi.org/10.1172/jci46110.
4. Kalos, M., Levine, B.L., Porter, D.L. et al. (2011). T cells with chimeric antigen receptors have potent antitumor effects and can establish memory in patients with advanced leukemia. *Sci Transl Med* 3 (95): 95ra73. https://doi.org/10.1126/scitranslmed.3002842.
5. Pegram, H.J., Lee, J.C., Hayman, E.G. et al. (2012). Tumor-targeted T cells modified to secrete IL-12 eradicate systemic tumors without the need for prior conditioning. *Blood* 119 (18): 4133–4141. https://doi.org/10.1182/blood-2011-12-400044.
6. Chmielewski, M., Kopecky, C., Hombach, A.A., and Abken, H. (2011). IL-12 release by engineered T cells expressing chimeric antigen receptors can effectively muster an antigen-independent macrophage response on tumor cells that have shut down tumor antigen expression. *Cancer Res* 71 (17): 5697–5706. https://doi.org/10.1158/0008-5472.CAN-11-0103.
7. Zhang, L., Morgan, R.A., Beane, J.D. et al. (2015). Tumor-infiltrating lymphocytes genetically engineered with an inducible gene encoding interleukin-12 for the immunotherapy of metastatic melanoma. *Clin Cancer Res* 21 (10): 2278–2288. https://doi.org/10.1158/1078-0432.CCR-14-2085.
8. Chmielewski, M. and Abken, H. (2017). CAR T cells releasing IL-18 convert to T-Bet(high) FoxO1(low) effectors that exhibit augmented activity against advanced solid tumors. *Cell Rep* 21 (11): 3205–3219. https://doi.org/10.1016/j.celrep.2017.11.063.

9. Svoboda, J., Gerson, J.N., Landsburg, D.J. et al. (2022). Interleukin-18 secreting autologous anti-CD19 CAR T-cells (huCART19-IL18) in patients with non-Hodgkin lymphomas relapsed or refractory to prior CAR T-cell therapy. *Blood* 140 (Supplement 1): 4612–4614. https://doi.org/10.1182/blood-2022-162393.
10. Klebanoff, C.A., Surman, D.R., Finkelstein, S.E. et al. (2004). IL-15 enhances the in vivo antitumor activity of tumor-reactive CD8+ T cells. *Proc Natl Acad Sci USA* 101 (7): 1969–1974. https://doi.org/10.1073/pnas.0307298101.
11. Merchant, R., Galligan, C., Munegowda, M.A., et al. (2022). Fine-tuned long-acting interleukin-2 superkine potentiates durable immune responses in mice and non-human primate. *J Immunother Cancer* 10 (1): e003155. http://doi.org/10.1136/jitc-2021-003155.
12. Caux, C., Massacrier, C., Vanbervliet, B. et al. (1994). Activation of human dendritic cells through CD40 cross-linking. *J Exp Med* 180 (4): 1263–1272. https://doi.org/10.1084/jem.180.4.1263.
13. Kuhn, N.F., Purdon, T.J., van Leeuwen, D.G. et al. (2019). CD40 ligand-modified chimeric antigen receptor T cells enhance antitumor function by eliciting an endogenous antitumor response. *Cancer Cell* 35 (3): 473–488 e6. https://doi.org/10.1016/j.ccell.2019.02.006.
14. Stephan, M.T., Ponomarev, V., Brentjens, R.J. et al. (2007). T cell-encoded CD80 and 4-1BBL induce auto- and transcostimulation, resulting in potent tumor rejection. *Nat Med* 13 (12): 1440–1449. https://doi.org/10.1038/nm1676.
15. Rafiq, S., Yeku, O.O., Jackson, H.J. et al. (2018). Targeted delivery of a PD-1-blocking scFv by CAR-T cells enhances antitumor efficacy in vivo. *Nat Biotechnol* 36 (9): 847–856. https://doi.org/10.1038/nbt.4195.
16. Adachi, K., Kano, Y., Nagai, T. et al. (2018). IL-7 and CCL19 expression in CAR-T cells improves immune cell infiltration and CAR-T cell survival in the tumor. *Nat Biotechnol* 36 (4): 346–351. https://doi.org/10.1038/nbt.4086.
17. Kershaw, M.H., Wang, G., Westwood, J.A. et al. (2002). Redirecting migration of T cells to chemokine secreted from tumors by genetic modification with CXCR2. *Hum Gene Ther* 13 (16): 1971–1980. https://doi.org/10.1089/10430340260355374.
18. Moon, E.K., Carpenito, C., Sun, J. et al. (2011). Expression of a functional CCR2 receptor enhances tumor localization and tumor eradication by retargeted human T cells expressing a mesothelin-specific chimeric antibody receptor. *Clin Cancer Res* 17 (14): 4719–4730. https://doi.org/10.1158/1078-0432.CCR-11-0351.
19. Di Stasi, A., De Angelis, B., Rooney, C.M. et al. (2009). T lymphocytes coexpressing CCR4 and a chimeric antigen receptor targeting CD30 have improved homing and antitumor activity in a Hodgkin tumor model. *Blood* 113 (25): 6392–6402. https://doi.org/10.1182/blood-2009-03-209650.
20. Zhang, L., Kerkar, S.P., Yu, Z. et al. (2011). Improving adoptive T cell therapy by targeting and controlling IL-12 expression in the tumor environment. *Mol Ther* 19 (4): 751–759. https://doi.org/10.1038/mt.2010.313.
21. Kunert, A., Chmielewski, M., Wijers, R. et al. (2017). Intra-tumoral production of IL18, but not IL12, by TCR-engineered T cells is non-toxic and counteracts immune evasion of solid tumors. *Oncoimmunology* 7 (1): e1378842. https://doi.org/10.1080/2162402x.2017.1378842.
22. Chen, A.X.Y., Yap, K.M., Kim, J.S. et al. (2025, https://doi.org/10.1038/s41586-025-09212-7). Rewiring endogenous genes in CAR T cells for tumour-restricted payload delivery. *Nature* 644: 241–251.
23. Nitta, T., Sato, K., Yagita, H. et al. (1990). Preliminary trial of specific targeting therapy against malignant glioma. *Lancet* 335 (8686): 368–371. https://doi.org/10.1016/0140-6736(90)90205-j.
24. Choi, B.D., Yu, X., Castano, A.P., et al. (2019). CAR-T cells secreting BiTEs circumvent antigen escape without detectable toxicity. *Nat Biotechnol* 37 (9): 1049–1058.

25. Cao, G., Zhang, G., Liu, M. et al. (2022). GPC3-targeted CAR-T cells secreting B7H3-targeted BiTE exhibit potent cytotoxicity activity against hepatocellular carcinoma cell in the in vitro assay. *Biochem Biophys Rep* 31: 101324. https://doi.org/10.1016/j.bbrep.2022.101324.
26. Mun, S.S., Meyerberg, J., Peraro, L. et al. (2023). Dual targeting ovarian cancer by Muc16 CAR T cells secreting a bispecific T cell engager antibody for an intracellular tumor antigen WT1. *Cancer Immunol Immunother* 72 (11): 3773–3786. https://doi.org/10.1007/s00262-023-03529-w.
27. von Scheidt, B., Wang, M., Oliver, A.J. et al. (2019). Enterotoxins can support CAR T cells against solid tumors. *Proc Natl Acad Sci USA* 116 (50): 25229–25235. https://doi.org/10.1073/pnas.1904618116.
28. Chan, J.D., von Scheidt, B., Zeng, B. et al. (2020). Enhancing chimeric antigen receptor T-cell immunotherapy against cancer using a nanoemulsion-based vaccine targeting cross-presenting dendritic cells. *Clin Transl Immunology* 9 (7): e1157. https://doi.org/10.1002/cti2.1157.
29. Shapir Itai Y, Barboy O, Salomon R, et al. (2024). Bispecific dendritic-T cell engager potentiates anti-tumor immunity. *Cell* 187 (2): 375–389 e18, 10.1016/j.cell.2023.12.011
30. Ma, L., Hostetler, A., Morgan, D.M. et al. (2023). Vaccine-boosted CAR T crosstalk with host immunity to reject tumors with antigen heterogeneity. *Cell* 186 (15): 3148–3165 e20. https://doi.org/10.1016/j.cell.2023.06.002.
31. Lai, J., Mardiana, S., House, I.G. et al. (2020). Adoptive cellular therapy with T cells expressing the dendritic cell growth factor Flt3L drives epitope spreading and antitumor immunity. *Nat Immunol* 21 (8): 914–926. https://doi.org/10.1038/s41590-020-0676-7.
32. Ma, S., Ming, Y., Wu, J., and Cui, G. (2024). Cellular metabolism regulates the differentiation and function of T-cell subsets. *Cell Mol Immunol* 21 (5): 419–435. https://doi.org/10.1038/s41423-024-01148-8.
33. van Bruggen, J.A.C., Martens, A.W.J., Fraietta, J.A. et al. (2019). Chronic lymphocytic leukemia cells impair mitochondrial fitness in CD8(+) T cells and impede CAR T-cell efficacy. *Blood* 134 (1): 44–58. https://doi.org/10.1182/blood.2018885863.
34. Frauwirth, K.A., Riley, J.L., Harris, M.H. et al. (2002). The CD28 signaling pathway regulates glucose metabolism. *Immunity* 16 (6): 769–777. https://doi.org/10.1016/s1074-7613(02)00323-0.
35. Sullivan MR, Danai LV, Lewis CA, et al. Quantification of microenvironmental metabolites in murine cancers reveals determinants of tumor nutrient availability. *Elife* 2019;8(https://doi.org/10.7554/eLife.44235
36. Nanjireddy, P.M., Olejniczak, S.H., and Buxbaum, N.P. (2023). Targeting of chimeric antigen receptor T cell metabolism to improve therapeutic outcomes. *Front Immunol* 14: 1121565. https://doi.org/10.3389/fimmu.2023.1121565.
37. Guerrero, J.A., Klysz, D.D., Chen, Y. et al. (2024). GLUT1 overexpression in CAR-T cells induces metabolic reprogramming and enhances potency. *Nat Commun* 15 (1): 8658. https://doi.org/10.1038/s41467-024-52666-y.
38. Toledano Zur, R., Atar, O., Barliya, T. et al. (2024). Genetically engineering glycolysis in T cells increases their antitumor function. *J Immunother Cancer* 12 (7): https://doi.org/10.1136/jitc-2023-008434.
39. Li, W., Chen, J., Li, J. et al. (2025). Envirotune-CAR-T: a hypoxia-responsive and glutamine-enhanced CAR-T cell therapy for overcoming tumor microenvironment-mediated suppression. *J Immunother Cancer* 13 (10): https://doi.org/10.1136/jitc-2025-012321.
40. Abbott KL, Ali A, Reinfeld BI, Deik A, et al. Metabolite profiling of human renal cell carcinoma reveals tissue-origin dominance in nutrient availability. *Elife* 2024;13. https://doi.org/10.7554/eLife.95652
41. Giuffrida, L., Sek, K., Henderson, M.A. et al. (2021). CRISPR/Cas9 mediated deletion of the adenosine A2A receptor enhances CAR T cell efficacy. *Nat Commun* 12 (1): 3236. https://doi.org/10.1038/s41467-021-23331-5.

42. Sek, K., Chen, A.X.Y., Cole, T. et al. (2025). Tumor site-directed A1R expression enhances CAR T cell function and improves efficacy against solid tumors. *Nat Commun* 16 (1): 6123. https://doi.org/10.1038/s41467-025-59021-9.
43. Frisch, A.T., Wang, Y., Xie, B. et al. (2025). Redirecting glucose flux during in vitro expansion generates epigenetically and metabolically superior T cells for cancer immunotherapy. *Cell Metab* 37 (4): 870–885.e8. https://doi.org/10.1016/j.cmet.2024.12.007.
44. Hercend, T., Farace, F., Baume, D. et al. (1990). Immunotherapy with lymphokine-activated natural killer cells and recombinant interleukin-2: a feasibility trial in metastatic renal cell carcinoma. *J Biol Response Mod* 9 (6): 546–555.
45. Zhang, S., Liu, W., Hu, B. et al. (2020). Prognostic significance of tumor-infiltrating natural killer cells in solid tumors: a systematic review and meta-analysis. *Front Immunol* 11: 1242. https://doi.org/10.3389/fimmu.2020.01242.
46. Ruggeri, L., Capanni, M., Urbani, E. et al. (2002). Effectiveness of donor natural killer cell alloreactivity in mismatched hematopoietic transplants. *Science* 295 (5562): 2097–2100. https://doi.org/10.1126/science.1068440.
47. Coca, S., Perez-Piqueras, J., Martinez, D. et al. (1997). The prognostic significance of intratumoral natural killer cells in patients with colorectal carcinoma. *Cancer* 79 (12): 2320–2328.
48. Liu, E., Marin, D., Banerjee, P. et al. (2020). Use of CAR-transduced natural killer cells in CD19-positive lymphoid tumors. *N Engl J Med* 382 (6): 545–553. https://doi.org/10.1056/NEJMoa1910607.
49. Teng, K.Y., Mansour, A.G., Zhu, Z. et al. (2022). Off-the-shelf prostate stem cell antigen-directed chimeric antigen receptor natural killer cell therapy to treat pancreatic cancer. *Gastroenterology* 162 (4): 1319–1333. https://doi.org/10.1053/j.gastro.2021.12.281.
50. Shanley, M., Daher, M., Dou, J. et al. (2024). Interleukin-21 engineering enhances NK cell activity against glioblastoma via CEBPD. *Cancer Cell* 42 (8): 1450–1466.e11. https://doi.org/10.1016/j.ccell.2024.07.007.
51. Slattery, K. and Gardiner, C.M. (2019). NK cell metabolism and TGFβ - implications for immunotherapy. *Front Immunol* 10: 02915. https://doi.org/10.3389/fimmu.2019.02915.
52. Rea, A., Santana-Hernández, S., Villanueva, J. et al. (2025). Enhancing human NK cell antitumor function by knocking out SMAD4 to counteract TGFβ and activin A suppression. *Nat Immunol* 26 (4): 582–594. https://doi.org/10.1038/s41590-025-02103-z.
53. Ren, Y., Xue, M., Hui, X. et al. (2025). Chimeric cytokine receptor TGF-β RII/IL-21R improves CAR-NK cell function by reversing the immunosuppressive tumor microenvironment of gastric cancer. *Pharmacol Res* 212: 107637. https://doi.org/10.1016/j.phrs.2025.107637.
54. Shin, S.H., Lee, Y.E., Yoon, H.N. et al. (2025). An innovative strategy harnessing self-activating CAR-NK cells to mitigate TGF-β1-driven immune suppression. *Biomaterials* 314: 122888. https://doi.org/10.1016/j.biomaterials.2024.122888.
55. Bonanni, V., Antonangeli, F., Santoni, A., and Bernardini, G. (2019). Targeting of CXCR3 improves anti-myeloma efficacy of adoptively transferred activated natural killer cells. *J Immunother Cancer* 7 (1): 290. https://doi.org/10.1186/s40425-019-0751-5.
56. Ng, Y.Y., Tay, J.C.K., and Wang, S. (2020). CXCR1 Expression to improve anti-cancer efficacy of intravenously injected CAR-NK cells in mice with peritoneal xenografts. *Mol Ther Oncolytics* 16: 75–85, https://doi.org/10.1016/j.omto.2019.12.006.
57. Delconte, R.B., Kolesnik, T.B., Dagley, L.F. et al. (2016). CIS is a potent checkpoint in NK cell-mediated tumor immunity. *Nat Immunol* 17 (7): 816–824. https://doi.org/10.1038/ni.3470.
58. Bernard, P.L., Delconte, R., Pastor, S. et al. (2022). Targeting CISH enhances natural cytotoxicity receptor signaling and reduces NK cell exhaustion to improve solid tumor immunity. *J Immunother Cancer* 10 (5): https://doi.org/10.1136/jitc-2021-004244.
59. Rafei, H., Basar, R., Acharya, S. et al. (2025). CREM is a regulatory checkpoint of CAR and IL-15 signalling in NK cells. *Nature* 643 (8073): 1076–1086. https://doi.org/10.1038/s41586-025-09087-8.

60. Slattery, K., Yao, C.H., Mylod, E. et al. (2025). Uptake of lipids from ascites drives NK cell metabolic dysfunction in ovarian cancer. *Sci Immunol* 10 (107): eadr4795. https://doi.org/10.1126/sciimmunol.adr4795.
61. Slattery, K., Woods, E., Zaiatz-Bittencourt, V. et al. (2021). TGFβ drives NK cell metabolic dysfunction in human metastatic breast cancer. *J Immunother Cancer* 9 (2): https://doi.org/10.1136/jitc-2020-002044.
62. Daher, M., Basar, R., Gokdemir, E. et al. (2021). Targeting a cytokine checkpoint enhances the fitness of armored cord blood CAR-NK cells. *Blood* 137 (5): 624–636. https://doi.org/10.1182/blood.2020007748.
63. Poznanski, S.M., Singh, K., Ritchie, T.M. et al. (2021). Metabolic flexibility determines human NK cell functional fate in the tumor microenvironment. *Cell Metab* 33 (6): 1205–1220.e5. https://doi.org/10.1016/j.cmet.2021.03.023.
64. Kobayashi, T., Lam, P.Y., Jiang, H. et al. (2020, https://doi.org/10.1182/blood.2020005602). Increased lipid metabolism impairs NK cell function and mediates adaptation to the lymphoma environment. *Blood* 136: 3004–3017.
65. Young, A., Ngiow, S.F., Gao, Y. et al. (2018). A2AR Adenosine Signaling Suppresses Natural Killer Cell Maturation in the Tumor Microenvironment. *Cancer Res* 78 (4): 1003–1016. https://doi.org/10.1158/0008-5472.can-17-2826.
66. Chambers, A.M., Wang, J., Lupo, K.B. et al. (2018). Adenosinergic signaling alters natural killer cell functional responses. *Front Immunol* 9: 2533. https://doi.org/10.3389/fimmu.2018.02533.
67. Bimbo, J.F., van Diest, E., Murphy, D.E. et al. (2025). T cell-specific non-viral DNA delivery and in vivo CAR-T generation using targeted lipid nanoparticles. *J Immunother Cancer* 13 (7): https://doi.org/10.1136/jitc-2025-011759.

7

Therapeutic Cancer Vaccines: Challenges and Successes in Cancer Immunotherapy

RICCARDO DOLCETTI[1,2,3]
[1] Peter MacCallum Cancer Centre, Melbourne, Victoria, Australia
[2] Peter MacCallum Department of Oncology, The University of Melbourne, Melbourne, Victoria, Australia
[3] Department of Microbiology and Immunology, The University of Melbourne, Melbourne, Victoria, Australia

LEARNING OBJECTIVES

- Recent advances in the mechanism of action of cancer vaccines with a focus on the involvement of recently identified immune cell subsets.
- Challenges and new perspectives in the identification, validation, and exploitation of clinically relevant antigens for cancer vaccines.
- Describe the main vaccine platforms, highlighting advantages and disadvantages.
- Discuss the current challenges and future perspectives for a broad application of cancer vaccines.

7.1 INTRODUCTION

Building on the early immunotherapy developments described in Chapter 1, cancer vaccines have re-emerged as a central pillar of tumour immunology through advances in antigen discovery and mRNA technology. Immunotherapy now represents an important treatment option for several cancers, offering a more favourable safety profile than conventional therapies and the potential for durable clinical responses. Among these approaches, cancer vaccines are particularly promising because they stimulate the immune system to selectively target malignant cells while sparing normal tissues. The immune responses they elicit can act against both primary and metastatic lesions and, unlike chemotherapy or radiotherapy, can generate long-lasting immune memory that supports sustained tumour surveillance. Despite earlier setbacks and the failure of several Phase III trials, interest in cancer vaccine development has accelerated, supported by major advances in antigen discovery, vaccine design, delivery technologies, genomic sequencing, artificial intelligence (AI)-guided prediction, and combination strategies with other immunotherapies.

This chapter outlines the essential requirements for effective therapeutic cancer vaccine development, including the selection of appropriate antigens, engagement of optimal immune effectors, and the integration of emerging delivery platforms. It aims to provide readers with a clear understanding of the key considerations and challenges in vaccine design while encouraging critical reflection and new ideas.

7.2 MECHANISM OF ACTION

Cancer vaccines aim to generate robust tumour-specific immunity by delivering antigens to dendritic cells (DCs), which must efficiently uptake, process, and present these antigens while receiving appropriate adjuvant-mediated activation signals [1, 2]. Mature DCs migrate to draining lymph nodes, upregulate major histocompatibility complex (MHC) and costimulatory molecules, and prime naïve T cells. The resulting antigen-specific T cells then expand, enter the circulation, and infiltrate tumours. For therapeutic vaccines, the key effector population is **$CD8^+$ cytotoxic T cells** [3], which mediate the direct killing of tumour cells. However, **$CD4^+$ T-cell help** is now recognised as essential for durable responses [4]. $CD4^+$ T cells promote DC activation and cytokine production (licencing) to support the durability and functionality of $CD8^+$ T-cell responses [4] and can also directly recognise MHC class II-expressing tumour cells. Vaccines that include class II tumour antigens outperform those relying on unrelated helper epitopes [5].

Beyond magnitude, several **qualitative features** of the T-cell response strongly influence vaccine efficacy:

- **TCR repertoire breadth**, enabling recognition of heterogeneous tumour antigens.
- **Polyfunctionality**, with vaccine-induced T cells producing multiple cytokines [6].
- **Stem-like T cells (progenitor exhausted T cells (Tpex))**, which reside primarily in tumour-draining lymph nodes, express TCF1 and provide a renewable source of effector cells during chronic antigen exposure. Supporting Tpex expansion is critical for durable control and synergy with checkpoint blockade [7, 8].
- **Tissue-resident memory T cells (T_{RM})**, identified by markers such as CD69 and CD103, which localise within tumours and provide rapid on-site effector function [9]. Vaccines capable of promoting T_{RM} formation may enhance local tumour control, although T_{RM} dysfunction can occur in suppressive microenvironments [10].

Although T cells remain the central effectors of cancer vaccine activity, **B cells** also contribute. Through tumour-specific antibody production, antigen presentation, and the formation of **tertiary lymphoid structures (TLSs)**, B cells can enhance local immune activation and sustain T-cell responses [11]. The presence of mature intratumoral TLSs has been associated with improved outcomes following vaccination [12, 13].

Together, these cellular mechanisms highlight that effective cancer vaccines must do more than generate cytotoxic T cells: they must orchestrate coordinated $CD8^+$, $CD4^+$, B cell, and memory-supportive responses that persist over time and operate within both lymphoid and tumour sites.

7.3 THE CRITICAL CHOICE OF THE BEST ANTIGENS FOR VACCINE DEVELOPMENT

Immune surveillance is fundamentally based on the ability to discriminate self from non-self. Whereas viruses are unequivocally perceived as foreign, tumours arise from normal cells and therefore retain many self-features, creating a major obstacle for vaccine design [14]. The key challenge is to identify tumour-specific antigens (TSAs) that are absent from normal cells and can be selectively and effectively targeted by the immune system. Ideally, such antigens should not only be highly immunogenic but also essential for tumour survival, thereby minimising the risk of immune escape due to antigen loss or downregulation. Defining the most effective antigen formulations for therapeutic cancer vaccines remains a major challenge. However, advances in high-throughput technologies, including next-generation sequencing, tandem mass spectrometry, immunopeptidomics, and computational antigen prediction models, have greatly enhanced the ability to identify clinically relevant targets. Tumour antigens can be broadly classified as tumour-associated antigens (TAAs) or TSAs (neoantigens) [2], although new classes of actionable antigens, such as cryptic and bacterial peptides, are emerging as promising targets for next-generation cancer vaccines (Figure 7.1).

Type of cancer vaccine				
	Off-the-shelf			Personalised
Class of antigens	TAAS	"Public" neoantigens	"Cryptic" neoantigens	"Private" neoantigens
Type of antigens	Self-antigen highly expressed on cancer cells	Neoantigens generated by mutations in coding regions	Neoantigens generated by mutations in non-coding regions	Unique neoantigens from individual tumours
Antigen discovery	Known antigens Es. Survivin, telomerase, cancer testis antigens, etc.	DNA sequencing RNA sequencing AI Prediction	Immunopeptidomics Ribosome sequencing	DNA sequencing RNA sequencing AI Prediction
Specificity	Low	High	High	Very high
Immunogenicity	Low	Moderate	High	High
Heterogeneity	High	Low	Moderate	Patient-specific
Clonal expression	No	Yes	Sometimes	Patient-specific
Patient coverage	Broad → Individual			

FIGURE 7.1 The key characteristics of off-the-shelf and personalised cancer vaccines. It focuses on the antigens used across various vaccine types, including tumour specificity, immunogenicity, heterogeneity, and clonality. This diversity in antigen types enables the development of cancer vaccines catering to different patient populations.

7.3.1 Tumour-Associated Antigens (TAAs)

Early cancer vaccine efforts primarily focused on TAAs, which are derived from non-mutated self-proteins that are: (i) overexpressed in cancer compared with healthy tissues, (ii) expressed during lineage differentiation and aberrantly expressed by tumour cells, or (iii) restricted in expression to germ cells and aberrantly expressed by cancer cells (such as the cancer testis antigens, or cancer-testis antigens (CTAs). TAAs are attractive candidates for "off-the-shelf" cancer vaccines because of their shared expression across patients and tumour types (Figure 7.1). Notable examples of TAA-targeted vaccines that have advanced into clinical evaluation include HER2, tested in breast cancer patients [15]; mesothelin, investigated in pancreatic cancer and mesothelioma [16]; and human telomerase, assessed across multiple cancer types [17, 18]. However, their limited tumour specificity poses challenges, as this can lead to on-target or off-target toxicity and may also limit their immunogenicity. Indeed, the clinical translation of cancer vaccines targeting TAAs has been limited, primarily because lymphocyte clones with the highest affinity for these widely expressed self-antigens are deleted during central tolerance in the thymus [19]. Of the many TAA-targeted vaccines evaluated clinically, only sipuleucel-T has demonstrated a clear overall survival (OS) benefit [20]. This autologous DC-based vaccine targets prostatic acid phosphatase in prostate cancer and extends survival by approximately four months. However, its adoption in routine practice has been limited, largely due to the high cost and complexity of autologous manufacturing and its modest efficacy. Although still suboptimal, the relatively better clinical outcomes achieved with sipuleucel-T compared with other TAA-based vaccines may reflect its nature as a DC-based product, functioning less as a conventional therapeutic vaccine and more like an adoptive cell therapy through modulation of DC populations. Moreover, unlike many other vaccine studies, sipuleucel-T was evaluated in patients with relatively indolent and asymptomatic prostate cancer, a setting that likely afforded sufficient time for vaccine-induced immune responses to influence survival outcomes.

7.3.2 Tumour-Specific Antigens (TSAs)

TSAs are uniquely expressed by cancer cells and absent from healthy tissues, making them highly attractive targets for therapeutic vaccination (Figure 7.1). Viral antigens represent the clearest example: they are entirely foreign to the host, highly immunogenic, and restricted to virus-driven tumours, as illustrated by the success of Human Papilloma Virus (HPV) vaccination [21] and Epstein-Barr Virus (EBV)-directed T-cell therapies [22]. In non-viral cancers, the major source of TSAs is **mutation-associated neoantigens**, which arise from tumour-specific genetic alterations that generate novel peptides not found in the normal human proteome. Neoantigens can originate from somatic mutations in coding regions, such as missense mutations, indels, or gene fusions, or from non-canonical processes, including abnormal splicing or atypical translation [23]. Tumours with high mutational burden typically generate more neoantigens, whereas low-mutational-burden cancers may offer fewer vaccine targets. Neoantigens are recognised by both $CD8^+$ and $CD4^+$ tumour-infiltrating T cells, and higher neoantigen load is consistently associated with stronger immune infiltration, improved prognosis, and better responses to immune checkpoint inhibitors (ICIs) [24, 25]. Although spontaneous T-cell responses emerge in many patients, they are generally insufficient for tumour control. Vaccines that amplify these responses or induce de novo neoantigen-specific immunity can therefore enhance tumour clearance and synergise with ICIs.

Neoantigens offer several advantages over TAAs:

- **Potent immunogenicity**, often resulting from mutation-driven increases in peptide- Human Leukocyte Antigen (HLA) affinity.
- **Lack of central tolerance**, enabling high-affinity T cells to persist in the periphery.
- **Tumour-restricted expression**, which minimises the risk of autoimmunity.

This safety profile is supported by recent trials in which personalised neoantigen vaccines combined with PD-1 blockade did not increase immune-related toxicities [26].

TSAs can be categorised into **shared (public)** and **personalised (private)** neoantigens (Figure 7.1). Public neoantigens arise from recurrent oncogenic mutations, such as *KRAS* G12D/G12V or *BRAF* V600E, and may support the development of off-the-shelf vaccines applicable across multiple patients (Figure 7.2). Their biological relevance also makes immune escape less likely. However, their utility depends on efficient antigen processing and presentation by common HLA alleles, a requirement often unmet, limiting the proportion of patients who can benefit [27]. Nevertheless, recent clinical evidence shows that public neoantigen vaccines can elicit potent $CD4^+$ and $CD8^+$ responses and delay recurrence, highlighting their potential in minimal-residual-disease settings. In particular, the recently concluded Phase I AMPLIFY-201 clinical trial demonstrated that a lymph-node targeting vaccine exploiting the G12D and G12R KRAS mutations induced potent, polyfunctional $CD4^+$ and $CD8^+$ T-cell immunity to mutated KRAS, alongside frequent antigen spreading that delayed tumour recurrence in patients with pancreatic and colorectal cancer with minimal residual disease [28] (Table 7.1). A randomised Phase II study (NCT05726864) is ongoing in the adjuvant setting of pancreatic cancer.

The majority of neoantigens are **private**, generated by patient-specific mutations (Figure 7.1). Their identification typically integrates genomic and transcriptomic profiling to detect expressed tumour mutations, followed by computational prediction of peptide-HLA presentation. Although prediction tools have improved, with models now incorporating antigen processing, presentation, and sometimes TCR-recognition features, their accuracy remains limited, and only a small fraction of predicted neoepitopes prove immunogenic [29, 30]. Immunopeptidomics can confirm natural presentation of some candidate peptides [31], but most HLA-bound peptides do not elicit T-cell responses, and only 1–2% of tumour mutations typically generate spontaneous T-cell recognition [32]. Large-scale datasets and high-throughput antigen screening platforms are helping refine prediction rules, but functional assays remain essential to validate immunogenicity. Despite these challenges, rapid progress in sequencing, antigen prediction, and scalable manufacturing has enabled the development of personalised vaccines tailored to each patient's tumour. Early-phase trials, including in highly aggressive cancers such as pancreatic cancer, have shown encouraging T-cell responses, evidence of antigen spreading, delayed recurrence, and prolonged survival in selected patients (reviewed in [25] (Table 7.1)). However, personalised vaccines remain limited by time- and

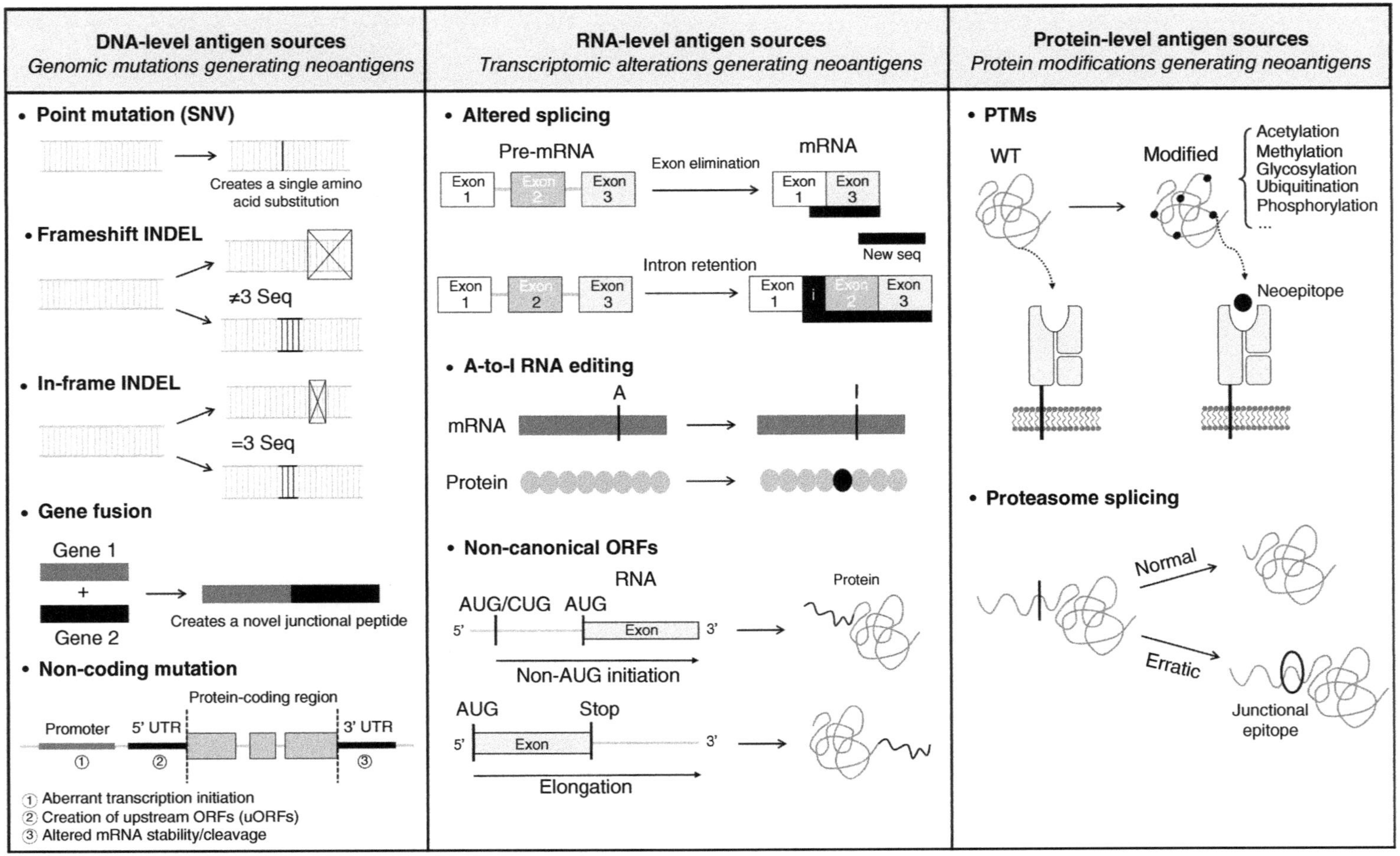

FIGURE 7.2 The figure schematically illustrates the most common tumour antigen sources arising from genomic alterations and transcriptional and post-transcriptional modifications (PTMs).

TABLE 7.1 Characteristics of clinical trials exploiting different cancer vaccine platforms.

Vaccine Platform	Trial/Ref.	Phase	tumour type	Antigen/ Formulation	Combination	Key Immunologic / Clinical Outcomes
Cell-based (whole-cell)	GVAX platform	Phase I/II	Pancreatic adenocarcinoma	Allogeneic whole-cell GM-CSF-secreting	± anti-PD-1 ± anti-CD137	Induced TLS, enhanced $CD4^+$/$CD8^+$ infiltration; immunologic responses met, but no significant OS difference
Cell-based (DC vaccine)	DCVax-L (NCT00045968)	Phase III	Glioblastoma (newly diagnosed/recurrent)	Autologous DCs loaded with tumour lysate	–	Improved median OS vs external controls (19.3 vs 16.5 mo newly diagnosed; 13.2 vs 7.8 mo recurrent); long-term survivors; safe
Cell-based (DC vaccine)	NCT02956551	Phase I/II	Metastatic lung cancer	Autologous DCs	–	Median OS 7.9 mo; safe; elicited durable immune responses
Cell-based (DC vaccine)	NCT02111941	Early phase	Ovarian cancer	DC-based	–	Potential prevention of recurrence; immunologic responses observed
Cell-based (-loaded DCs)	NCT04078269	Early phase	NSCLC	Neoantigen-loaded DCs	–	Durable systemic T-cell responses up to 19 mo
Cell-based (CD137L-DCs)	NCT03282617	Phase I	Nasopharyngeal carcinoma	EBV-antigen-loaded CD137L-DCs	–	Well tolerated; prolonged survival; strong cytotoxic T-cell responses

Peptide-based (neoantigen SLPs)	[113]	Phase I/Ib	Glioblastoma	Poly-ICLC-adjuvanted neoantigen SLPs	–	Induced durable $CD4^+$/$CD8^+$ T-cell memory; intra-tumoural T cells upregulated inhibitory molecules
Peptide-based (neoantigen SLPs + ICI)	[65]	Phase I	Melanoma, NSCLC, bladder cancer	Poly-ICLC-adjuvanted neoantigen SLPs	+ Nivolumab	Durable neoantigen-specific $CD8^+$ T cells, epitope spreading, and correlated with longer PFS
Peptide-based (HPV16 SLPs)	[114]	Early phase	HPV16-positive premalignancies	HPV16-derived SLPs linked to the TLR2 ligand	–	Strong T-cell responses; minimal adverse effects
Peptide-based (mutant KRAS SLPs)	–	Early phase	Solid tumours	Mutant KRAS peptide + CpG + albumin-binding lipids	–	Epitope-specific T cells in 84% of patients; tumour biomarker responses; 24% complete clearance; delayed recurrence correlated with T-cell responses
DNA vaccine (neoantigen)	GNOS-PV02 / [53]	Phase I/II	Hepatocellular carcinoma (TKI-refractory/intolerant)	Personalised neoantigen DNA + IL-12 plasmid	+ Pembrolizumab	Safe; robust $CD4^+$/$CD8^+$ T-cell responses; ORR 30.6% (CR 8.3%); confirmatory Phase III planned
RNA vaccine (mRNA)	[97]	Phase I	Stage III/IV melanoma	Personalised mRNA encoding up to 10 neoantigens	–	Induced robust $CD4^+$/$CD8^+$ T-cell responses; sustained PFS

(*Continued*)

TABLE 7.1 (Continued)

Vaccine Platform	Trial/Ref.	Phase	tumour type	Antigen/ Formulation	Combination	Key Immunologic / Clinical Outcomes
RNA vaccine (mRNA + ICI)	[26, 52]	Early phase	Resected melanoma and PDAC	Personalised neoantigen mRNA	+ ICI	Promising early clinical outcomes; enhanced T-cell immunity
Bacterial vector (Listeria-based)	[115]	Early phase	Prostate cancer	Listeria expressing PSA	± ICI	Safe; immunogenic; early signs of tumour regression
Bacterial vector (Listeria-based)	[116]	Early phase	Solid tumours	Listeria expressing mesothelin	–	Demonstrated anti-tumour activity; safety confirmed
Bacterial vector (Listeria-based)	[117]	Early phase	Solid tumours	Listeria expressing MAGE-B	–	Induced immune responses; preclinical efficacy translated to early clinical trials
Bacterial vector (Listeria-based)	[118]	Early phase	HPV-associated cancers	Listeria expressing HPV E7	–	Demonstrated immunogenicity; tumour regression in early-phase studies

resource-intensive production, high cost, and reduced applicability in rapidly progressing or low-mutational-burden tumours.

Overall, TSAs, particularly mutation-associated neoantigens, represent the most promising targets for cancer vaccine development. Their unique specificity, high immunogenic potential, and synergy with immune checkpoint blockade position them at the forefront of next-generation immunotherapy strategies.

7.3.3 Non-conventional or Cryptic Antigens: A New Class of Immunogenic Targets for Cancer Vaccines

Recent discoveries dispute the long-held assumption that mutated neoantigens are the primary or most readily exploitable immunogenic targets in cancer [33, 34]. High-resolution immunopeptidomic profiling, combined with ribosome profiling and cross-tissue comparisons, has revealed a repertoire of cancer-restricted non-canonical HLA class I-presented peptides, often referred to as *cryptic antigens* [33] (Figure 7.1). These peptides arise from unconventional genomic regions or aberrant RNA processing events, rather than from the standard protein-coding exome, including alternative reading frames, intron retention events, and unannotated open reading frames (ORF) [35]. In particular, alternative splicing events, including back-splicing circularisation that generates circular RNAs (circRNAs), are more frequent in cancers than in normal tissues and have been identified as important sources of cryptic antigens [35, 36] (Figure 7.2). Notably, cryptic antigens constitute a significant portion of the cancer-associated immunopeptidome [37, 38], and their absence from healthy tissues and the thymus allows them to escape central tolerance. Moreover, cryptic antigens have been shown to be highly immunogenic, being capable of eliciting specific cytotoxic T-cell responses and effective tumour cell killing. These findings broaden the landscape of tumour antigen discovery by implicating dysregulated RNA processing and translation as critical sources of novel immunogenic peptides. Strikingly, many of these cryptic antigens were recurrent across patients carrying common HLA alleles, underscoring their potential as broadly applicable targets for the development of "off-the-shelf" vaccines and TCR-based therapies. Epitopes provided by human endogenous retroviruses (HERVs) may also be considered tumour-associated cryptic antigens. HERVs are remnants of ancient viral infections integrated into the human genome, many of which are transcriptionally silenced in normal tissues but can become aberrantly expressed in cancer [39, 40]. These tumour-associated HERV proteins can be processed and presented as neoantigenic epitopes on MHC class I and II molecules, eliciting both $CD8^+$ and $CD4^+$ T-cell responses. HERV-derived epitopes are particularly attractive as immunotherapy targets because they are largely absent from healthy tissues, reducing the risk of autoimmunity, yet are broadly shared across patients within certain tumour types. Emerging evidence suggests that HERV-specific T cells contribute to spontaneous anti-tumour immunity and may enhance the efficacy of therapeutic cancer vaccines or checkpoint blockade [39, 40], highlighting HERVs as a promising source of actionable epitopes for vaccine development.

Post-translational modifications associated with cancer-specific signalling pathways add an additional layer of complexity to the tumour antigen repertoire and may lead to the generation of cryptic antigens (Figure 7.2). In particular, the proteasome can generate spliced peptides through the ligation of non-contiguous peptide fragments from the same (*cis*-spliced peptides) or different proteins (*trans*-spliced peptides) [41]. Until recently, the absence of dedicated tools for spliced peptide prediction in immunopeptidomics made it challenging to accurately determine the true prevalence of proteasome-generated spliced peptides. Recent findings indicate that although HLA class I-spliced peptides constitute a small fraction of the immunopeptidome (<3–5%), they outnumber other categories of aberrant peptides identified to date [42, 43]. Moreover, several *cis*-spliced peptides were shown to be immunogenic and shared across multiple patients with melanoma or colorectal cancer [42, 44]. Overall, these findings broaden the landscape of tumour antigen discovery by implicating dysregulated RNA processing and translation as critical sources of novel immunogenic peptides. Strikingly, many of these cryptic antigens are recurrent across patients carrying common HLA alleles, underscoring their potential as broadly applicable targets for the development of "off-the-shelf" vaccines and TCR-based therapies.

7.3.4 Bacterial Peptides

An emerging paradigm highlights metagenome-derived peptides as a novel immunotherapeutic target. Microbial peptides from the gut microbiota, translocated to tumour sites, can be presented by both tumour cells and antigen-presenting cells (APCs) via HLA class I and II pathways, eliciting robust $CD8^+$ and $CD4^+$ T-cell responses [45, 46]. Moreover, tumour-infiltrating lymphocytes can recognise a broad array of peptide-HLA complexes derived from pathogenic and commensal bacteria, amplifying antitumour immunity [45, 46]. Clinically, these mechanisms are reflected in patient outcomes, as specific gut microbiota compositions correlate with improved responses to ICIs in patients with different cancers [47–49]. Beyond directly activating specific T cells, bacterial peptides can induce cross-reactive T-cell responses through structural or sequence similarity with tumour antigens, a phenomenon known as molecular mimicry [50, 51]. These findings suggest that bacterial peptides could complement conventional neoantigen-based vaccines, broaden the repertoire of targetable antigens and potentially improve anti-tumour immunity, particularly in tumours with low mutational burden. Careful selection of peptides is, however, required to maximise efficacy while minimising the risk of off-target immune reactions.

7.4 VACCINE DELIVERY PLATFORMS

Multiple delivery platforms have been explored, each with distinct advantages, limitations, and clinical applicability. While no single platform has yet emerged as universally superior, advances in neoantigen discovery, vector design, and combination immunotherapy are rapidly shaping the landscape of translational and clinical development [52, 53].

7.4.1 Cell-Based Vaccines

Cell-based vaccines utilise whole tumour cells, lysates, or defined cellular components to present a broad repertoire of tumour antigens, bypassing the need to predefine epitopes [54, 55]. Whole-cell vaccines provide both MHC class I- and II-restricted antigens, stimulating $CD8^+$ cytotoxic and $CD4^+$ helper T cells for durable antitumor immunity. Autologous vaccines derived from resected tumour tissue deliver patient-specific neoantigens, while allogeneic formulations enable off-the-shelf use with lower cost and broader feasibility but reduced personalisation. Tumour heterogeneity, however, can limit efficacy by facilitating immune evasion.

Strategies to enhance cell-based vaccine efficacy include combination with pro-inflammatory cytokines (e.g. GM-CSF, IL-2, IL-12, IFN-α). GVAX, an allogeneic granulocyte-macrophage colony-stimulating factor (GM-CSF)-secreting whole-cell vaccine, has been tested in multiple trials, including pancreatic cancer [56, 57]. GVAX alone induced TLSs and, when combined with anti-PD-1 or anti-CD137, enhanced intra-tumoural $CD4^+$ and $CD8^+$ T-cell infiltration, though survival outcomes were not significantly improved [56, 58] (Table 7.1). These studies highlight that effector T-cell expansion alone may be insufficient and point to the need for combination strategies.

Tumour cell lysates provide 'anonymous' antigen sources, often loaded onto DCs [55]. DCVax-L (NCT00045968), a Phase III trial in glioblastoma, showed improved median survival versus external controls and a favourable safety profile, particularly in biomarker-defined subgroups, though reliance on historical controls limits causal interpretation (Table 7.1). Several strategies have been explored to enhance the immunogenicity of tumour cell lysates. These include repeated freeze–thaw cycles or hypochlorous acid oxidation to induce necrosis; ultraviolet B irradiation to promote apoptosis; heat treatment to increase MHC class I expression and upregulate heat shock proteins; and exposure to immunogenic cell death inducers to boost antigenicity [55, 59, 60]. Although promising, these approaches still rely on the availability of tumour cells for clinical application.

DC-based vaccines exploit the antigen-presenting capacity of autologous DCs, generated from monocytes or $CD34^+$ progenitors, matured *ex vivo*, and loaded with tumour antigens. Sipuleucel-T remains the only FDA-approved DC vaccine, demonstrating safety and modest benefit in prostate cancer. Ongoing trials in lung, ovarian, and non-small cell lung cancer (NSCLC) have shown durable T-cell responses, prevention of recurrence, and long-term immune memory (reviewed in [61]) (Table 7.1). Novel DC subsets, such as CD137L-DCs, exhibit enhanced cytotoxic potential, as demonstrated in nasopharyngeal carcinoma patients [62], while cDC1 cells, specialised for cross-presenting exogenous antigens to $CD8^+$ T cells, represent a promising avenue for next-generation vaccines [63, 64].

Overall, cell-based vaccines offer the advantage of presenting a wide antigenic repertoire and engaging both innate and adaptive immunity, but challenges remain in standardisation, cost, and ensuring clinically meaningful responses (Table 7.2).

7.4.2 Peptide-Based Vaccines

Peptide vaccines use short or long synthetic peptides (SLPs) representing tumour-associated or neoantigens, often delivered with adjuvants to enhance immunogenicity. Short peptides (8–11 amino acids) bind MHC-I on non-professional APCs but may induce transient responses or tolerance, whereas SLPs (20–30 amino acids) contain both MHC-I and II epitopes, promoting robust $CD4^+$ and $CD8^+$ T-cell responses with durable memory [65]. Early SLP trials showed good safety but limited clinical efficacy, likely due to suboptimal antigens, adjuvants, and delivery. Recent neoantigen-based

TABLE 7.2 Advantages and limitations of cancer vaccine platforms.

Vaccine Platform	Key Features/ Mechanism	Clinical Advantages	Limitations/ Challenges
Cell-based (whole-cells, lysates, DCs)	Whole tumour antigens or DCs loaded with patient-specific or shared antigens	Broad antigen repertoire; stimulates both $CD4^+$ and $CD8^+$ T cells; autologous vaccines personalize therapy; some FDA-approved examples (e.g. sipuleucel-T)	Labour-intensive and costly; tumour heterogeneity may reduce efficacy; variable immunogenicity; dependence on the availability of patient tumour material
Peptide-based (short peptides, SLPs, heteroclitic peptides)	Synthetic peptides representing TAAs or neoantigens	Easy and cost-effective production; excellent safety; can induce epitope spreading; compatible with neoantigen personalisation	HLA restriction limits applicability; short peptides may induce tolerance; need for adjuvants; limited clinical efficacy if $CD8^+$ T-cell induction is weak; dose optimisation required
DNA-based	Plasmid DNA encoding tumour antigens, optionally with immunomodulatory elements	Safe, modular, and stable; can target multiple antigens; potential for combination with checkpoint inhibitors	Poor intrinsic immunogenicity; requires specialised delivery (e.g. electroporation); limited clinical efficacy as monotherapy
RNA-based (mRNA, saRNA, circRNA, taRNA)	*In vivo* translation of tumour antigens; advanced platforms allow prolonged expression	Rapid manufacturing induces both $CD4^+$ and $CD8^+$ T-cell responses; personalised therapy is feasible; non-integrating into the host genome	mRNA instability; delivery barriers; preclinical stage for advanced RNA platforms (saRNA, circRNA, taRNA); large antigens may be challenging for circRNA; long-term efficacy data limited
Bacteria-based (Listeria, Salmonella, Clostridium)	Live-attenuated bacteria or bacterial components deliver antigens and activate innate immunity	Strong innate and adaptive stimulation; preferentially target hypoxic/ necrotic tumours; synergistic with checkpoint inhibitors	Variable tumour colonisation; safety concerns; limited clinical experience; standardisation and strain selection critical

studies in glioblastoma, melanoma, NSCLC, and bladder cancer demonstrated polyfunctional, tumour-infiltrating T-cell responses, epitope spreading, and correlations with prolonged progression-free survival. Vaccines targeting shared tumour antigens, such as HPV16 SLPs or mutant KRAS peptides, also elicited potent T-cell responses and objective biomarker effects (Table 7.1).

Heteroclitic peptides, modified to enhance MHC binding, further improve immunogenicity [66], though clinical trials indicate a predominance of $CD4^+$ Th1 responses, suggesting that strategies to enhance $CD8^+$ T-cell induction may be required [65, 67] (Table 7.1). Since SLPs present both MHC class I and II epitopes, careful evaluation of inhibitory $CD4^+$ T-cell populations, including regulatory T cells, is also critical, as these can dampen anti-tumour immunity. Interestingly, a recent study in mouse models demonstrated that high-dose peptide vaccination (15 μg) induced a novel inhibitory $CD4^+$ T-cell subset, whereas ultra-low doses (1.5 ng) avoided this suppression and achieved superior tumour control [68]. While validation in humans is needed, these findings underscore the importance of dose optimisation and single-cell phenotyping in clinical trials to fully characterise the functionality and durability of vaccine-induced T-cell responses.

7.4.3 DNA-Based Vaccines

DNA vaccines deliver plasmids encoding tumour antigens, enabling host cells to produce antigens and stimulate both humoral and cellular immunity. Advantages include cost-effective manufacturing, stability, modularity, and the ability to incorporate costimulatory or immunomodulatory elements [2, 69]. The clinical translation of optimised DNA vaccines has been limited by poor immunogenicity, resulting in little progress in clinical trials, but recent trials have demonstrated promise (Table 7.1). For example, a personalised neoantigen DNA vaccine (GNOS-PV02) co-delivered with an IL-12 plasmid and pembrolizumab in hepatocellular carcinoma induced robust $CD4^+$ and $CD8^+$ T-cell responses with a 30.6% objective response rate, including complete responses [53]. A confirmatory Phase III trial assessing OS is planned. In addition to these encouraging findings, DNA vaccines have recently seen significant advances that enhance their potency, safety, and precision. Innovations such as synthetic gene circuits, self-amplifying DNA, and DNA-encoded monoclonal antibodies allow programmable antigen expression and strong immune activation. Compared with mRNA vaccines, DNA vaccines offer advantages in thermal stability, manufacturability, and long-term storage. Additionally, the use of novel adjuvants, electroporation techniques, and formulation strategies such as lyophilisation or encapsulation further expands their therapeutic potential [70].

7.4.4 RNA-Based Vaccines

RNA vaccines have emerged as a versatile platform for cancer immunotherapy due to their safety, rapid manufacturability, and ability to induce strong $CD4^+$ and $CD8^+$ T-cell responses. Unlike DNA vaccines, mRNA does not require nuclear entry and carries no risk of genomic integration, while its transient expression profile minimises toxicity (Table 7.2). These features, combined with the capacity to encode multiple neoantigens, make mRNA particularly well suited for personalised cancer vaccines.

Conventional mRNA consists of a 5′ cap, untranslated regions (UTRs), an antigen-encoding ORF, and a poly(A) tail. Although mRNA is inherently unstable and susceptible to innate sensing, advances in sequence engineering and nucleoside modification have enabled more efficient and less inflammatory constructs tailored for therapeutic use [71, 72]. Modern design approaches increasingly rely on high-throughput screening and machine learning to optimise antigen expression and improve vaccine potency, supporting their integration into individualised cancer vaccine pipelines.

Beyond conventional mRNA, next-generation RNA platforms aim to extend antigen expression and enhance antitumor efficacy. **Self-amplifying RNA (saRNA)** encodes alphavirus replicase machinery, allowing intracellular RNA replication and prolonged antigen production [73, 74]. Early cancer-focused preclinical studies have shown enhanced immunogenicity [75], and first-in-human studies are underway. **Trans-amplifying RNA (taRNA)** separates the replicase and antigen onto two cooperative RNA molecules, improving safety and reducing competition with host translation; its simplified formats have demonstrated high potency in preclinical models and are being explored for cancer applications [74]. **circRNA** offers greater stability and prolonged protein expression due to its covalently closed structure [76, 77]. Recent work in melanoma, colon carcinoma, and metastatic models has shown that circRNA vaccines can induce robust $CD4^+$ and $CD8^+$ T-cell responses, synergise with adoptive T-cell therapy, and overcome tumour immune suppression [78]. Newer 'small circRNA' constructs further reduce innate immune activation and support durable antitumor immunity [79], though their ability to encode large or multivalent antigens remains limited.

Effective delivery remains a defining requirement for clinical performance. Lipid nanoparticles (LNPs) are currently the most advanced system, providing protection from RNases, enabling efficient uptake and endosomal escape, and contributing intrinsic adjuvant activity [80]. Their clinical feasibility is illustrated by personalised mRNA neoantigen vaccines, which induced robust T-cell responses and prolonged progression-free survival in early melanoma trials (Table 7.1). More recently, individualised mRNA vaccines combined with checkpoint blockade have shown encouraging early outcomes in resected melanoma and pancreatic ductal adenocarcinoma (PDAC), supporting ongoing development in the adjuvant setting (Table 7.1).

Overall, RNA-based platforms combine flexibility, speed, and potent immunogenicity, positioning them as central technologies in the next generation of personalised and off-the-shelf cancer vaccines.

7.4.5 Bacteria-Based Vaccines

Bacteria-based vaccines exploit the strong innate and adaptive immune activation triggered by bacterial vectors to enhance antitumour immunity. Live-attenuated strains such as *Listeria monocytogenes*, *Salmonella typhimurium*, and *Clostridium novyi-NT* can preferentially accumulate in tumours, particularly in hypoxic or necrotic regions where other platforms perform poorly, and can be engineered to deliver tumour antigens directly to professional APCs. Their intrinsic pathogen-associated molecular patterns provide potent adjuvant activity, enabling efficient priming of $CD8^+$ T-cell responses [81, 82]. Engineered *Listeria* strains have shown the greatest clinical progress, demonstrating robust preclinical activity across multiple tumour models and antigens, including prostate-specific antigen (PSA), mesothelin, MAGE-B, and HPV E7 [83]. Several constructs have advanced into clinical testing, where they have shown acceptable safety, strong immunogenicity, and early signs of therapeutic benefit, particularly in combination with ICIs, which can augment the inflammation and T-cell recruitment triggered by bacterial vaccination [83] (Table 7.1). Beyond live vectors, non-replicating bacterial platforms such as bacterial ghosts and outer membrane vesicles offer flexible, modular systems for antigen delivery with improved safety profiles. These platforms retain immunostimulatory components while avoiding systemic infection risk and are under active investigation for use as off-the-shelf tumour antigen carriers [84]. Despite their promise, bacteria-based vaccines face challenges that include inconsistent tumour colonisation across cancer types, variable responses linked to the tumour microenvironment, and the need for careful strain attenuation to ensure safety (Table 7.2). Standardised, clinically scalable platforms will be essential to fully translate bacterial vaccines into effective immunotherapies capable of converting immunologically 'cold' tumours into responsive ones.

7.5 CASE STUDIES

7.5.1 ISA101 + PD-1 Blockade in Incurable HPV16-Related Cancer

Patients with HPV-positive oropharyngeal cancer often mount strong spontaneous HPV-specific T-cell responses, but PD-1 blockade alone benefits only a minority with recurrent disease. ISA101, a synthetic long-peptide vaccine targeting HPV-16 E6/E7, previously showed durable responses in high-grade VIN but limited activity in advanced cervical cancer [85], suggesting that combining vaccination with PD-1 inhibition could improve efficacy. In a Phase II trial (NCT02426892), 24 patients with incurable HPV16-positive cancers received ISA101 plus nivolumab. Treatment yielded a 33% overall response rate (ORR), with a median response duration of ~11 months and a median OS of ~15 months. Toxicities were manageable [86]. Long-term follow-up showed that 38% of responders remained progression-free at 3 years. Responders had higher intratumoral $CD8^+$ T-cell infiltration and upregulation of immune and interferon-signalling genes [87] (Table 7.1).

Significance: The combination showed greater activity than expected from PD-1 blockade alone, supporting therapeutic vaccination as a strategy to boost anti-tumour immunity. A randomised trial is underway.

7.5.2 KEYNOTE-942: Personalised Neoantigen mRNA Vaccine (mRNA-4157/V940)

Personalised neoantigen vaccines have historically been limited by slow, complex manufacturing. KEYNOTE-942 tested mRNA-4157, an individualised mRNA vaccine encoding up to 34 neoantigens, combined with pembrolizumab in high-risk resected melanoma. In this Phase IIb trial, the vaccine was well tolerated, with mostly grade 1–2 AEs. Among 157 patients, the combination reduced the risk of recurrence or death by ~44% compared with pembrolizumab alone [26] (Table 7.1).

Significance: This study provided the first randomised evidence that personalised neoantigen mRNA vaccines are feasible, scalable, and clinically effective. It established synergy between neoantigen vaccination and PD-1 blockade and accelerated the development of a confirmatory Phase III trial (V940–001).

7.5.3 Autogene Cevumeran in Resected Pancreatic Cancer

PDAC rarely responds to checkpoint inhibitors despite evidence that long-term survivors generate neoantigen-specific T-cell responses [88]. A Phase I study evaluated autogene cevumeran, an individualised mRNA lipoplex vaccine (up to 20 neoantigens), given sequentially with atezolizumab and mFOLFIRINOX after PDAC resection [52]. The vaccine was well tolerated and elicited strong neoantigen-specific $CD8^+$ T-cell responses in 8 of 16 patients, with vaccine-expanded clones comprising up to 10% of circulating T cells and showing long-term persistence. Responders had markedly prolonged recurrence-free survival, and recurrent tumours lacked the vaccine-targeted clones, indicating effective immune pressure [89] (Table 7.1).

Significance: Autogene cevumeran can induce durable, high-magnitude $CD8^+$ T-cell responses in a poorly immunogenic tumour type, supporting the feasibility of personalised mRNA vaccines in early-stage settings and motivating larger trials.

7.6 CURRENT CHALLENGES AND FUTURE PERSPECTIVES

Therapeutic cancer vaccines continue to face several challenges that hinder their widespread clinical application.

7.6.1 Antigen Selection and Validation: Are We Focusing on the Right Class of Antigens?

Identifying truly immunogenic TSAs that are naturally presented on HLA molecules remains challenging, particularly in low TMB cancers. Although neoantigen-specific T cells can be detected in these tumours, the overall density of actionable mutations is often low [90, 91], and only a small fraction of predicted peptides prove immunogenic in functional assays. The Tumour Neoantigen Selection Alliance recently reported that only ~6% of top-ranked predictions elicit T-cell responses, underscoring the limitations of current prioritisation pipelines [92]. Advances in neoantigen prediction, including transformer, transfer-learning, and graph-based models [30], offer improved performance, but their clinical utility is hindered by heterogeneous datasets, lack of standardised benchmarks, and inconsistent generalisability across tumour types. More integrated approaches that combine AI-driven prediction with multi-omics data (e.g. TCR repertoire, immunopeptidomics, tumour microenvironment signatures) may more accurately capture both peptide-HLA binding and TCR-peptide interactions. In parallel, scalable high-throughput functional assays remain essential for validating immunogenicity and narrowing candidate lists. While most clinical efforts have focused on predicted neoantigens, **cryptic antigens** represent a complementary class of naturally processed, shared, and highly immunogenic targets. Their systematic discovery has lagged behind, but integrating cryptic antigens into platforms such as mRNA vaccines, viral vectors, or TCR-based therapies may broaden applicability, especially in tumours with limited mutational landscapes. A further challenge is **immunodominance,** the tendency of the immune system to mount strong responses against only a limited subset of available epitopes while ignoring others. Personalised vaccines often include numerous predicted neoantigens, yet patients typically respond to only a small subset. For example, in a recent mRNA vaccine trial in pancreatic cancer, patients vaccinated against up to 20 neoantigens mounted responses to a median of two [52]; in an off-the-shelf KRAS/p53 vaccine, p53 epitopes dominated at the expense of KRAS-specific responses [93]. These observations suggest that simply increasing antigen number may dilute responses to clinically meaningful targets. Strategies such as sequential antigen delivery or combining personalised and off-the-shelf vaccines targeting complementary epitopes may help optimise both breadth and potency. Collectively, these challenges highlight the need for integrated antigen-discovery pipelines that combine robust prediction, functional validation, and rational antigen selection. Such approaches will be critical to improving the precision, scalability, and clinical efficacy of next-generation cancer vaccines.

7.6.2 Tumour Heterogeneity

Tumour heterogeneity remains a major obstacle to identifying robust neoantigens and designing effective vaccines [94]. Because mutations vary across regions of the primary tumour and between metastases, antigen selection must account for **clonality**. Multi-region sequencing can help determine whether candidate neoantigens are broadly shared, but this approach is often impractical in routine clinical settings. Neoantigens from **passenger mutations** are particularly vulnerable to immune-mediated elimination, as they do not confer a growth advantage and can be lost during tumour evolution. In contrast, neoantigens arising from **driver mutations** are more likely to be consistently retained and therefore represent more reliable vaccine targets, although they remain uncommon and subject to HLA restriction [25]. When tissue sampling is limited, **liquid biopsies** combined with sequencing of matched normal samples offer a minimally invasive strategy to capture the tumour's mutational landscape. However, current technologies have limited sensitivity for low-frequency variants and are often restricted to predefined mutation panels, underscoring the need for more comprehensive platforms [95]. Tumour evolution further complicates neoantigen prediction. Immune pressure can selectively eliminate highly immunogenic clones, reshaping the neoantigen landscape over time and favouring immune-evasive populations. Longitudinal monitoring through serial liquid biopsies or multi-omics profiling may help track these dynamics and identify emerging targets. Integrating such approaches with AI-driven prediction tools could enable more adaptive, accurate neoantigen selection for next-generation vaccine strategies [96].

7.6.3 Route of Administration and DC Targeting

Route of administration is a key determinant of cancer vaccine efficacy, influencing biodistribution, the magnitude and quality of immune responses, and ultimately antitumor activity. A wide range of delivery routes have been explored in clinical [97] and preclinical [98, 99] studies, including intravenous, intranodal, subcutaneous, intramuscular and intranasal administration. Preclinical models clearly demonstrate that the site of vaccine delivery shapes the conditions of T-cell priming: localised administration generally restricts antigen presentation to draining lymph nodes, whereas systemic delivery allows targeting of the spleen, a major secondary lymphoid organ enriched in DCs and T cells. These differences can profoundly affect the breadth and durability of immune responses. Moreover, intranodal delivery has been proposed to enhance direct access to professional APCs, while intravenous administration may favour broader systemic distribution. Understanding how distinct administration routes influence immune cell engagement, trafficking, and functional polarisation is therefore critical for optimising vaccine strategies. Future approaches may combine novel formulations (e.g. nanoparticle-based vaccines) with route-specific delivery to maximise antigen presentation and T-cell priming in both local and systemic compartments.

As discussed above, selectively targeting antigens to highly immunogenic DC subsets offers a promising strategy to enhance the efficacy of cancer vaccines. This can be achieved through antibody–antigen conjugates or nanoparticle formulations engineered with ligands that bind cross-presenting cDC1-specific receptors, including DEC-205 (CD205), XCR1, and CLEC9A [100–102]. By directing antigens to these specialised DCs, which are particularly effective at initiating cytotoxic T-cell responses, vaccine formulations may achieve more robust and durable antitumour immunity.

7.6.4 Immunosuppressive Tumour Microenvironment

Tumours employ multiple mechanisms (e.g. regulatory T cells, myeloid-derived suppressor cells, immune checkpoint pathways, and metabolic barriers) that blunt vaccine-induced immune responses (reviewed in [103, 104]). In 'cold' tumours, the immunosuppressive microenvironment limits effective immune responses through a combination of low neoantigen availability, impaired antigen presentation, immunosuppressive APCs, dense stroma that hinders infiltration, and inhibitory signalling that prevents T-cell recruitment and activation. Dysregulated chemokines further promote the accumulation of suppressive cell populations, while exhausted effector cells and regulatory subsets restrict antitumour immunity. Overcoming these barriers requires a multi-pronged immunotherapy strategy targeting different stages of the immune response. TSA availability can be increased by immunogenic chemotherapy, radiotherapy, oncolytic viruses, or cancer vaccines, while cytokines, cGAS-STING agonists, and epigenetic drugs enhance antigen processing and APC activation. Stromal modulators, T-cell agonists, CAR-T cells, and checkpoint blockade therapies facilitate T-cell trafficking and infiltration, enabling stronger immune engagement. Finally, checkpoint inhibitors and therapies targeting suppressive pathways restore the function of infiltrating effector cells, maximising antitumour activity.

7.6.5 Need for Reliable Surrogate Markers for Clinical Efficacy

Randomised Phase III trials remain the gold standard for evaluating clinical endpoints, but they are costly, time-consuming, and poorly suited to testing the many variables involved in cancer vaccine development, such as delivery platforms, antigen selection, adjuvants, and combination strategies. Traditional radiological markers, typically used for cytotoxic therapies, are also inadequate for immunotherapies, as cancer vaccines often require more time to induce measurable tumour shrinkage and may initially cause apparent progression due to immune infiltration (pseudo-progression). A promising alternative is the use of immune responses as surrogate markers of efficacy, similar to immunobridging trials in infectious disease vaccines [101]. However, identifying reliable immunological surrogates for cancer vaccines is particularly challenging given the diversity of anti-tumour immune mechanisms, cancer heterogeneity, and the immunosuppressive tumour microenvironment. In particular, identifying predictive biomarkers to select patients most likely to benefit from cancer vaccines is critical. Early-phase trials of neoantigen-based vaccines have shown that some patients develop strong T-cell responses accompanied by prolonged survival. However, it remains unclear whether this T-cell activation directly drives survival benefits or instead reflects preexisting antitumor immunity and an inherent responsiveness to vaccination [52]. Clinical evidence indicates that while cancer vaccines in unselected populations often fail to demonstrate significant survival gains, they may provide substantial benefit to patient subgroups defined by specific biomarkers or favourable physiological conditions.

Unlike infectious diseases, where antibody titres can serve as universal correlates of protection, no single cross-applicable marker is likely to exist for therapeutic cancer vaccines. Instead, composite measures of immune activity may be required, tailored to each vaccine candidate. Recent advances in 'omic' technologies, including integrated proteomic, transcriptomic, genomic, and spatial profiling, provide opportunities to capture immune responses more comprehensively and support the development of more accurate surrogates. These approaches could make early-phase (I/II) trials more informative, enabling the detection of immunological changes prior to clinical benefit. Ultimately, clinical endpoints such as OS or responses assessed by immune response evaluation criteria in solid tumours (iRECIST) will be essential for validating candidate surrogates. Progress will also depend on the adoption of standardised protocols, consistent specimen preservation, and robust data sharing across trials to enable pooled datasets that can be mined with advanced statistical methods and AI. Clearer regulatory guidance on the evidence required to validate surrogate markers and their clinical application will be critical to encourage their use.

Validated correlates of protection could provide early evidence of vaccine efficacy, streamline regulatory approval, and reduce reliance on large Phase III trials. They would also facilitate adaptive trial designs, allowing real-time adjustment of dosing, assessment of likely clinical response, and optimisation of combination therapies based on patient-specific immune readouts.

7.6.6 Integration of Cancer Vaccines with Standard Therapies

Cancer vaccines can prime or amplify anti-tumour T-cell responses, but they rarely induce complete tumour regression as monotherapy. Consequently, increasing attention has turned to integrating vaccines into multimodal treatment strategies. Because tumour immune evasion involves multiple barriers, combinations that engage different steps of the cancer-immunity cycle generally offer the greatest therapeutic potential. Several standard therapies can enhance vaccine efficacy by increasing tumour antigen availability. Chemotherapy, radiotherapy, targeted therapies, photodynamic therapy, and oncolytic viruses can induce immunogenic cell death, release neoantigens, and improve antigen presentation [105–107]. Additional immune stimulation can be achieved with cytokines and innate agonists (e.g. IFN-α, GM-CSF, CD40, TLR, and STING agonists), which promote DC activation and more efficient T-cell priming [104]. Strategies that remodel the tumour microenvironment [104] or deliver intra-tumoural immunostimulants [108] can further enhance immune-cell infiltration. Checkpoint inhibitors (reviewed in Chapter 5) and other agents targeting immunosuppressive pathways can then sustain and amplify vaccine-induced T-cell activity. Vaccines may also promote epitope spreading [109], broadening antitumour immunity and improving the effectiveness of combination regimens. **Therapeutic timing** is emerging as a critical determinant of combination success. Preclinical and clinical studies show that vaccination should precede or coincide with PD-1 blockade; administering PD-1 inhibitors before antigen priming can drive dysfunctional $CD8^+$ T-cell states and diminish therapeutic outcomes [110]. Concurrent administration has proven more effective in both murine models and clinical trials [111, 112], supporting coordinated scheduling rather than sequential therapy.

Recent studies indicate that neoantigen vaccines are particularly effective in the **adjuvant setting**, where low tumour burden and a less suppressive microenvironment permit strong vaccine-induced T cell control and reduce recurrence risk. In contrast, vaccination in advanced, unresectable disease often elicits robust peripheral T-cell responses but limited clinical benefit, largely due to inadequate tumour infiltration and microenvironmental suppression. Future approaches must therefore pair vaccination with strategies that reshape the tumour microenvironment to allow vaccine-induced T cells to function intra-tumourally. Despite clear promise, combination therapies introduce new complexities. Layering multiple immunomodulatory agents increases the risk of immune-related adverse events, requiring careful optimisation of dosing, sequencing, and monitoring to ensure safety while preserving therapeutic potency. Identifying the most effective combinations and defining the optimal timing for vaccination within each clinical context remains a central challenge for the next generation of cancer vaccine development.

7.7 CONCLUDING REMARKS

Cancer vaccines hold significant promise for harnessing the immune system to prevent or treat malignancies, yet their clinical success remains limited by tumour heterogeneity, the immunosuppressive microenvironment, and challenges in optimising antigen selection, delivery, and combination strategies. Advances in the identification and validation of personalised and shared neoantigens, immunomonitoring, and rational combination therapies offer opportunities to overcome these barriers. Moving forward, integrating robust biomarkers, adaptive trial designs, and strategies to remodel the tumour microenvironment will be key to translating cancer vaccines into effective and durable therapies.

KEY TERMS & DEFINITIONS SIDEBAR

Antigen-presenting cell (APC) Specialised immune cells that capture, process, and display antigens on their surface bound to major histocompatibility complex (MHC) molecules, enabling the activation of T lymphocytes. Professional APCs, such as dendritic cells, macrophages, and B cells, are essential for initiating and regulating adaptive immune responses.

Cancer-testis antigens (CTAs) A group of tumour-associated proteins normally expressed only in germ cells of the testis (and occasionally in the ovary or placenta) but aberrantly activated in various cancers. CTAs are largely absent from other normal tissues, making them highly tumour-specific antigens. They can be recognised by the immune system, particularly T cells, and are considered promising targets for cancer immunotherapy and vaccine development.

Central tolerance The process by which developing T cells and B cells that recognise self-antigens with high affinity are eliminated or inactivated during their maturation in primary lymphoid organs, the thymus for T cells and the bone marrow for B cells. Central tolerance prevents the emergence of self-reactive lymphocytes, thereby reducing the risk of autoimmunity and ensuring that the adaptive immune system can distinguish self from non-self.

Cryptic tumour antigens Peptides derived from tumour proteins that are normally hidden from the immune system under physiological conditions due to low expression, inefficient processing, or limited presentation on MHC molecules. In cancer, these antigens can become exposed and elicit T-cell responses, making them potential targets for cancer immunotherapy, particularly when conventional TAAs are absent or poorly immunogenic.

Driver/passenger mutations Driver mutations are genetic alterations that directly contribute to cancer development and progression by conferring growth or survival advantages to tumour cells. These mutations affect key oncogenes or tumour suppressor genes and are essential for tumour initiation and maintenance. Passenger mutations are genetic alterations that do not contribute to cancer development but occur alongside driver mutations due to the high mutational burden in tumour cells. They are largely neutral in terms of tumour growth and serve as a record of genomic instability rather than a functional advantage.

Heteroclitic peptides Modified versions of naturally occurring peptides in which one or more amino acids are intentionally altered to increase their binding affinity to MHC molecules or enhance recognition by T-cell receptors. These peptides are used in vaccines and immunotherapy to boost T-cell responses against the original (native) antigen, thereby improving the magnitude and quality of the immune response without altering the tumour or pathogen target itself.

Immunoediting The dynamic process by which the immune system interacts with developing tumours, shaping tumour immunogenicity over time. It consists of three phases: elimination (immune-mediated destruction of tumour cells), equilibrium (selection of tumour variants that survive immune pressure), and escape (emergence of tumour cells that evade immune detection or suppression). Immunoediting explains how tumours can evolve mechanisms to avoid immune recognition while influencing the quality and intensity of anti-tumour immune responses.

Immunogenicity The ability of a substance, such as an antigen, vaccine, or therapeutic protein, to provoke an immune response. This includes the activation of humoral immunity (antibody production) and/or cellular immunity (T-cell responses). High immunogenicity is desired for vaccines to induce protective immunity, whereas in some biologic therapies, it can lead to unwanted immune reactions.

Immunopeptidomics The study and characterisation of the repertoire of peptides, known as immunopeptides, presented by MHC molecules on the surface of cells. Immunopeptidomic analyses, typically using mass spectrometry, identify the specific peptides derived from self, mutated, or pathogen proteins that are displayed to T cells, providing insights into antigen presentation, immune recognition, and potential targets for vaccines or immunotherapies.

Licencing (of antigen-presenting cells, APC) A process by which APCs, particularly dendritic cells, acquire the ability to effectively activate $CD8^+$ cytotoxic T lymphocytes. This occurs after the APCs receive stimulatory signals, often through interaction with activated $CD4^+$ helper T cells via CD40–CD40L engagement or through inflammatory cues, which enhance their expression of costimulatory molecules and cytokines. Licenced APCs can then provide the necessary signals to prime and sustain robust cytotoxic T-cell responses.

Off-the-shelf vaccine A pre-manufactured vaccine designed for broad use in multiple patients without the need for individual customisation. Unlike personalised vaccines, which are tailored to a patient's specific tumour antigens or genetic profile, off-the-shelf vaccines target shared TAAs or common pathogen epitopes, enabling rapid administration and standardised production for larger patient populations.

Polyfunctional immunity An immune response characterised by the ability of individual immune cells, particularly T cells, to simultaneously perform multiple functions, such as producing several cytokines (e.g. IFN-γ, TNF, IL-2), exhibiting cytotoxic activity, and proliferating. Polyfunctional T cells are considered a hallmark of effective and durable immune protection, as their multifunctional nature enhances pathogen or tumour control compared to monofunctional responses.

Progenitor-exhausted (T_{pex}) T cells A subset of exhausted T cells that retain self-renewal capacity and the potential to differentiate into terminally exhausted effector T cells. Progenitor-exhausted T cells play a critical role in maintaining long-term immune responses during chronic infection and cancer, serving as the main population that can be reinvigorated by immune checkpoint blockade therapies (e.g. anti-PD-1).

Tertiary lymphoid structures (TLSs) Organised aggregates of immune cells that form *de novo* in non-lymphoid tissues during chronic inflammation, infection, or cancer. TLSs resemble secondary lymphoid organs (such as lymph nodes) in their cellular composition and architecture, often containing B-cell follicles, T-cell zones, follicular dendritic cells, and high endothelial venules. They serve as local sites for antigen presentation, T- and B-cell activation, and adaptive immune responses. In tumours, the presence of TLSs is generally associated with improved immune infiltration and favourable clinical outcomes.

Tissue-resident memory T (T_{RM}) cells A subset of memory T cells that permanently reside within non-lymphoid tissues, such as the skin, lungs, gut, or brain, without recirculating through the bloodstream. They are characterised by the expression of markers like CD69 and CD103, which promote tissue retention. T_{RM} cells provide rapid, localised immune protection upon re-exposure to pathogens or tumour antigens by producing cytokines and cytotoxic molecules. They play a crucial role in frontline defence, immune surveillance, and long-term tissue-specific immunity.

LIST OF ABBREVIATIONS

AI	artificial intelligence
APC	antigen-presenting cell
circRNA	circular RNA
CMV	cytomegalovirus
DC	dendritic cell
EBV	Epstein-Barr Virus
HBV	hepatitis B virus
HERV	human endogenous retrovirus

HLA	human leukocyte antigen
HPV	human papilloma virus
ICI	immune checkpoint inhibitor
iRECIST	Immune Response Evaluation Criteria in Solid Tumours
LNP	lipid nanoparticle
MHC	major histocompatibility complex
MoDC	monocyte-derived dendritic cell
NK	natural killer
NSCLC	non-small cell lung cancer
ORF	open reading frame
ORR	overall response rate
OS	overall survival
PDAC	pancreatic ductal adenocarcinoma
PSA	prostate-specific antigen
saRNA	self-amplifying RNA
SLP	synthetic long peptide
TAA	tumour-associated antigen
taRNA	trans-amplifying RNA
TCR	T-cell receptor
TLS	tertiary lymphoid structure
T_{pex}	progenitor-exhausted T cells
T_{RM}	tissue-resident memory T cells
TSA	tumour-specific antigen
UTR	untranslated region
WES	whole-exome sequencing

REVIEW QUESTIONS

1. Which are the qualitative features of T-cell responses that are critical for cancer vaccine efficacy?
2. What are the advantages of exploiting cryptic antigens instead of private neoantigens for the development of cancer vaccines?
3. What are the main challenges to broaden the applicability and enhance the efficacy of therapeutic cancer vaccines?
4. Which are the main factors to be considered for an effective integration of cancer vaccines within standard therapy?

REFERENCES

1. Del Prete, A., Salvi, V., Soriani, A. et al. (2023). Dendritic cell subsets in cancer immunity and tumor antigen sensing. *Cell Mol Immunol* 20 (5): 432–447.
2. Saxena, M., van der Burg, S.H., Melief, C.J.M., and Bhardwaj, N. (2021). Therapeutic cancer vaccines. *Nat Rev Cancer* 21 (6): 360–378.

3. Raskov, H., Orhan, A., Christensen, J.P., and Gögenur, I. (2021). Cytotoxic CD8+ T cells in cancer and cancer immunotherapy. *Br J Cancer* 124 (2): 359–367.
4. Montauti, E., Oh, D.Y., and Fong, L. (2024). CD4+ T cells in antitumor immunity. *Trends Cancer* 10 (10): 969–985.
5. Ninmer, E.K., Zhu, H., Chianese-Bullock, K.A. et al. (2024). Multipeptide vaccines for melanoma in the adjuvant setting: long-term survival outcomes and post-hoc analysis of a randomized phase II trial. *Nat Commun* 15 (1): 2570.
6. Makedonas, G. and Betts, M.R. (2006). Polyfunctional analysis of human t cell responses: importance in vaccine immunogenicity and natural infection. *Springer Semin Immunopathol* 28 (3): 209–219.
7. Siddiqui, I., Schaeuble, K., Chennupati, V. et al. (2019). Intratumoral Tcf1+PD-1+CD8+ T cells with stem-like properties promote tumor control in response to vaccination and checkpoint blockade immunotherapy. *Immunity* 50 (1): 195–211.e10.
8. Connolly, K.A., Kuchroo, M., Venkat, A. et al. (2021). A reservoir of stem-like $CD8^+$ T cells in the tumor-draining lymph node preserves the ongoing antitumor immune response. *Sci Immunol* 6 (64): eabg7836.
9. Wei, H., Wang, Y., Jiang, S. et al. (2025). The roles of tissue-resident memory T cells (TRMs) in diseases and vaccine development: a comprehensive review. *Vaccine* 62: 127605.
10. Chude, C.F., Uzonna, J.E., and Arsenio, J. (2025). Tissue resident memory cells: friend or foe? *Immunology* https://doi.org/10.1111/imm.70024.
11. Conejo-Garcia, J.R., Lopez-Bailon, L.U., and Anadon, C.M. (2024). Unraveling spontaneous humoral immune responses against human cancer: a road to novel immunotherapies. *J Leukoc Biol* 116 (5): 919–926.
12. Fridman, W.H., Meylan, M., Pupier, G. et al. (2023). Tertiary lymphoid structures and B cells: an intratumoral immunity cycle. *Immunity* 56 (10): 2254–2269.
13. Shu, D.H., Ho, W.J., Kagohara, L.T. et al. (2024). Immunotherapy response induces divergent tertiary lymphoid structure morphologies in hepatocellular carcinoma. *Nat Immunol* 25 (11): 2110–2123.
14. Haen, S.P., Löffler, M.W., Rammensee, H.G., and Brossart, P. (2020). Towards new horizons: characterization, classification and implications of the tumour antigenic repertoire. *Nat Rev Clin Oncol* 17 (10): 595–610.
15. Zhou, Y. (2023). HER2/neu-based vaccination with li-Key hybrid, GM-CSF immunoadjuvant and trastuzumab as a potent triple-negative breast cancer treatment. *J Cancer Res Clin Oncol* 149 (9): 6711–6718.
16. Tsujikawa, T., Crocenzi, T., Durham, J.N. et al. (2020). Evaluation of cyclophosphamide/GVAX pancreas followed by Listeria-Mesothelin (CRS-207) with or without Nivolumab in patients with pancreatic cancer. *Clin Cancer Res* 26 (14): 3578–3588.
17. Haakensen, V.D., Öjlert, Å.K., Thunold, S. et al. (2024). UV1 telomerase vaccine with ipilimumab and nivolumab as second line treatment for pleural mesothelioma – a phase II randomised trial. *Eur J Cancer* 202: 113973.
18. Brandt, A., Klinghammer, K., Schultheiss, C. et al. (2025). UV1 vaccination in pembrolizumab-treated patients with recurrent or metastatic head and neck cancer: a randomized multicenter phase 2 trial. *Medicine* 6 (7): 100647.
19. Leko, V. and Rosenberg, S.A. (2020). Identifying and targeting human tumor antigens for T cell-based immunotherapy of solid tumors. *Cancer Cell* 38 (4): 454–472.
20. Rastogi, I., Muralidhar, A., and McNeel, D.G. (2023). Vaccines as treatments for prostate cancer. *Nat Rev Urol* 20 (9): 544–559.
21. Gupta, C., Dolma, K.G., Sherpa, M.L. et al. (2025). Human papillomavirus vaccine: success and challenges. *J Biosci* 50: 51.
22. Gottschalk, S. and Rooney, C.M. (2015). Adoptive t-cell immunotherapy. *Curr Top Microbiol Immunol* 391: 427–454.
23. Xie, N., Shen, G., Gao, W. et al. (2023). Neoantigens: promising targets for cancer therapy. *Signal Transduct Target Ther* 8 (1): 9.

24. Puig-Saus, C., Sennino, B., Peng, S. et al. (2023). Neoantigen-targeted CD8+ T cell responses with PD-1 blockade therapy. *Nature* 615 (7953): 697–704.
25. Zaidi, N., Jaffee, E.M., and Yarchoan, M. (2025). Recent advances in therapeutic cancer vaccines. *Nat Rev Cancer* 25 (7): 517–533.
26. Weber, J.S., Carlino, M.S., Khattak, A. et al. (2024). Individualised neoantigen therapy mRNA-4157 (V940) plus pembrolizumab versus pembrolizumab monotherapy in resected melanoma (KEYNOTE-942): a randomised, phase 2b study. *Lancet* 403 (10427): 632–644.
27. Pearlman, A.H., Hwang, M.S., Konig, M.F. et al. (2021). Targeting public neoantigens for cancer immunotherapy. *Nat Cancer* 2 (5): 487–497.
28. Wainberg, Z.A., Weekes, C.D., Furqan, M. et al. (2025). Lymph node-targeted, mKRAS-specific amphiphile vaccine in pancreatic and colorectal cancer: phase 1 AMPLIFY-201 trial final results. *Nat Med* 31 (11): 3648–3653.
29. Zeng, J., Lin, Z., Zhang, X. et al. (2025). Leveraging artificial intelligence for neoantigen prediction. *Cancer Res* 85 (13): 2376–2387.
30. Wang, Z., Gu, Y., Sun, X., and Huang, H. (2025). Computation strategies and clinical applications in neoantigen discovery towards precision cancer immunotherapy. *Biomark Res* 13 (1): 96.
31. Pongcharoen, S., Kaewsringam, N., Somaparn, P. et al. (2024). Immunopeptidomics in the cancer immunotherapy era. *Explor Target Antitumor Ther* 5 (4): 801–817.
32. Lang, F., Schrörs, B., Löwer, M. et al. (2022). Identification of neoantigens for individualized therapeutic cancer vaccines. *Nat Rev Drug Discov* 21 (4): 261–282.
33. Ely, Z.A., Kulstad, Z.J., Gunaydin, G. et al. (2025). Pancreatic cancer-restricted cryptic antigens are targets for T cell recognition. *Science* 388 (6747): eadk3487.
34. Goncalves, G., Dolcetti, R., Ooi, J.D., and Faridi, P. (2025). Cryptic but critical: noncanonical antigens in cancer immunotherapy. *Trends Immunol* 46 (7): 499–501.
35. Wright, B.W., Yi, Z., Weissman, J.S., and Chen, J. (2022). The dark proteome: translation from noncanonical open reading frames. *Trends Cell Biol* 32 (3): 243–258.
36. Huang, D., Zhu, X., Ye, S. et al. (2024). Tumour circular RNAs elicit anti-tumour immunity by encoding cryptic peptides. *Nature* 625 (7995): 593–602.
37. Ruiz Cuevas, M.V., Hardy, M.P., Hollý, J. et al. (2021). Most non-canonical proteins uniquely populate the proteome or immunopeptidome. *Cell Rep* 34 (10): 108815.
38. Ouspenskaia, T., Law, T., Clauser, K.R. et al. (2022). Unannotated proteins expand the MHC-I-restricted immunopeptidome in cancer. *Nat Biotechnol* 40 (2): 209–217.
39. Petrizzo, A., Ragone, C., Cavalluzzo, B. et al. (2021). Human endogenous retrovirus reactivation: implications for cancer immunotherapy. *Cancers (Basel)* 13 (9): 1999.
40. Müller, M.D., Holst, P.J., and Nielsen, K.N. (2022). A systematic review of expression and immunogenicity of human endogenous retroviral proteins in cancer and discussion of therapeutic approaches. *Int J Mol Sci* 23 (3): 1330.
41. Liepe J, Marino F, Sidney J, et al. A large fraction of HLA class I ligands are proteasome-generated spliced peptides. *Science* 2016 354(6310):354–358.
42. Faridi, P., Woods, K., Ostrouska, S. et al. (2020). Spliced peptides and cytokine-driven changes in the immunopeptidome of melanoma. *Cancer Immunol Res* 8 (10): 1322–1334.
43. Levy, R., Alter Regev, T., Paes, W. et al. (2023). Large-scale immunopeptidome analysis reveals recurrent posttranslational splicing of cancer- and immune-associated genes. *Mol Cell Proteomics* 22 (4): 100519.
44. Dolcetti, R., Zeng, B., Ye, J. et al. (2024). Targeting alternative classes of tumor antigens to improve immunotherapy for microsatellite stable, mismatch repair-proficient colorectal cancer. *Cancer Res* 84 (6_Supplement): 4095.
45. Kalaora, S., Nagler, A., Nejman, D. et al. (2021). Identification of bacteria-derived HLA-bound peptides in melanoma. *Nature* 592 (7852): 138–143.
46. Naghavian, R., Faigle, W., Oldrati, P. et al. (2023). Microbial peptides activate tumour-infiltrating lymphocytes in glioblastoma. *Nature* 617 (7962): 807–817.

47. Gopalakrishnan, V., Spencer, C.N., Nezi, L. et al. (2018). Gut microbiome modulates response to anti-PD-1 immunotherapy in melanoma patients. *Science* 359 (6371): 97–103.
48. Routy, B., Le Chatelier, E., Derosa, L. et al. (2018). Gut microbiome influences efficacy of PD-1-based immunotherapy against epithelial tumors. *Science* 359 (6371): 91–97.
49. Zheng, Y., Wang, T., Tu, X. et al. (2019). Gut microbiome affects the response to anti-PD-1 immunotherapy in patients with hepatocellular carcinoma. *J Immunother Cancer* 7 (1): 193.
50. Bessell, C.A., Isser, A., Havel, J.J. et al. (2020). Commensal bacteria stimulate antitumor responses via T cell cross-reactivity. *JCI Insight* 5 (8): e135597.
51. Tagliamonte, M. and Buonaguro, L. (2022). The impact of antigenic molecular mimicry on anti-cancer T-cell immune response. *Front Oncol* 12: 1009247.
52. Rojas, L.A., Sethna, Z., Soares, K.C. et al. (2023). Personalized RNA neoantigen vaccines stimulate T cells in pancreatic cancer. *Nature* 618 (7963): 144–150.
53. Yarchoan, M., Gane, E.J., Marron, T.U. et al. (2024). Personalized neoantigen vaccine and pembrolizumab in advanced hepatocellular carcinoma: a phase 1/2 trial. *Nat Med* 30 (4): 1044–1053.
54. Diao, L. and Liu, M. (2023). Rethinking antigen source: cancer vaccines based on whole tumor cell/tissue lysate or whole tumor cell. *Adv Sci (Weinh)* 10 (22): e2300121.
55. Pérez-Baños, A., Gleisner, M.A., Flores, I. et al. (2023). Whole tumour cell-based vaccines: tuning the instruments to orchestrate an optimal antitumour immune response. *Br J Cancer* 129 (4): 572–585.
56. Heumann, T., Judkins, C., Li, K. et al. (2023). A platform trial of neoadjuvant and adjuvant antitumor vaccination alone or in combination with PD-1 antagonist and CD137 agonist antibodies in patients with resectable pancreatic adenocarcinoma. *Nat Commun* 14 (1): 3650.
57. Le, D.T., Lutz, E., Uram, J.N. et al. (2013). Evaluation of ipilimumab in combination with allogeneic pancreatic tumor cells transfected with a GM-CSF gene in previously treated pancreatic cancer. *J Immunother* 36 (7): 382–389.
58. Li, K., Tandurella, J.A., Gai, J. et al. (2022). Multi-omic analyses of changes in the tumor microenvironment of pancreatic adenocarcinoma following neoadjuvant treatment with anti-PD-1 therapy. *Cancer Cell* 40 (11): 1374–1391.e7.
59. Foley, C.R., Swan, S.L., and Swartz, M.A. (2024). Engineering challenges and opportunities in autologous cellular cancer immunotherapy. *J Immunol* 212 (2): 188–198.
60. Montico, B., Lapenta, C., Ravo, M. et al. (2017). Exploiting a new strategy to induce immunogenic cell death to improve dendritic cell-based vaccines for lymphoma immunotherapy. *Oncoimmunology* 6 (11): e1356964.
61. Heras-Murillo, I., Adán-Barrientos, I., Galán, M. et al. (2024). Dendritic cells as orchestrators of anticancer immunity and immunotherapy. *Nat Rev Clin Oncol* 21 (4): 257–277.
62. Nickles, E., Dharmadhikari, B., Yating, L. et al. (2022). Dendritic cell therapy with CD137L-DC-EBV-VAX in locally recurrent or metastatic nasopharyngeal carcinoma is safe and confers clinical benefit. *Cancer Immunol Immunother* 71 (6): 1531–1543.
63. Blander, J.M., Yee Mon, K.J., Jha, A., and Roycroft, D. (2023). The show and tell of cross-presentation. *Adv Immunol* 159: 33–114.
64. Hussain, Z., Zhang, Y., Qiu, L. et al. (2025). Exploring Clec9a in dendritic cell-based tumor immunotherapy for molecular insights and therapeutic potentials. *NPJ Vaccines* 10 ((1)): 27.
65. Ott, P.A., Hu-Lieskovan, S., Chmielowski, B. et al. (2020). A phase Ib trial of personalized neoantigen therapy plus anti-PD-1 in patients with advanced melanoma, non-small cell lung cancer, or bladder cancer. *Cell* 183 (2): 347–362.e24.
66. Tagliamonte, M., Cavalluzzo, B., Mauriello, A. et al. (2023). Molecular mimicry and cancer vaccine development. *Mol Cancer* 22 (1): 75.
67. Braun, D.A., Moranzoni, G., Chea, V. et al. (2025). A neoantigen vaccine generates antitumour immunity in renal cell carcinoma. *Nature* 639 (8054): 474–482.

68. Sultan, H., Takeuchi, Y., Ward, J.P. et al. (2024). Neoantigen-specific cytotoxic Tr1 CD4 T cells suppress cancer immunotherapy. *Nature* 632 (8023): 182–191.
69. Vishweshwaraiah, Y.L. and Dokholyan, N.V. (2022). Toward rational vaccine engineering. *Adv Drug Deliv Rev* 183: 114142.
70. Neeli, P., Chai, D., Roy, D. et al. (2025). DNA vaccines in the post-mRNA era: engineering, applications, and emerging innovations. *Int J Mol Sci* 26 (17): 8716.
71. Yao, R., Xie, C., and Xia, X. (2024 Dec 31). Recent progress in mRNA cancer vaccines. *Hum Vaccin Immunother* 20 (1): 2307187.
72. Jin, L., Zhou, Y., Zhang, S., and Chen, S.J. (2025). mRNA vaccine sequence and structure design and optimization: advances and challenges. *J Biol Chem* 301 (1): 108015.
73. Lundstrom, K. (2021). Self-replicating RNA viruses for vaccine development against infectious diseases and cancer. *Vaccines (Basel)* 9 (10): 1187.
74. Perenkov, A.D., Sergeeva, A.D., Vedunova, M.V., and Krysko, D.V. (2023). In vitro transcribed RNA-based platform vaccines: past, present, and future. *Vaccines (Basel)* 11 (10): 1600.
75. Ramos da Silva, J., Bitencourt Rodrigues, K., Formoso Pelegrin, G. et al. (2023). Single immunizations of self-amplifying or non-replicating mRNA-LNP vaccines control HPV-associated tumors in mice. *Sci Transl Med* 15 (686): eabn3464.
76. Das, U., Banerjee, S., Sarkar, M. et al. (2025). Circular RNA vaccines: pioneering the next-gen cancer immunotherapy. *Cancer Pathog Ther* 3 (4): 309–321.
77. Gong, Z., Hu, W., Zhou, C. et al. (2025). Recent advances and perspectives on the development of circular RNA cancer vaccines. *NPJ Vaccines* 10 (1): 41.
78. Li, H., Peng, K., Yang, K. et al. (2022). Circular RNA cancer vaccines drive immunity in hard-to-treat malignancies. *Theranostics* 12 (14): 6422–6436.
79. Zhang, Y., Liu, X., Shen, T. et al. (2025). Small circular RNAs as vaccines for cancer immunotherapy. *Nat Biomed Eng* 9 (2): 249–267.
80. Zong, Y., Lin, Y., Wei, T., and Cheng, Q. (2023). Lipid nanoparticle (LNP) enables mRNA delivery for cancer therapy. *Adv Mater* 35 (51): e2303261.
81. Zhou, M., Tang, Y., Xu, W. et al. (2023). Bacteria-based immunotherapy for cancer: a systematic review of preclinical studies. *Front Immunol* 14: 1140463.
82. Zhang, S., Li, R., Xu, Y. et al. (2025). Engineered bacteria: Strategies and applications in cancer immunotherapy. *Fundam Res* 5 (3): 1327–1345.
83. Yang, M., Zhong, P., and Wei, P. (2025). Living bacteria: a new vehicle for vaccine delivery in cancer immunotherapy. *Int J Mol Sci* 26 (5): 2056.
84. Garling, A., Auvray F., Epardaud M. et al. (2025). Outer membrane vesicles as a versatile platform for vaccine development: engineering strategies, applications and challenges. *J Extracell Vesicles* 14 (9): e70150.
85. Kenter, G.G., Welters, M.J., Valentijn, A.R. et al. (2009). Vaccination against HPV-16 oncoproteins for vulvar intraepithelial neoplasia. *N Engl J Med* 361 (19): 1838–1847.
86. Massarelli, E., William, W., Johnson, F. et al. (2019). Combining immune checkpoint blockade and tumor-specific vaccine for patients with incurable human papillomavirus 16-related cancer: a phase 2 clinical trial. *JAMA Oncol* 5 (1): 67–73.
87. Sousa, L.G., Rajapakshe, K., Rodriguez Canales, J. et al. (2022). ISA101 and nivolumab for HPV-16+ cancer: updated clinical efficacy and immune correlates of response. *J Immunother Cancer* 10 (2): e004232.
88. Yarchoan, M., Hopkins, A., and Jaffee, E.M. (2017). Tumor mutational burden and response rate to PD-1 inhibition. *N Engl J Med* 377 (25): 2500–2501.
89. Sethna, Z., Guasp, P., Reiche, C. et al. (2025). RNA neoantigen vaccines prime long-lived CD8+ T cells in pancreatic cancer. *Nature* 639 (8056): 1042–1051.
90. Cieri, N. and Wu, C.J. (2021 Apr 13). Splice it up: atypical transcripts to boost leukemia immunotherapy. *Immunity* 54 (4): 608–610.
91. Ehx, G., Larouche, J.D., Durette, C. et al. (2021). Atypical acute myeloid leukemia-specific transcripts generate shared and immunogenic MHC class-I-associated epitopes. *Immunity* 54 (4): 737–752.e10.

92. Wells, D.K., van Buuren, M.M., Dang, K.K. et al. (2020). Key parameters of tumor epitope immunogenicity revealed through a consortium approach improve neoantigen prediction. *Cell* 183 (3): 818–834.e13.
93. Rappaport, A.R., Kyi, C., Lane, M. et al. (2024). A shared neoantigen vaccine combined with immune checkpoint blockade for advanced metastatic solid tumors: phase 1 trial interim results. *Nat Med* 30 (4): 1013–1022.
94. Pounraj, S., Chen, S., Ma, L. et al. (2024). Targeting tumor heterogeneity with neoantigen-based cancer vaccines. *Cancer Res* 84 (3): 353–363.
95. Chen, M. and Zhao, H. (2019). Next-generation sequencing in liquid biopsy: cancer screening and early detection. *Hum Genomics* 13 (1): 34.
96. Faghfuri, E. (2024). Recent advances in personalized cancer immunotherapy with immune checkpoint inhibitors, T cells and vaccines. *Per Med* 21 (1): 45–57.
97. Sahin, U., Derhovanessian, E., Miller, M. et al. (2017). Personalized RNA mutanome vaccines mobilize poly-specific therapeutic immunity against cancer. *Nature* 547 (7662): 222–226.
98. Baharom, F., Ramirez-Valdez, R.A., Tobin, K.K.S. et al. (2021). Intravenous nanoparticle vaccination generates stem-like TCF1+ neoantigen-specific CD8+ T cells. *Nat Immunol* 22 (1): 41–52.
99. James, A., Vajrashree, P.S., Meghana, G.S. et al. (2025). Beyond the blood-brain barrier: intranasal vaccines in cancer immunotherapy. *Crit Rev Oncol Hematol* 216: 104938.
100. Zeng, B., Middelberg, A.P., Gemiarto, A. et al. (2018). Self-adjuvanting nanoemulsion targeting dendritic cell receptor Clec9A enables antigen-specific immunotherapy. *J Clin Invest* 128 (5): 1971–1984.
101. Hussain, A., Moxley-Wyles, B., Bryan, M. et al. (2025). Cancer vaccine trial evaluations: immunobridging and potential immunological endpoints. *Immunother Adv* 5 (1): ltaf016.
102. Rhee, I. (2025). Refining dendritic cell-based cancer vaccines: subset targeting, translational barriers, and emerging strategies. *J Microbiol Biotechnol* 35: e2506021.
103. Verma, N.K., Wong, B.H.S., Poh, Z.S. et al. (2022). Obstacles for T-lymphocytes in the tumour microenvironment: therapeutic challenges, advances and opportunities beyond immune checkpoint. *EBioMedicine* 83: 104216.
104. Baharom, F., Hermans, D., Delamarre, L., and Seder, R.A. (2025). Vax-Innate: improving therapeutic cancer vaccines by modulating T cells and the tumour microenvironment. *Nat Rev Immunol* (3): 195–211.
105. Gomez-Randulfe, I., Lavender, H., Symeonides, S., and Blackhall, F. (2025). Impact of systemic anticancer therapy timing on cancer vaccine immunogenicity: a review. *Ther Adv Med Oncol* 17: 17588359251316988.
106. Wang, J., Ma, J., Xie, F. et al. (2024). Immunogenic cell death-based cancer vaccines: promising prospect in cancer therapy. *Front Immunol* 29 (15): 1389173.
107. Rosenthal, I. and Padler-Karavani, V. (2025). Current landscape of therapeutic cancer vaccines. *Methods Mol Biol* 2926: 1–14.
108. Milhem, M.M., Wise-Draper, T.M., Chandra, S. et al. (2025). Phase 1b/2 study evaluating safety, efficacy and immune effects of TLR9 agonist cavrotolimod with anti-PD-1 antibodies among patients with advanced solid tumors. *J Immunother Cancer* 13 (7): e011651.
109. Hu, Z., Leet, D.E., Allesøe, R.L. et al. (2021). Personal neoantigen vaccines induce persistent memory T cell responses and epitope spreading in patients with melanoma. *Nat Med* 27 (3): 515–525.
110. Verma, V., Shrimali, R.K., Ahmad, S. et al. (2019). PD-1 blockade in subprimed CD8 cells induces dysfunctional PD-1+CD38hi cells and anti-PD-1 resistance. *Nat Immunol* 20 (9): 1231–1243.
111. Vavolizza, R.D., Petroni, G.R., Mauldin, I.S. et al. (2022). Phase I/II clinical trial of a helper peptide vaccine plus PD-1 blockade in PD-1 antibody-naïve and PD-1 antibody-experienced patients with melanoma (MEL64). *J Immunother Cancer* 10 (9): e005424.

112. McNeel, D.G., Eickhoff, J.C., Wargowski, E. et al. (2018). Concurrent, but not sequential, PD-1 blockade with a DNA vaccine elicits antitumor responses in patients with metastatic, castration-resistant prostate cancer. *Oncotarget* 9 (39): 25586–25596.
113. Keskin, D.B., Anandappa, A.J., Sun, J. et al. (2019). Neoantigen vaccine generates intratumoral T cell responses in phase Ib glioblastoma trial. *Nature* 565 (7738): 234–239.
114. Zom, G.G., Welters, M.J., Loof, N.M. et al. (2016). TLR2 ligand-synthetic long peptide conjugates effectively stimulate tumor-draining lymph node T cells of cervical cancer patients. *Oncotarget* 7 (41): 67087–67100.
115. Stein MN, Fong L, Tutrone Ret al. ADXS31142 immunotherapy ± pembrolizumab treatment for metastatic castration-resistant prostate cancer: open-label phase I/II KEYNOTE-046 study. *Oncologist* 2022 27(6):453–461. doi: https://doi.org/10.1093/oncolo/oyac048.
116. Le, D.T., Brockstedt, D.G., Nir-Paz, R. et al. (2012). A live-attenuated Listeria vaccine (ANZ-100) and a live-attenuated Listeria vaccine expressing mesothelin (CRS-207) for advanced cancers: phase I studies of safety and immune induction. *Clin Cancer Res* 18 (3): 858–868.
117. Kim, S.H., Castro, F., Gonzalez, D. et al. (2008). Mage-b vaccine delivered by recombinant *Listeria monocytogenes* is highly effective against breast cancer metastases. *Br J Cancer* 99 (5): 741–749.
118. Duan, F., Chen, J., Yao, H. et al. (2021). Enhanced therapeutic efficacy of Listeria-based cancer vaccine with codon-optimized HPV16 E7. *Hum Vaccin Immunother* 17 (6): 1568–1577.

PART III

Immunotherapy in Infectious Diseases

CHAPTER 8

Immunotherapy for Viral Infections: Mechanisms, Clinical Applications, and Future Directions

STEPHANIE JOST, CORDELIA MANICKAM, AND R. KEITH REEVES
Division of Innate and Comparative Immunology, Centre for Human Systems Immunology, Department of Surgery, Duke University School of Medicine, Durham, NC, USA

LEARNING OBJECTIVES

- Understand the various challenges associated with the treatment of chronic viral infections or severe acute infections caused by respiratory viruses.
- Recognise how distinct immunotherapeutic strategies can be applied to specific viral infections based on the mechanism of action.
- Be cognisant of successes achieved so far with immunotherapies for viral infections and identify the major roadblocks limiting their use or efficacy, including toxicities and viral escape.
- Synthesise the future directions of immunotherapies for viral infections, including clinical evaluation of combination therapies and development or optimisation of new or existing products, respectively.

8.1 INTRODUCTION

Viral infections continue to be a major global cause of mortality and morbidity [1]. As of this writing, human immunodeficiency virus (HIV), hepatitis C virus (HCV), and hepatitis B virus (HBV) remain top contributors to premature mortality worldwide, along with respiratory viruses like influenza, severe acute respiratory syndrome coronavirus 2 (SARS-CoV-2), and respiratory syncytial virus (RSV) (Table 8.1).

In immunocompetent hosts, infections typically resolve through coordinated immune responses, yet certain viruses can establish chronic infections by evading or subverting these defences. For instance, RNA viruses (e.g. HIV, HCV) exhibit high mutation rates that facilitate the emergence of escape mutants, enabling evasion of host immune responses and antiretroviral therapies. Interference with innate immune signalling pathways and establishment of reservoirs or niches

TABLE 8.1 Top global viral pathogens.

Pathogen	Global burden	Estimated mortality	Economic impact
COVID-19/ SARS-CoV-2	779 million (since 2020)*	6.9 million (since 2020)*	>3 trillion
HIV/AIDS	40.8 million#	630,000/year#	> 20 billion/year
Hepatitis B & C viruses	304 million*	1.3 million/year*	>40 billion/year[a]
Influenza virus	Approx. billion cases*	0.29–0.65 million/year*	>100 billion/year[b]
Dengue virus	100–400 million*	Approx. 52,000/year*	8 billion/year*

* World Health Organisation information sheet.
# UNAIDS report 2024.
[a] Wang et al. [129].
[b] Walsh and Maher [130].

poorly accessible to immune cells represent other major mechanisms by which viruses, such as HIV, HCV, or HBV, persist despite an otherwise functional immune system. HIV also directly targets and depletes $CD4^+$ T cells, progressively weakening immune surveillance.

Untreated, chronic viral infections can lead to progressive disease, partly driven by active viral replication that promotes chronic immune activation, inflammation, and tissue damage. In contrast to HIV, HCV, and HBV, other viruses, such as herpesviruses or polyomaviruses, typically establish latent infections with minimal replication and immune evasion, allowing them to persist without causing overt disease in healthy hosts. These viruses are usually controlled by the immune system and cause significant pathology only in immunocompromised hosts.

Acute infections, including those caused by respiratory viruses like influenza, RSV, and coronaviruses, can also result in severe morbidity and mortality, particularly in vulnerable populations. The host immune response, while essential for viral clearance, can become dysregulated, leading to excessive production of pro-inflammatory cytokines and chemokines – a phenomenon known as a 'cytokine storm'. This hyperinflammatory state contributes to widespread tissue injury, increased vascular permeability, and pulmonary oedema. In severe cases, these processes culminate in acute respiratory distress syndrome (ARDS), a potentially fatal lung condition associated with breathing difficulties and low blood oxygen levels. Secondary bacterial infections and multi-organ dysfunction further compound the risk of death. Host age, comorbidities, immune status, viral burden, and virulence influence disease severity.

Antiviral treatments help prevent severe disease, decrease complication risks, and improve overall clinical outcomes. However, effective antiviral therapies are not available for all viral infections. When they are, frequent viral genome mutations lead to drug resistance and increased virulence, necessitating continual development of new antivirals. Several challenges are linked to the development of effective antiviral therapies. First, suppressing factors crucial for viral replication broadly implies targeting the host cell machinery that viruses rely on, making treatments potentially toxic. Few unique viral antigens are essential for replication, limiting the number of non-host drug targets. Developing drugs that inhibit viral assembly or release rather than replication is feasible but requires detailed knowledge of viral structure and life cycle, which is often unavailable. Finally, despite helping contain viral replication, antiviral drugs do not necessarily allow viral clearance. In the case of HIV, antiretroviral therapy (ART) significantly reduces mortality among people living with HIV (PLWH) by effectively suppressing plasma viremia [2, 3]. However, ART does not cure HIV infection due to persistent tissue reservoirs of replication-competent latent HIV that can rapidly rebound following ART interruption or failure. Moreover, chronic HIV infection, despite long-term ART use, is associated with persistent inflammation, premature ageing, and increased risk of chronic disease [4]. Similarly, complete eradication of HBV infection is rarely achievable with available treatments. However, antiviral therapy effectively mitigates viral replication and disease progression in individuals with chronic infection, protecting against cirrhosis and hepatocellular carcinoma. Thus, the development of effective strategies to eliminate persistent viral reservoirs or achieve long-term immunological control is critical to attain drug-free remission of viral infection and curtail the detrimental consequences of viral-associated comorbidities and/or complications.

Managing established or emerging viral infections remains a significant challenge, underscoring the critical need for innovative therapeutic approaches. Immunotherapies are particularly attractive because they enhance or restore the immune system's ability to recognise and eliminate viruses, especially when traditional antiviral treatments are insufficient or resistance has developed. They also offer potential durable control or even eradication of chronic viral infections by targeting latent reservoirs and modulating immune exhaustion. This chapter presents a comprehensive overview of immunotherapeutic approaches for viral infectious diseases (Table 8.2; Figure 8.1), emphasising strategies targeting HIV (Figure 8.2) and other major viruses. We will explore modalities such as antibodies, cytokines, Toll-like receptor (TLR) agonists, adoptive cell therapies, and therapeutic vaccines, as well as emerging innovations to improve the efficacy and safety of immunotherapies.

8.2 IMMUNOTHERAPIES FOR VIRAL INFECTIONS IN THE CLINIC

8.2.1 Anti-viral Antibodies

Antibodies have been used to prevent and treat viral infections for over 100 years. The first passive immunisation strategies consisted of injecting convalescent plasma as emergency treatments during viral outbreaks, when effective vaccines or antivirals were lacking. This stopgap therapy was widely used during the 1918 influenza pandemic and the 2014 Ebola outbreak and was rapidly deployed at the beginning of the SARS-CoV-2 pandemic. Intravenous immunoglobulin (IVIG) represents another antibody-based therapy comprising pooled immunoglobulin (Ig) from healthy donors [5], providing antibodies against diverse antigens. IVIG is a preventive and therapeutic option for several viruses, including RSV, particularly in immunocompromised populations. Beyond IVIG, hyperimmune globulin preparations

TABLE 8.2 Traditional and emerging immunotherapeutic approaches to viral infections.

	Immunomodulators	Passive immunizations	Cellular therapies	Vaccine strategies
Traditional approaches	■ Adjuvants e.g. Alum, BCG ■ Cytokine infusions e.g. Interferon-alpha, IL-2	■ Convalescent plasma/serum ■ Purified immunoglobulins ■ Antiserum	■ Adoptive T cell transfer ■ Unmodified NK cell infusions ■ Donor lymphocyte infusions	■ Live attenuated e.g. Measles virus vaccine ■ Inactivated (killed) e.g. Inactivated Polio vaccine ■ Subunit
Emerging strategies	■ TLR agonists e.g. TLR7 agonist (vestalimod) ■ Cytokine superagonists e.g. N-803 ■ Immune exhaustion blockade e.g. PD-1/CTLA4 blockade	■ Monoclonal Abs (mAb) e.g. broadly neutralizing antibodies (BNAbs) ■ Engineered antibodies e.g. bi-specific, tri-specific	■ Chimeric antigen receptor (CAR) or TCR-engineered immune cells e.g. CAR-T cells, CAR-NK cells ■ Gene-edited immune cells e.g. CCR5 deleted T cells, tissue homing receptor expressing cells	■ mRNA based e.g. SARS-Cov-2 mRNA vaccine ■ Viral vector-based e.g. Adenovirus-based vaccines ■ DNA/RNA-based ■ Nanoparticle/viral-like particle ■ Germline targeting

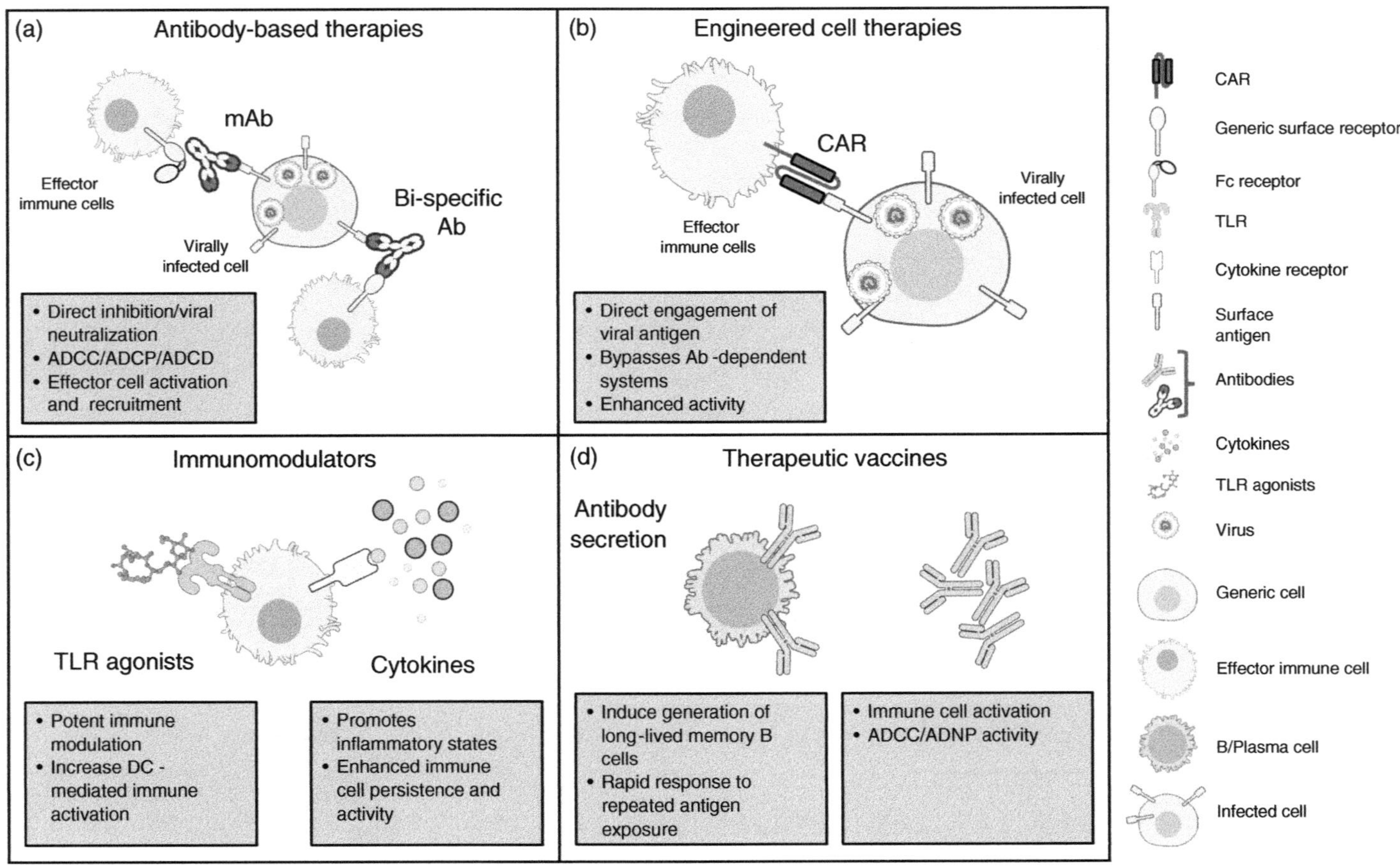

FIGURE 8.1 Immunotherapeutics for viral infections. Four broad categories of emerging immune-based strategies include: (a) antibody-based therapies – ranging from monoclonal antibodies, broadly neutralizing antibodies, and Fc-engineered antibodies in mono-, bi- and multivalent formats that induce neutralizing and Fc-mediated effector functions; (b) engineered cell-based therapies such as CAR-T cells, CAR-NK cells, and gene-edited lymphocytes for autologous/allogenic/off-the-shelf therapies; (c) immunomodulating agents such as cytokines, checkpoint inhibitors, and TLR agonists that enhance viral immunity or dampen immune exhaustion; and (d) therapeutic vaccines, designed to boost virus-specific T-cell and B-cell responses through platforms such as DNA, mRNA, viral vectors, and nanoparticle immunogens. In practice, combinations of these strategies are employed to achieve a more effective and durable antiviral response. Ab, antibody; ADCC, antibody-dependent cellular cytotoxicity; ADCD, antibody-dependent complement deposition; ADCP, antibody-dependent cellular phagocytosis; CAR, chimeric antigen receptor; mAb, monoclonal antibody; TLR, Toll-like receptor.

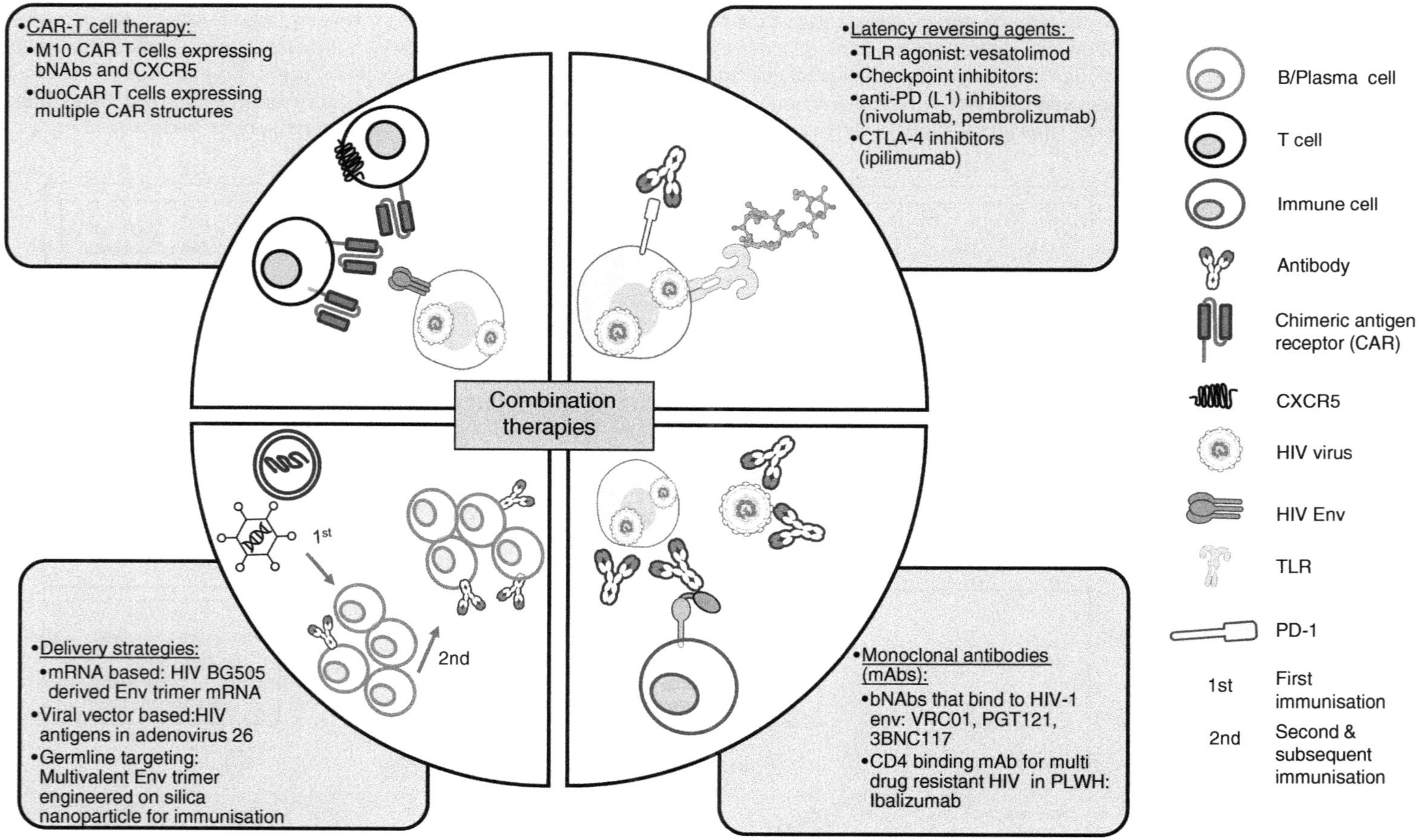

FIGURE 8.2 HIV-specific immunotherapeutics. Examples of immune-based therapeutics against HIV, based on the mode of action, are represented in the figure.

are derived from the plasma of donors with high antibody titres against a specific pathogen, providing targeted passive immunity. Examples include post-exposure prophylaxis scenarios where immediate protection against HBV is needed and for preventing HCV or HBV recurrence post-transplantation.

Since the early trials with convalescent plasma, substantial progress has been made in isolating and engineering virus-specific monoclonal antibodies (mAbs) that offer higher specificity, reproducibility, and scalability. In general, antibodies inhibit virus replication at multiple steps in the virus life cycle through diverse mechanisms [6] including: (i) prevent attachment of the virus to its cognate cell surface receptor(s), (ii) block viral entry into target cells by interrupting fusion between the virus and cell membrane, (iii) block the egress of new viral particles from infected cells, and (iv) recruit and engage Fc receptor (FcR)-bearing cells, thereby promoting elimination of infected cells by immune effectors such as natural killer (NK) cells and monocytes/macrophages.

Of particular interest for strategies aimed at controlling HIV in the absence of ART, a specialised class of mAbs known as broadly neutralising antibodies (bNAbs) was identified. bNAbs target conserved regions of HIV envelope proteins and neutralise a broad spectrum of HIV strains. Since the 2010s, treatment with second-generation bNAbs (i.e. VRC01, 3BNC117), which demonstrate enhanced potency against even more HIV strains, has improved durability of viral control upon ART interruption [7]. While passive administration of a single bNAb is insufficient to maintain long-term viral control, combining two or more bNAbs has demonstrated improved viral suppression and delayed rebound during analytical treatment interruption in individuals with HIV strains sensitive to antibody targeting. In addition, bNAb combinations are a promising tool to reduce the latent HIV reservoir. When administered in conjunction with latency-reversing agents (LRAs), which prompt HIV to resume expression of the Env protein on infected cells, bNAbs can target latently infected cells for elimination by FcR-bearing immune effector cells.

The decline in plasma antibody levels over time and the emergence of resistance continue to pose significant obstacles to bNAb therapy, with nonresponders often carrying viral variants inherently resistant to the administered antibodies before infusion. Several strategies are being explored to circumvent these limitations, including the repeated administration of multiple bNAbs and the engineering of bNAbs with extended half-lives and/or improved effector functions [8, 9]. In 2018, the FDA approved the use of ibalizumab, an mAb administered with other antiretroviral agents for the treatment of PLWH with multidrug-resistant HIV. This antibody prevents HIV entry into the cell after HIV attaches to CD4 by targeting CD4 itself.

Several antibody-based strategies for HBV have entered clinical trials to complement or replace long-term antiviral therapy in patients with chronic HBV infection. This includes HepB mAb19 and VIR-3434, two mAbs that bind conserved regions of HBsAg, and GIGA-2339, a recombinant polyclonal antibody therapy that broadly targets HBV epitopes. These antibodies block viral entry and efficiently engage Fc-mediated immune effector functions, enhancing elimination of infected cells. In contrast, mAbs targeting HCV remain primarily in preclinical or exploratory stages, largely due to the success of direct-acting antivirals (DAAs), which achieve high cure rates.

mAbs are a valuable strategy in preventing and treating respiratory infections, particularly for high-risk populations. For RSV, FDA-approved mAbs like palivizumab and the more recent nirsevimab offer effective prophylaxis in infants and young children, with efforts to expand coverage to older adults and immunocompromised individuals. In the case of SARS-CoV-2, several mAbs were granted emergency use authorisation during the pandemic, though many lost efficacy due to viral evolution and emerging variants. Pemivibart, among the few mAbs still authorised in 2025, is administered as pre-exposure prophylaxis in immunocompromised individuals unlikely to mount an adequate response to vaccination. For influenza, mAb development remains largely investigational, with current candidates focusing on conserved epitopes to achieve broader and more durable protection. Some mAbs under investigation [10, 11] include viral entry inhibitors targeting the haemagglutinin (HA) head, membrane fusion inhibitors targeting the HA stem (NCT02603952, NCT02623322, and NCT04033406), and viral budding disruptors targeting matrix protein 2 or endosomal trafficking component TSG101 (NCT01390025 and NCT01299142).

In summary, the clinical use of antibodies currently presents several limitations: viral resistance, limited durability, high production costs, and risks such as antibody-dependent enhancement, potentially exacerbating disease. However, antibody-based therapies have shown remarkable success in neutralising viruses during outbreaks and hold tremendous potential to achieve functional cures in people with chronic infections and as a critical adjunct to vaccines and antivirals in managing respiratory viral diseases.

8.2.2 Immunomodulatory Antibodies

Similarly to cancer, sustained antigenic activation in chronic infections like HIV, HCV, or HBV promotes exhaustion of T and NK cells [12]. This dysfunctional state is characterised by diminished antiviral and proliferative activity and increased expression of inhibitory receptors, all of which compromise efficient viral suppression by T and NK cells. In this respect, and based on their extensive use as cancer immunotherapies, mAbs that inhibit checkpoint pathways, or immune checkpoint inhibitors (ICIs), hold promise for reinvigorating immunity to chronic viruses [13–15]. In PLWH, emerging data indicate that HIV-specific T-cell responses are boosted by ICI, especially under sustained antigenic stimulation. The benefits go beyond reversing immune exhaustion; ICIs, particularly mAbs targeting PD-1/PD-L1, specifically target the HIV reservoir. Indeed, latent HIV is predominantly localised within resting memory T cells exhibiting high expression of immune checkpoint receptors, including PD-1, LAG-3, and/or TIGIT [16–19]. Moreover, a large fraction of the HIV reservoir in lymphoid tissues resides in T follicular helper cells, which express high levels of PD-1 [20–23]. Accordingly, ICI induces HIV latency reversal [24, 25], likely enabling immune detection of reservoir cells. However, studies examining how ICI influences the latent HIV reservoir and viral control following ART interruption are limited and report inconsistent findings. Several clinical trials in PLWH – both with and without cancer – are currently in progress and will clarify the therapeutic benefits of ICI, expected to be significantly enhanced in combination with other approaches. Sparse data are available on the ability of ICI to improve control of HBV and HCV, as studies have mainly focused on the safety of ICI treatment in patients with chronic HBV/HCV infection and cancer.

In contrast to immune exhaustion observed in chronic infections, severe respiratory infections are characterised by harmful immune hyperactivation, necessitating therapeutic strategies that precisely suppress aberrant immune pathways. Several mAbs approved to treat chronic inflammatory conditions and autoimmune diseases have been investigated as therapeutic options for severe COVID-19 cases. Elevated levels of proinflammatory cytokines, such as TNF-α and IL-6, are associated with poor clinical outcomes in severe SARS-CoV-2 infection [26, 27]. While TNF-α inhibitors (i.e. infliximab, etanercept) or mAbs targeting the IL-6 receptor (i.e. tocilizumab, sarilumab) have demonstrated efficacy in reducing disease severity and mortality among specific subsets of patients with COVID-19, further investigations would advance our understanding of the therapeutic mechanisms and clinical utility of these mAbs in SARS-CoV-2 treatment.

Genetic studies have revealed associations between genetic variants in the chemokine receptor CCR5 and the development of severe COVID-19 [28, 29], which is further supported by elevated levels of CCR5 ligands, including CCL3 and CCL5 [30, 31], in patients with severe SARS-CoV-2 infection. Based on these observations, leronlimab, an mAb that blocks CCR5 on immune cells, was evaluated for its ability to prevent inflammatory cell recruitment to the lungs and mitigate inflammation associated with severe COVID-19. While clinical benefits of leronlimab treatment have been reported in severely ill patients, its exact role in COVID-19 management remains unelucidated. Before its assessment in COVID-19 patients, leronlimab had been investigated as a therapeutic agent for HIV infection, based on its ability to block CCR5-mediated entry of a broad range of HIV strains into $CD4^+$ T cells [32]. Clinical trials have demonstrated its ability to significantly reduce viral load in PLWH with multidrug-resistant HIV strains [33] and mediate potent and prolonged antiretroviral activity in ART-free viremic PLWH [34]. Its favourable safety profile and potential for monotherapy or pre-exposure prophylaxis make it a promising candidate in the evolving HIV treatment landscape. Among these immunomodulatory mAbs, only tocilizumab is currently FDA-approved to treat viral infections, exclusively in hospitalised adults with severe COVID-19. While the immunosuppressive effect of mAbs offers a plausible therapeutic rationale for severe cytokine-driven respiratory viral infections beyond SARS-CoV-2, their use in influenza or RSV infection remains unexplored in clinical trials.

8.2.3 Interferons

Pegylated interferon-alpha (peg-IFN-α), a modified IFN-α with an extended *in vivo* half-life, remains a clinically relevant antiviral therapy, particularly for chronic HBV infection management. Peg-IFN-α is associated with modest response rates, even when administered with antiviral drugs, with limited tolerability and contraindications in patients with advanced liver disease. Yet, it remains a valuable therapeutic option in specific patient populations with favourable baseline characteristics. Peg-IFN-α also offers potential for a functional cure [35], especially in combination with emerging therapies, including DAAs and immune modulators aimed at reviving or stimulating HBV-specific immune responses.

Peg-IFN-α combined with ribavirin was the cornerstone of antiviral therapy for chronic HCV infection before the advent of DAAs. Despite its finite treatment course and lack of viral resistance, Peg-IFN-α therapy was limited by significant adverse effects. DAAs have largely supplanted their use due to superior efficacy, tolerability, and safety profiles, though Peg-IFN-α is considered in resource-limited settings or select clinical scenarios.

Peg-IFN-α has also been explored as a potential adjunct in HIV cure strategies due to its ability to activate innate immune responses and reduce viral reservoirs [36, 37]. Studies in HIV/HCV coinfected individuals undergoing Peg-IFN-α and ribavirin therapy have demonstrated significant reductions in HIV DNA levels in $CD4^+$ T cells, suggesting a reservoir-modulating effect. This reduction was strongly associated with NK cell activation [38, 39] rather than HIV-specific $CD8^+$ T-cell responses. Specific IFN-α subtypes, IFN-α8 and IFN-α14, have shown potent anti-HIV activity with minimal immune activation, while others enhance NK cell function, indicating potential combination approaches with LRAs, bNAbs, or therapeutic vaccines.

Interferon-lambda (IFN-λ) plays a specialised role in antiviral immunity at epithelial barrier surfaces such as the respiratory and gastrointestinal tracts and has been evaluated as an alternative to IFN-α for the treatment of chronic HBV and HCV [40]. These trials generated encouraging data supporting the use of IFN-λ combined with antiviral drugs in supporting immune-mediated control of HBV. When administered early, peg-IFN-λ has demonstrated antiviral efficacy and safety by reducing severe outcomes in COVID-19 outpatients. Improved clinical outcomes were also reported in patients with moderate SARS-CoV-2 infection receiving Peg-IFN-α combined with standard of care [41, 42]. Its use in influenza and RSV remains experimental, with no clinical data currently available [43].

8.2.4 Interleukins

Interleukins (ILs) represent promising candidates for therapeutic interventions against viral infections [44, 45]. High-dose IL-2 immunotherapy, valued for its ability to activate and expand cytotoxic effector cells, was primarily investigated in HIV infection. However, enthusiasm waned after large trials showed limited impact on viral control and survival, coupled with significant toxicity and complex dosing requirements. Recent research has focused on engineering IL-2 variants with enhanced efficacy and reduced toxicity, as well as investigating how low-dose IL-2 modulates immune responses and may promote viral clearance [46–48].

The interleukin-15 (IL-15) superagonist, N-803, represents an innovative therapeutic approach to enhance immune cell function and potentially address viral reservoirs [49, 50]. N-803 has been found to reduce the HIV viral reservoir in lymphoid tissue, as evidenced by decreases in viral RNA^+ and DNA^+ cells and reductions in ileal infected cells [51]. N-803 can achieve these antiviral effects by enhancing the function, proliferation, activation, and mobilisation of immune cells, including $CD4^+$ T cells, $CD8^+$ T cells, and NK cells [50, 52]. A Phase I study of N-803 [NCT02191098] identified a maximum tolerated dose and observed mild primary adverse events, as well as encouraging immunological activity, including peak immune cell proliferation at four days post-dosing [49]. However, only a limited direct reduction in viral reservoir was observed in the context of SHIV infection, suggesting that therapeutic applications of N-803 likely require combination with LRAs to be both safe and effective [52].

IL-22 has shown promise in clinical trials, shortening hospital stays for individuals with severe COVID-19 and reducing RSV production [53, 54]. The IL-6 family, including IL-6, IL-11, IL-27, and IL-31, exhibits clinical relevance in respiratory diseases, and IL-6 inhibitors such as tocilizumab are useful to control overt immune activation [55, 56]. Similarly, therapeutic inhibition of IL-1β has been shown to prolong survival and reduce inflammation during influenza infections [57].

The most exciting developments in IL therapeutics research lie in combination immunotherapy strategies involving bNAbs and LRAs [58]. For example, the LRA vorinostat has demonstrated clinical relevance by enabling IL-15-treated NK cells to clear latently HIV-infected cells successfully [59]. However, a challenge to these combinational therapies remains their inability to reactivate a substantial proportion of the latent HIV reservoir, indicating the need for continued research and more sophisticated therapeutic approaches [58].

8.2.5 TLR Agonists

TLRs are key innate immune proteins and members of the pattern recognition receptor family. TLRs are critical in host defence against microbial pathogens, recognising pathogen-associated molecular patterns and self-derived damage-associated molecular patterns, thereby activating specific downstream signalling pathways that direct and modulate immune responses [60]. Due to their potent immunomodulatory functions, TLRs are promising adjuvants for vaccination against HIV, HBV, HCV, SARS-CoV-2, and others [61–65] or as components of HIV cure strategies.

The therapeutic potential of TLR7 and TLR8 agonists is being actively explored for HIV and HBV infections. TLR7/8 have a broad range of immunomodulatory functions, including (i) stimulating dendritic cells to upregulate co-stimulatory receptors and produce proinflammatory cytokines [61, 64], (ii) stimulating Ig and cytokine secretion by B cells [64, 66], (iii) activating NK cells to produce IFN-y [64, 67], and (iv) stimulating cytokine and IL secretion by T cells [64, 68].

In nonhuman primate models of HIV infection, the TLR7 agonist GS-9620 (vesatolimod) combined with a therapeutic vaccine and/or bNAbs delayed viral rebound, lowered setpoint, and achieved remission after ART interruption [69–75]. Human studies confirmed that GS-9620 induces strong immune activation, although clinical trials in PLWH have not consistently translated these benefits into durable ART-free remission [76–79].

In chronic HBV infection, the TLR8 agonist GS-9688 (selgantolimod) yielded promising early-phase clinical results, with strong innate immune activation, including IL-12 production and NK/T-cell stimulation [80]. However, these studies have not shown consistent improvements in viral clearance or HBsAg loss, highlighting the need for combination strategies with antivirals, therapeutic vaccines, or other immunomodulators to achieve a functional cure.

8.2.6 Immune Cell Therapies

Immune cell therapies are rapidly emerging as a transformative frontier in viral disease treatment, surpassing their established cancer therapy roles [81]. One cell therapeutic strategy in cancer immunotherapy involves the use of engineered T cells that target tumour or viral antigens. During HIV infection, predominant T-cell engineering approaches include transduction of T cells with a lentiviral vector encoding either a TCR that recognises conserved HIV epitopes or a CAR specific to HIV envelope proteins. However, a comparison study by Zhou et al. [82] indicated that HIV-specific CAR T cells were superior to HIV-specific TCR-mediated T cells due to their rapid target recognition and killing of HIV-infected cells, as evidenced by caspase-3 release in infected cells. In addition, there are several ways to improve the potency of the CAR-T construct [83], including (i) a co-stimulatory signal domain such as CD28 and

4-1BB, (ii) multiple domains specific for HIV Env peptide and CD4 receptor leading to bispecific and trispecific CARs, (iii) modifications that enhance tissue trafficking and persistence such as CXCR5 for migration to lymph nodes (key HIV reservoir sites), (iv) additional armouring with bNAbs or cytokines such as IL-15, (v) modifications to prevent exhaustion such as PD-1 inhibitors, and (vi) safety switches or tuneable systems to minimise off-target toxicity. HIV-specific CAR T cells in clinical trials include anti-HIV duo CAR T cells targeting multiple highly conserved HIV gp120 Env glycoprotein epitopes using a two-molecule CAR structure [NCT04648046], which has already received FDA approval [84, 85]; bNAb-derived CAR T cells [NCT03240328] [86]; anti-HIV CAR-expressing CMV-specific T cells [NCT06252402]; $CD4^+CAR^+$ zinc finger nuclease-modified T cells [NCT03617198]; and M10 cells, which are anti-HIV CAR T cells armed with endogenic bNAbs and the follicle homing receptor CXCR5 [87].

As a therapy for severe SARS-CoV-2 infection, partially HLA-matched, convalescent donor-derived SARS-CoV-2-specific T cells are being investigated in a Phase I/II clinical trial [NCT05447013] [88]. Another Phase I trial [NCT05141058] is currently underway to assess the safety of coronavirus-specific T cells for preventing SARS-CoV-2 infection, specifically in immunocompromised haematopoietic stem cell transplantation patients [89]. For HBV, a Phase I trial [NCT06885710] is underway to test the safety and efficacy of autologous T cells transfected with mRNA encoding HBV-specific TCR in combination with nucleos(t)ide analogues (called HBV LioCyx-M) in HBeAg-positive and negative chronic HBV patients [90].

In addition to T cells, CAR engineering techniques are also being applied to NK cells, although few are in clinical trials for the treatment of viral infections. Indeed, autologous and allogenic primary NK cells and NK-932 cell lines are suitable for genetic modification for immunotherapy due to their potent antiviral and antitumoural roles [91, 92]. Further, NK cell therapies have a more manageable safety profile than T-cell therapies and do not necessarily require autologous transfer [92]. In a Phase I/II clinical trial [NCT04324996], universal, off-the-shelf, NKG2D ACE-2 CAR NK cells secreting IL-15 super agonists and GM-CSF neutralising single-chain variable fragments were investigated in early-stage COVID-19 patients. In a Phase I clinical trial of six PLWH, a single infusion of haploidentical NK cells, given with either IL-2 [NCT03346499] or N-803 [NCT0389940], was well tolerated and led to a moderate decrease in HIV-producing cells in lymph nodes [93], providing proof-of-principle that CAR-NK cells can mediate viral control.

CAR T and NK cell therapies for viral diseases are expanding but still face significant and unique challenges compared to cancer therapy. Viral diversity and rapid mutation rate, such as in HIV, lead to the emergence of immune escape variants, requiring additional therapeutic components such as bNAbs and immune modulators. Practical concerns about cost, scalability, and whether such complex therapies are needed compared to effective antiviral drugs persist, although they offer unique potential to target latent reservoirs.

8.2.7 Therapeutic Vaccines

Therapeutic vaccines for chronic viral infections stimulate host immune responses to control or eliminate persistent pathogens, such as HIV and HBV. However, unlike prophylactic vaccines, therapeutic vaccines are used to enhance virus-specific immune responses in persons already living with the infection and are often combined with other antiviral therapies.

Therapeutic vaccination for HIV has long been a strategy to control virus replication and/or reduce latent reservoirs. Momentum is building around clinical trials exploring novel vaccine platforms combined with traditional and new adjuvants or other immunomodulators. A Phase I trial [NCT06680479] evaluating the CH505 TF chTrimer vaccine with 3M-052-AF and aluminium hydroxide in individuals on suppressive ART aims to elicit HIV envelope-specific B-cell responses [94]. A Phase I/IIa trial [NCT06071767] investigates a triple regimen combining conserved mosaic T-cell vaccines (ChAdOx1 and MVA), the TLR7 agonist vesatolimod, and bNAbs to induce HIV control during analytical treatment interruption in acutely treated individuals [95]. Additionally, [NCT05217641] is assessing the soluble and membrane-bound HIV BG505 isolate-derived envelope trimer mRNA, designed to stimulate bNAb precursors through germline-targeting strategies [96]. These trials reflect a shift towards multicomponent immunotherapies that synergise innate and adaptive responses to achieve durable viral suppression.

Parallel advances in HBV therapeutic vaccine development evaluate independent but related strategies. A Phase Ia trial [NCT05727267] evaluates a heterologous prime-boost approach using HEPLISAV B followed by TherVacB, a therapeutic vaccine based on HBV surface and core antigens delivered via protein and MVA vectors [97]. This strategy aims to elicit robust, sustained HBV-specific T-cell responses capable of controlling or eliminating chronic HBV infection. Separately, a randomised clinical trial of εPA-44 [NCT00869778], a liposome-based lipopeptide vaccine, demonstrated enhanced HBeAg seroconversion and durable off-treatment effects in patients living with chronic HBV [98]. These studies highlight the potential of nanoparticle and vector-based platforms to overcome immune tolerance and restore antiviral immunity in persistent viral infections like HBV.

HIV and HBV therapeutic vaccine efforts aim to stimulate and redirect host immunity through similar approaches. However, subtle differences exist that may present unique challenges and opportunities, such as HIV persisting in the central nervous system and lymphoid tissues and HBV replicating in the liver, both of which may be poorly penetrated by ART and other immunotherapies [99–102]. Despite these differences, the convergence of immunological design principles and translational platforms suggests growing opportunities for cross-pathogen innovation against chronic viral infections.

8.2.8 Boxed Case Studies

CASE STUDY 8.1: TO INVESTIGATE THE SAFETY AND EFFICACY OF UB-421 MONOTHERAPY IN HIV-INFECTED ADULTS

HIV-specific bNAbs could incur resistant HIV in PLWH, leading to viral rebound in the absence of ART. To circumvent viral escape, investigators utilised UB-421 as an antiviral agent in a Phase II clinical study [NCT02369146] as a monotherapy in ART-stabilised individuals with HIV during structured treatment interruptions [103]. UB-421 is a humanised Fc-aglycosylated IgG1 mAb that binds to conformational epitopes on the HIV receptor complex, including the CD4 receptor, with high affinity, thus competitively blocking HIV entry without depleting $CD4^+$ T cells. Remarkably, viral suppression without rebound and emergence of resistant HIV variants was observed during 8–16 weeks of treatment. While $CD4^+$ T-cell counts remained stable, UB-421 administration significantly reduced the frequency of T regulatory cells, which can harbour high levels of HIV proviral DNA. Further, in another case study [104], a 58-year-old male living with multidrug-resistant HIV and Kaposi sarcoma was treated with UB-421 and the capsid inhibitor lenacapavir, resulting in delayed but sustained suppression of plasma viremia and elevated $CD4^+$ T-cell count. The individual was also treated with pembrolizumab for Kaposi sarcoma. No evidence of viral evolution or UB-421-resistant viruses was reported. An *ex vivo* study of 93 infectious viral isolates derived from 11 PLWH harbouring multidrug-resistant HIV found no resistance to UB-421 but did show resistance to at least two of the eight bNAbs tested [105]. These findings underscore the promise of receptor-targeted antibodies as an alternative or adjunctive treatment for PLWH harbouring multidrug- or pan-resistant viruses. However, the durability and long-term safety of UB-421 remain open questions.

CASE STUDY 8.2: HUMAN PAPILLOMAVIRUS (HPV) DIRECTED IMMUNOTHERAPY

HPV belongs to the family Papillomaviridae and is transmitted through sexual and skin-to-skin contact. High-risk HPV strains, including HPV16 and 18, are associated with malignancies, including cervical, oropharyngeal, anal, and other anogenital cancers. HPV serves as both a viral pathogen and driver of tumorigenesis (specifically the HPV oncoproteins E6 and E7); therefore, immunotherapeutic strategies intersect both virology and oncology. These strategies include:

- Preclinical therapeutic lipid nanoparticle that encapsulates both mRNA vaccine encoding for HPV E7 oncoprotein and a tumour-specific antigen of HPV-positive oropharyngeal squamous cell carcinoma has shown promising immunogenicity in mice and nonhuman primate models [106, 107].
- Phase 1/2 nonrandomised clinical trial (NCT04287868) [108] shows improved overall survival and an acceptable safety profile when patients with HPV-positive tumours were given a combination of PDS0101, a micellar therapeutic vaccine that targets the HPV 16 subtype E6 and E7 oncoproteins; PDS01ADC, a tumour-targeting IL-12 antibody drug conjugate; and Binatrafusp alpha (BA), a fusion protein that sequesters TGF-b and blocks PD-1.
- Phase III clinical trial showed clinically meaningful improvements in overall survival of patients with metastatic cervical cancer when treated with pembrolizumab and chemotherapy (NCT03635567) [109].

CASE STUDY 8.3: IN NEED OF UNIVERSAL INFLUENZA VACCINES

Influenza causes seasonal epidemics worldwide and thus represents a significant global health care burden. Its high mutation rate and frequent antigenic shift and drift undermine influenza vaccine efficacy and promote antiviral resistance. It is imperative to develop universal vaccines/immunotherapies less vulnerable to viral variability. There are several candidates under clinical and preclinical development. In a mouse model of IAV, recombinant adenovirus-based vaccines expressing influenza nucleoprotein, HA, and the ectodomain of matrix protein 2 showed efficacy and safety when administered intranasally [110]. In a Phase III clinical trial, a quadrivalent nucleoside-modified RNA influenza vaccine was found to have superior efficacy but also more reactogenicity events over the control quadrivalent inactivated vaccine against A/H3N2 and A/H1N1 strains (NCT05540522) [111]. A mosaic nanoparticle vaccine that co-displays four HA of licensed quadrivalent influenza vaccines (FluMos v-1), developed as a universal vaccine, awaits results from the completed clinical trial (NCT04896086) [112]. While several candidates are being tested, a universal influenza vaccine remains elusive. Incremental advances in influenza immunotherapeutics will nevertheless reduce overall influenza-related mortality and hospitalisations.

8.3 CHALLENGES AND CONTROVERSIES

There are several scientific and clinical hurdles to the development of immunotherapeutics for viral infections. One of the biggest challenges is viral diversity, driven by rapid mutation rates and antigenic shifts, as seen in HIV and influenza infections. High viral diversity and viral latency lead to immune escape and limit the durability and efficacy of therapeutic responses. Safety and immunopathological concerns persist in some of the immunotherapeutic strategies due to enhanced immune activation. For example, CAR-T-cell therapy can trigger severe toxicities, including cytokine release syndrome and immune effector-associated neurotoxicity syndrome [113]. While most immunotherapies demonstrate reduced viral load and efficacy, sterilising immunity has not been achieved in chronic infections, including HIV and HBV. Effective tissue trafficking of immunotherapeutics remains a major challenge, since most infections are tissue-specific, as in respiratory viral infections or HIV infection and latency at mucosal sites and lymphoid organs.

Treatment cost is another challenge [114]. Most antibody-based, cytokine-based, and engineered T-cell therapies are more expensive than conventional antimicrobial drugs due to the complex development process and infrastructure required before administration. Treatment costs could be several hundred thousand dollars per patient, limiting their use in economically limited or low-income groups [114]. Globally, the economic burden of expensive immunotherapeutics can exacerbate economic disparities, leading to a heavier burden of infectious diseases in low- and middle-income countries than in developed countries. For global health burdens such as HIV, influenza, and COVID-19, it is imperative to develop universal immunotherapeutics rather than individualised therapies [115], except for specific clinical phenotypes, such as PLWH with advanced multidrug-resistant HIV conditions. Overall, immunotherapy is a promising and versatile platform for combating viral infections; however, future strategies need to counter viral diversity, chronicity, toxicity, complex tissue microenvironments, and cost-effective implementation.

8.4 FUTURE DIRECTIONS

A new wave of immunotherapies is reshaping the antiviral landscape, with strategies that extend beyond classical neutralisation to harness innate and adaptive immune pathways in highly tailored ways, aiming for durable control and cure. Most of the emerging therapies against viral diseases target chronic and currently incurable diseases like HIV and HBV, among others. Preclinical studies introducing CCR5delta32 alleles into $CD34^+$ IPSCs have resulted in genetically engineered HIV-resistant haematopoietic progenitors that could reduce reservoir seeding and offer durable protection against HIV [116]. Gene editing strategies and antibody engineering techniques are rapidly evolving from first-generation to third-generation CAR T cells, from monospecific to bispecific and trispecific bNAb formats, and towards germline-targeting vaccine designs [117]. Third-generation bNAb-derived CAR-T cells have shown promise in reducing the viral reservoir in PLWH undergoing analytical treatment interruption [86]. Preliminary findings from MC-M113 and GS-8588 studies indicate that combining multiple Env-targeting specificities into a single molecule broadens coverage across viral strains and simultaneously enhances Fc-mediated effector functions [118]. Further refinement of antibody isotypes for antiviral defence, including the exploitation of IgA for mucosal protection, will expand treatment efficacy at key mucosal sites of entry, notably the gut and genital tract, where HIV transmission and persistence intersect.

For HBV, mAbs are being optimised for neutralisation and Fc effector functions, while IAP antagonists may sensitise infected hepatocytes to immune clearance. Further T-cell-based therapies, including HBV-specific CAR T cells [119], are also under study to directly target HBV-infected cells. In addition, cytokine-based interventions, such as IL-15 superagonists, remain of interest for boosting T and NK cells and for reducing latent virus reservoirs [49].

In respiratory infections such as influenza and RSV, consideration of the intranasal route/oropharyngeal delivery is essential for developing mucosa-relevant immunotherapeutics, since the respiratory mucosa is the primary site of infection. In addition, creating a universal vaccine targeting multiple respiratory viruses will entail high costs and substantial health benefits. A Phase III clinical trial (NCT6097273) showed mRNA-1083, combining an HA-based influenza vaccine with SARS-CoV-2 spike and receptor-binding domain proteins, demonstrated immunogenicity and safety equivalent to the recommended standard care influenza and COVID-19 vaccines [120]. The development of such multicomponent platforms with the flexibility to rapidly update vaccine compositions will help improve coverage, regulate compliance, and reduce the burden of seasonal respiratory hospitalisations.

Beyond T cells and antibody-based therapies, NK cells are emerging as central players in next-generation antiviral strategies [121]. Memory-like NK cells, including cytokine-induced memory-like NK cells and HLA-E-dependent adaptive NK populations, exhibit adaptive features, such as enhanced recall responses and antiviral potency [122]. Indeed, antigen-specific memory and memory-like responses have been demonstrated against CMV, HIV, and influenza [123–125]. Furthermore, allogeneic NK cells can be expanded *ex vivo* as universal, off-the-shelf therapies with lower side effects than their T-cell counterparts [126]. In parallel, gamma delta T cells, which bridge innate and adaptive immunity, are being explored as flexible effector cells due to their expression of TLRs, TCRs, and NK receptors. They are capable of broad pathogen recognition, tissue homing, and cytotoxicity, particularly in the mucosa [127, 128].

These therapeutic approaches underscore a major shift towards a multipronged, precision-engineered immunotherapy. As therapies evolve, tissue targeting will be critical for immunotherapy, since viral reservoirs often persist in lymphoid tissues, the liver, and mucosal sites. By coordinating platforms that modulate innate and adaptive immunity using gene-modified progenitors and designer antibodies, coupled with tissue-targeting strategies, future approaches aim to control chronic infections and recalibrate host immunity for durable remission and cure.

KEY TERMS & DEFINITIONS SIDEBAR

Broadly neutralising antibodies (bNAbs) Antibodies that recognise conserved regions across diverse viral strains, enabling them to neutralise the viral strains.

Convalescent plasma Plasma collected from individuals who have recovered from an infection that contains pathogen-specific antibodies that can be passively transferred to other individuals for immune protection against same pathogen.

Immunomodulatory antibodies Therapeutic antibodies that have been designed to alter immune responses by enhancing or suppressing specific immune pathways or cell functions.

Latency-reversal agent (LRA) A compound that induces expression of latent viral genomes in infected cells, making them detectable for recognition by antibody or immune cells.

Therapeutic vaccine A vaccine administered after infection to enhance antigen specific immune responses for the clearance of pathogen or functional cure of a disease.

Toll-like receptor (TLR) agonists Compounds/molecules that activate Toll- like receptors to stimulate innate immune signalling and downstream cascade of adaptive immune response.

Checkpoint inhibitors Agents that block inhibitory immune checkpoint pathways on immune cells, thereby restoring or enhancing immune activity against infected cells.

Natural killer (NK) cells Innate immune lymphocytes that recognise and kill virus infected and tumour cells.

Interferons (IFN) Proteins secreted by immune cells and epithelial cells that have antiviral functions and can modulate both innate and adaptive immune responses to infection.

Interleukin-15 (IL-15) superagonist An engineered IL-15- based molecule with enhanced stability and potency that promotes expansion and activation of NK cells and memory T cells

Bispecific/trispecific antibodies Engineered antibodies capable of binding to two or three distinct antigens, enabling coordinated targeting or immune cell redirection.

LIST OF ABBREVIATIONS

AIDS	Acquired Immunodeficiency Syndrome
ARDS	Acute Respiratory Distress Syndrome
ART	Antiretroviral Therapy
bNAb	Broadly Neutralising Antibody
CAR	Chimeric Antigen Receptor
CCR	C-C Chemokine Receptor CCL- C-C Chemokine Ligand
CD	Cluster of Differentiation COVID-19 – Coronavirus Disease 2019
DAA	Direct Acting Antiviral
Env	Envelope Protein
FcR	Fc Receptor
GM-CSF	Granulocyte-Macrophage Colony-Stimulating Factor
HA	Hemagglutinin
HBV	Hepatitis B Virus
HBsAg	Hepatitis B Surface Antigen
HBeAg	Hepatitis B e Antigen
HCV	Hepatitis C Virus
HIV	Human Immunodeficiency Virus
HLA	Human Leukocyte Antigen
ICI	Immune Checkpoint Inhibitor
IFN	Interferon
IFN-α	Interferon Alpha
IFN-λ	Interferon Lambda
IFN-γ	Interferon Gamma
Ig	Immunoglobulin
IL	Interleukin
IVIG	Intravenous Immunoglobulin
LAG-3	Lymphocyte Activation Gene 3
LRA	Latency-Reversing Agent
mAb	Monoclonal Antibody
MHC	Major Histocompatibility Complex
mRNA	Messenger RNA
NK	Natural Killer cell
NHP	Nonhuman Primate
PD-1	Programmed Cell Death Protein 1
PD-L1	Programmed Death Ligand 1
PLWH	People Living With HIV
RSV	Respiratory Syncytial Virus
SARS-CoV-2	Severe Acute Respiratory Syndrome Coronavirus 2

SHIV Simian-Human Immunodeficiency Virus
TCR T-cell Receptor
TIGIT T-cell Immunoreceptor with Ig and ITIM domains
TLR Toll-like Receptor
TNF-α Tumour Necrosis Factor Alpha

REVIEW QUESTIONS

1. Compare the mechanisms of action of monoclonal antibodies in antiviral therapy.
2. Discuss the rationale for using immune checkpoint inhibitors in chronic viral infections.
3. Discuss the benefits and risks of CAR T-cell and CAR-NK therapies in viral disease treatment.
4. Propose a combination immunotherapy strategy to achieve functional cure in HIV.
5. Discuss the challenges of targeting viral reservoirs and strategies to overcome them.

ACKNOWLEDGEMENTS

The authors would like to thank Kyle Kroll and Griffin Woolley for their contributions to the chapter.

REFERENCES

1. World Health Organization (2025). *World Health Statistics 2025: Monitoring Health for the SDGs, Sustainable Development Goals*. Geneva: World Health Organization.
2. Dybul, M., Attoye, T., Baptiste, S. et al. (2021). The case for an HIV cure and how to get there. *Lancet HIV* 8 (1): e51–e58.
3. Okesanya, O.J., Ayeni, R.A., Amadin, P. et al. (2025). Advances in HIV treatment and vaccine development: emerging therapies and breakthrough strategies for long-term control. *AIDS Res Treat* 2025: 6829446.
4. Nou, E., Lo, J., and Grinspoon, S.K. (2016). Inflammation, immune activation, and cardiovascular disease in HIV. *AIDS* 30 (10): 1495–1509.
5. Perricone, C., Triggianese, P., Bursi, R. et al. (2021). Intravenous immunoglobulins at the crossroad of autoimmunity and viral infections. *Microorganisms* 9 (1): 121.
6. Crowe, J.E. Jr. (2022). Human antibodies for viral infections. *Annu Rev Immunol* 40: 349–386.
7. Tebas, P. (2025). Future of bNAbs in HIV treatment. *Curr HIV/AIDS Rep* 22 (1): 34.
8. Fidler, S.L., Lee, M.J., Collins, S. et al. (2025) , RIO: a randomised placebo-controlled study of 2 LS-bNAbs in people treated in early HIV (Conference Abstract). *Conference on Retroviruses and Opportunistic Infections*, San Francisco, CA.
9. Dong, K.A., Govender, V., Pillay, V. et al., (2025). Evaluation of 2 bNAbs plus Vesatolimod in early-treated South African women with HIV-1 during ATI (Conference Abstract). *Conference on Retroviruses and Opportunistic Infections*, San Francisco, CA.
10. Mota, K.G. and Moro, A.M. (2025). Monoclonal antibodies against influenza viruses: a clinical trials review. *Front Immunol* 16: 1669073.

11. Bonomini, A., Mercorelli, B., and Loregian, A. (2025). Antiviral strategies against influenza virus: an update on approved and innovative therapeutic approaches. *Cell Mol Life Sci* 82 (1): 75.
12. Merino, A., Zhang, B., Dougherty, P. et al. (2019). Chronic stimulation drives human NK cell dysfunction and epigenetic reprograming. *J Clin Invest* 129 (9): 3770–3785.
13. Gubser, C. and Kaufmann, D.E. (2025). Understanding the HIV-specific T-cell response to immune checkpoint blockade: what can we learn from cancer immunotherapy? *Curr Opin HIV AIDS* 20 (5): 441–448.
14. Bai, R. and Cui, J. (2022). Burgeoning exploration of the role of natural killer cells in anti-PD-1/PD-L1 therapy. *Front Immunol* 13: 886931.
15. Khan, M., Arooj, S., and Wang, H. (2020). NK cell-based immune checkpoint inhibition. *Front Immunol* 11: 167.
16. Evans, V.A., van der Sluis, R., Solomon, A. et al. (2018). Programmed cell death-1 contributes to the establishment and maintenance of HIV-1 latency. *AIDS* 32 (11): 1491–1497.
17. Xie, G., Luo, X., Ma, T. et al. (2021). Characterization of HIV-induced remodeling reveals differences in infection susceptibility of memory CD4(+) T cell subsets in vivo. *Cell Rep* 35 (4): 109038.
18. Fisher, K., Schlub, T.E., Boyer, Z. et al. (2023). Unequal distribution of genetically-intact HIV-1 proviruses in cells expressing the immune checkpoint markers PD-1 and/or CTLA-4. *Front Immunol* 14: 1064346.
19. Gubser, C., Chiu, C., Lewin, S.R. et al. (2022). Immune checkpoint blockade in HIV. *EBioMedicine* 76: 103840.
20. Banga, R., Procopio, F.A., Noto, A. et al. (2016). PD-1(+) and follicular helper T cells are responsible for persistent HIV-1 transcription in treated aviremic individuals. *Nat Med* 22 (7): 754–761.
21. Perreau, M. et al. (2013). Follicular helper T cells serve as the major CD4 T cell compartment for HIV-1 infection, replication, and production. *J Exp Med* 210 (1): 143–156.
22. Fukazawa, Y., Lum, R., Okoye, A.A. et al. (2015). B cell follicle sanctuary permits persistent productive simian immunodeficiency virus infection in elite controllers. *Nat Med* 21 (2): 132–139.
23. Kohler, S.L., Pham, M.N., Folkvord, J.M. et al. (2016). Germinal center T follicular helper cells are highly permissive to HIV-1 and alter their phenotype during virus replication. *J Immunol* 196 (6): 2711–2722.
24. Fromentin, R., DaFonseca, S., Costiniuk, C.T. et al. (2019). PD-1 blockade potentiates HIV latency reversal ex vivo in CD4(+) T cells from ART-suppressed individuals. *Nat Commun* 10 (1): 814.
25. Uldrick, T.S., Adams, S.V., Fromentin, R. et al. (2022). Pembrolizumab induces HIV latency reversal in people living with HIV and cancer on antiretroviral therapy. *Sci Transl Med* 14 (629): eabl3836.
26. Janosi, A., Bódy, B., Nagy, R. et al. (2025). Tumour necrosis factor-alpha inhibitors decrease mortality in COVID-19: a systematic review and meta-analysis. *Crit Care* 29 (1): 232.
27. Bakkari, M.A., Ghoal, G., Sabei, F. et al. (2025). Exploring interleukin-6 inhibitor antibodies in combatting SARS-CoV-2 and its mutated variants: challenges and future directions. *J Pharmacol Pharmacother* 16 (4): 0976500X251316939.
28. Severe Covid-19 GWAS Group, Ellinghaus, D., Degenhardt, F. et al. (2020). Genomewide association study of severe Covid-19 with respiratory failure. *N Engl J Med* 383 (16): 1522–1534.
29. Cuesta-Llavona, E., Gómez, J., Albaiceta, G.M. et al. (2021). Variant-genetic and transcript-expression analysis showed a role for the chemokine-receptor CCR5 in COVID-19 severity. *Int Immunopharmacol* 98: 107825.
30. Harrison, C. (2020). Focus shifts to antibody cocktails for COVID-19 cytokine storm. *Nat Biotechnol* 38 (8): 905–908.

31. Patterson, B.K., Seethamraju, H., Dhody, K. et al. (2021). CCR5 inhibition in critical COVID-19 patients decreases inflammatory cytokines, increases CD8 T-cells, and decreases SARS-CoV2 RNA in plasma by day 14. *Int J Infect Dis* 103: 25–32.
32. Trkola, A., Ketas, T.J., Nagashima, K.A. et al. (2001). Potent, broad-spectrum inhibition of human immunodeficiency virus type 1 by the CCR5 monoclonal antibody PRO 140. *J Virol* 75 (2): 579–588.
33. Gathe, J.C., Dejesus, E., Ramgopal, M.N. et al. (2025). Leronlimab treatment for multidrug-resistant HIV-1 (OPTIMIZE): a randomized, double-blind, placebo-controlled trial. *J Acquir Immune Defic Syndr* 99 (2): 185–194.
34. Jacobson, J.M., Thompson, M.A., Lalezari, J.P. et al. (2010). Anti-HIV-1 activity of weekly or biweekly treatment with subcutaneous PRO 140, a CCR5 monoclonal antibody. *J Infect Dis* 201 (10): 1481–1487.
35. Jeng, W.J. and Lok, A.S.F. (2023). What will it take to cure hepatitis B? *Hepatol Commun* 7 (4): e0084.
36. Papasavvas, E., Azzoni, L., Pagliuzza, A. et al. (2021). Safety, immune, and antiviral effects of pegylated interferon alpha 2b administration in antiretroviral therapy-suppressed individuals: results of pilot clinical trial. *AIDS Res Hum Retroviruses* 37 (6): 433–443.
37. Azzoni, L., Foulkes, A.S., Papasavvas, E. et al. (2013). Pegylated Interferon alfa-2a monotherapy results in suppression of HIV type 1 replication and decreased cell-associated HIV DNA integration. *J Infect Dis* 207 (2): 213–222.
38. Papasavvas, E., Azzoni, L., Kossenkov, A.V. et al. (2019). NK response correlates with HIV decrease in pegylated IFN-alpha2a-treated antiretroviral therapy-suppressed subjects. *J Immunol* 203 (3): 705–717.
39. Hua, S., Vigano, S., Tse, S. et al. (2018). Pegylated interferon-alpha-induced natural killer cell activation is associated with human immunodeficiency virus-1 DNA decline in antiretroviral therapy-treated HIV-1/hepatitis C virus-coinfected patients. *Clin Infect Dis* 66 (12): 1910–1917.
40. Chronopoulou, S. and Tsochantaridis, I. (2025). Interferon Lambda: the next frontier in antiviral therapy? *Pharmaceuticals (Basel)* 18 (6).
41. Bhushan, B.L.S., Wanve, S., Koradia, P. et al. (2021). Efficacy and safety of pegylated interferon-alpha2b in moderate COVID-19: a phase 3, randomized, comparator-controlled, open-label study. *Int J Infect Dis* 111: 281–287.
42. Pandit, A., Bhalani, N., Bhushan, B.L.S. et al. (2021). Efficacy and safety of pegylated interferon alfa-2b in moderate COVID-19: a phase II, randomized, controlled, open-label study. *Int J Infect Dis* 105: 516–521.
43. Dunning, J., Baillie, J.K., Cao, B. et al. (2014). Antiviral combinations for severe influenza. *Lancet Infect Dis* 14 (12): 1259–1270.
44. Justiz Vaillant, A.A. and Qurie, A. (2025). Interleukin. Treasure Island, FL: StatPearls.
45. Paul, P., Choong, C., Heinemann, J. et al. (2025). The lasting impact of IL-2: approaching 50 years of advancing immune tolerance, cancer immunotherapies, and autoimmune diseases. *Immunol Invest* 54 (5): 589–603.
46. Im, S.J., Lee, K., and Ha, S.J. (2024). Harnessing IL-2 for immunotherapy against cancer and chronic infection: a historical perspective and emerging trends. *Exp Mol Med* 56 (9): 1900–1908.
47. Raeber, M.E., Sahin, D., Karakus, U. et al. (2023). A systematic review of interleukin-2-based immunotherapies in clinical trials for cancer and autoimmune diseases. *EBioMedicine* 90: 104539.
48. Su, R., Zhang, T., Wang, H. et al. (2024). New sights of low dose IL-2: restoration of immune homeostasis for viral infection. *Immunology* 171 (3): 324–338.
49. Miller, J.S., Davis, Z.B., Helgeson, E. et al. (2022). Safety and virologic impact of the IL-15 superagonist N-803 in people living with HIV: a phase 1 trial. *Nat Med* 28 (2): 392–400.

50. Harwood, O. and O'Connor, S. (2021). Therapeutic potential of IL-15 and N-803 in HIV/SIV infection. *Viruses* 13 (9).
51. Rhein, J., Chipman, J.G., Beilman, G.J. et al. (2025). Impact of the IL-15 superagonist N-803 on lymphatic reservoirs of HIV. *JCI Insight* 10 (13): e190831.
52. Webb, G.M., Molden, J., Busman-Sahay, K. et al. (2020). The human IL-15 superagonist N-803 promotes migration of virus-specific CD8+ T and NK cells to B cell follicles but does not reverse latency in ART-suppressed, SHIV-infected macaques. *PLoS Pathog* 16 (3): e1008339.
53. Fang, S., Ju, D., Lin, Y. et al. (2022). The role of interleukin-22 in lung health and its therapeutic potential for COVID-19. *Front Immunol* 13: 951107.
54. Das, S., St Croix, C., Good, M. et al. (2020). Interleukin-22 inhibits respiratory syncytial virus production by blocking virus-mediated subversion of cellular autophagy. *iScience* 23 (7): 101256.
55. Ji, T., Huang, G., Cao, Y. et al. (2025). Advances in interleukin-6 family cytokines and the role in respiratory diseases. *J Inflamm Res* 18: 3125–3141.
56. Dawson, R.E., Jenkins, B.J., and Saad, M.I. (2021). IL-6 family cytokines in respiratory health and disease. *Cytokine* 143: 155520.
57. Bawazeer, A.O., Rosli, S., Harpur, C.M. et al. (2021). Interleukin-1beta exacerbates disease and is a potential therapeutic target to reduce pulmonary inflammation during severe influenza A virus infection. *Immunol Cell Biol* 99 (7): 737–748.
58. Nel, C. and Frater, J. (2024). Enhancing broadly neutralising antibody suppression of HIV by immune modulation and vaccination. *Front Immunol* 15: 1478703.
59. Garrido, C., Abad-Fernandez, M., Tuyishime, M. et al. (2018). Interleukin-15-stimulated natural killer cells clear HIV-1-infected cells following latency reversal ex vivo. *J Virol* 92 (12): e00235-18.
60. Kawai, T., Ikegawa, M., Ori, D. et al. (2024). Decoding Toll-like receptors: recent insights and perspectives in innate immunity. *Immunity* 57 (4): 649–673.
61. Kayesh, M.E.H., Kohara, M., and Tsukiyama-Kohara, K. (2023). TLR agonists as vaccine adjuvants in the prevention of viral infections: an overview. *Front Microbiol* 14: 1249718.
62. Kayesh, M.E.H., Kohara, M., and Tsukiyama-Kohara, K. (2023). Toll-like receptor response to human immunodeficiency virus type 1 or co-infection with hepatitis B or C virus: an overview. *Int J Mol Sci* 24 (11): 9624.
63. Liu, Z.M., Yang, M.H., Yu, K. et al. (2022). Toll-like receptor (TLRs) agonists and antagonists for COVID-19 treatments. *Front Pharmacol* 13: 989664.
64. Steinhagen, F., Kinjo, T., Bode, C. et al. (2011). Tlr-based immune adjuvants. *Vaccine* 29 (17): 3341–3355.
65. Wang, W., Mu, S., Yan, D. et al. (2025). Comprehending toll-like receptors: pivotal element in the pathogenesis of sepsis and its complications. *Front Immunol* 16: 1591011.
66. Bishop, G.A., Hsing, Y., Hostager, B.S. et al. (2000). Molecular mechanisms of B lymphocyte activation by the immune response modifier R-848. *J Immunol* 165 (10): 5552–5557.
67. Hart, O.M., Athie-Morales, V., O'Connor, G.M. et al. (2005). TLR7/8-mediated activation of human NK cells results in accessory cell-dependent IFN-gamma production. *J Immunol* 175 (3): 1636–1642.
68. Caron, G., Duluc, D., Frémaux, I. et al. (2005). Direct stimulation of human T cells via TLR5 and TLR7/8: flagellin and R-848 up-regulate proliferation and IFN-gamma production by memory CD4+ T cells. *J Immunol* 175 (3): 1551–1557.
69. Borducchi, E.N., Liu, J., Nkolola, J.P. et al. (2018). Antibody and TLR7 agonist delay viral rebound in SHIV-infected monkeys. *Nature* 563 (7731): 360–364.
70. Cong, Z., Sun, Y., Dang, C. et al. (2023). TLR7 agonist GS-9620 combined with nicotinamide generate viral reactivation in seronegative SHIV(SF162P3)-infected rhesus monkeys. *Biomedicines* 11 (6): 1707.

71. Lim, S.Y., Osuna, C.E., Hraber, P.T. et al. (2018). TLR7 agonists induce transient viremia and reduce the viral reservoir in SIV-infected rhesus macaques on antiretroviral therapy. *Sci Transl Med* 10 (439): eaao4521.
72. Moldt, B., Chandrashekar, A. et al. (2022). HIV envelope antibodies and TLR7 agonist partially prevent viral rebound in chronically SHIV-infected monkeys. *PLoS Pathog* 18 (4): e1010467.
73. Ventura, J.D., Nkolola, J.P., Chandrashekar, A. et al. (2022). Therapeutic efficacy of an Ad26/MVA vaccine with SIV gp140 protein and vesatolimod in ART-suppressed rhesus macaques. *NPJ Vaccines* 7 (1): 53.
74. Walker-Sperling, V.E.K., Mercado, N.B., Chandrashekar, A. et al. (2022). Therapeutic efficacy of combined active and passive immunization in ART-suppressed, SHIV-infected rhesus macaques. *Nat Commun* 13 (1): 3463.
75. Borducchi, E.N., Cabral, C., Stephenson, K.E. et al. (2016). Ad26/MVA therapeutic vaccination with TLR7 stimulation in SIV-infected rhesus monkeys. *Nature* 540 (7632): 284–287.
76. Bam, R.A., Hansen, D., Irrinki, A. et al. (2017). TLR7 agonist GS-9620 is a potent inhibitor of acute HIV-1 infection in human peripheral blood mononuclear cells. *Antimicrob Agents Chemother* 61 (1): e01369-16.
77. Bailon, L., Moltó, J., Curran, A. et al. (2025). Safety, immunogenicity and effect on viral rebound of HTI vaccines combined with a TLR7 agonist in early-treated HIV-1 infection: a randomized, placebo-controlled phase 2a trial. *Nat Commun* 16 (1): 2146.
78. Riddler, S.A., Para, M., Benson, C.A. et al. (2021). Vesatolimod, a toll-like receptor 7 agonist, induces immune activation in virally suppressed adults living with human immunodeficiency virus-1. *Clin Infect Dis* 72 (11): e815–e824.
79. SenGupta, D., Brinson, C., DeJesus, E. et al. (2021). The TLR7 agonist vesatolimod induced a modest delay in viral rebound in HIV controllers after cessation of antiretroviral therapy. *Sci Transl Med* 13 (599): eabg3071.
80. Gane, E.J., Dunbar, P.R., Brooks, A.E. et al. (2023). Safety and efficacy of the oral TLR8 agonist selgantolimod in individuals with chronic hepatitis B under viral suppression. *J Hepatol* 78 (3): 513–523.
81. Kourti, M., Evangelidis, P., Roilides, E. et al. (2025). Chimeric antigen receptor immunotherapy for infectious diseases: current advances and future perspectives. *Pathogens* 14 (8): 774.
82. Zhou, Y., Jadlowsky, J., Baiduc, C. et al. (2023). Chimeric antigen receptors enable superior control of HIV replication by rapidly killing infected cells. *PLoS Pathog* 19 (12): e1011853.
83. Su, H., Mueller, A., and Goldstein, H. (2024). Recent advances on anti-HIV chimeric antigen receptor-T-cell treatment to provide sustained HIV remission. *Curr Opin HIV AIDS* 19 (4): 169–178.
84. Anthony-Gonda, K., Bardhi, A., Ray, A. et al. (2019). Multispecific anti-HIV duoCAR-T cells display broad in vitro antiviral activity and potent in vivo elimination of HIV-infected cells in a humanized mouse model. *Sci Transl Med* 11 (504): eaav5685.
85. Anthony-Gonda, K., Ray, A., Su, H. et al. (2022). In vivo killing of primary HIV-infected cells by peripheral-injected early memory-enriched anti-HIV duoCAR T cells. *JCI Insight* 7 (21): e161698.
86. Liu, B., Zhang, W., Xia, B. et al. (2021). Broadly neutralizing antibody-derived CAR T cells reduce viral reservoir in individuals infected with HIV-1. *J Clin Invest* 131 (19): e150211.
87. Mao, Y., Liao, Q., Zhu, Y. et al. (2024). Efficacy and safety of novel multifunctional M10 CAR-T cells in HIV-1-infected patients: a phase I, multicenter, single-arm, open-label study. *Cell Discov* 10 (1): 49.

88. Papadopoulou, A. et al. (2023). SARS-CoV-2-specific T cell therapy for severe COVID-19: a randomized phase 1/2 trial. *Nat Med* 29 (8): 2019–2029.
89. Hasnani, Z., Armstrong, E., Abbas, A. et al. (2025). Donor-derived sars-cov-2-specific T cells to prevent COVID-19 early post allogeneic hematopoietic stem cell transplant. *Blood* 146 (1): 6028. https://doi.org/10.1182/blood-2025-6028.
90. Guangzhou Lion (ed.) (2025). Safety and efficacy of hepatitis B virus (HBV)-specific T cell receptor (TCR)-T cell therapy combined with nucleos(t)ide analogues (NAs) in HBeAg-positive chronic hepatitis B patients. T.C.R.C.L.
91. Lin, M.H., Hu, L.J., Miller, J.S. et al. (2025). CAR-NK cell therapy: a potential antiviral platform. *Sci Bull (Beijing)* 70 (5): 765–777.
92. Kalathil, S.G. and Thanavala, Y. (2021). Natural killer cells and T cells in hepatocellular carcinoma and viral hepatitis: current status and perspectives for future immunotherapeutic approaches. *Cells* 10 (6): 1332.
93. Miller, J.S., Rhein, J., Davis, Z.B. et al. (2024). Safety and virologic impact of haploidentical NK cells plus interleukin 2 or N-803 in HIV infection. *J Infect Dis* 229 (5): 1256–1265.
94. U. Duke and I. Access to Advanced Health (eds.) (2024). Safety and immunogenicity of stabilized CH505 TF chTrimer vaccination in adults living with HIV-1 on suppressive antiretroviral therapy.
95. O. University of and S. Gilead (eds.) (2023). A phase I/IIa randomized, placebo-controlled trial of conserved-mosaic T-cell vaccine in a regimen with vesatolimod and broadly neutralizing antibodies in adults initiated on suppressive antiretroviral therapy during acute HIV-1.
96. Ramezani-Rad, P., Cottrell, C.A., Marina-Zárate, E. et al. (2025). Vaccination with mRNA-encoded membrane-bound HIV envelope trimer induces neutralizing antibodies in animal models. *Sci Transl Med* 17 (809): eadw0721.
97. R. German Center for Infection et al. (eds.) (2022). TherVacB_Phase1a: open phase 1a trial to assess the safety and immunogenicity of a heterologous protein prime/MVA boost therapeutic hepatitis B vaccine candidate in healthy volunteers.
98. Wei, L., Zhao T., Zhang J. et al., Efficacy and safety of a nanoparticle therapeutic vaccine in patients with chronic hepatitis B: a randomized clinical trial. *Hepatology*, 2022. 75(1): p. 182–195.
99. Lewin, S.R. and Mellors, J.W. (2016). HIV persistence in the CNS: the final frontier for a cure? *J Virus Erad* 2 (4): 242.
100. Hoogeveen, R.C. and Boonstra, A. (2020). Checkpoint inhibitors and therapeutic vaccines for the treatment of chronic HBV infection. *Front Immunol* 11: 401.
101. Barnes, E. (2015). Therapeutic vaccines in HBV: lessons from HCV. *Med Microbiol Immunol* 204 (1): 79–86.
102. Papadopoulos, A.O., Mvaya, L., Khaba, T. et al. (2025). Spatial regulation of CD8(+) T cells at the HLA-E-NKG2A axis drives HIV persistence in lymph node B cell follicles. *Cell Rep* 44 (9): 116181.
103. Wang, C.Y., Wong, W.W., Tsai, H.C. et al. (2019). Effect of anti-CD4 antibody UB-421 on HIV-1 rebound after treatment interruption. *N Engl J Med* 380 (16): 1535–1545.
104. Rai, M.A., Blazkova, J., Kardava, L. et al. (2025). Sustained virologic suppression of multidrug-resistant HIV in an individual treated with anti-CD4 domain 1 antibody and lenacapavir. *Nat Med* 31 (2): 427–432.
105. Rai, M.A., Blazkova, J., Justement, J.S. et al. (2024). Ex vivo sensitivity to broadly neutralizing antibodies and anti-CD4 antibody UB-421 of infectious viral isolates from people living with multidrug-resistant HIV. *EBioMedicine* 104: 105151.

106. Qiu, K., Duan, X., Mao, M. et al. (2023). mRNA-LNP vaccination-based immunotherapy augments CD8(+) T cell responses against HPV-positive oropharyngeal cancer. *NPJ Vaccines* 8 (1): 144.
107. Lee, S., Yoon, H., Hong, S.H. et al. (2023). mRNA-HPV vaccine encoding E6 and E7 improves therapeutic potential for HPV-mediated cancers via subcutaneous immunization. *J Med Virol* 95 (12): e29309.
108. Floudas, C.S., Goswami, M., Donahue, R.N. et al. (2025). Novel combination immunotherapy and clinical activity in patients with HPV-associated cancers: a nonrandomized clinical trial. *JAMA Oncol* 11 (4): 394–399.
109. Colombo, N., Dubot, C., Lorusso, D. et al. (2021). Pembrolizumab for persistent, recurrent, or metastatic cervical cancer. *N Engl J Med* 385 (20): 1856–1867.
110. Kim, J. and Chang, J. (2024). Cross-protective efficacy and safety of an adenovirus-based universal influenza vaccine expressing nucleoprotein, hemagglutinin, and the ectodomain of matrix protein 2. *Vaccine* 42 (15): 3505–3513.
111. Fitz-Patrick, D., McVinnie, D., Jackson, L.A. et al. (2025). Efficacy, immunogenicity, and safety of modified mRNA influenza vaccine. *N Engl J Med* 393 (20): 2001–2011.
112. Yang, R.S., Traver, M., Barefoot, N. et al. (2024). Mosaic quadrivalent influenza vaccine single nanoparticle characterization. *Sci Rep* 14 (1): 4534.
113. Luo, J. and Zhang, X. (2024). Challenges and innovations in CAR-T cell therapy: a comprehensive analysis. *Front Oncol* 14: 1399544.
114. Ramamurthy, D., Nundalall, T. et al. (2021). Recent advances in immunotherapies against infectious diseases. *Immunother Adv* 1 (1): ltaa007.
115. Wallis, R.S., O'Garra, A., Sher, A. et al. (2023). Host-directed immunotherapy of viral and bacterial infections: past, present and future. *Nat Rev Immunol* 23 (2): 121–133.
116. Morvan, M.G., Teque, F., Ye, L. et al. (2021). Genetically edited CD34(+) cells derived from human iPS cells in vivo but not in vitro engraft and differentiate into HIV-resistant cells. *Proc Natl Acad Sci USA* 118 (20): e2102404118.
117. Nkolola, J.P. and Barouch, D.H. (2024). Prophylactic HIV-1 vaccine trials: past, present, and future. *Lancet HIV* 11 (2): e117–e124.
118. Board, N.L., Yuan, Z., Wu, F. et al. (2024). Bispecific antibodies promote natural killer cell-mediated elimination of HIV-1 reservoir cells. *Nat Immunol* 25 (3): 462–470.
119. Wang, Y., Li, Q., Li, C. et al. (2024). Chimeric antigen receptors of HBV envelope proteins inhibit hepatitis B surface antigen secretion. *Gut* 73 (4): 668–681.
120. Rudman Spergel, A.K., Wu, I., Deng, W. et al. (2025). Immunogenicity and safety of influenza and COVID-19 multicomponent vaccine in adults >/=50 years: a randomized clinical trial. *JAMA* 333 (22): 1977–1987.
121. Smith, D.M., Schafer, J.R., Tullius, B. et al. (2023). Natural killer cells for antiviral therapy. *Sci Transl Med* 15 (677): eabl5278.
122. Bjorkstrom, N.K., Strunz, B., and Ljunggren, H.G. (2022). Natural killer cells in antiviral immunity. *Nat Rev Immunol* 22 (2): 112–123.
123. Jost, S., Lucar, O., Lee, E. et al. (2023). Antigen-specific memory NK cell responses against HIV and influenza use the NKG2/HLA-E axis. *Sci Immunol* 8 (90): eadi3974.
124. Wijaya, R.S., Read, S.A., Truong, N.R. et al. (2021). HBV vaccination and HBV infection induce HBV-specific natural killer cell memory. *Gut* 70 (2): 357–369.
125. Sheppard, S. and Sun, J.C. (2021). Virus-specific NK cell memory. *J Exp Med* 218 (4): e20201731.
126. Vivier, E., Rebuffet, L., Narni-Mancinelli, E. et al. (2024). Natural killer cell therapies. *Nature* 626 (8000): 727–736.

127. Bordoni, V., Guarracino, F., Galaverna, F. et al. (2025). Antiviral potential of Vdelta2 T cells in children given TCR alphabeta/CD19 cell-depleted HLA-haploidentical HSCT. *Blood Adv* 9 (5): 990–1002.

128. Caron, J., Ridgley, L.A., and Bodman-Smith, M. (2021). How to train your dragon: harnessing Gamma Delta T cells' antiviral functions and trained immunity in a pandemic era. *Front Immunol* 12: 666983.

129. Wang, X., Ren, N., Liu, H., et al. (2025). Global disease and economic burden of noncommunicable diseases attributable to hepatitis B infection: a health economic evaluation study. *J Med Virol* 97(8): e70519. 10.1002/jmv.70519.

130. Walsh, J.A. and Maher, C. (2010). Economic implications of influenza and influenza vaccine. In *Influenza Vaccines for the Future*, 425–440. 10.1007/978-3-0346-0279-2_19.

CHAPTER 9

Immunotherapy for Microbial Infections: Addressing Bacterial Resistance and Parasitic Infections with Immunotherapy

CHRISTIAN R. ENGWERDA AND JESSICA A. ENGEL
Division of Infection and Inflammation, QIMR Berghofer Medical Research Institute, Brisbane, Queensland, Australia

LEARNING OBJECTIVES

- Understand the immunological basis for treating microbial infections with immunotherapy.
- Explore how immune-based therapies can counter AMR.
- Assess current and emerging clinical applications for bacterial and parasitic infections.
- Evaluate challenges in implementing immunotherapy in infectious diseases.
- Identify future directions and opportunities for innovation in the field.

9.1 INTRODUCTION

Infectious diseases caused by bacteria and parasites continue to pose major global health challenges, despite decades of advances in antimicrobial therapy and public health interventions. The World Health Organization (WHO) has identified antimicrobial resistance (AMR) as one of the top 10 global public health threats, with bacterial resistance rendering once-effective antibiotics increasingly obsolete [1]. Concurrently, parasitic diseases such as malaria, leishmaniasis, and schistosomiasis persist in large parts of the world, often in resource-limited settings where access to diagnosis and treatment remains inadequate. These infections not only contribute to substantial morbidity and mortality but also perpetuate poverty and socioeconomic disparity in affected communities [2].

Historically, the control of microbial infections has relied on the use of small-molecule antimicrobial agents. However, the increasing emergence of resistant strains, the stagnation in antibiotic discovery pipelines, and the frequent failure of antiparasitic drugs to induce sterile cures highlight the urgent need for alternative therapeutic strategies. Furthermore, many parasitic infections are chronic in nature, characterised by complex host-pathogen interactions and immune evasion strategies that blunt or misdirect protective immune responses. These features complicate both therapeutic and vaccine-based approaches.

Immunotherapy can be broadly defined as the modulation of the immune system to prevent or treat disease. It offers a promising avenue for addressing these challenges because, rather than directly targeting the pathogen, it harnesses the host immune response to control infection and/or limit/cure disease. While immunotherapy has gained significant traction in oncology, where immune checkpoint inhibitors and cellular therapies have transformed clinical outcomes, its application in infectious diseases remains limited but promising. In microbial infections, immunotherapy holds the potential to enhance host immunity, overcome immune suppression, and provide durable protection through the promotion of immunological memory. Critically, it can also complement traditional antimicrobial agents, boosting efficacy or restoring sensitivity in the context of drug resistance. This is particularly relevant when pathogens develop partial resistance or tolerance to antimicrobial drugs, allowing the involvement of the host immune response to tip the balance in favour of host control.

This chapter explores the potential of immunotherapeutic strategies to address two major types of microbial infections: those caused by drug-resistant bacteria and those caused by parasitic organisms. These distinct but overlapping areas of infection share key challenges, including immune evasion, chronicity, and the limitations of current treatment approaches. Importantly, they also share opportunities for immune-based interventions, including monoclonal antibodies targeting bacterial virulence factors, cytokine therapies that enhance host resistance, immune checkpoint blockade to reverse pathogen-induced T cell exhaustion, and host-directed therapies (HDTs) that improve dysfunctional or ineffective immune responses.

The use of immunotherapy in microbial infections requires a comprehensive understanding of host-pathogen interactions, particularly the ways in which microbial agents manipulate the immune response to ensure their survival. For example, intracellular pathogens such as *Mycobacterium tuberculosis* (TB), *Plasmodium falciparum*, and *Leishmania donovani* create immunosuppressive environments both within host cells and in surrounding tissue niches that facilitate persistence and disease progression. Immunotherapies targeting these suppressive pathways offer new approaches for promoting protective immunity. Likewise, therapies that activate or expand key immune populations, such as stem-like T cells, B cells, and monocytes, are being investigated for their ability to boost long-term immunity following infection or vaccination.

This chapter starts by reviewing the immunological foundations that underpin host defence against bacterial and parasitic infections. It then examines the current and emerging clinical applications of immunotherapy in these settings. Real-world examples, such as the use of recombinant IFN-γ to treat drug-resistant TB, will be discussed to highlight the translational potential of these approaches.

We also address the key challenges and limitations in the field, including the risk of immunopathology, the difficulty of predicting individual responses to immune-based treatments, and the limited pipeline for developing and approving such therapies in infectious disease settings. Finally, we look ahead to the future, considering how advances in systems immunology, spatial transcriptomics, single-cell analysis, and synthetic biology are likely to shape the development of next-generation immunotherapies for microbial infections.

By applying both immunological principles and recent translational advances, this chapter aims to provide a comprehensive overview of how immunotherapy can be leveraged to address two of the most urgent challenges in global infectious diseases: bacterial resistance and parasitic infection. By doing this, we hope to stimulate further research and innovation in the field and to contribute to the development of more effective, durable, and equitable strategies for controlling and eliminating microbial threats.

9.2 IMMUNOTHERAPY FOR MICROBIAL INFECTIONS

9.2.1 Immunological Background

The concept of leveraging the immune system to combat microbial infections has a long history [3]. In the late nineteenth and early twentieth centuries, serum therapy was pioneered by Emil von Behring, using antibodies from immune animals or convalescent humans. Protective antibodies contained within serum were able to neutralise toxins and bind pathogens, thereby mediating disease control with help from the recipient's own immune system, including complement components and phagocytic cells. This was among the first attempts at immunotherapy for infectious diseases, notably against diphtheria and pneumococcal pneumonia [4]. However, the development of antibiotics in the mid-twentieth century shifted therapeutic focus, relegating immune-based approaches to the background. The resurgence of interest in immunotherapy, driven largely by advances in cancer treatment, has now reinvigorated efforts to apply similar strategies to infectious diseases. The development of monoclonal antibody (mAb) technology in the 1970s was a key turning point, enabling highly specific targeting of microbial antigens or host immune modulators [5]. These tools have since matured into clinically relevant therapies, including mAbs against respiratory syncytial virus (RSV), *Clostridioides difficile* toxins, and, more recently, SARS-CoV-2 spike protein to prevent binding to the host cell angiotensin-converting enzyme 2 (ACE2) receptor [6].

The effectiveness of immunotherapy for microbial infections depends on the interplay between innate and adaptive immunity. The innate immune system provides the first line of defence, mediated by pattern recognition receptors (PRRs) such as Toll-like receptors (TLRs), which detect conserved microbial structures and initiate inflammatory cascades. Activation of dendritic cells and macrophages leads to the release of pro-inflammatory cytokines and the presentation of antigens to T cells, bridging the innate and adaptive responses. Cluster of differentiation 4 positive ($CD4^+$) T helper cells are crucial for coordinating cellular immunity, while cluster of differentiation 8 positive ($CD8^+$) cytotoxic T lymphocytes recognise and kill target cells expressing pathogen peptides on major histocompatibility complex (MHC) I molecules. B cells produce antibodies that can neutralise toxins or bind pathogens to contribute to direct killing and clearance by phagocytic cells and provide long-term protection.

Several immunological pathways and checkpoints are now recognised as therapeutic targets in microbial infections. Interferon-gamma (IFN-γ) plays a central role in activating macrophages to kill intracellular pathogens such as *L. donovani* and *M. tuberculosis*. Conversely, regulatory cytokines like interleukin-10 (IL-10) suppress inflammation to protect tissue but can also impede pathogen clearance. Manipulating these pathways, either enhancing IFN-γ signalling or blocking IL-10, has shown promise in preclinical models of infection. Immune checkpoint receptors such as programmed cell death protein 1 (PD-1) and cytotoxic T-lymphocyte antigen 4 (CTLA-4), and co-stimulatory molecules like 4-1BB, also regulate T cell function and are increasingly studied for their roles in chronic infection. Therapeutic blockade of PD-1, for example has demonstrated reversal of T cell exhaustion in both chronic viral and parasitic infections, raising the possibility of immune stimulation in patients with persistent microbial burdens [7].

Host-pathogen interactions are dynamic and shaped by mutual evolutionary pressures. Pathogens have evolved diverse strategies to evade or suppress host immunity. Bacteria can secrete immunomodulatory toxins, mask antigens, or form biofilms to avoid immune detection. Parasites such as *P. falciparum* and *Trypanosoma spp.* exhibit genetic diversity, making it difficult for the immune system to recognise all infecting parasites. They also manipulate host immune signalling pathways to create anti-inflammatory environments that support chronic infection. *P. falciparum*, for instance, induces expression of Type I interferons (IFN-I) that promote IL-10 production, which can blunt effective $CD4^+$ T-cell responses [8]. *L. donovani* has been shown to stimulate IL-10 production and, like many chronic bacterial and parasitic infections, drive T-cell suppression and skew myeloid cell function towards a regulatory phenotype [9].

Understanding these immunological foundations is critical for the rational design of immunotherapies that can either enhance protective responses or remove suppressive constraints. By targeting specific pathways and cell types, immunotherapy can be tailored to overcome microbial immune evasion while minimising the risk of immunopathology (see Figure 9.1).

9.2.2 Clinical Applications

The application of immunotherapy in microbial infections has advanced significantly in recent years, with approaches increasingly tailored to the immunopathology and evasion strategies of specific pathogens. In bacterial infections, mAbs have been at the forefront of clinical development. These include anti-toxin mAbs, such as bezlotoxumab, which neutralises *Clostridioides difficile* toxin B and is approved to prevent recurrent infection [10]. Other candidates target virulence factors rather than bacterial viability, aiming to disarm the pathogen without applying direct selective pressure for resistance. For example, mAbs against *Staphylococcus aureus* adhesins or *Pseudomonas aeruginosa* biofilm components are in clinical trials. These strategies offer adjunctive benefits to antibiotics, particularly in immunocompromised patients or those with recurrent infections [11].

Beyond passive immunity, immune checkpoint inhibitors, originally developed for cancer, are being investigated to enhance host responses to persistent bacterial infections. Blockade of PD-1 or CTLA-4 may restore effector T cell function in settings of chronic immune suppression, such as TB [12] (see Figure 9.2). However, despite CTLA-4 blockade improving immune responses against *M. tuberculosis* in a preclinical model, it did not protect against disease [13], highlighting the nuanced responses to these types of interventions in infectious diseases. Although these

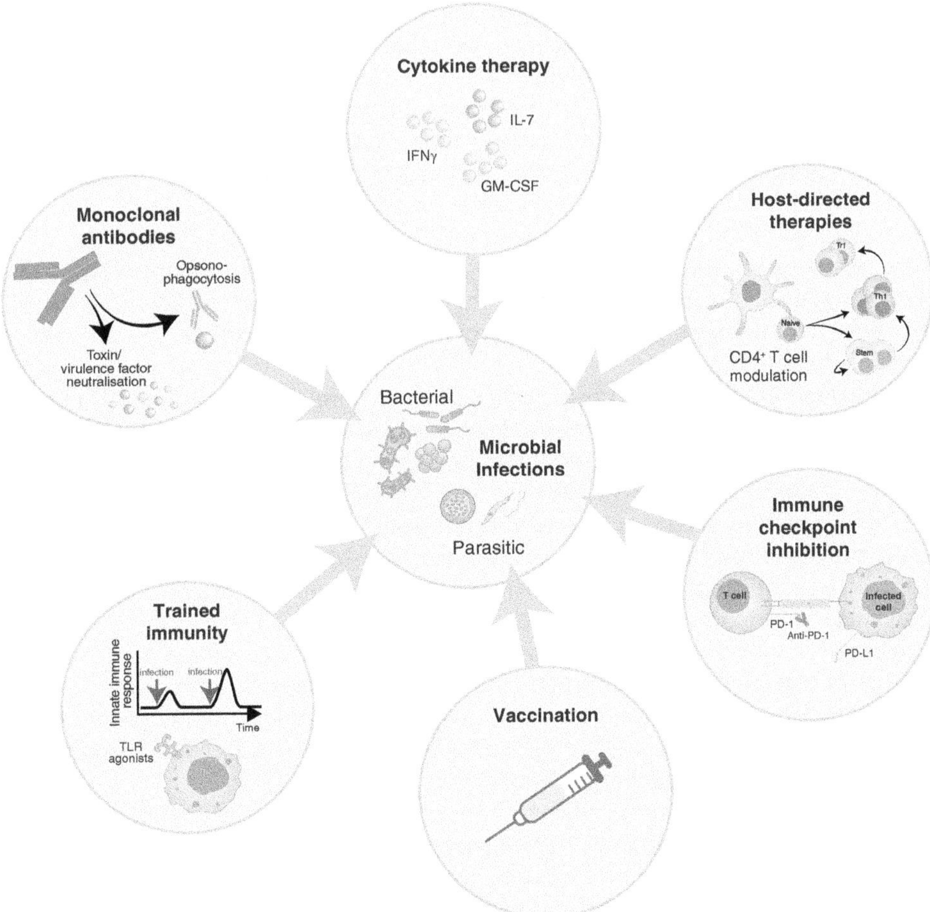

FIGURE 9.1 Diagram of immunotherapy approaches for microbial infections.

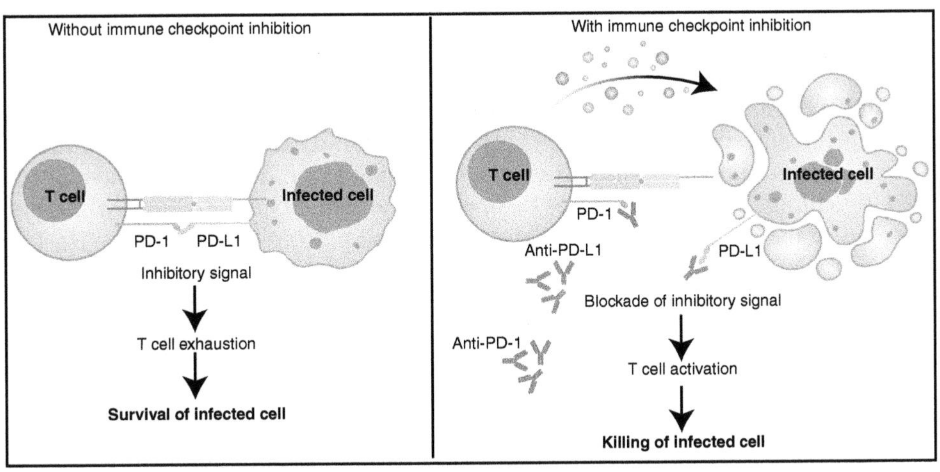

FIGURE 9.2 Mechanism of immune checkpoint inhibition in chronic microbial infections.

treatment approaches are still experimental in infectious diseases, early-phase studies suggest that checkpoint blockade can augment immunity without exacerbating inflammation when used judiciously [14].

Another promising area is trained immunity, whereby innate immune cells are epigenetically reprogrammed to respond more robustly to subsequent infections. Bacillus Calmette–Guérin (BCG) vaccination has demonstrated non-specific protective effects in multiple contexts, including respiratory infections (see Figure 9.1). Pharmacological inducers of trained immunity, including TLR agonists, are being investigated as vaccine adjuvants and stand-alone immunostimulants. TLR4 and TLR7/8 agonists, for example enhance the maturation and activation of dendritic cells and macrophages, potentially improving microbial clearance and enhancing vaccine efficacy [15].

In parasitic infections, clinical applications of immunotherapy are still in early stages but show considerable promise [14]. Therapeutic vaccines designed not only to prevent infection but also to modulate immune responses during chronic disease are a key focus. Adjuvanted subunit vaccines for malaria, such as RTS, S/AS01 and R21/Matrix-M, aim to enhance protective antibody and T cell responses. In leishmaniasis, experimental vaccines seek to elicit strong T helper type 1 (Th1) cell immunity, which is critical for effective parasite control ([16]). Importantly, the use of novel adjuvants that promote tissue-resident memory or stem-like T-cell formation may be necessary for long-term efficacy (Figure 9.1). An active area of research to try to achieve these goals is modulating cytokine signalling pathways that regulate immune cell metabolism. For example, transforming growth factor beta (TGFβ) promotes the establishment of quiescent or stem-like physiological states in T cells by suppression of mammalian target of rapamycin (mTOR) [17].

T cell-based strategies are also emerging, particularly in the context of chronic or recurrent parasitic infections. For instance, modulation of $CD4^+$ T cell responses through immune checkpoint blockade or cytokine therapy has been shown to reverse T cell exhaustion in leishmaniasis and improve parasite control ([18]). Controlled human malaria infection (CHMI) studies have revealed that exposure to parasites drives the development of $CD4^+$ T cell-mediated immune regulation, even after a single infection [19]. Similar responses are observed in young children living in malaria-endemic areas [8]. Thus, interventions that manipulate this response to improve anti-parasitic immune responses could offer new prophylactic or therapeutic tools.

HDT represents a paradigm shift in treating parasitic diseases, focusing on modulating the host response rather than targeting the pathogen directly. One example is the use of ruxolitinib, a Janus Kinase (JAK) 1/2 inhibitor, to suppress maladaptive IFN-I signalling. This approach has been shown to reduce inflammation while preserving or enhancing protective immunity, providing proof of concept for HDT in malaria and leishmaniasis clinical settings [20, 21].

Importantly, these immunotherapies are not envisioned as replacements for antimicrobial agents but as complementary tools. By integrating immunotherapy with standard treatments, it may be possible to improve pathogen clearance, prevent recurrence, and reduce the emergence of resistance. Rational combination therapies, whereby agents that modulate immune responses against pathogens are paired with antimicrobial drugs, will be central to future clinical applications and should be designed based on the immunological landscape of each infection.

9.3 CHALLENGES AND LIMITATIONS

Despite growing enthusiasm for immunotherapy in infectious diseases, its clinical application faces substantial scientific, translational, and regulatory challenges. Infectious diseases involve a diverse array of pathogens that actively manipulate host immunity in dynamic and tissue-specific ways. This complexity complicates the design, evaluation, and deployment of HDTs across microbial infections.

One major challenge is the limited translational pipeline. While preclinical studies using mouse models or *ex vivo* human immune systems have yielded promising results, relatively few immunotherapeutic agents have advanced to late-phase clinical trials for infectious diseases. This gap reflects both scientific uncertainty and structural disincentives: the cost of immunotherapy development is high, the return on investment for infectious disease indications is often limited, and regulatory pathways remain underdeveloped for non-traditional anti-infective agents, such as HDTs. Additionally, immunotherapies rarely meet the classical criteria for microbiological efficacy (e.g. reduction in pathogen load), making it difficult to demonstrate benefit using traditional endpoints. These limitations contribute to bottlenecks in translation from bench to bedside.

Another key concern is the risk of immunopathology. Immune activation, while essential for clearing pathogens, can cause tissue damage if unchecked. This is particularly relevant in infections where inflammation contributes significantly to morbidity, such as TB, cerebral malaria, or visceral leishmaniasis. Immunotherapies that boost T cell responses or inhibit regulatory pathways (e.g. PD-1, IL-10) may tip the balance towards excessive inflammation, exacerbating rather than alleviating disease. Although this is also a risk in oncology, these treatments are usually conducted in clinical settings where careful monitoring and interventions can occur, thereby reducing risks associated with these adverse events. Identifying the appropriate timing, dosage, and patient population for these interventions remains a central challenge for infectious diseases.

This leads to a core challenge: how to balance immune stimulation with immune regulation. While enhancing immunity is desirable in chronic or immunosuppressive infections, excessive stimulation may precipitate autoimmunity or worsen bystander tissue injury. HDTs must walk a fine line between suppressing deleterious inflammation and preserving protective immune responses. Clinical decision-making in this context is further complicated by the lack of reliable biomarkers to predict immunological trajectories or treatment responses in individual patients. The lack of such biomarkers remains a major unmet need to advance the development and clinical testing of HDTs in AMR bacterial infections and parasitic diseases.

A related limitation lies in our incomplete understanding of host heterogeneity. Immune responses to infection vary widely between individuals due to factors such as age, sex, nutritional status, coinfections, comorbidities (e.g. diabetes), prior exposure, and host genetic background. These variables influence not only susceptibility to infection but also responsiveness to immunotherapy. For example, older adults and immunocompromised patients may have blunted responses to vaccines or immune checkpoint inhibitors, while others may be predisposed to hyperinflammation [22]. Most preclinical models do not capture this diversity, and clinical trials often exclude populations most at risk of infection or severe disease.

Addressing these challenges will require a multidisciplinary approach that integrates systems immunology, personalised medicine, and context-specific trial design, including the development of appropriate controlled human infection models. While immunotherapy holds great promise for infectious diseases, realising its full potential demands a more nuanced and data-driven understanding of immune variation, risk thresholds, and optimal therapeutic windows across diverse patient populations.

9.4 FUTURE DIRECTIONS

The next decade promises to be transformative for immunotherapy in infectious diseases, driven by converging advances in systems immunology, multi-omics technologies, gene editing, and precision medicine. These innovations are enabling a shift from empirical, population-based approaches towards rational, individualised strategies that target specific immune pathways disrupted during infection (see Figure 9.3).

One of the most powerful developments is the application of systems immunology, particularly single-cell and spatial omics, to dissect immune responses at unprecedented resolution. Technologies such as single-cell RNA sequencing (scRNA-seq), mass cytometry, and spatial transcriptomics are revealing the cellular heterogeneity, functional states, and tissue localisation of immune cells during infection [23]. These approaches are uncovering novel targets for immunotherapy, such as stem-like or tissue-resident memory T cells, and identifying immunosuppressive niches that could be reversed by HDTs [24, 25]. In parasitic infections, spatial mapping of splenic and hepatic immune microenvironments during *Leishmania* or *Plasmodium* infection, for example may reveal immune checkpoint molecules or cytokine networks amenable to intervention for promotion of disease resolution, as well as durable, protective immunity.

Gene-editing tools such as Clustered Regularly Interspaced Short Palindromic Repeats (CRISPR)/Cas9 are also beginning to reshape infectious disease research. Beyond basic target discovery, CRISPR is being explored to engineer T cells, macrophages, or dendritic cells with enhanced antimicrobial activity or resistance to immunosuppression [26]. At the same time, nanoparticle-based delivery systems are being optimised to transport immunomodulatory molecules, such as cytokines, immune checkpoint inhibitors, small interfering RNAs, or viral vectors directly to infected tissues, minimising systemic toxicity [27]. The messenger ribonucleic acid (mRNA) platform, which rose to prominence during the COVID-19 pandemic, holds enormous promise for infectious disease immunotherapy. mRNA-based vaccines and immunomodulators can be rapidly designed, modified, and deployed to elicit targeted immune responses or induce protective cytokine environments [28].

Together, these technologies lay the foundation for precision immunotherapy, where treatments are tailored to an individual's immune profile, infection history, genetic background, and disease stage. Predictive algorithms incorporating omics data, clinical parameters, and machine learning will help stratify patients most likely to benefit from specific immunotherapies while minimising risk. For example, patients with elevated IL-10 or PD-1 expression during *Leishmania* infection may be selected for checkpoint blockade, while those with dominant IFN-I signatures in malaria might benefit from JAK–STAT inhibitors. This personalised approach could also guide the use of immunomodulatory adjuvants in vaccine design or determine

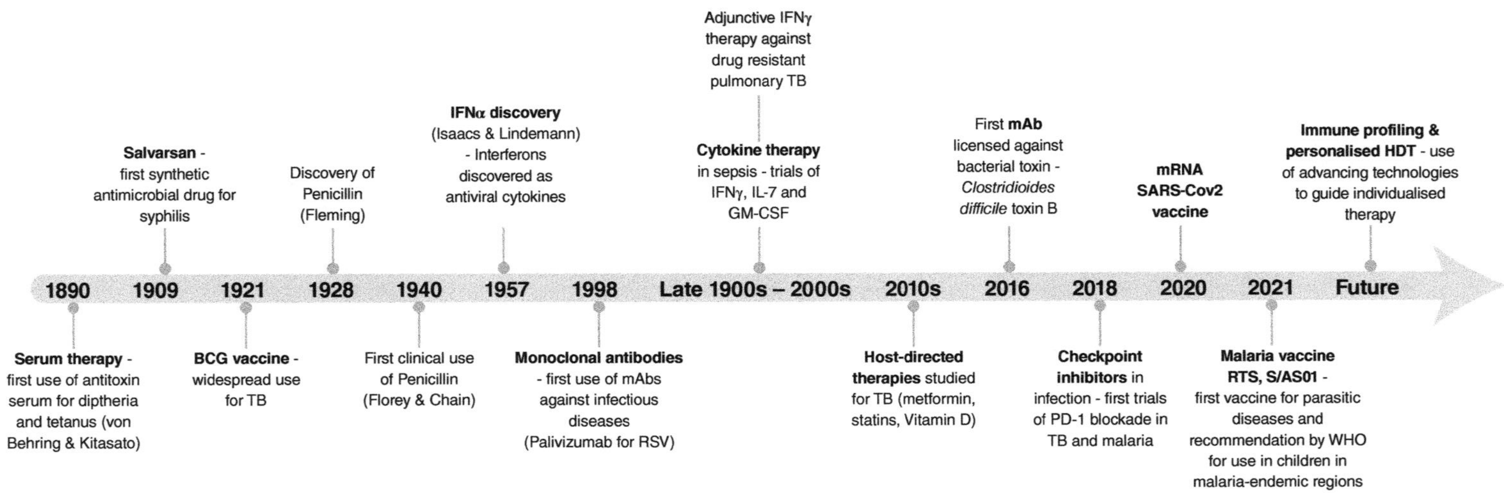

FIGURE 9.3 Timeline of immunotherapy development in infectious disease.

optimal timing for immunotherapy in relation to antimicrobial treatment. However, these personalised approaches will be limited by the scale of affected people and associated costs. One approach to address this issue could be to sort patients into specific groups based on readily available biomarker assays that could direct the best approaches to treating a population with maximum impact.

Realising this vision will require robust collaboration between academia, biotechnology companies, and global health organisations. Translating cutting-edge immunological insights into scalable therapies demands not only innovation but also investment, infrastructure, and coordination. Public–private partnerships will be critical in bridging the translational gap, particularly for neglected tropical diseases where market incentives are limited. Collaborative clinical trial networks, shared biorepositories, and harmonised data platforms can accelerate the development and evaluation of immunotherapies across diverse global settings.

In summary, the future of immunotherapy in infectious diseases is poised to harness technological convergence and collaborative science to deliver more effective, durable, and equitable treatments. With continued investment and integration of immunological insight into clinical decision-making, the field stands at the threshold of a new era in infection control.

9.5 CASE STUDIES AND REAL-WORLD EXAMPLES

9.5.1 Monoclonal Antibody Bezlotoxumab Neutralising Clostridioides Difficile Toxin B and Preventing Recurrent Infection [10, 11]

9.5.1.1 Disease Context

Recurrent *Clostridioides difficile* infection (rCDI) is a major clinical problem, particularly in elderly and immunocompromised patients. Following initial therapy, up to one in four patients experience recurrence, often associated with persistent toxin production, microbiome disruption, and prolonged morbidity. The risk of relapse increases with each episode, and available treatments have a limited ability to prevent recurrence.

9.5.1.2 Mechanism

Bezlotoxumab is a human mAb specifically targeting toxin B, a key virulence factor responsible for mucosal damage and disease recurrence. Administered as a single intravenous infusion alongside standard-of-care antibiotic treatment (e.g. vancomycin, fidaxomicin, or metronidazole), bezlotoxumab binds circulating toxin B and neutralises its cytotoxic effects. This prevents ongoing epithelial injury and modulates inflammatory responses in the gut, allowing the microbiota to recover and reducing conditions that favour relapse.

9.5.1.3 Impact

In placebo-controlled clinical trials, patients receiving bezlotoxumab plus standard antibiotics had significantly lower rates of *Clostridioides difficile* recurrence compared to antibiotics alone (from approximately 25% down to 10–15%). The benefit was particularly pronounced in high-risk individuals, such as older adults, people with severe disease, or those with multiple prior episodes. Rates of sustained clinical cure improved, with longer-term protection over a 12-week follow-up. Bezlotoxumab was generally well tolerated, with adverse effects comparable to placebo and no significant systemic toxicity. This targeted immunotherapy represents the first approved strategy specifically designed to prevent recurrent *Clostridioides difficile infection* and has been integrated into clinical guidelines as adjunctive therapy for high-risk patients.

This case demonstrates how antibody-based immunotherapy to neutralise microbial toxins can shift outcomes in infections where recurrence is driven by persistent virulence factors rather than active bacterial load.

9.5.2 Adjunctive Interferon-γ in Drug-Resistant Pulmonary Tuberculosis [29]

9.5.2.1 *Disease Context*

Drug-resistant pulmonary TB, including multidrug-resistant (MDR) cases, presents a major therapeutic challenge due to limited treatment options, prolonged therapy, and poor outcomes. In a Cuban pilot open-label clinical trial, eight patients with drug-resistant pulmonary TB were enrolled to evaluate an adjunctive immunotherapy approach in combination with tailored anti-TB chemotherapy.

9.5.2.2 *Mechanism*

Patients received recombinant human interferon-γ (IFN-γ) at a dose of 1×10^6 international units (IU) intramuscularly daily for 4 weeks, followed by three times weekly for an additional 20 weeks. IFN-γ enhances macrophage activation and supports the Th1 cell-mediated immune response, which is essential for controlling *M. tuberculosis*. By boosting cell-mediated immunity, IFN-γ aims to improve bacterial clearance in patients whose immune systems are insufficiently controlling infection despite antimicrobial treatment.

9.5.2.3 *Impact*

All eight patients achieved sputum smear and culture conversion within three months. Radiological imaging showed reduced pulmonary lesions in all participants, with complete resolution in one case. Clinical recovery was evidenced by weight gain and improved general health. Importantly, IFN-γ therapy was well tolerated, with only mild adverse events such as low-grade fever and joint pain. These outcomes support the potential of IFN-γ as a safe and effective host-directed adjunctive therapy for enhancing treatment outcomes in drug-resistant TB, warranting further investigation in larger controlled trials.

9.5.3 BCG Vaccination and Trained Immunity for Protection Against Bacterial and Parasitic Infections [30, 31]

9.5.3.1 *Disease Context*

The BCG vaccine, originally developed to protect against TB, has been observed to confer broader, non-specific protection against a range of infectious diseases. This unexpected benefit has been reported in both bacterial and parasitic infection settings, particularly in low-resource environments where BCG is routinely administered. Epidemiological studies suggest reduced mortality and infection rates in BCG-vaccinated individuals, even in the absence of *M. tuberculosis* exposure, prompting investigations into the underlying immunological mechanisms.

9.5.3.2 Mechanism

BCG vaccination induces a form of innate immune memory known as trained immunity. This process involves the functional reprogramming of monocytes and other innate immune cells, mediated through PRRs such as nucleotide-binding oligomerisation domain 2 (NOD2). Following BCG exposure, these cells undergo epigenetic and metabolic changes that enhance their responsiveness to subsequent infections. As a result, upon reexposure to unrelated pathogens, these trained innate cells produce higher levels of pro-inflammatory cytokines, enabling more effective microbial control.

9.5.3.3 Impact

The ability of BCG to enhance innate immunity beyond its intended target opens new avenues for preventing infections, especially in populations at high risk of bacterial or parasitic disease. This has practical implications for global health, suggesting that BCG and similar live-attenuated vaccines could serve as low-cost, broadly protective interventions. The concept of trained immunity is now being explored as a platform for novel immunotherapies and adjuvant strategies, particularly in settings where rapid, broad-spectrum protection is needed.

9.5.4 Anti-IL-10 Receptor Antibody Therapy in Visceral Leishmaniasis (Preclinical)

9.5.4.1 Disease Context

Visceral leishmaniasis is a parasitic disease characterised by infection of internal organs, especially the spleen, liver, and bone marrow, often leading to fatal outcomes if left untreated. In experimental mouse models, chronic infection results in high parasite burdens and suppressed cellular immunity. Chemotherapy can clear parasites slowly and incompletely. Researchers investigated whether targeting host immune regulation could improve treatment efficacy and disease resolution.

9.5.4.2 Mechanism

In this disease, IL-10 plays a central role in limiting protective immune responses, allowing parasites to survive within host macrophages. Administration of antagonistic antibodies against the IL-10 receptor (IL-10R) blocks IL-10 signalling, releasing the brake on the immune system. Blockade of IL-10R unleashes IFN-γ-driven macrophage activation and promotes Th1 cell responses. When combined with anti-leishmanial drugs, anti-IL-10R therapy accelerates parasite killing by enhancing cell-mediated immunity, while chemotherapy targets the parasite directly.

9.5.4.3 Impact

Mice treated with the combination of anti-IL-10R antibody and chemotherapy show reduced organ parasite loads compared to chemotherapy alone. Immune reactivation results in enhanced Th1 cell responses, increased macrophage leishmanicidal activity, and faster clearance of infection. These results suggest that modulating host immune regulation can convert an inefficient or failed treatment into an effective one. The study demonstrates that strategic immunotherapy, targeting regulatory pathways like those stimulated by IL-10, can synergise with conventional drugs and may improve outcomes in visceral leishmaniasis, especially where drug efficacy is limited by host immune suppression.

9.5.5 Immune Checkpoint Blockade (PD-1/PD-L1) in Malaria (Preclinical/Translational) [34]

9.5.5.1 Disease Context

During blood-stage malaria infection, *Plasmodium* parasites provoke a strong yet dysfunctional immune response. In established infections, $CD4^+$ and $CD8^+$ T cell subsets become exhausted and express elevated levels of inhibitory receptors such as PD-1 and lymphocyte-activation gene 3 (LAG-3). This exhausted state impairs their capacity to produce cytokines and perform effective pathogen clearance, allowing the parasite to persist and maintain high parasitaemia.

9.5.5.2 Mechanism

Immune checkpoint blockade targeting PD-1/programmed death-ligand 1 (PD-L1) and LAG-3 was employed in murine models with ongoing blood-stage malaria. The therapeutic approach involved administering antibodies that bind and inhibit these inhibitory pathways, increasing T cell activation. Blockade of PD-L1 (combined in this study with LAG-3 blockade) leads to improved activation of exhausted T cells, enhancing their proliferation and cytokine production. This restored effector function in pathogen-specific T cells, enabling a more robust adaptive immune response against *Plasmodium.*

9.5.5.3 Impact

Combined blockade of PD-L1 and LAG-3 resulted in accelerated clearance of established parasitaemia in mice, with many animals achieving rapid resolution of the infection. Treated mice demonstrated restored T cell activity, elevated levels of inflammatory cytokines, and enhanced parasite-specific immune responses. The intervention significantly shortened infection duration compared to controls and improved disease outcomes without obvious immunopathology. These results suggest that immune checkpoint blockade can reverse immune exhaustion in chronic malaria, offering a promising host-directed strategy to improve parasite clearance and potentially inform adjunctive therapies or vaccine enhancement in human malaria.

9.5.6 Type I Interferon Signalling Blockade in Malaria (Preclinical/Translational) [21, 35, 36]

9.5.6.1 Disease Context

In malaria, especially during initial and recurring infections, persistent or excessive Type I interferon (IFN) signalling is increasingly recognised as detrimental. Rather than aiding clearance, sustained IFN-I responses can suppress effective adaptive immunity, hinder germinal centre (GC) formation, and impair protective T cell function. This immunoregulatory imbalance limits immune memory development and can contribute to severe disease manifestations, underscoring the need to modulate IFN-I signalling to improve immunity.

9.5.6.2 Mechanism

Preclinical and human challenge studies demonstrate that therapeutic modulation of the IFN-I axis through inhibitors of downstream signalling can enhance immune responses. In animal models, drugs like JAK1/2 inhibitors reduce IFN-I–mediated inflammation and restore Th1 cell activity, improving $CD4^+$ T cell responses. In CHMI studies, transient inhibition of JAK/STAT signalling (a key pathway downstream of IFN-I) using the small-molecule ruxolitinib has been shown to attenuate inflammatory biomarkers while enhancing antigen-specific memory responses. These interventions effectively recalibrate immune activation, balancing pathogen control with minimised immunosuppression.

9.5.6.3 Impact

Results in mouse malaria models reveal that blocking IFN-I signalling leads to lower parasitaemia, improved survival, and reduced immunopathology. In experimental human malaria, ruxolitinib was safe and well tolerated, dampened inflammatory markers (like C-reactive protein (CRP), intercellular adhesion molecule 1 (ICAM-1), and angiopoietin-2), and on re-exposure enhanced markers of GC activation and immune memory (e.g. human leukocyte antigen – DR isotype (HLA-DR) and chemokine (C-X-C motif) ligand 13 (CXCL13)). Overall, these findings point towards an emerging therapeutic strategy whereby targeted modulation, rather than wholesale suppression of IFN-I pathways, boosts effective immunity and holds promise for adjunctive treatment against severe malaria syndromes and could improve vaccine responses in malaria-endemic settings.

KEY TERMS & DEFINITIONS SIDEBAR

Antimicrobial Resistance (AMR) The ability of microorganisms (e.g. bacteria, parasites) to survive and grow despite exposure to drugs designed to kill them or stop their growth.

Checkpoint Blockade A therapy that inhibits immune checkpoint receptors (e.g. PD-1, CTLA-4) to restore or enhance immune cell activity, particularly T cell function.

Cytokine Storm A harmful, excessive immune response characterised by the rapid release of large amounts of inflammatory cytokines, often leading to tissue damage.

Host-Directed Therapy (HDT) An approach that targets the host's immune or physiological pathways – rather than the pathogen itself – to improve disease outcomes.

Immunotherapy A treatment strategy that modifies or harnesses the immune system to prevent, control, or eliminate disease.

Monoclonal Antibody (mAb) A laboratory-produced antibody that binds to a specific antigen, used for diagnostics or to neutralise pathogens or modulate immune responses.

Trained Immunity A form of immune memory in innate immune cells that leads to enhanced responses upon re-exposure to pathogens, independent of adaptive immunity.

LIST OF ABBREVIATIONS

Abbreviation	Full Term	Definition
ACE2	Angiotensin-converting enzyme 2	A receptor on host cells used by some viruses, including SARS-CoV-2, for entry.
AMR	Antimicrobial resistance	The ability of microbes to resist the effects of drugs previously effective against them.
BCG	Bacillus Calmette–Guérin	A live-attenuated vaccine is primarily used to prevent tuberculosis.
$CD4^+$	Cluster of differentiation 4 positive	A marker on T helper cells that is important for orchestrating immune responses.
$CD8^+$	Cluster of differentiation 8 positive	A marker on cytotoxic T lymphocytes that kill infected or cancerous cells.
CHMI	Controlled human malaria infection	A research method involving intentional infection of human volunteers with malaria under controlled conditions.
CRISPR	Clustered regularly interspaced short palindromic repeats	A gene-editing technology that enables precise modifications to DNA.
CRP	C-reactive protein	An acute-phase protein and marker of systemic inflammation.
CXCL13	Chemokine (C-X-C motif) ligand 13	A cytokine that recruits B cells to GCs.
CTLA-4	Cytotoxic T-lymphocyte antigen 4	An immune checkpoint receptor that inhibits T cell activation.
DNA	Deoxyribonucleic acid	The molecule that carries genetic instructions in organisms.

Abbreviation	Full Term	Definition
DOTS	Directly observed therapy, short-course	A TB treatment strategy involving supervised administration of medication.
GC	Germinal Centre	A site within lymphoid tissue where B cells mature and undergo affinity maturation.
HDT	Host-directed therapy	A therapeutic approach that targets host mechanisms rather than the pathogen directly.
HIV	Human immunodeficiency virus	A virus that attacks the immune system and causes AIDS.
HLA-DR	Human leukocyte antigen – DR isotype	A MHC class II molecule is involved in antigen presentation.
ICAM-1	Intercellular adhesion molecule 1	A protein that facilitates leukocyte endothelial transmigration.
IFN-γ	Interferon Gamma	A cytokine critical for innate and adaptive immunity, especially macrophage activation.
IFN-I	Type I interferons	A group of cytokines, including IFN-α and IFN-β, is involved in antiviral responses and immune modulation.
IFNAR	Interferon alpha/beta receptor	The receptor for IFN-Is.
IL-10	Interleukin 10	An anti-inflammatory cytokine that regulates immune responses.
IL-10R	Interleukin 10 receptor	The receptor through which IL-10 exerts its immunoregulatory effects.
IU	International units	A unit of measurement for the amount of a substance based on its biological activity.
JAK	Janus kinase	A family of enzymes involved in cytokine signalling via the JAK–STAT pathway.
LAG-3	Lymphocyte-activation gene 3	An immune checkpoint receptor that downregulates T cell activity.
mAb	Monoclonal antibody	Lab-engineered antibodies are designed to bind specific antigens.
mRNA	Messenger ribonucleic acid	A type of RNA used to produce proteins and, in vaccines, to instruct cells to make immune-targeted proteins.
mTOR	Mammalian target of rapamycin	A kinase that regulates cell growth, metabolism, and immune function.

Abbreviation	Full Term	Definition
NOD2	Nucleotide-binding oligomerisation domain 2	A pattern recognition receptor involved in innate immune responses.
PD-1	Programmed cell death protein 1	An immune checkpoint receptor that inhibits T cell activity.
PD-L1	Programmed death-ligand 1	A ligand for PD-1 that downregulates immune responses.
PRR	Pattern recognition receptor	Receptors of the innate immune system that recognise pathogen-associated molecular patterns.
RNA	Ribonucleic acid	A nucleic acid involved in the coding, decoding, regulation, and expression of genes.
RSV	Respiratory syncytial virus	A common virus that causes respiratory infections.
rCDI	Recurrent *Clostridioides difficile* infection	The recurrence of infection by *C. difficile* often occurs after initial treatment.
rIFN-γ	Recombinant interferon gamma	A synthetic form of IFN-γ is used therapeutically.
SARS-CoV-2	Severe acute respiratory syndrome coronavirus 2	The virus responsible for COVID-19.
scRNA-seq	Single-cell RNA sequencing	A technique to analyse gene expression at the single-cell level.
TB	Tuberculosis	A bacterial infection caused by *Mycobacterium tuberculosis.*
TCR	T-cell receptor	The molecule on T cells that recognises antigens presented by MHC molecules.
TGFβ	Transforming growth factor beta	A cytokine involved in immune regulation and tissue repair.
Th1	T Helper type 1 cell	A subtype of T helper cells that promotes cellular immunity.
TLR	Toll-like receptor	A class of PRRs that detect microbial components and activate immune responses.
Treg	Regulatory T cell	A T cell subset involved in suppressing immune responses and maintaining tolerance.
WHO	World Health Organization	A UN agency responsible for global public health.

REVIEW QUESTIONS

1. What are the key mechanisms by which parasites evade host immunity?
2. How do immune checkpoint inhibitors enhance immune responses to chronic infections?
3. What are the potential risks associated with immunotherapy in infectious diseases?
4. Describe a clinical application of host-directed therapy in a parasitic infection.
5. What technological advances are driving future innovations in immunotherapy for infection?

REFERENCES

1. Murray, C.J.L., Ikuta, K.S., Sharara, F. et al. (2022). Global burden of bacterial antimicrobial resistance in 2019: a systematic analysis. *Lancet* 399 (10325): 629–655. https://doi.org/10.1016/S0140-6736(21)02724-0.
2. Kaminsky, R. and Mäser, P. (2025). Global impact of parasitic infections and the importance of parasite control. *Front Parasitol* 4: e13. https://doi.org/10.3389/fpara.2025.1546195.
3. Bordon, Y. (2016). The many sides of Paul Ehrlich. *Nat Immunol* 17 (1): S6–S6. https://doi.org/10.1038/ni.3601.
4. Graham, B.S. and Ambrosino, D.M. (2015). History of passive antibody administration for prevention and treatment of infectious diseases. *Curr Opin HIV AIDS* 10 (3): 129–134. https://doi.org/10.1097/coh.0000000000000154.
5. Liu, J.K. (2014). The history of monoclonal antibody development – progress, remaining challenges and future innovations. *Ann Med Surg (Lond)* 3 (4): 113–116. https://doi.org/10.1016/j.amsu.2014.09.001.
6. Esposito, S., Amirthalingam, G., Bassetti, M. et al. (2023). Monoclonal antibodies for prophylaxis and therapy of respiratory syncytial virus, SARS-CoV-2, human immunodeficiency virus, rabies and bacterial infections: an update from the World Association of Infectious Diseases and Immunological Disorders and the Italian Society of Antinfective Therapy. *Front Immunol* 14: 1162342. https://doi.org/10.3389/fimmu.2023.1162342.
7. Pauken, K.E. and Wherry, E.J. (2015). Overcoming T cell exhaustion in infection and cancer. *Trends Immunol* 36 (4): 265–276. https://doi.org/10.1016/j.it.2015.02.008.
8. Boyle, M.J., Engwerda, C.R., and Jagannathan, P. (2024). The impact of *Plasmodium*-driven immunoregulatory networks on immunity to malaria. *Nat Rev Immunol* https://doi.org/10.1038/s41577-024-010.1-5 24: 637–653.
9. Kaye, P.M., Svensson, M., Ato, M. et al. (2004). The immunopathology of experimental visceral leishmaniasis. *Immunol Rev* 201: 239–253. https://doi.org/10.1111/j.0105-2896.2004.00188.x.
10. Wilcox, M.H., Gerding, D.N., Poxton, I.R. et al. (2017). Bezlotoxumab for prevention of recurrent *Clostridium difficile* infection. *N Engl J Med* 376 (4): 305–317. https://doi.org/10.1056/NEJMoa1602615.
11. Motley, M.P., Banerjee, K., and Fries, B.C. (2019). Monoclonal antibody-based therapies for bacterial infections. *Curr Opin Infect Dis* 32 (3): 210–216. https://doi.org/10.1097/qco.0000000000000539.
12. Kauffman, K.D., Sakai, S., Lora, N.E. et al. (2021). PD-1 blockade exacerbates *Mycobacterium tuberculosis* infection in rhesus macaques. *Sci Immunol* 6 (55): eabf3861. https://doi.org/10.1126/sciimmunol.abf3861.
13. Kirman, J., McCoy, K., Hook, S. et al. (1999). CTLA-4 blockade enhances the immune response induced by mycobacterial infection but does not lead to increased protection. *Infect Immun* 67 (8): 3786–3792. https://doi.org/10.1128/iai.67.8.3786-3792.1999.

14. Wykes, M.N. and Lewin, S.R. (2018). Immune checkpoint blockade in infectious diseases. *Nat Rev Immunol* 18 (2): 91–104. https://doi.org/10.1038/nri.2017.112.
15. Mulder, W.J.M., Ochando, J., Joosten, L.A.B. et al. (2019). Therapeutic targeting of trained immunity. *Nat Rev Drug Discov* 18 (7): 553–566. https://doi.org/10.1038/s41573-019-0025-4.
16. Kumar, R. and Engwerda, C. (2014). Vaccines to prevent leishmaniasis. *Clin Transl Immunol* 3 (3): e13. https://doi.org/10.1038/cti.2014.4.
17. Gabriel, S.S., Tsui, C., Chisanga, D. et al. (2021). Transforming growth factor-beta-regulated mTOR activity preserves cellular metabolism to maintain long-term T cell responses in chronic infection. *Immunity* 54 (8): 1698–1714.e5. https://doi.org/10.1016/j.immuni.2021.06.007.
18. Kumar, R., Chauhan, S.B., Ng, S.S. et al. (2017). Immune checkpoint targets for host-directed therapy to prevent and treat leishmaniasis. *Front Immunol* 8: 1492. https://doi.org/10.3389/fimmu.2017.01492.
19. Montes de Oca, M., Kumar, R., Rivera, F.L. et al. (2016). Type I interferons regulate immune responses in humans with blood-stage *Plasmodium falciparum* infection. *Cell Rep* 17 (2): 399–412. https://doi.org/10.1016/j.celrep.2016.09.015.
20. Kumar, R., Bunn, P.T., Singh, S.S. et al. (2020). Type I interferons suppress anti-parasitic immunity and can be targeted to improve treatment of visceral Leishmaniasis. *Cell Rep* 30 (8): 2512–2525.e2519. https://doi.org/10.1016/j.celrep.2020.01.099.
21. Webster, R., Oyong, D.A., Abd-Rahman, A.N. et al. (2025). Adjunctive ruxolitinib attenuates inflammation and enhances antiparasitic immunity in human volunteers experimentally infected with *Plasmodium falciparum*. *Sci Transl Med.* 17: eaea2531. https://doi: 10.1126/scitranslmed.aea2531.
22. Goronzy, J.J. and Weyand, C.M. (2013). Understanding immunosenescence to improve responses to vaccines. *Nat Immunol* 14 (5): 428–436. https://doi.org/10.1038/ni.2588.
23. Molla Desta, G. and Birhanu, A.G. (2025). Advancements in single-cell RNA sequencing and spatial transcriptomics: transforming biomedical research. *Acta Biochim Polon* 72: 13922. https://doi.org/10.3389/abp.2025.13922.
24. Kunzli, M. and Masopust, D. (2023). CD4(+) T cell memory. *Nat Immunol* 24 (6): 903–914. https://doi.org/10.1038/s41590-023-01510-4.
25. Zou, D., Yin, Z., Yi, S.G. et al. (2024). CD4(+) T cell immunity is dependent on an intrinsic stem-like program. *Nat Immunol* 25 (1): 66–76. https://doi.org/10.1038/s41590-023-01682-z.
26. Li, T., Yang, Y., Qi, H. et al. (2023). CRISPR/Cas9 therapeutics: progress and prospects. *Signal Transd Target Therapy* 8 (1): 36. https://doi.org/10.1038/s41392-023-01309-7.
27. Mitchell, M.J., Billingsley, M.M., Haley, R.M. et al. (2021). Engineering precision nanoparticles for drug delivery. *Nat Rev Drug Disc* 20 (2): 101–124. https://doi.org/10.1038/s41573-020-0090-8.
28. Parhiz, H., Atochina-Vasserman, E.N., and Weissman, D. (2024). mRNA-based therapeutics: looking beyond COVID-19 vaccines. *Lancet* 403 (10432): 1192–1204. https://doi.org/10.1016/S0140-6736(23)02444-3.
29. Suárez-Méndez, R., García-García, I., Fernández-Olivera, N. et al. (2004). Adjuvant interferon gamma in patients with drug-resistant pulmonary tuberculosis: a pilot study. *BMC Infect Dis* 4 (1): 44. https://doi.org/10.1186/1471-2334-4-44.
30. Kleinnijenhuis, J., Quintin, J., Preijers, F. et al. (2012). Bacille Calmette-Guérin induces NOD2-dependent nonspecific protection from reinfection via epigenetic reprogramming of monocytes. *Proc Natl Acad Sci* 109 (43): 17537–17542. https://doi.org/10.1073/pnas.1202870109.
31. Netea, M.G., Joosten, L.A.B., Latz, E. et al. (2016). Trained immunity: a program of innate immune memory in health and disease. *Science* 352 (6284): aaf1098. https://doi.org/10.1126/science.aaf1098.
32. Murray, H.W., Moreira, A.L., Lu, C.M. et al. (2003). Determinants of response to interleukin-10 receptor blockade immunotherapy in experimental visceral leishmaniasis. *J Infect Dis* 188 (3): 458–464. https://doi.org/10.1086/376510.

33. Nylén, S. and Sacks, D. (2007). Interleukin-10 and the pathogenesis of human visceral leishmaniasis. *Trends Immunol* 28 (9): 378–384. https://doi.org/10.1016/j.it.2007.07.004.
34. Butler, N.S., Moebius, J., Pewe, L.L. et al. (2012). Therapeutic blockade of PD-L1 and LAG-3 rapidly clears established blood-stage *Plasmodium* infection. *Nature Immunol* 13 (2): 188–195. https://doi.org/10.1038/ni.2180.
35. Bukali, L., Oyong, D., de Labastida Rivera, F. et al. (2025). Transient JAK/STAT inhibition by ruxolitinib modulates malaria-specific CD4+ T cell responses and enhances recall immunity in volunteers experimentally infected with *Plasmodium falciparum*. *medRxiv* https://doi.org/10.1101/2025.04.09.25325416.
36. Wang, Y, De Labastida Rivera, F., Edwards, C. L. et al. (2023). STING activation promotes autologous type I interferon-dependent development of type 1 regulatory T cells during malaria. *J Clin Invest* 133: e169417. https://doi: 10.1172/JCI169417.

CHAPTER 10

Vaccine Development and Immune Response Optimisation

LIMIN ZHAO[1,2], JINGRU GONG[1], IAN H. FRAZER[1], AND ZHIAN CHEN[1]

[1] Frazer Institute, The University of Queensland, Brisbane, Queensland, Australia

[2] Department of Otolaryngology Head and Neck Surgery, Beijing TongRen Hospital, Capital Medical University, Beijing, China

LEARNING OBJECTIVES

- Describe the historical evolution of vaccine platforms, from live-attenuated and inactivated vaccines to modern nucleic acid and recombinant approaches.
- Explain the immunological principles underlying vaccine-induced protection, including innate immune cell activation, germinal centre (GC) responses, T follicular helper (T_{FH}) cell function, and plasma cell (PC) differentiation.
- Analyse how vaccine platforms such as virus-like particles (VLPs), viral vectors, and mRNA–LNP platforms induce strong immune responses.

10.1 INTRODUCTION

Vaccines are among the most effective public health interventions. Traditional platforms such as live-attenuated, inactivated, and subunit vaccines have enabled the control, and in some cases, elimination of major pathogens such as smallpox, polio, measles, and hepatitis B viruses (HBVs) [1]. Many of these vaccines have provided decades of durable protection worldwide, particularly several developed nearly a century ago, including diphtheria, tetanus, and Bacillus Calmette-Guérin (BCG) vaccines, which continue to serve as the backbone of routine immunisation programmes today.

A common feature of early vaccine development was the extensive culture and serial passage of infectious organisms, either to attenuate their pathogenicity or to generate sufficient material for inactivation while retaining immunogenicity. The advent of the genomic era then revolutionised vaccine design by enabling the use of genetic information to guide antigen selection. A landmark achievement was the cloning and expression of the HBV surface antigen, which self-assembles into virus-like particles (VLPs) and led to the first licenced recombinant vaccine in 1986 [2]. Recombinant DNA technology subsequently paved the way for a new generation of vaccines, including VLP-based human papillomavirus (HPV) vaccines and transgenetically detoxified, protein extract-based acellular pertussis vaccines [3].

However, traditional vaccine development has been time-consuming and largely dependent on empirical, trial-and-error approaches. Recent pandemics have exposed the limitations of these platforms, particularly their inability to scale rapidly or adapt to newly emerging pathogens. In addition, while some conventional vaccines generate long-lasting immunity, others exhibit rapid waning or limited effectiveness against rapidly evolving microbes. These challenges have accelerated the shift towards next-generation platforms designed to enable faster production, greater adaptability, and improved breadth and durability of immune protection.

Building on advances in genomics, protein engineering, and biomaterials, modern vaccinology now leverages deep immunological insight to improve antigen presentation, fine-tune innate activation, and sustain long-term immunity. This chapter highlights the innovations that reshaped vaccine design and the immunological principles that underpin effective protection against infectious diseases.

10.2 HOW THE IMMUNE SYSTEM RESPONDS TO VACCINES

Essentially, vaccines introduce harmless mimics of pathogens to elicit immunological memory, enabling rapid and effective responses upon pathogen re-exposure. Most vaccines (with the BCG vaccine as a notable exception, acting primarily through T-cell immunity) protect by eliciting pathogen-specific antibodies that recognise microbial epitopes [4, 5]. Circulating and mucosal antibodies neutralise pathogens by blocking their interaction with host cells and preventing dissemination, which serves as the principal mechanism of protection against viral infections [6]. For bacterial pathogens, antibodies also mediate opsonophagocytic and complement-dependent lysis, facilitating pathogen clearance [6]. Antibodies are secreted by plasma cells (PCs), a subtype of terminally differentiated B cells whose generation depends on finely coordinated innate and adaptive immune responses [7].

Following subcutaneous or intramuscular vaccination, antigens drain from the injection site to secondary lymphoid organs, where adaptive immunity is initiated. Particle size determines trafficking route [8]: specifically, small antigens or nanoparticles (20–200 nm) drain to lymph nodes directly via lymphatic vessels, whereas larger particles (>200 nm) rely on uptake and transport by migratory dendritic cells (DCs). Innate immune cells like DCs can engulf and process antigens into peptides presented on major histocompatibility complex (MHC) molecules and present antigen peptides to T cells, functioning as specialised antigen-presenting cells (APCs). APCs recognise pathogen-associated molecular patterns (PAMPs) or damage-associated molecular patterns (DAMPs) via pattern recognition receptors (PRRs), such as Toll-like receptors (TLRs), and become activated and migrate to draining lymph nodes. In addition to antigen presentation, activated APCs also provide costimulatory signals for T-cell activation [8]. Notably, B cells can also function as APCs. They may be activated in a T-cell-dependent manner via cognate B-cell receptor (BCR)-antigen engagement or independently through TLR-mediated pathways triggered by PAMPs [9].

Live-attenuated and some inactivated whole-pathogen vaccines effectively activate APCs through their abundant PAMPs. But purified subunit antigens lack sufficient PAMPs, so adjuvants are essential to potentiate innate activation. For most of the twentieth century, the traditional aluminium-based adjuvants ('alum') were the only licenced adjuvants, which have now been complemented by new adjuvants like liposomes and TLR agonists that stimulate PRRs or induce cell stress and DAMP release [10].

Within lymph nodes, small antigens can directly access B-cell follicles, whereas larger ones are captured by subcapsular macrophages or DCs [11, 12]. B cells recognise antigens via their BCR, internalise and present them on MHC class II molecules, and receive 'help signals' from $CD4^+$ T cells at the T–B border [13]. Depending on the signals received, activated B cells either differentiate into short-lived PCs or enter germinal centres (GCs) for affinity maturation [7].

In parallel, $CD4^+$ T cells are activated by T-cell receptor (TCR) recognition of peptide–MHC class II complexes on APCs, particularly DCs, along with costimulatory signals provided by APCs (e.g. CD80/CD86-CD28 signalling) [14]. The activated $CD4^+$ T cells differentiate into various effector phenotypes, among which T follicular helper (T_{FH}) cells are critical for humoral immunity. Localising within B-cell follicles, T_{FH} cells provide CD40 ligand (CD40L) and cytokines such as interleukin-21 (IL-21) to support B-cell proliferation, isotype switching, and differentiation [15–17].

During early responses, extrafollicular PCs arise with support from T helper cells. Some live-attenuated vaccines can also trigger extrafollicular antibody responses independently of T cells, for example via bacterial lipopolysaccharide (LPS) [7]. The extrafollicular PCs produce immunoglobulin G (IgG) or IgM with low-affinity maturation and short-lived protection [7].

Durable vaccine-induced protection depends on GC responses. Within GCs, B cells undergo somatic hypermutation (SHM) of Ig genes [7, 18]. B cells compete for antigens retained on follicular dendritic cells (FDCs) and then present them to T_{FH} cells for helper signals [19]. Through multiple rounds of selection and a process termed affinity maturation, clones with high antigen affinity are preferentially expanded. Ultimately, selected GC B cells differentiate into long-lived plasma cells (LLPCs) or memory B cells [7, 20, 21]. The molecular cues governing these fates remain incompletely defined, but BCR's affinity to bind antigens and T_{FH} interactions are central determinants [7, 21].

Moreover, $CD8^+$ T cells complement humoral immunity by killing infected cells and limiting viral spread. Notably, in SARS-CoV-2 infection, individuals with impaired antibody responses can still exhibit substantial vaccine-mediated protection, underscoring the important contribution of T-cell immunity [22]. In vaccination, they are activated through cross-presentation of antigens on MHC class I molecules by DCs [23]. Upon activation, naïve $CD8^+$ T cells proliferate into effector and memory subsets: most effector cells are short-lived, while memory $CD8^+$ T cells persist long-term and mount rapid recall responses upon re-exposure [23]. However, in humans, only live-attenuated vaccines efficiently induce cytotoxic $CD8^+$ T-cell responses, highlighting a key unmet goal for next-generation vaccine platforms [24].

With booster vaccination or natural infection, long-lived memory B cells rapidly differentiate into PCs, producing high-affinity antibodies. Because these memory B cells arise from GC reactions and have undergone affinity maturation, the secondary response is faster and stronger than the primary response [24]. Therefore, many vaccines use a prime–boost regimen to amplify antibody protection. However, high levels of circulating neutralising antibodies during boosting can limit antigen access for memory B cells [25]. To overcome this, longer intervals between doses are often applied. For example, the common '0–1–6' schedule, with boosters at 1 and 6 months after the primary immunisation.

In summary, vaccine efficacy relies on the precise orchestration of innate sensing, T–B collaboration, and memory formation. These principles provide the mechanistic foundation for the rational design of next-generation vaccines.

10.3 NEXT-GENERATION VACCINE PLATFORMS AND THE IMMUNOLOGICAL ADVANTAGES

10.3.1 VLP

The advent of genomics and high-throughput sequencing in the 1990s profoundly accelerated immunology and virology research. As viral genomes were rapidly decoded and recombinant expression systems became widely accessible, vaccine development shifted from empirical methods towards more rational, sequence-guided design. A landmark success of this genomics-enabled era is the HPV vaccines.

CASE STUDY: GARDASIL: TRANSLATING VLP TECHNOLOGY INTO GLOBAL CANCER PREVENTION

HPVs are a family of over 40 closely related DNA viruses that induce hyperproliferation of epithelial and mucosal cells [26]. Although most infections resolve spontaneously, persistent infection with high-risk HPV subtypes is the primary cause of the majority of cervical cancer and leads to several other anogenital and oropharyngeal malignancies. Therefore, effective vaccination against HPV represents a critical strategy for cervical cancer prevention.

In 1991, using wild-type HPV16 L1 capsid genes cloned from a precancerous lesion, Frazer and Zhou successfully expressed recombinant L1 capsid protein in eukaryotic cells and showed that the L1 protein self-assembled into VLPs [27]. VLPs utilise the intrinsic properties of viral capsid or envelope proteins to self-assemble into virus-like structures. They closely mimic native virions in size, shape, and epitope presentation but lack viral DNA or RNA, making them non-infectious[1, 29]. In principle, VLP vaccines can elicit immune responses without adjuvants, but co-formulation with adjuvants further optimises their efficacy [30]. The strong immunogenicity of VLP vaccines is not yet fully understood, but their capacity to target B cells is considered a key factor. As mentioned earlier, their nanoscale size (20–200 nm) facilitates efficient lymphatic drainage, allowing them to reach B-cell follicles directly [31]. Furthermore, their large surface-to-volume ratio enhances interactions with APCs (Figure 10.1). More importantly, VLPs display dense, repetitive arrays of epitopes; for example, HPV VLPs present 72 copies of the L1 protein [28]. In vitro observation showed this multivalent arrangement and viral-like geometry promote extensive cross-linking of BCRs, resulting in strong activation signals and more efficient antigen presentation via MHC class II molecules compared to soluble monomeric antigens [32–34]. In vivo studies in mouse models using HIV-engineered outer domain germline-targeting

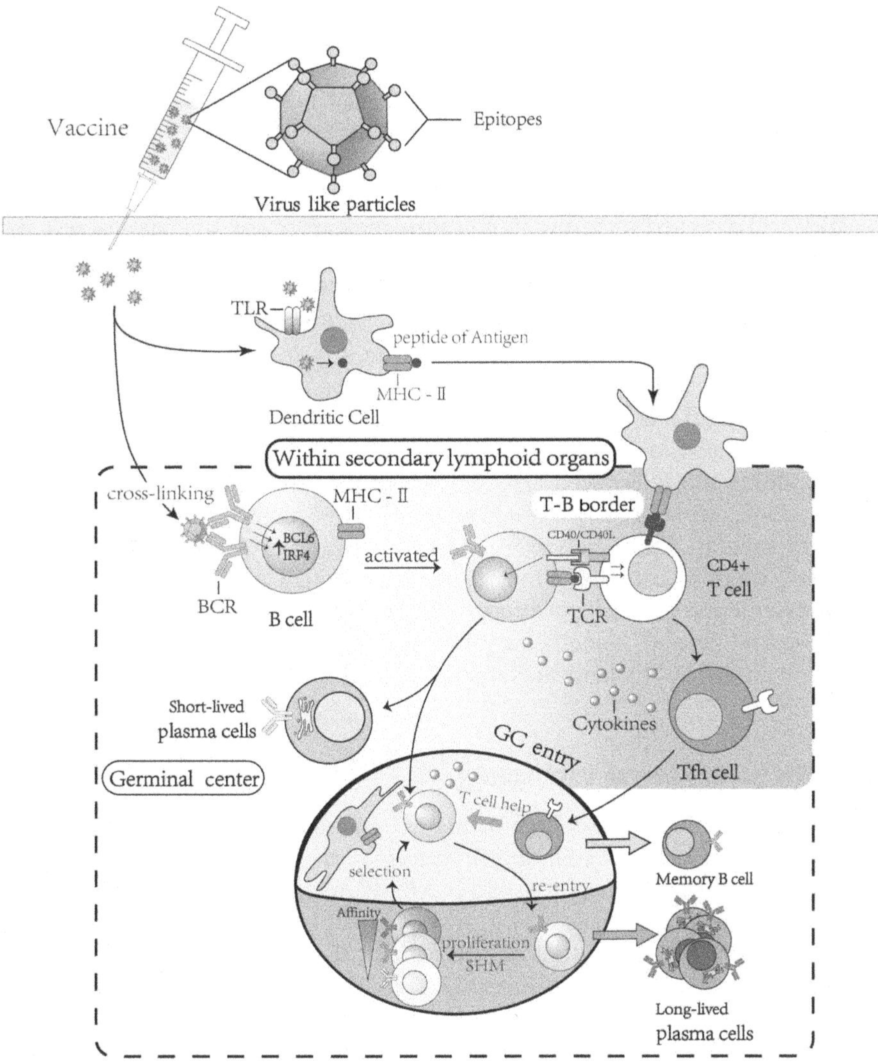

FIGURE 10.1 The immune response induced by VLP vaccines. Following VLP immunisation, dendritic cells (DCs) process and present antigens via major MHC class II to prime CD4$^+$ T cells. Antigen-specific B cells are activated through BCR cross-linking. Cognate interactions between activated B and CD4$^+$ T cells at the T–B border promote the differentiation of T_{FH} cells and B cells entering the GC. Within the GC, T_{FH} cells provide help for somatic hypermutation, affinity maturation, and selection, resulting in the generation of memory B cells and long-lived plasma cells.

(eOD-GT) antigens with varying valency showed that higher antigen valence and BCR cross-linking enhance B-cell activation. This was marked by enhanced expression of the transcription factors BCL6 and IRF4, driving greater B-cell expansion, elevated extrafollicular PC output, and more robust GC formation in a T_{FH}-dependent manner [35]. HPV-VLPs can effectively activate DCs via TLR4 signalling, promoting antigen presentation [36, 37]. Interestingly, in vivo mouse models immunised with RNA phage Qβ-derived VLPs also showed that B cells themselves can act as the primary APCs, directly priming cognate $CD4^+$ T cells. In this context, TLR–myeloid differentiation primary response protein 88 (MyD88) signalling was essential in B cells but dispensable in DCs, as $CD4^+$ T-cell activation was unaffected in DC-depleted mice [38].

HPV VLPs proved to be highly immunogenic, forming the basis of vaccines to prevent infection with the cervical cancer-associated HPV genotypes. The first licenced HPV vaccine ('Gardasil') was approved by the Australian Therapeutic Goods Administration in 2006 and, together with Cervarix, has since been incorporated into national immunisation programmes in more than 140 countries by 2023. The impact on cervical cancer prevention has been profound: vaccination before age 17 could reduce the risk of cervical cancer by around 10-fold compared with unvaccinated individuals [39].

In addition to the licenced HBV, HPV vaccines, and a later Hepatitis E Virus (HEV) vaccine, numerous VLP-based vaccines have been in clinical development for pathogens such as chikungunya virus, Zika virus, and SARS-CoV-2 [40]. In summary, VLP vaccines combine strong safety with potent immunogenicity, making them a versatile and promising platform with broad applications in infectious disease prevention and beyond. Nonetheless, their application as a universal vaccine platform is still limited by challenges in large-scale production, purification, and stability.

10.3.2 The Era of Reverse Vaccinology

Advances in sequencing and bioinformatics enabled 'next-generation' strategies for rational vaccine design. A landmark example was the development of a vaccine against *Neisseria meningitidis* serogroup B (MenB), a leading cause of meningococcal disease in developed countries [41]. Conventional polysaccharide capsule-targeted strategies for other *N. meningitidis* groups were unsuitable; this is because the MenB polysaccharide is structurally similar to human glycoproteins, raising a serious risk of autoimmune cross-reactivity [42]. To identify suitable vaccine antigens, the MenB genome was analysed. Unlike viruses, which encode relatively few proteins, bacteria present many more potential antigens, and eventually, ~350 putative surface proteins were identified [42]. These were expressed and tested for immunisation in mice. The generated antibodies were screened, and five antigen targets were identified as meeting key criteria: immunogenicity and conservation across different MenB strains. These proteins were combined to form a multivalent vaccine [42]. Clinical trials demonstrated strong immunogenicity and protection, leading to its licensure in 2013. The vaccine is now widely used worldwide. Based on this reverse genetics approach, the concept of 'reverse vaccinology' has established the foundation for modern vaccine development.

As seen in the development of MenB vaccines, modern vaccinology increasingly relies on systematic, large-scale antigen discovery. Looking ahead, the integration of artificial intelligence (AI) and machine learning (ML) shows promise to fundamentally transform this process [43]. These technologies could enable enhanced prediction of epitopes, exemplified by advances in identifying MHC-presented T-cell epitopes using deep learning frameworks [44, 45]. AI-driven protein modelling tools such as AlphaFold and RoseTTAFold now enable high-precision prediction of protein structures from amino acid sequences [46, 47]. These innovations accelerate structure-guided antigen design (as discussed below), including stabilising key antigen conformation and mRNA sequence optimisation, paving the way for a future paradigm in which vaccine design becomes increasingly data-driven, predictive, and systematically optimised.

10.3.3 Synthetic Nucleotide Vaccines

Recombinant protein vaccines, while safe and widely used, often show low immunogenicity and rapidly waning protection, as seen with influenza vaccines [48]. Moreover, their production and characterisation remain time-consuming, limiting responsiveness to emerging pathogens [49].

The next conceptual leap in vaccinology came with the idea of directly using nucleic acids as vaccines, based on the discovery that injected DNA or mRNA could drive in vivo protein expression [50]. A landmark study in 1992 demonstrated that plasmids encoding human growth hormone, delivered into mouse skin by microprojectiles, elicited growth hormone-specific antibody responses. Early studies in mice showed that both DNA and mRNA could induce antibody production, but most efforts focused on DNA vaccines, as mRNA was considered unstable and overly inflammatory [50].

In practice, DNA vaccines proved only modestly immunogenic in humans [51]. Approaches such as electroporation and plasmid-encoded adjuvants were tested to improve efficacy, but enthusiasm eventually shifted to mRNA vaccines following their remarkable success during the COVID-19 pandemic. Within 11 months of the SARS-CoV-2 genome being sequenced, mRNA vaccines were designed, tested, approved, and deployed worldwide. These vaccines transformed global vaccine development [52].

mRNA became a viable vaccine platform only after major breakthroughs addressed its instability and innate immune recognition. In the early 2000s, Karikó and Weissman discovered that RNA sensors distinguish self from foreign RNA through modified nucleosides [53]. Substituting uridine with pseudouridine (Ψ) reduces recognition by TLR3, TLR7, TLR8, and cytosolic sensors such as retinoic acid-inducible gene I (RIG-I) and melanoma differentiation-associated protein 5 (MDA5), thereby diminishing inflammation and enhancing translation. These modifications underpin the design of SARS-CoV-2 mRNA vaccines [54–57].

Both DNA and mRNA vaccines rely on somatic cells and APCs to express antigens in situ, allowing native folding and post-translational modification before presentation to the immune system. Yet, only one DNA vaccine – ZyCoV-D for SARS-CoV-2 – has been licenced, showing roughly 30% lower efficacy than mRNA vaccines and requiring 30–100-fold higher nucleic acid doses [58, 59]. The key difference might be attributed to the delivery hurdles: DNA must traverse both plasma and nuclear membranes to access the nucleus, whereas mRNA functions after cytoplasmic entry.

Efficient cytoplasmic delivery of mRNA is enabled by lipid nanoparticles (LNPs). LNPs comprise ionisable lipids – critical for endosomal escape – alongside structural, helper, and PEG-lipids. Ionisable lipids remain neutral at physiological pH to avoid rapid clearance but become protonated in endosomes, destabilising membranes and releasing mRNA into the cytoplasm [60].

Beyond delivery, LNPs also provide adjuvanticity. mRNA vaccines rapidly activate macrophages and DCs in draining lymph nodes, inducing cytokines such as IL-6, CXCL10, and IFN-γ within hours [61]. In humans, these innate signatures peak 24 hours postinjection and are amplified after boosting. Fine-needle aspirates reveal persistent GC and T_{FH} cell responses, consistent with strong and durable humoral immunity [62, 63] (Figure 10.2).

Interestingly, in mice, the potent antibody responses elicited by the BNT162b2 SARS-CoV-2 mRNA vaccine appear independent of classical innate sensors, including TLR2–5, TLR7, inflammasome components ASC and NLRP3, or the cGAS–STING pathway [61]. However, compensatory activation of parallel pathways in knockout models cannot be excluded. In contrast, an influenza haemagglutinin (HA) mRNA–LNP vaccine showed partial dependence on MyD88, an adaptor for

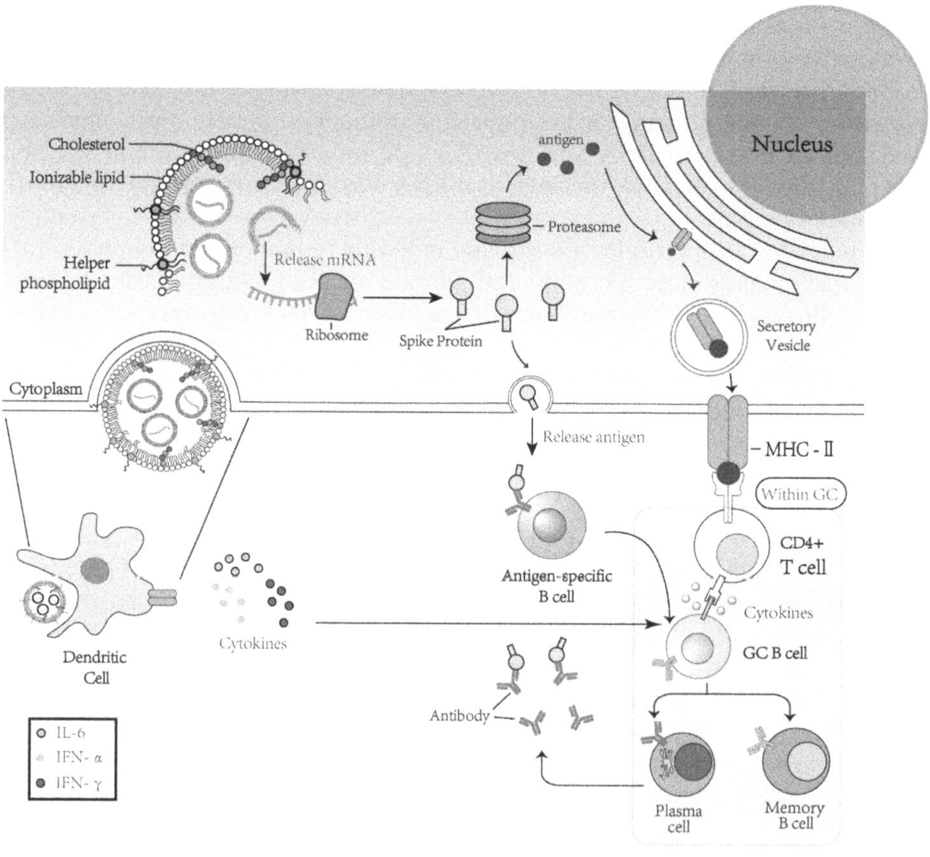

FIGURE 10.2 The immune response induced by mRNA vaccine. Lipid nanoparticles deliver mRNA into host cells, where it is translated into antigen proteins. The released antigen is then captured and processed by antigen-presenting cells, enabling MHC-II presentation to CD4⁺ T cells in the germinal centre. Cognate CD4⁺ T-cell help drives germinal centre formation, B-cell selection, isotype switching, and differentiation into long-lived PCs and memory B cells. Original figure; copyright held by the chapter contributors.

several TLRs, suggesting context- and formulation-specific innate engagement [64]. Importantly, LNPs lacking mRNA did not reproduce these effects, indicating that innate immune activation arises from the mRNA–LNP complex rather than lipids alone [64].

Evidence from SARS-CoV-2 mRNA vaccination suggests that LNPs trigger release of DAMPs without engaging canonical programmed cell-death pathways such as necroptosis or pyroptosis [61]. Nonetheless, the precise mechanisms underlying LNP-induced innate activation remain unclear and appear highly formulation-dependent: for example certain heterocyclic-lipid LNPs activate STING, while others signal via TLR4 [65].

10.3.4 Viral Vector Vaccine

Beyond mRNA vaccines, other innovative approaches, particularly those enabled by reverse vaccinology, have also demonstrated substantial value. Among them, viral-vector vaccines represented the second major class to gain emergency authorisation during the COVID-19 pandemic. Interest in these platforms had been growing since the early 2000s, paralleling the rise of mRNA vaccines following the decline in enthusiasm for DNA-based systems [66].

Viral-vector vaccines employ non-replicating viruses to deliver antigen-encoding DNA into host cells, enabling endogenous antigen expression and presentation. Prior to 2020, five such vaccines were licenced for human use, including a yellow fever virus (YFV)-based Japanese encephalitis vaccine and an adenovirus 26-based Ebola vaccine [66]. During the COVID-19 pandemic, five adenoviral vector vaccines were approved, demonstrating potent immunogenicity without the need for additional adjuvants, owing to the vector's intrinsic ability to engage innate sensors and drive strong adaptive responses [66].

Adenoviral vectors enter host cells via receptors such as the Coxsackievirus and Adenovirus Receptor, triggering endocytosis [67]. Both viral capsid components and released DNA activate multiple PRRs, inducing type I interferon and proinflammatory cytokine production [66, 68]. This innate activation promotes Th1-biased antibody responses and robust $CD8^+$ T-cell priming through MHC-I antigen presentation by transfected DCs [69, 70].

However, rare but serious adverse events – most notably thrombosis with thrombocytopenia syndrome (TTS) – emerged during large-scale deployment [71]. These effects, linked to interactions between the viral capsid and platelet factor 4, prompted the discontinuation of adenoviral SARS-CoV-2 vaccines in several countries. This experience highlights that the structural and biochemical properties of both antigen and delivery platform profoundly shape vaccine efficacy and safety, guiding future refinements of viral-vector and other next-generation systems.

10.3.5 Structure-Guided Vaccine Design

It is important to recognise that even with 'next-generation' vaccine platforms that enable in situ expression of antigens in their native conformation, many proteins do not naturally elicit potent antibody responses. To address such challenges, structure-guided antigen engineering is essential. A prominent example is the development of vaccines against the respiratory syncytial virus (RSV). RSV infects nearly all children under age three and is a leading cause of hospitalisation and death in infants under one year [72]. Yet despite its prevalence, RSV vaccine development faced setbacks for over half a century.

The crystal structure of an RSV fusion (F) protein-neutralising antibody complex revealed the reason: potent neutralising epitopes (i.e. those that induce strong neutralising antibody responses), termed antigenic sites Ø and V, are exposed only in the metastable pre-fusion conformation of the F protein. In contrast, the protein tends to adopt a stable post-fusion form that masks these sites [72, 73]. Engineering mutations to stabilise the F protein in the pre-fusion state produced antigens that elicited far stronger neutralising responses [73], ultimately enabling the successful licensure of highly protective RSV vaccines in 2023, now available for infants worldwide. Recently, researchers at the University of Queensland developed a 'molecular clamp' protein scaffold to stabilise the pre-fusion F protein even without mutations. Prototype vaccines based on this approach have shown efficacy comparable to, or exceeding, current RSV vaccines [73] and were recently licenced.

10.4 OUTSTANDING QUESTIONS IN IMPROVING VACCINE IMMUNITY

Next-generation vaccine platforms hold immense promise for controlling emerging infectious diseases, yet key challenges persist.

While some vaccines, such as YFV-17D, induce lifelong immunity, others, including mRNA-based SARS-CoV-2 vaccines, show waning protection within a year [74]. Efficacy also varies across individuals due to host heterogeneity shaped by age, metabolism, and genetics. In older adults, immunosenescence, which is marked by loss of naïve T cells, mature B cells, and impaired innate cell function [75], leads to diminished vaccine responsiveness [76]. Extending protection and improving efficacy in vulnerable populations thus remain central goals in vaccinology.

Innate immune activation profoundly shapes adaptive responses. Live-attenuated vaccines such as YFV-17D engage multiple TLRs (TLRs 2, 7, 8, and 9), driving DC activation, robust $CD4^+$ T-cell-dependent antibody production, and potent $CD8^+$ T-cell responses [74]. In contrast, mRNA vaccines stimulate these pathways relatively less efficiently, contributing to weaker long-term immunity [60]. Yet, live-attenuated vaccines are not universally preferred, as attenuated pathogens may rarely revert to virulence, posing risks to pregnant or immunocompromised individuals [49]. Furthermore, attenuation can reduce safety and productivity, and viral evolution risks immune escape. Ongoing efforts to engineer genetically stabilised, safer live-attenuated platforms – such as proteolysis-targeting influenza vaccines – highlight a promising direction [49].

Non-live vaccines, though safer, often require adjuvants to boost innate activation. Modern adjuvants like TLR agonists complement classical aluminium salts by stimulating PRRs or releasing DAMPs. Beyond adjuvants, the kinetics of antigen delivery are crucial: in nonhuman primate HIV models, slow-release systems prolonged germinal-centre reactions and diversified antibody repertoires. Nanoparticle formulations combining TLR7 agonists with sustained-release systems elicited stronger and more durable antibody responses than alum-based adjuvants, underscoring the importance of antigen persistence in shaping immunity [77].

Another major challenge in modern vaccinology is eliciting broadly neutralising antibodies (bnAbs) against variable pathogens such as HIV. BnAbs neutralise diverse strains by recognising conserved epitopes, yet vaccination rarely induces them because their naïve B-cell precursors are scarce and bind weakly to native antigens [78, 79]. Germline-targeting (GT) strategies use engineered immunogens to activate these rare precursors and recruit them into GC responses. The eOD-GT8 60mer – a nanoparticle displaying 60 modified gp120 outer-domain copies – successfully primed VRC01-class bnAb precursors in 97% of participants in a Phase I trial, providing the first clinical proof-of-concept for GT vaccines [80]. Sequential immunisation, starting with a high-affinity GT priming antigen followed by progressively native-like boosters, has been shown in preclinical models to guide bnAb maturation and breadth [81]. Similar strategies are being applied to influenza, where engineered stem-focused or sequential head-variant immunogens elicit cross-strain bnAbs, advancing the pursuit of a 'universal influenza vaccine' [82].

Together, these advances suggest that the long-standing goal of universal, cross-protective vaccines is increasingly within reach. Guided by deep immunological understanding and supported by innovations in delivery and design, next-generation platforms promise vaccines that are safer, longer-lasting, and more broadly protective – ready to meet the challenges of future pandemics.

KEY TERMS & DEFINITIONS SIDEBAR

Antigen-presenting cells (APCs) Immune cells, such as DCs, macrophages, and B cells that capture, process, and present antigens to T cells to initiate adaptive immunity.

Damage-associated molecular patterns (DAMPs) Endogenous molecules released from damaged or dying cells that activate PRRs and induce sterile inflammation.

Germinal centre (GC) A lymphoid microenvironment where activated B cells proliferate, mutate, and mature into high-affinity plasma and memory cells.

Lipid nanoparticles (LNPs) Lipid-based carriers that encapsulate nucleic acids, protect them from degradation, and enable efficient cytoplasmic delivery for antigen expression.

Pathogen-associated molecular patterns (PAMPs) Conserved microbial motifs (e.g. LPS, dsRNA) recognised by PRRs to trigger innate immune responses.

Pattern recognition receptors (PRRs) Innate immune sensors that detect PAMPs or DAMPs and activate inflammatory and antiviral signalling pathways.

Somatic hypermutation (SHM) A mutation process in germinal-centre B cells that diversifies Ig genes and enables affinity maturation.

Toll-like receptors (TLRs) A major class of PRRs that recognise pathogen- or damage-derived ligands at the cell surface or within endosomes to induce cytokine production.

Virus-like particles (VLPs) Non-infectious nanostructures that mimic native viral architecture but lack genetic material, eliciting strong immune responses with excellent safety.

LIST OF ABBREVIATIONS

AI	artificial intelligence
APCs	antigen-presenting cells
BCG	Bacillus Calmette-Guérin
BCR	B-cell receptor
bnAbs	Broadly neutralising antibodies
DAMPs	damage-associated molecular patterns
DCs	dendritic cells
CD40L	CD40 ligand
eOD-GT	outer domain germline-targeting
FDCs	follicular dendritic cells
GC	germinal centre
GT	Germline-targeting
HBV	hepatitis B virus
HPV	human papillomavirus
HEV	Hepatitis E Virus
IgG	immunoglobulin G
IL-21	interleukin-21
LLPCs	long-lived plasma cells
LNPs	lipid nanoparticles
LPS	lipopolysaccharide
MenB	meningitidis serogroup B
MDA5	melanoma differentiation-associated protein 5
MHC	major histocompatibility complex
ML	machine learning
MyD88	myeloid differentiation primary response protein 88
PAMPs	pathogen-associated molecular patterns
PCs	plasma cells
PRRs	pattern recognition receptors
RIG-I	retinoic acid-inducible gene I
RSV	respiratory syncytial virus
SHM	somatic hypermutation
TCR	T-cell receptor
T_{FH}	T follicular helper
TLRs	toll-like receptors
TTS	thrombocytopenia syndrome
VLPs	virus-like particles
YFV	yellow fever virus

REVIEW QUESTIONS

1. What are the key limitations of conventional vaccine platforms, and how have next-generation technologies addressed them?
2. How does vaccine particle size influence the nature and magnitude of immune responses?
3. Compared with other vaccines, what are the advantages of mRNA vaccines? And how to estimate its value for vaccinology?
4. How might future vaccine design integrate insights from systems immunology, structural biology, and AI-based antigen prediction?

REFERENCES

1. Gupta, A., Rudra, A., Reed, K. et al. (2024). Advanced technologies for the development of infectious disease vaccines. *Nat Rev Drug Discov* 23 (12): 914–938.
2. McAleer, W.J., Buynak, E.B., Maigetter, R.Z. et al. (1984). Human hepatitis B vaccine from recombinant yeast. *Nature* 307 (5947): 178–180.
3. Kuchar, E., Karlikowska-Skwarnik, M., Han, S., and Nitsch-Osuch, A. (2016). Pertussis: history of the disease and current prevention failure. *Adv Exp Med Biol* 934: 77–82.
4. Plotkin, S.A. (2010). Correlates of protection induced by vaccination. *Clin Vaccine Immunol* 17 (7): 1055–1065.
5. Andersen, P. and Kaufmann, S.H. (2014). Novel vaccination strategies against tuberculosis. *Cold Spring Harb Perspect Med* 4 (6): a018523.
6. Lu, L.L., Suscovich, T.J., Fortune, S.M., and Alter, G. (2018). Beyond binding: antibody effector functions in infectious diseases. *Nat Rev Immunol* 18 (1): 46–61.
7. Cyster, J.G. and Allen, C.D.C. (2019). B cell responses: cell interaction dynamics and decisions. *Cell* 177 (3): 524–540.
8. Bachmann, M.F. and Jennings, G.T. (2010). Vaccine delivery: a matter of size, geometry, kinetics and molecular patterns. *Nat Rev Immunol* 10 (11): 787–796.
9. Coffman, R.L., Sher, A., and Seder, R.A. (2010). Vaccine adjuvants: putting innate immunity to work. *Immunity* 33 (4): 492–503.
10. Pulendran, B., Prabhu, S.A., and O'Hagan, D.T. (2021). Emerging concepts in the science of vaccine adjuvants. *Nat Rev Drug Discov* 20 (6): 454–475.
11. Phan TG, Grigorova I, Okada T, Cyster JG. Subcapsular encounter and complement-dependent transport of immune complexes by lymph node B cells. *Nat Immunol* 2007;8(9):992–1000.
12. Carrasco, Y.R. and Batista, F.D. (2007). B cells acquire particulate antigen in a macrophage-rich area at the boundary between the follicle and the subcapsular sinus of the lymph node. *Immunity* 27 (1): 160–171.
13. Krogsgaard, M. and Davis, M.M. (2005). How T cells 'see' antigen. *Nat Immunol* 6 (3): 239–245.
14. Chen, L. and Flies, D.B. (2013). Molecular mechanisms of T cell co-stimulation and co-inhibition. *Nat Rev Immunol* 13 (4): 227–242.
15. Vinuesa, C.G., Linterman, M.A., Yu, D., and MacLennan, I.C. (2016). Follicular helper T cells. *Annu Rev Immunol* 34: 335–368.
16. Yu, D., Walker, L.S.K., Liu, Z. et al. (2022). Targeting T(FH) cells in human diseases and vaccination: rationale and practice. *Nat Immunol* 23 (8): 1157–1168.
17. Chen, Z., Cui, Y., Yao, Y. et al. (2023). Heparan sulfate regulates IL-21 bioavailability and signal strength that control germinal center B cell selection and differentiation. *Sci Immunol* 8 (80): eadd1728.

18. Elsner, R.A. and Shlomchik, M.J. (2020). Germinal center and extrafollicular B cell responses in vaccination, immunity, and autoimmunity. *Immunity* 53 (6): 1136–1150.
19. Shulman, Z., Gitlin, A.D., Targ, S. et al. (2013). T follicular helper cell dynamics in germinal centers. *Science* 341 (6146): 673–677.
20. Inoue, T. and Kurosaki, T. (2024). Memory B cells. *Nat Rev Immunol* 24 (1): 5–17.
21. Victora, G.D. and Nussenzweig, M.C. (2022). Germinal centers. *Annu Rev Immunol* 40: 413–442.
22. Wherry, E.J. and Barouch, D.H. (2022). T cell immunity to COVID-19 vaccines. *Science* 377 (6608): 821–822.
23. Jameson, S.C. and Masopust, D. (2018). Understanding subset diversity in T cell memory. *Immunity* 48 (2): 214–226.
24. Ellebedy, A.H. and Ahmed, R. (2012). Re-engaging cross-reactive memory B cells: The influenza puzzle. *Front Immunol* 3: 53.
25. Ellebedy, A.H., Jackson, K.J., Kissick, H.T. et al. (2016). Defining antigen-specific plasmablast and memory B cell subsets in human blood after viral infection or vaccination. *Nat Immunol* 17 (10): 1226–1234.
26. Chesson, H.W., Dunne, E.F., Hariri, S., and Markowitz, L.E. (2014). The estimated lifetime probability of acquiring human papillomavirus in the United States. *Sex Transm Dis.* 41 (11): 660–664.
27. Zhou, J., Sun, X.Y., Stenzel, D.J., and Frazer, I.H. (1991). Expression of vaccinia recombinant HPV 16 L1 and L2 ORF proteins in epithelial cells is sufficient for assembly of HPV virion-like particles. *Virology* 185 (1): 251–257.
28. Zhou, J., Sun, X.Y., Davies, H. et al. (1992). Definition of linear antigenic regions of the HPV16 L1 capsid protein using synthetic virion-like particles. *Virology* 189 (2): 592–599.
29. Ghattas, M., Dwivedi, G., Lavertu, M., and Alameh, M.G. (2021). Vaccine technologies and platforms for infectious diseases: current progress, challenges, and opportunities. *Vaccines (Basel)* 9 (12): 1490.
30. Mohsen, M.O., Zha, L., Cabral-Miranda, G., and Bachmann, M.F. (2017). Major findings and recent advances in virus-like particle (VLP)-based vaccines. *Semin Immunol* 34: 123–132.
31. Manolova, V., Flace, A., Bauer, M. et al. (2008). Nanoparticles target distinct dendritic cell populations according to their size. *Eur J Immunol* 38 (5): 1404–14013.
32. Dempsey, L.A. (2023). Multivalent virus-like epitope display amplifies BCR signaling independent of avidity. *Nat Immunol* 24 (10): 1610–1611.
33. Bachmann, M.F. and Jennings, G.T. (2010). Vaccine delivery: a matter of size, geometry, kinetics and molecular patterns. *Nat Rev Immunol* 10 (11): 787–796.
34. Batista, F.D., Iber, D., and Neuberger, M.S. (2001). B cells acquire antigen from target cells after synapse formation. *Nature* 411 (6836): 489–494.
35. Kato, Y., Abbott, R.K., Freeman, B.L. et al. (2020). Multifaceted effects of antigen valency on B cell response composition and differentiation *in vivo*. *Immunity* 53 (3): 548–563.e8.
36. Mohsen, M.O. and Bachmann, M.F. (2022). Virus-like particle vaccinology, from bench to bedside. *Cell Mol Immunol* 19 (9): 993–1011.
37. Yan, M., Peng, J., Jabbar, I.A. et al. (2005). Activation of dendritic cells by human papillomavirus-like particles through TLR4 and NF-kappaB-mediated signalling, moderated by TGF-beta. *Immunol Cell Biol* 83 (1): 83–91.
38. Hong, S., Zhang, Z., Liu, H. et al. (2018). B cells are the dominant antigen-presenting cells that activate naive CD4(+) T cells upon immunization with a virus-derived nanoparticle antigen. *Immunity* 49 (4): 695–708.e4.
39. Lei, J., Ploner, A., Elfström, K.M. et al. (2020). HPV vaccination and the risk of invasive cervical cancer. *N Engl J Med* 383 (14): 1340–1348.
40. Laxmi, B., Devi, P.U.M., Naveen, T., and Buddolla, V. (2025). Virus-like particles: innovative strategies for combatting emerging and re-emerging viral threats. *The Microbe* 7: 100351.

41. Pizza, M., Scarlato, V., Masignani, V. et al. (2000). Identification of vaccine candidates against serogroup B meningococcus by whole-genome sequencing. *Science* 287 (5459): 1816–1820.
42. Shea, M.W. (2013). The long road to an effective vaccine for meningococcus group B (MenB). *Ann Med Surg* 2 (2): 53–56.
43. Gasperini, G., Baylor, N., Black, S. et al. (2025). Vaccinology in the artificial intelligence era. *Sci Transl Med* 17 (794): eadu3791.
44. Chen, B., Khodadoust, M.S., Olsson, N. et al. (2019). Predicting HLA class II antigen presentation through integrated deep learning. *Nat Biotechnol* 37 (11): 1332–1343.
45. Wohlwend, J., Nathan, A., Shalon, N. et al. (2025). Deep learning enhances the prediction of HLA class I-presented CD8(+) T cell epitopes in foreign pathogens. *Nat Mach Intell* 7 (2): 232–243.
46. Abramson, J., Adler, J., Dunger, J. et al. (2024). Accurate structure prediction of biomolecular interactions with AlphaFold 3. *Nature* 630 (8016): 493–500.
47. Baek, M., DiMaio, F., Anishchenko, I. et al. (2021). Accurate prediction of protein structures and interactions using a three-track neural network. *Science* 373 (6557): 871–876.
48. Davis, C.W., Jackson, K.J.L., McCausland, M.M. et al. (2020). Influenza vaccine–induced human bone marrow plasma cells decline within a year after vaccination. *Science* 370 (6513): 237–241.
49. Rappuoli, R., Alter, G., and Pulendran, B. (2024). Transforming vaccinology. *Cell* 187 (19): 5171–5194.
50. Pardi, N., Hogan, M.J., Porter, F.W., and Weissman, D. (2018). mRNA vaccines — a new era in vaccinology. *Nat Rev Drug Discov* 17 (4): 261–279.
51. Pagliari, S., Dema, B., Sanchez-Martinez, A. et al. (2023). DNA vaccines: history, molecular mechanisms and future perspectives. *J Mol Biol* 435 (23): 168297.
52. Pardi, N. and Krammer, F. (2024). mRNA vaccines for infectious diseases - advances, challenges and opportunities. *Nat Rev Drug Discov* 23 (11): 838–861.
53. Karikó, K., Buckstein, M., Ni, H., and Weissman, D. (2005). Suppression of RNA recognition by Toll-like receptors: the impact of nucleoside modification and the evolutionary origin of RNA. *Immunity* 23 (2): 165–175.
54. Karikó, K., Muramatsu, H., Welsh, F.A. et al. (2008). Incorporation of pseudouridine into mRNA yields superior nonimmunogenic vector with increased translational capacity and biological stability. *Mol Ther* 16 (11): 1833–1840.
55. Anderson, B.R., Muramatsu, H., Nallagatla, S.R. et al. (2010). Incorporation of pseudouridine into mRNA enhances translation by diminishing PKR activation. *Nucl Acids Res* 38 (17): 5884–5892.
56. Kauffman, K.J., Mir, F.F., Jhunjhunwala, S. et al. (2016). Efficacy and immunogenicity of unmodified and pseudouridine-modified mRNA delivered systemically with lipid nanoparticles *in vivo*. *Biomaterials* 109: 78–87.
57. Young, A.P. and Kanneganti, T.D. (2025). For "U" the bell tolls: pseudouridine evades TLR detection. *Mol Cell* 85 (17): 3206–3208.
58. Khobragade, A., Bhate, S., Ramaiah, V. et al. (2022). Efficacy, safety, and immunogenicity of the DNA SARS-CoV-2 vaccine (ZyCoV-D): the interim efficacy results of a phase 3, randomised, double-blind, placebo-controlled study in India. *Lancet* 399 (10332): 1313–1321.
59. Polack, F.P., Thomas, S.J., Kitchin, N. et al. (2020). Safety and efficacy of the BNT162b2 mRNA Covid-19 vaccine. *N Engl J Med* 383 (27): 2603–2615.
60. Verbeke, R., Hogan, M.J., Loré, K., and Pardi, N. (2022). Innate immune mechanisms of mRNA vaccines. *Immunity* 55 (11): 1993–2005.
61. Li, C., Lee, A., Grigoryan, L. et al. (2022). Mechanisms of innate and adaptive immunity to the Pfizer-BioNTech BNT162b2 vaccine. *Nat Immunol* 23 (4): 543–555.
62. Turner, J.S., O'Halloran, J.A., Kalaidina, E. et al. (2021). SARS-CoV-2 mRNA vaccines induce persistent human germinal centre responses. *Nature* 596 (7870): 109–113.

63. Mudd, P.A., Minervina, A.A., Pogorelyy, M.V. et al. (2022). SARS-CoV-2 mRNA vaccination elicits a robust and persistent T follicular helper cell response in humans. *Cell* 185 (4): 603–613.e15.
64. Alameh, M.G., Tombácz, I., Bettini, E. et al. (2021). Lipid nanoparticles enhance the efficacy of mRNA and protein subunit vaccines by inducing robust T follicular helper cell and humoral responses. *Immunity* 54 (12): 2877–2892.e7.
65. Zhang, H., You, X., Wang, X. et al. (2021). Delivery of mRNA vaccine with a lipid-like material potentiates antitumor efficacy through Toll-like receptor 4 signaling. *Proc Natl Acad Sci USA* 118 (6): e2005191118.
66. McCann, N., O'Connor, D., Lambe, T., and Pollard, A.J. (2022). Viral vector vaccines. *Curr Opi Immunol* 77: 102210.
67. Atasheva, S., Yao, J., and Shayakhmetov, D.M. (2019). Innate immunity to adenovirus: lessons from mice. *FEBS Lett* 593 (24): 3461–3483.
68. Van Doremalen, N., Lambe, T., Spencer, A. et al. (2020). ChAdOx1 nCoV-19 vaccine prevents SARS-CoV-2 pneumonia in rhesus macaques. *Nature* 586 (7830): 578–582.
69. Keeton, R., Tincho, M.B., Ngomti, A. et al. (2022). T cell responses to SARS-CoV-2 spike cross-recognize Omicron. *Nature* 603 (7901): 488–492.
70. Ewer, K.J., Barrett, J.R., Belij-Rammerstorfer, S. et al. (2021). T cell and antibody responses induced by a single dose of ChAdOx1 nCoV-19 (AZD1222) vaccine in a phase 1/2 clinical trial. *Nat Med* 27 (2): 270–278.
71. Cines, D.B. and Bussel, J.B. (2021). SARS-CoV-2 vaccine-induced immune thrombotic thrombocytopenia. *N Engl J Med* 384 (23): 2254–2256.
72. McLellan, J.S., Chen, M., Leung, S. et al. (2013). Structure of RSV fusion glycoprotein trimer bound to a prefusion-specific neutralizing antibody. *Science* 340 (6136): 1113–1117.
73. McLellan, J.S., Chen, M., Joyce, M.G. et al. (2013). Structure-based design of a fusion glycoprotein vaccine for respiratory syncytial virus. *Science* 342 (6158): 592–598.
74. Querec, T., Bennouna, S., Alkan, S. et al. (2006). Yellow fever vaccine YF-17D activates multiple dendritic cell subsets via TLR2, 7, 8, and 9 to stimulate polyvalent immunity. *J Exp Med* 203 (2): 413–424.
75. Liu, Z., Liang, Q., Ren, Y. et al. (2023). Immunosenescence: molecular mechanisms and diseases. *Signal Transduct Target Ther* 8 (1): 200.
76. Hofer, S.J., Rapp, S., Klenerman, P., and Simon, A.K. (2025). Understanding and improving vaccine efficacy in older adults. *Nat Aging* 5 (8): 1455–1470.
77. Yin, Q., Luo, W., Mallajosyula, V. et al. (2023). A TLR7-nanoparticle adjuvant promotes a broad immune response against heterologous strains of influenza and SARS-CoV-2. *Nat Mater* 22 (3): 380–390.
78. Burton, D.R., Poignard, P., Stanfield, R.L., and Wilson, I.A. (2012). Broadly neutralizing antibodies present new prospects to counter highly antigenically diverse viruses. *Science* 337 (6091): 183–186.
79. Jardine, J., Julien, J.P., Menis, S. et al. (2013). Rational HIV immunogen design to target specific germline B cell receptors. *Science* 340 (6133): 711–716.
80. Leggat, D.J., Cohen, K.W., Willis, J.R. et al. (2022). Vaccination induces HIV broadly neutralizing antibody precursors in humans. *Science* 378 (6623): eadd6502.
81. Chen, X., Zhou, T., Schmidt, S.D. et al. (2021). Vaccination induces maturation in a mouse model of diverse unmutated VRC01-class precursors to HIV-neutralizing antibodies with >50% breadth. *Immunity* 54 (2): 324–339.e8.
82. Puente-Massaguer, E., Vasilev, K., Beyer, A. et al. (2023). Chimeric hemagglutinin split vaccines elicit broadly cross-reactive antibodies and protection against group 2 influenza viruses in mice. *Sci Adv* 9 (37): eadi4753.

PART

IV

Immunotherapy in Transplantation Settings, Autoimmune, and Inflammatory Diseases

11

Engineering Regulatory T Cells: Applications for Autoimmune Disorders

LEONARDO M.R. FERREIRA[1,2] AND RUSSELL W. COCHRANE[1,2]
[1] Department of Pharmacology and Immunology, Medical University of South Carolina, Charleston, SC, USA
[2] Hollings Cancer Center, Medical University of South Carolina, Charleston, SC, USA

LEARNING OBJECTIVES

After reading this chapter, the reader should be able to:

- Explain the role of Tregs in maintaining immune tolerance and how their dysfunction can contribute to autoimmune disease.
- Describe the cellular and molecular mechanisms by which Tregs suppress immune responses, including contact-dependent and contact-independent pathways.
- Compare outcomes of preclinical studies and clinical trials using polyclonal versus antigen-specific Treg therapies across autoimmune disease indications.
- Evaluate emerging engineering strategies, such as TCR- and CAR-modified Tregs, and their potential to enhance specificity, stability, survival, and suppression for maximum therapeutic efficacy and safety.
- Identify current challenges and future directions in developing Treg-based therapies.

11.1 INTRODUCTION

Autoimmune diseases are caused by the recognition and destruction of self-tissues by the patients' immune system. While individual autoimmune diseases are relatively rare, there are over 80 different autoimmune disorders currently described, together affecting 4–10% of the world's population. The incidence of autoimmune disease is on the rise, and most cases have unknown causes and cannot be cured [1–4]. According to the current paradigm, autoimmunity arises due to defects in self-immune tolerance, that is unresponsiveness of the immune system towards self-antigens. As a result, autoimmune disease patients' B cells produce antibodies against self-proteins, and T cells recognise and eliminate their own cells. For example, type 1 diabetes (T1D) patients harbour antibodies and T cells that target insulin-producing pancreatic beta cells for elimination, whereas non-diabetics do not [5].

First described in 1982, IPEX (immune dysregulation, polyendocrinopathy, X-linked) is a devastating syndrome where patients suffer from several autoimmune disorders, including T1D [6, 7]. At the turn of the millennium, IPEX was found to be caused by mutations in forkhead box protein P3 (FOXP3) [8]. The Nobel Prize in Medicine or Physiology 2025 was awarded jointly to Mary Brunkow, Fred Ramsdell, and Shimon Sakaguchi for their discoveries in peripheral immune tolerance. In 2001, Brunkow and Ramsdell discovered FOXP3 to be the gene defective in scurfy mice, which develop uncontrolled T-cell proliferation and widespread inflammation [9]. FOXP3 was revealed shortly after to be a master transcription factor essential for the development of a lineage of immunosuppressive cells called regulatory T cells (Tregs) [10–12]. Dedicated to inhibiting overt immune responses and maintaining immune homeostasis, Tregs were first described in mice by Sakaguchi in 1995 as thymically derived $CD4^+CD25^+$ cells [13]. The existence of Tregs in humans was confirmed in 2001 [14, 15]. Since this collective 'Eureka!' moment in immunology, manipulating Tregs has been pursued feverishly with the hope of re-establishing immune tolerance in autoimmune and inflammatory diseases, as well as in transplant rejection and graft-versus-host disease (GvHD) [16].

11.2 MECHANISMS OF TREG-MEDIATED SUPPRESSION

Tregs establish immunological tolerance by directly suppressing the activation, expansion, and function of effector immune cells. Tregs suppress through a diverse set of molecular mechanisms that fall under two broad categories: infectious tolerance and bystander suppression. Infectious tolerance consists of the transfer of suppressive capacity from one cell population to another. It is believed to occur mainly by blocking dendritic cell (DC) maturation, polarising DCs towards a tolerogenic phenotype, and/or driving naïve T-cell differentiation into induced Tregs (iTregs) [17, 18]. In bystander suppression, Tregs target an unrelated antigen and indirectly inhibit immune responses within the same microenvironment [19]. Both processes involve combinations of contact-dependent and contact-independent mechanisms.

11.2.1 Contact-Dependent Suppression

Contact-dependent suppression requires direct physical interaction between Tregs and their target cells. These mechanisms can result in the blockade or even removal of costimulatory molecules, modulation of antigen presentation machinery, induction of apoptosis, and/or direct delivery of inhibitory second messengers (Table 11.1).

11.2.2 Contact-Independent Suppression

Contact-independent suppression employs soluble factors to regulate immune responses at a distance or within the immediate microenvironment (Table 11.2). These mechanisms are especially relevant in inflammatory environments where cell-to-cell contact is spatially restricted.

These suppressive mechanisms enable Tregs to exert context-specific control over a variety of immune responses. Each mechanism's relative contribution varies by

TABLE 11.1 Contact-dependent mechanisms employed by Tregs.

Mechanism	Description	References
CTLA-4	CTLA-4 on Tregs competes for and removes CD80 and CD86 from antigen-presenting cells (APCs), such as DCs, via trogocytosis and trans-endocytosis, reducing CD28 costimulation of conventional T cells (Tconv). CTLA-4 binding also induces indoleamine 2,3-dioxygenase (IDO) expression in DCs, depleting tryptophan essential for T-cell activation in the microenvironment.	[20–24]
Granzyme B delivery	Tregs induce apoptosis in Tconv by releasing granzyme B, which binds to cation-independent mannose-6-phosphate receptor (CI-M6PR) on Tconv cells and is internalised via receptor-mediated endocytosis.	[25]
Perforin-dependent cytotoxicity	Tregs lyse target cells, such as DCs, by releasing perforin, which forms pores in the target cell's membrane and delivers granzymes.	[26, 27]
TIGIT	TIGIT on Tregs interacts with CD155 on DCs to promote tolerogenic DC polarisation.	[28, 29]
cAMP transfer	Tregs transfer cyclic AMP to Tconv cells via gap junctions, disrupting Tconv activation.	[30, 31]
LAG-3	LAG-3 on Tregs binds to MHC-II, inhibiting DC activation and maturation.	[32, 33]
Membrane-bound TGF-β (LAP-TGF-β)	Tregs display latency-associated peptide transforming growth factor beta (LAP-TGF-β) on their surface, polarising activated T cells to become iTregs.	[34]
NRP1	Neuropilin-1 (NRP1) increases Treg binding time to immature DCs, preventing Tconv from attaching to DCs.	[35]
Antigen-specific peptide–MHC trogocytosis	Tregs remove cognate peptide–MHC complexes from antigen-presenting cells, reducing their ability to activate antigen-specific Tconv.	[36]

TABLE 11.2 Contact-independent mechanisms employed by Tregs.

Mechanism	Description	References
IL-2 sequestration via CD25	Tregs constitutively express high levels of CD25 and outcompete Tconv cells for IL-2, limiting Tconv survival and proliferation.	[37, 38]
IL-10 secretion	IL-10 dampens APC activation and inflammatory cytokine production.	[39–41]
TGF-β secretion	TGF-β inhibits Tconv proliferation and supports the induction of iTregs from naïve T cells.	[42]
IL-35 secretion	IL-35 is a heterodimeric cytokine (EBI3/IL12A) that suppresses Tconv proliferation and supports the induction of IL-35-producing iTregs.	[43, 44]
IL-1R2 decoy receptor	Tregs express both membrane-bound and soluble IL-1R2, which bind to IL-1β and prevent its engagement with IL-1R1 expressed on effector immune cells.	[45, 46]
CD39/CD73-mediated adenosine production	Extracellular ATP is enzymatically converted into adenosine by cell surface ectoenzymes CD39 and CD73, inhibiting Tconv and APC function via the adenosine receptor A2A.	[47–49]
miRNA-containing extracellular vesicles (EVs)	Tregs release EVs containing microRNAs (miRNAs) to modulate gene expression in target cells, leading to decreased effector activity.	[50]

tissue, Treg subset, and extent of inflammation. Collectively, they reinforce tolerance in both steady-state and inflammatory settings. This adaptable, multifaceted suppressive activity has caused Tregs to be viewed as a potential cellular therapy for autoimmunity.

11.3 CLINICAL APPLICATIONS ACROSS AUTOIMMUNE DISEASES

Treg-based therapies have been tested in several autoimmune indications [51, 52]. Yet, clinical progress has been uneven, with most efforts concentrated in T1D. All completed Treg-based autoimmune clinical trials to date have utilised polyclonal

Tregs expanded *ex vivo*. They have been shown to be safe and well-tolerated but with disappointing efficacy. The lacklustre disease-modifying activity has spawned a new wave of preclinical research into antigen-specific Treg-based approaches, which promise more potent suppression. But this avenue is not without challenges. Antigen-specific Tregs are exceedingly rare, with frequencies as low as one in ten million cells in circulation [53, 54]. Simply carrying out multiple rounds of activation and expansion might not be an adequate approach, however, as it can result in Tregs losing FOXP3 expression and becoming effector-like cells [55]. These hurdles prompted the field to embrace technology to synthetically impart antigen specificity to Tregs using engineered TCRs and chimeric antigen receptors (CARs). Composed of an extracellular antigen-binding domain, typically antibody-based, and an intracellular signalling domain, often CD28-CD3ζ, CARs redirect Tregs to any desired cell surface antigen, not only major histocompatibility complex (MHC)–peptide complexes [56, 57]. Below is a summary of the current state of Treg-based therapeutic development across representative autoimmune diseases.

11.3.1 Type 1 Diabetes

Gene variants conferring susceptibility to T1D can almost invariably be mapped to pathways crucial to Treg development and function, such as T-cell receptor (TCR) signalling, IL-2 signalling, insulin peptide presentation in the thymus, and FOXP3 itself [58]. Mutations in FOXP3, which lead to loss of Tregs and IPEX syndrome, almost always cause T1D [6]. Interestingly, while in bulk the frequency of $FOXP3^+$ $CD4^+$ Tregs in peripheral blood is not different between T1D patients and their relatives or unrelated healthy controls [59, 60] and Tregs isolated from the peripheral blood of patients with T1D expand as much and suppress as well *in vitro* as those from healthy controls [61], T1D patients have an increased frequency of $FOXP3^+$ Tregs that lack HELIOS expression, display a methylated at the Treg-specific demethylated region (TSDR) locus, secrete interferon gamma (IFN-γ), and are less suppressive *in vitro* [60], potentially arising from persistent exposure to inflammation. This cumulative evidence suggests that Tregs can play a key role in treating T1D. Indeed, adoptive transfer of murine islet antigen-specific BDC2.5 TCR transgenic Tregs, but not control polyclonal Tregs, was shown to prevent and even reverse autoimmune diabetes in the nonobese diabetic (NOD) mice in the early 2000s [62]. A phase I clinical trial demonstrated that infusing up to 3 billion polyclonal Tregs in T1D patients is safe, and infused Tregs remain stable and do not convert into effector T cells [63]. A pilot study with paediatric patients within 2 months of T1D diagnosis reported that a small number of patients experienced disease improvement and increased circulating c-peptide (a more stable correlate of insulin) levels following polyclonal Treg infusion, with some even becoming exogenous insulin independent [64]. However, a phase II clinical trial with over 100 patients found that polyclonal Tregs have no effect on T1D progression [65]. These results have led to the deployment of combination therapies and antigen-specific Treg therapies. For instance, PolTreg recently finished a phase I/II clinical trial testing polyclonal Tregs in combination with rituximab (an anti-CD20 antibody that eliminates B cells) in stage 3 presymptomatic paediatric patients. They found that the combination resulted in better C-peptide preservation and delay in T1D incidence than polyclonal Tregs. There was, however, no difference in disease remission between the groups 2 years after treatment [66, 67]. In contrast, teplizumab, a now U.S. Food and Drug Administration (FDA) approved non-Fc receptor binding anti-CD3 antibody, delays the onset of T1D by 2 years [68], making it a potential agent to use in combination with Tregs in the future. PolTreg has received permission from the FDA in August 2025 to carry out a phase II/III clinical trial, including stage 1 and 2 diabetic patients. Antigen-specific Tregs for T1D currently in development all use engineered TCRs and exist only in the preclinical space. PolTreg has 3 TCR Tregs in their preclinical pipeline; Abata Therapeutics has developed preproinsulin (PPI) specific TCR Tregs (ABA-201) to test in new onset T1D patients with an Investigational New Drug (IND) under review, and GentiBio has islet-specific glucose-6-phosphatase catalytic subunit-related protein (IGRP)-specific TCR Tregs (GNTI-122) [69] for which an IND has been approved and phase I clinical trials are slated to start soon.

CASE STUDY: REGULATORY T CELL AND STEM CELL-BASED STRATEGIES TO CURE TYPE 1 DIABETES

T1D is an autoimmune disease at the forefront of cell and gene therapy. As T1D is caused by immune destruction of beta cells, there are immunomodulatory and cell replacement-centric therapeutic strategies being developed. On the immunomodulatory front, human islet antigen-specific Tregs for T1D have been generated by transducing Tregs with a TCR specific for the islet epitope $IGRP_{305}$ [69] and, more recently, with a CAR specific for the islet antigen ENTPD3 [70] (Figure 11.1). But what can be done for patients who no longer have enough beta cell mass to protect? Transplant of pancreatic islets, obtained by digestion of cadaveric pancreases, via the portal vein into the liver, has been carried out for over two decades [71] and approved by the FDA as a treatment for T1D since 2023. Ongoing trials by Vertex yielded positive results using human pluripotent stem cell (hPSC)-derived beta cell transplants in the clinic, potentially addressing the shortage and variable quality of primary islets for transplant. A weakness of both these cell replacement approaches, however, is the reliance on broad immunosuppressive drugs, which cause many toxic side effects and inhibit the immune system systemically, not only the immune responses against the transplanted beta cells. One solution being developed to address this is the use of gene editing to make hPSCs and primary islets hypoimmune, that is, almost invisible to the immune system [72, 73]. Currently, the most advanced such strategy, pushed forward by Sana Biotechnology, involves ablating surface expression of MHC class I and class II by deleting the B2M and CIITA genes, respectively, to prevent T-cell-mediated rejection, while constitutively expressing CD47 to inhibit NK cells and macrophages. This approach has been tested in humanised mice [74] and in non-human primates [73], and there is an ongoing study in one T1D patient. A potential weakness of this approach is that eliminating MHC surface expression could pose a safety hazard in the event of viral infection or cancer formation. Utilising Tregs to specifically protect transplanted beta cells could circumvent this weakness. One strategy is to use HLA-A2 CAR Tregs to protect HLA-A2-positive islets transplanted into HLA-A2-negative recipients [75], while a more recent strategy

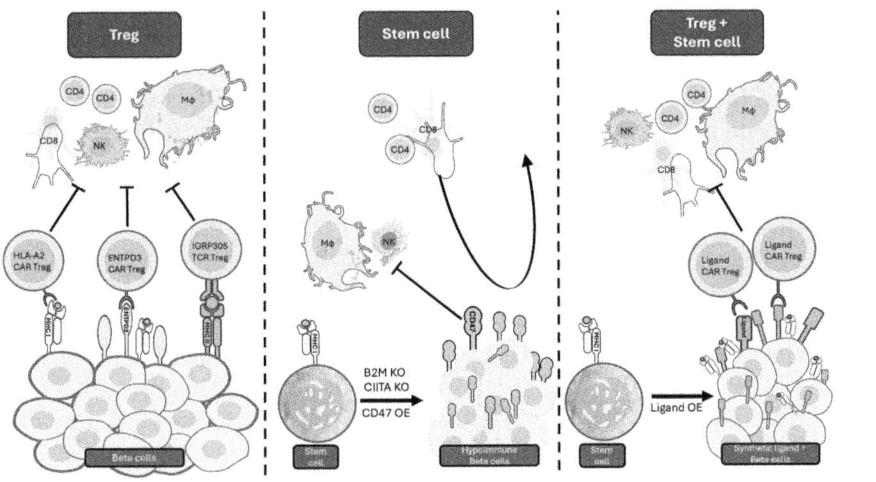

FIGURE 11.1 Overview of therapeutics using engineered regulatory T cells, engineered stem cell-derived beta cells, and combinations to cure type 1 diabetes. Some approaches to cure type 1 diabetes (T1D) involve engineering antigen-specific regulatory T cells (Tregs) by introducing islet-specific T-cell receptor (TCR) or chimeric antigen receptor (CAR) ('Treg'). Alternatively, human pluripotent stem cells (hPSCs), later differentiated into beta cells, and primary islets are gene edited to be rendered hypoimmune, escaping immune recognition ('Stem cell'). Combination approaches employing both engineered hPSC-derived beta cells and CAR Tregs, such that the CAR Tregs uniquely recognise the hPSC-derived beta cells via a CAR-ligand pair, could provide specific local protection of transplanted beta cells in T1D patients without eliminating immune recognition ('Treg + Stem cell').

involves combining engineered hPSC-derived beta cells expressing a unique surface ligand with CAR Tregs specific for that ligand, providing an MHC allele-independent and hence more broadly applicable approach to provide specific local protection of transplanted beta cells [76].

11.3.2 Systemic Lupus Erythematosus

Systemic lupus erythematosus (SLE) is a highly heterogeneous B-cell-mediated systemic autoimmune disease characterised by widespread organ damage and the presence of autoantibodies targeting nucleic acids [77]. Tregs in SLE patients frequently exhibit numerical deficiencies and impaired suppressive function compared to healthy individuals [78, 79]. Despite promising preclinical data using Tregs [80], clinical translation remains limited due to the systemic and polyclonal nature of SLE. A single-patient case study demonstrated that an autologous polyclonal Treg infusion led to increased activation of FOXP3$^+$ Tregs within the lesional skin [81]. However, the associated clinical trial (NCT02428309) was terminated prematurely due to enrolment constraints. Progressing to antigen-specific Treg approaches is particularly difficult due to the absence of shared targets across patients. Despite this, recent preclinical work has taken a more systematic approach by using CD19 CAR Tregs in a humanised mouse SLE model. Researchers showed suppression of autoantibody production [82], establishing proof of concept for engineered Treg approaches for SLE. Yet this raises the concern of suppressing all B cells, which would possibly result in an immunocompromised patient. While this Treg-based strategy has not yet progressed into human studies, conventional CD19 CAR T cells, the same exact therapeutic used to treat leukaemia and lymphoma [56], have been tested in phase I clinical trials and shown to be safe and potentially efficacious using both autologous [83] and allogeneic CAR T cells [84].

11.3.3 Inflammatory Bowel Disease

Inflammatory bowel disease (IBD), including Crohn's disease and ulcerative colitis, has been associated with local Treg dysfunction in the intestinal mucosa. Preclinical studies have suggested that adoptive transfer of polyclonal Tregs can attenuate disease in murine models of colitis [85]. Capitalising on these observations, 2 phase I clinical trials (NCT04691232 and NCT03185000) have tested autologous polyclonal Tregs in patients with IBD [86, 87]. While these trials demonstrated safety and biomarker modulation, clinical improvement was modest. An additional phase I clinical trial by type 1 regulatory T cells (Tr1)X Bio (NCT06721962) is currently evaluating allogeneic polyclonal Tr1, a subset of $CD4^{+}FOXP3^{-}$ cells that secrete high levels of interleukin-10 (IL-10) [88, 89]. Antigen-specific engineering efforts remain encumbered by limited universal disease targets, akin to SLE. Despite this, strategies like targeting gut-homing chemokines or mucosal antigen-presenting cells (APCs) have emerged: interleukin-23 receptor (IL23R) CAR Tregs [90] and flagellin-specific CAR Tregs [91] have both shown promising suppressive activity in preclinical mouse models. Sonoma Biotherapeutics, in partnership with Regeneron, and Quell Therapeutics, in partnership with AstraZeneca, have CAR Treg candidates to treat IBD in development, signalling growing momentum for Treg therapy in this disease indication.

11.3.4 Rheumatoid Arthritis

In rheumatoid arthritis (RA), a B-cell-mediated autoimmune disease affecting the joints, Tregs appear decreased in number in the blood but increased in the synovial fluid [92]. However, some reports suggest that Tregs are functionally impaired at sites of inflammation, though this remains controversial [93]. Polyclonal Treg adoptive transfer showed promising results in a preclinical mouse model called collagen-induced arthritis (CIA), where mice are immunised with collagen to develop disease [94]. Yet, antigen-specific strategies for RA, such as targeting citrullinated proteins, have yet to yield published CAR or TCR constructs [95]. Nevertheless, a first-in-human trial of CAR Tregs in RA (NCT06201416) is currently recruiting patients, marking a significant step towards clinical testing of antigen-specific Treg therapies for this indication.

11.3.5 Multiple Sclerosis

Multiple sclerosis (MS) is a chronic demyelinating disorder of the central nervous system (CNS) in which Treg dysfunction has been implicated [96, 97]. Indeed, similar to T1D [60], MS patients have also been found to have increased frequencies of

IFN-γ-producing FOXP3+ Tregs in circulation [97]. In the preclinical mouse model for MS, called experimental autoimmune encephalomyelitis (EAE) and often induced by immunisation with either myelin basic protein (MBP) or myelin oligodendrocyte glycoprotein (MOG) peptides, adoptive transfer of myelin-reactive Tregs, but not polyclonal Tregs, has been shown to delay disease onset and reduce CNS inflammation [98]. These findings are consistent with results from PolTreg's European clinical study, where polyclonal Tregs infused intravenously (IV) were well-tolerated but showed no therapeutic benefit in patients with relapsing–remitting MS [99]. PolTreg has since initiated a U.S. phase I clinical trial administering polyclonal Tregs via intrathecal injection. Of note, antigen-specific engineered Treg strategies for MS were among the earliest to be developed and tested *in vivo*. In 2005, a study introduced a chimeric receptor consisting of an MHC–peptide complex, specifically an I-A^s molecule fused to MBP_{89-101}, linked to CD3ζ into mouse Tregs. Transfer of these engineered Tregs prevented MBP_{89-101}-induced EAE and reversed established disease after epitope spreading, demonstrating bystander suppression [100]. Moreover, the engineered Tregs induced IL-10-producing MBP_{89-101} T cells, which in turn prevented EAE when transferred into new recipient mice, indicating that these engineered Tregs also induced infectious tolerance [101]. Over the past decade, several studies have reported mouse MOG- and MBP-directed TCR and CAR Tregs that suppress EAE [102–104]. More recently, human MOG CAR Tregs have been successfully generated from Tregs isolated from MS patients [105]. In parallel, Abata Therapeutics has developed MBP-specific TCR Tregs (ABA-101) for progressive MS, currently in an active phase I clinical trial (NCT06566261).

11.3.6 Non-Treg-Based Cell Therapies

While Tregs remain the leading candidate for restoring immune tolerance, alternative cellular strategies have emerged for autoimmune disorders primarily driven by autoreactive B cells such as systemic sclerosis (SSc) and SLE. In these disorders, the humoral arm of immunity plays a central role, with autoreactive B cells perpetuating inflammation through autoantibody production and antigen presentation. Consequently, direct elimination of pathogenic B cells has been explored as an alternative cellular approach for inducing an immune reset.

In 2021, the first human reports of adoptive transfer of CD19 CAR T cells in patients suffering from refractory SLE demonstrated that deep depletion of B cells can induce long-term disease remission, leading to normalisation of autoantibody titres and restoration of naïve B cell repertoires [84]. CAR T-cell therapy has since been expanded to several autoimmune diseases, including SSc, idiopathic inflammatory myopathy, myasthenia gravis, and MS, with promising preclinical and clinical results [106]. To further broaden cell therapy strategies and improve safety, CAR natural killer (NK) cells are also being investigated. Unlike autologous T cells, allogeneic NK cells do not cause GvHD, making them attractive for off-the-shelf cell therapies, and lack long-term engraftment, which is advantageous here since sustained persistence is unnecessary; once the target autoreactive B cells are cleared, persistent B cell depletion would be unfavourable [107, 108]. Early clinical data support this strategy, with a dual targeting CD19/B-cell maturation antigen (BCMA)-induced pluripotent stem cell (iPSC)-derived CAR NK cell product achieving significant clinical improvement in an SSc patient with minimal toxicity [109].

Together, these advances are rapidly driving a new paradigm: instead of managing autoimmunity with indefinite immunosuppression, we may purge the autoreactive immune repertoire and allow regeneration of a self-tolerant immune repertoire. Given the recent deployment of these methods, durability and its long-term implications for autoimmune relapse remain active areas of investigation [110].

11.4 CHALLENGES AND FUTURE DIRECTIONS

Despite increasing enthusiasm around Treg therapy, several key barriers remain unresolved. A recurring challenge in human Tregs is *in vivo* survival after infusion. Multiple studies suggest that Tregs are short-lived after infusion [63, 111, 112], which could be attributed to suboptimal IL-2 availability, poor tissue homing, immune-mediated clearance, or loss of FOXP3, although the available limited data suggest that surviving infused Tregs do not destabilise [63] and sampling peripheral blood alone may offer an incomplete picture of Treg survival if the cells are sequestered in tissues and hence inaccessible to liquid biopsy.

A related major focus is improving the isolation and identification of Tregs. There is currently no truly unique surface marker to distinguish Tregs from conventional T (Tconv) cells. Comprehensive transcriptomic and proteomic studies profiled human Tregs and Tconv cells to discover new Treg markers. Surprisingly, only three molecules were significantly higher in Tregs simultaneously at the mRNA and protein levels: all intracellular proteins (FOXP3, SHMT2, SWAP70). Still, from 22 proteins overexpressed in human Tregs compared with T_{conv}, one was a surface molecule: inducible T-cell co-stimulator (ICOS) [113]. Indeed, $ICOS^+$ Tregs have been reported to be more potent suppressors [113]. Most recently, it was reported that GPA33 surface expression marks a subset of thymically derived human Tregs that are highly suppressive and lack effector cytokine secretion [49]. Efforts to find new markers for human Tregs will certainly continue. The value of such efforts is at least twofold: better purification of Tregs for research and therapy, and more accurate identification and quantification of Tregs in blood and tissue samples.

Functional assays are also a weak point. *In vitro* suppression assays are commonly used for testing Tregs before infusion, but their ability to predict *in vivo* performance is limited [114]. This disconnect is especially problematic for engineered Tregs, where subtle changes in function may not be detected without more context-specific readouts. Standardising more predictive functional metrics remains an open need. Additionally, model systems for testing human Tregs preclinically have their own limitations. Humanised NOD SCID IL2RG-deficient (NSG) mouse models are widely used but do not fully recapitulate human immune microenvironments, cytokine networks, or APC diversity that Tregs depend on for functional context. Even with advances like HLA-transgenic or MHC-null mouse hosts [115, 116], there are still significant gaps in modelling the complexity of human autoimmunity *in vivo* [117]. Given these difficulties, preclinical studies often utilise xenogeneic GvHD and organ transplant rejection models instead. For GvHD, immunodeficient NSG mice are preconditioned by radiation or lymphodepleting drugs and injected IV with human peripheral blood mononuclear cells (PBMCs) with or without human Tregs (from the same donor or a different one) at different PBMC: Treg ratios. Mice receiving PBMCs alone lose weight, suffer multi-organ damage, and eventually perish over the course of weeks, whereas those co-infused with therapeutic Tregs remain healthy and alive for longer [75]. It remains a workhorse in preclinical studies with human Tregs to this day. Interestingly, it was found that performing this experiment with PBMCs from MS patients resulted in exacerbated GvHD that was resistant to prevention by Tregs from healthy controls; co-injection of the FDA-approved anti-IL-6 antibody tocilizumab significantly ameliorated disease [118]. For organ transplant rejection, human skin grafts and human pancreatic islet transplantation under the kidney capsule are the most well-described paradigms to study solid organ transplant protection by human Tregs *in vivo* [75, 76, 119, 120]. These humanised models are helpful for obtaining proof of concept but are arguably limited in their ability to predict clinical efficacy in autoimmune disease patients.

Another barrier pertains to engineering Treg specificity. In spite of the moderate popularity of using CAR to redirect Treg specificity, studies are reporting that CAR signalling can diminish suppressive function and elicit inflammatory cytokine secretion relative to endogenous TCR stimulation [27, 121]. More studies need to focus on tailoring synthetic immunology approaches to Treg biology and maximising what we like to call the 5S's of Treg therapy: stability, specificity, survival, suppression, and safety [16] (Table 11.3). For example, overexpressing FOXP3 or inserting a constitutive promoter upstream of FOXP3 improves Treg stability [69, 122]; synthetic receptors other than TCRs and CARs are being explored to redirect human Treg specificity [123–126]; introducing an artificial chemically inducible signalling complex (CISC) that dimerises upon binding to

TABLE 11.3 Key engineering strategies to enhance Treg stability, specificity, survival, suppression, and safety.

Parameter	Strategies	References
Stability	FOXP3 overexpression Constitutive promoter knocked in upstream of the FOXP3 gene CAR signalling domain optimisation	[114, 122, 130, 131]
Specificity	CAR (chimeric antigen receptor) TCR (T-cell receptor) TRuC (T-cell receptor fusion construct) BAR (B-cell-targeting antibody receptor) CHAR (chimeric anti-HLA antibody receptor) AIR (artificial immune receptor sensing TNF family ligands)	[104, 124, 125, 132–137]
Survival	Receptor-tethered orthoIL-2 CISC (chemically inducible signalling complex for rapamycin-induced IL-2 signalling) CAR signalling domain optimisation Chemokine receptor overexpression	[114, 130, 138, 139]
Suppression	IL-10 induction by activation CAR antigen-binding domain optimisation CAR signalling domain optimisation	[27, 114, 127, 128]
Safety	Inducible safety switch FOXP3 overexpression FOXP3 promoter-controlled CAR expression Endogenous TCR deletion	[75, 122, 129–131, 140]

rapamycin analogues and mimics IL-2 signalling improves TCR Treg survival [69]; forcing IL-10 secretion has been shown to improve CAR Treg-mediated suppression [127, 128]; and utilising a FOXP3 promoter to drive CAR expression improves safety by preventing FOXP3 negative ex-Tregs from maintaining CAR function [129]. Collectively, these challenges underscore the need for deeper mechanistic insight into Treg biology and more predictive *in vitro* assays and preclinical *in vivo* models.

Continued integration and boosting of Treg suppressive mechanisms will be essential for making Treg therapy a viable platform across autoimmune diseases. The next phase of the engineering Treg field will rely less on proof of concept and more on rigorous optimisations of defined constructs and experimental models. Moving forward, progress in Treg therapy will depend on refining both our understanding of the underlying biology and our dexterity in genetic engineering.

KEY TERMS & DEFINITIONS SIDEBAR

Antigen specificity The selective recognition of a particular antigen peptide-major histocompatibility complex (pMHC) complex by a T cell, ensuring targeted immune responses.

Autoimmune disease A disorder in which the immune system mounts an immune response against self-antigens, leading to tissue inflammation and organ damage.

Bystander suppression The ability of Tregs activated by one antigen to suppress immune responses against unrelated antigens in the same local environment.

CAR (Chimeric Antigen Receptor) An engineered receptor that combines antibody-derived antigen recognition with intracellular T-cell signalling domains to redirect antigen specificity.

FOXP3 (Forkhead box protein P3) A transcription factor that defines the regulatory T-cell (Treg) lineage and controls genes necessary for suppressive function.

Immunosuppressive Describes any mechanism, molecule, or therapy that inhibits or downregulates immune activation or inflammatory function.

Infectious tolerance A process by which Tregs confer suppressive function to other immune cells, spreading tolerance beyond the original antigen-specific response.

Polyclonal Describes a heterogeneous T-cell population displaying multiple TCR specificities, collectively recognising diverse antigens rather than a single defined epitope.

TCR (T-Cell Receptor) A heterodimeric receptor on T cells that recognises a specific pMHC complex and determines antigen specificity of the immune response.

Treg (Regulatory T cell) A $CD4^{+}FOXP3^{+}$ T-cell subset that maintains immune tolerance by suppressing autoreactive and inflammatory immune responses.

Treg stability The capacity of Tregs to maintain lineage identity and suppressive function under inflammatory or stimulatory conditions.

LIST OF ABBREVIATIONS

AIR artificial immune receptor

APC antigen-presenting cell

ATP adenosine triphosphate

BAR	B-cell antibody targeting receptor
BCMA	B-cell maturation antigen
CAR	chimeric antigen receptor
CD	cluster of differentiation
CHAR	chimeric anti-HLA antibody receptor
CIA	collagen-induced arthritis
CISC	chemically inducible signalling complex
CNS	central nervous system
CTLA-4	cytotoxic T-lymphocyte-associated protein 4
DC	dendritic cell
EAE	experimental autoimmune encephalomyelitis
EBI3	Epstein–Barr virus-induced gene 3
EV	extracellular vesicle
FDA	U.S. Food and Drug Administration
FOXP3	forkhead box protein P3
GvHD	graft-versus-host disease
IKZF2 (HELIOS)	Ikaros family of zinc-finger proteins 2
ICOS	inducible T-cell co-stimulator
IDO	indoleamine 2,3-dioxygenase
IFN-γ	interferon gamma
IGRP	islet-specific glucose-6-phosphatase catalytic subunit-related protein
IL-1R/IL-1R2/IL-1R1	interleukin-1 receptor family members
IL-2R (CD25)	interleukin-2 receptor alpha chain
IL-10	interleukin-10
IL23R	interleukin-23 receptor
iTreg	induced regulatory T cell
iPSC	induced pluripotent stem cell
LAG-3	lymphocyte activation gene 3
LAP-TGF-β	latency-associated peptide transforming growth factor beta
MHC	major histocompatibility complex
MBP	myelin basic protein
MOG	myelin oligodendrocyte glycoprotein
MS	multiple sclerosis
NOD	nonobese diabetic mouse
NRP1	neuropilin-1
PBMC	peripheral blood mononuclear cells
PPI	preproinsulin
RA	rheumatoid arthritis
SLE	systemic lupus erythematosus
SSc	systemic sclerosis
T1D	type 1 diabetes

TCR T-cell receptor
Tconv conventional (non-regulatory) $CD4^+$ T cell
TGF-β transforming growth factor beta
TIGIT T-cell immunoreceptor with Ig and ITIM domains
Tr1 type 1 regulatory T cell
Treg regulatory T cell
TSDR Treg-specific demethylated region
TRuC T-cell receptor fusion construct

REVIEW QUESTIONS

1. What are the main differences between infectious tolerance and bystander suppression in Treg-mediated immune regulation? How are these relevant when designing Treg-based therapies?
2. Compare contact-dependent and contact-independent mechanisms of Treg suppression. Provide at least two examples of each and explain how they contribute to immune tolerance and in what context.
3. What are the major reasons for the limited success of polyclonal Tregs? How might engineering strategies to confer antigen specificity address these limitations?
4. Discuss the advantages and potential drawbacks of engineering Tregs with TCRs or CARs. What other receptor designs could be used to bestow new antigen specificity to Tregs?
5. There are five key features often summarised as the 5S's of Treg therapy: stability, specificity, survival, suppression, and safety. Select two of these and describe strategies that researchers are currently exploring to improve them in engineered Tregs.

REFERENCES

1. Gershteyn, I.M., Burov, A.A., Miao, B.Y. et al. (2020). Immunodietica: interrogating the role of diet in autoimmune disease. *Int Immunol* 32 (12): 771–783.
2. Pisetsky, D.S. (2023). Pathogenesis of autoimmune disease. *Nat Rev Nephrol* 19 (8): 509–524.
3. Conrad, N., Misra, S., Verbakel, J.Y. et al. (2023). Incidence, prevalence, and co-occurrence of autoimmune disorders over time and by age, sex, and socioeconomic status: a population-based cohort study of 22 million individuals in the UK. *Lancet* 401 (10391): 1878–1890.
4. Abend AH, He I, Bahroos N, et al. Estimation of prevalence of autoimmune diseases in the United States using electronic health record data. *J Clin Invest* 2024;135(4): e178722. https://doi.org/10.1172/JCI178722.
5. Bechi Genzano, C., Young, T., Bonami, R. et al. (2025). Autoimmune diabetes and targets for immunomodulation. *Semin Immunol* 79: 101983.
6. Barzaghi, F., Passerini, L., and Bacchetta, R. (2012). Immune dysregulation, polyendocrinopathy, enteropathy, x-linked syndrome: a paradigm of immunodeficiency with autoimmunity. *Front Immunol* 3: 211.
7. Powell, B.R., Buist, N.R., and Stenzel, P. (1982). An X-linked syndrome of diarrhea, polyendocrinopathy, and fatal infection in infancy. *J Pediatr* 100 (5): 731–737.

8. Bennett, C.L., Christie, J., Ramsdell, F. et al. (2001). The immune dysregulation, polyendocrinopathy, enteropathy, X-linked syndrome (IPEX) is caused by mutations of FOXP3. *Nat Genet* 27 (1): 20–21.
9. Brunkow, M.E., Jeffery, E.W., Hjerrild, K.A. et al. (2001). Disruption of a new forkhead/winged-helix protein, scurfin, results in the fatal lymphoproliferative disorder of the scurfy mouse. *Nat Genet* 27 (1): 68–73.
10. Fontenot, J.D., Gavin, M.A., and Rudensky, A.Y. (2003). Foxp3 programs the development and function of CD4+CD25+ regulatory T cells. *Nat Immunol* 4 (4): 330–336.
11. Khattri, R., Cox, T., Yasayko, S.A., and Ramsdell, F. (2003). An essential role for Scurfin in CD4+CD25+ T regulatory cells. *Nat Immunol* 4 (4): 337–342.
12. Ono, M., Yaguchi, H., Ohkura, N. et al. (2007). Foxp3 controls regulatory T-cell function by interacting with AML1/Runx1. *Nature* 446 (7136): 685–689.
13. Sakaguchi, S., Sakaguchi, N., Asano, M. et al. (1995). Immunologic self-tolerance maintained by activated T cells expressing IL-2 receptor alpha-chains (CD25). Breakdown of a single mechanism of self-tolerance causes various autoimmune diseases. *J Immunol* 155 (3): 1151–1164.
14. Baecher-Allan, C., Brown, J.A., Freeman, G.J., and Hafler, D.A. (2001). CD4+CD25high regulatory cells in human peripheral blood. *J Immunol* 167 (3): 1245–1253.
15. Levings, M.K., Sangregorio, R., and Roncarolo, M.G. (2001). Human cd25(+)cd4(+) t regulatory cells suppress naive and memory T cell proliferation and can be expanded in vitro without loss of function. *J Exp Med* 193 (11): 1295–1302.
16. Ferreira, L.M.R., Muller, Y.D., Bluestone, J.A., and Tang, Q. (2019). Next-generation regulatory T cell therapy. *Nat Rev Drug Discov* 18 (10): 749–769.
17. Gershon, R.K. and Kondo, K. (1971). Infectious immunological tolerance. *Immunology* 21 (6): 903–914.
18. Qin, S., Cobbold, S.P., Pope, H. et al. (1993). “Infectious” transplantation tolerance. *Science* 259 (5097): 974–977.
19. Homann, D., Holz, A., Bot, A. et al. (1999). Autoreactive CD4+ T cells protect from autoimmune diabetes via bystander suppression using the IL-4/Stat6 pathway. *Immunity* 11 (4): 463–472.
20. Read, S., Malmstrom, V., and Powrie, F. (2000). Cytotoxic T lymphocyte-associated antigen 4 plays an essential role in the function of CD25(+)CD4(+) regulatory cells that control intestinal inflammation. *J Exp Med* 192 (2): 295–302.
21. Grohmann, U., Orabona, C., Fallarino, F. et al. (2002). CTLA-4-Ig regulates tryptophan catabolism in vivo. *Nat Immunol* 3 (11): 1097–1101.
22. Wing, K., Onishi, Y., Prieto-Martin, P. et al. (2008). CTLA-4 control over Foxp3+ regulatory T cell function. *Science* 322 (5899): 271–275.
23. Sojka, D.K., Hughson, A., and Fowell, D.J. (2009). CTLA-4 is required by CD4+CD25+ Treg to control CD4+ T-cell lymphopenia-induced proliferation. *Eur J Immunol* 39 (6): 1544–1551.
24. Qureshi, O.S., Zheng, Y., Nakamura, K. et al. (2011). Trans-endocytosis of CD80 and CD86: a molecular basis for the cell-extrinsic function of CTLA-4. *Science* 332 (6029): 600–603.
25. Gondek, D.C., Lu, L.F., Quezada, S.A. et al. (2005). Cutting edge: contact-mediated suppression by CD4+CD25+ regulatory cells involves a granzyme B-dependent, perforin-independent mechanism. *J Immunol* 174 (4): 1783–1786.
26. Boissonnas, A., Scholer-Dahirel, A., Simon-Blancal, V. et al. (2010). Foxp3+ T cells induce perforin-dependent dendritic cell death in tumor-draining lymph nodes. *Immunity* 32 (2): 266–278.
27. Cochrane, R.W., Robino, R.A., Granger, B. et al. (2024). High-affinity chimeric antigen receptor signaling induces an inflammatory program in human regulatory T cells. *Mol Ther Methods Clin Dev* 32 (4): 101385.

28. Yu, X., Harden, K., Gonzalez, L.C. et al. (2009). The surface protein TIGIT suppresses T cell activation by promoting the generation of mature immunoregulatory dendritic cells. *Nat Immunol* 10 (1): 48–57.
29. Joller, N., Lozano, E., Burkett, P.R. et al. (2014). Treg cells expressing the coinhibitory molecule TIGIT selectively inhibit proinflammatory Th1 and Th17 cell responses. *Immunity* 40 (4): 569–581.
30. Bopp, T., Becker, C., Klein, M. et al. (2007). Cyclic adenosine monophosphate is a key component of regulatory T cell-mediated suppression. *J Exp Med* 204 (6): 1303–1310.
31. Bodor, J., Fehervari, Z., Diamond, B., and Sakaguchi, S. (2007). ICER/CREM-mediated transcriptional attenuation of IL-2 and its role in suppression by regulatory T cells. *Eur J Immunol* 37 (4): 884–895.
32. Huang, C.T., Workman, C.J., Flies, D. et al. (2004). Role of LAG-3 in regulatory T cells. *Immunity* 21 (4): 503–513.
33. Liang, B., Workman, C., Lee, J. et al. (2008). Regulatory T cells inhibit dendritic cells by lymphocyte activation gene-3 engagement of MHC class II. *J Immunol* 180 (9): 5916–5926.
34. Andersson, J., Tran, D.Q., Pesu, M. et al. (2008). CD4+ FoxP3+ regulatory T cells confer infectious tolerance in a TGF-beta-dependent manner. *J Exp Med* 205 (9): 1975–1981.
35. Sarris, M., Andersen, K.G., Randow, F. et al. (2008). Neuropilin-1 expression on regulatory T cells enhances their interactions with dendritic cells during antigen recognition. *Immunity* 28 (3): 402–413.
36. Akkaya, B., Oya, Y., Akkaya, M. et al. (2019). Regulatory T cells mediate specific suppression by depleting peptide-MHC class II from dendritic cells. *Nat Immunol* 20 (2): 218–231.
37. Barthlott, T., Moncrieffe, H., Veldhoen, M. et al. (2005). CD25+ CD4+ T cells compete with naive CD4+ T cells for IL-2 and exploit it for the induction of IL-10 production. *Int Immunol* 17 (3): 279–288.
38. Pandiyan, P., Zheng, L., Ishihara, S. et al. (2007). CD4+CD25+Foxp3+ regulatory T cells induce cytokine deprivation-mediated apoptosis of effector CD4+ T cells. *Nat Immunol* 8 (12): 1353–1362.
39. Asseman, C., Mauze, S., Leach, M.W. et al. (1999). An essential role for interleukin 10 in the function of regulatory T cells that inhibit intestinal inflammation. *J Exp Med* 190 (7): 995–1004.
40. Rubtsov, Y.P., Rasmussen, J.P., Chi, E.Y. et al. (2008). Regulatory t cell-derived interleukin-10 limits inflammation at environmental interfaces. *Immunity* 28 (4): 546–558.
41. Chaudhry, A., Samstein, R.M., Treuting, P. et al. (2011). Interleukin-10 signaling in regulatory T cells is required for suppression of Th17 cell-mediated inflammation. *Immunity* 34 (4): 566–578.
42. Nakamura, K., Kitani, A., Fuss, I. et al. (2004). TGF-beta 1 plays an important role in the mechanism of CD4+CD25+ regulatory T cell activity in both humans and mice. *J Immunol* 172 (2): 834–842.
43. Collison, L.W., Workman, C.J., Kuo, T.T. et al. (2007). The inhibitory cytokine IL-35 contributes to regulatory T-cell function. *Nature* 450 (7169): 566–569.
44. Collison, L.W., Chaturvedi, V., Henderson, A.L. et al. (2010). IL-35-mediated induction of a potent regulatory T cell population. *Nat Immunol* 11 (12): 1093–1101.
45. Mercer, F., Kozhaya, L., and Unutmaz, D. (2010). Expression and function of TNF and IL-1 receptors on human regulatory T cells. *PLoS One* 5 (1): e8639.
46. Nikolouli, E., Elfaki, Y., Herppich, S. et al. (2021). Recirculating IL-1R2(+) Tregs fine-tune intrathymic Treg development under inflammatory conditions. *Cell Mol Immunol* 18 (1): 182–193.
47. Kobie, J.J., Shah, P.R., Yang, L. et al. (2006). T regulatory and primed uncommitted CD4 T cells express CD73, which suppresses effector CD4 T cells by converting 5′-adenosine monophosphate to adenosine. *J Immunol* 177 (10): 6780–6786.

48. Deaglio, S., Dwyer, K.M., Gao, W. et al. (2007). Adenosine generation catalyzed by CD39 and CD73 expressed on regulatory T cells mediates immune suppression. *J Exp Med* 204 (6): 1257–1265.
49. Mandapathil, M., Hilldorfer, B., Szczepanski, M.J. et al. (2010). Generation and accumulation of immunosuppressive adenosine by human CD4+CD25highFOXP3+ regulatory T cells. *J Biol Chem* 285 (10): 7176–7186.
50. Okoye, I.S., Coomes, S.M., Pelly, V.S. et al. (2014). MicroRNA-containing T-regulatory-cell-derived exosomes suppress pathogenic T helper 1 cells. *Immunity* 41 (1): 89–103.
51. Ghobadinezhad, F., Ebrahimi, N., Mozaffari, F. et al. (2022). The emerging role of regulatory cell-based therapy in autoimmune disease. *Front Immunol* 13: 1075813.
52. Bluestone, J.A., McKenzie, B.S., Beilke, J., and Ramsdell, F. (2023). Opportunities for Treg cell therapy for the treatment of human disease. *Front Immunol* 14: 1166135.
53. Jenkins, M.K. and Moon, J.J. (2012). The role of naive T cell precursor frequency and recruitment in dictating immune response magnitude. *J Immunol* 188 (9): 4135–4140.
54. Menier, C., Meunier, S., Porcheddu, V. et al. (2024). Frequency of natural regulatory T cells specific for factor VIII in the peripheral blood of healthy donors. *Eur J Immunol* 54 (4): e2350506.
55. Hoffmann, P., Eder, R., Boeld, T.J. et al. (2006). Only the CD45RA+ subpopulation of CD4+CD25high T cells gives rise to homogeneous regulatory T-cell lines upon in vitro expansion. *Blood* 108 (13): 4260–4277.
56. June, C.H. and Sadelain, M. (2018). Chimeric antigen receptor therapy. *N Engl J Med* 379 (1): 64–73.
57. Zimmerman, C.M., Robino, R.A., Cochrane, R.W. et al. (2024). Redirecting human conventional and regulatory T cells using chimeric antigen receptors. *Methods Mol Biol* 2748: 201–241.
58. Bettini, M. and Bettini, M.L. (2021). Function, failure, and the future potential of Tregs in type 1 diabetes. *Diabetes* 70 (6): 1211–1219.
59. Brusko, T., Wasserfall, C., McGrail, K. et al. (2007). No alterations in the frequency of FOXP3+ regulatory T-cells in type 1 diabetes. *Diabetes* 56 (3): 604–612.
60. McClymont, S.A., Putnam, A.L., Lee, M.R. et al. (2011). Plasticity of human regulatory T cells in healthy subjects and patients with type 1 diabetes. *J Immunol* 186 (7): 3918–3926.
61. Putnam, A.L., Brusko, T.M., Lee, M.R. et al. (2009). Expansion of human regulatory T-cells from patients with type 1 diabetes. *Diabetes* 58 (3): 652–662.
62. Tang, Q., Henriksen, K.J., Bi, M. et al. (2004). In vitro-expanded antigen-specific regulatory T cells suppress autoimmune diabetes. *J Exp Med* 199 (11): 1455–1465.
63. Bluestone, J.A., Buckner, J.H., Fitch, M. et al. (2015). Type 1 diabetes immunotherapy using polyclonal regulatory T cells. *Sci Transl Med* 7 (315): 315ra189.
64. Marek-Trzonkowska, N., Mysliwiec, M., Dobyszuk, A. et al. (2012). Administration of CD4+CD25highCD127- regulatory T cells preserves beta-cell function in type 1 diabetes in children. *Diabetes Care* 35 (9): 1817–1820.
65. Bender, C., Wiedeman, A.E., Hu, A. et al. (2024). A phase 2 randomized trial with autologous polyclonal expanded regulatory T cells in children with new-onset type 1 diabetes. *Sci Transl Med* 16 (746): eadn2404.
66. Zielinski, M., Zalinska, M., Iwaszkiewicz-Grzes, D. et al. (2022). Combined therapy with CD4(+) CD25highCD127(−) T regulatory cells and anti-CD20 antibody in recent-onset type 1 diabetes is superior to monotherapy: Randomized phase I/II trial. *Diabetes Obes Metab* 24 (8): 1534–1543.
67. Zielinski, M., Sakowska, J., Iwaszkiewicz-Grzes, D. et al. (2024). PD-1 receptor (+) T cells are associated with the efficacy of the combined treatment with regulatory t cells and rituximab in type 1 diabetes children via regulatory t cells suppressive activity amelioration. *Int Immunopharmacol* 132: 111919.

68. Herold, K.C., Bundy, B.N., Long, S.A. et al. (2019). An anti-CD3 antibody, teplizumab, in relatives at risk for type 1 diabetes. *N Engl J Med* 381 (7): 603–613.
69. Uenishi GI, Repic M, Yam JY, et al. (2024). GNTI-122: an autologous antigen-specific engineered Treg cell therapy for type 1 diabetes. *JCI Insight* 9 (6): e171844. https://doi.org/10.1172/jci.insight.171844
70. Pieper, T., Riet, T., Saetzler, V. et al. (2024). ENTPD3-specific CAR regulatory T cells for local immune control in T1D. *bioRxiv* https://doi.org/10.1101/2024.11.12.622951
71. Rickels, M.R. and Robertson, R.P. (2019). Pancreatic islet transplantation in humans: recent progress and future directions. *Endocr Rev* 40 (2): 631–668.
72. Han, X., Wang, M., Duan, S. et al. (2019). Generation of hypoimmunogenic human pluripotent stem cells. *Proc Natl Acad Sci USA* 116 (21): 10441–10446.
73. Hu, X., White, K., Young, C. et al. (2024). Hypoimmune islets achieve insulin independence after allogeneic transplantation in a fully immunocompetent non-human primate. *Cell Stem Cell* 31 (3): 334–340.e5.
74. Hu, X., Gattis, C., Olroyd, A.G. et al. (2023). Human hypoimmune primary pancreatic islets avoid rejection and autoimmunity and alleviate diabetes in allogeneic humanized mice. *Sci Transl Med* 15 (691): eadg5794.
75. Muller, Y.D., Ferreira, L.M.R., Ronin, E. et al. (2021). Precision engineering of an anti-HLA-A2 chimeric antigen receptor in regulatory T cells for transplant immune tolerance. *Front Immunol* 12: 686439.
76. Barra, J.M., Robino, R.A., Castro-Gutierrez, R. et al. (2024). Combinatorial genetic engineering strategy for immune protection of stem cell-derived beta cells by chimeric antigen receptor regulatory T cells. *Cell Rep* 43 (11): 114994.
77. Dai, X., Fan, Y., and Zhao, X. (2025). Systemic lupus erythematosus: updated insights on the pathogenesis, diagnosis, prevention and therapeutics. *Signal Transduct Target Ther* 10 (1): 102.
78. Kamal, M., Gabr, H., Anwar, S. et al. (2022). The relation of CD4(+)CD25+Foxp3+ regulatory T cells concentration with disease activity and damage index in systemic lupus erythematosus. *Lupus* 31 (4): 463–471.
79. Li, W., Deng, C., Yang, H., and Wang, G. (2019). The regulatory T cell in active systemic lupus erythematosus patients: a systemic review and meta-analysis. *Front Immunol* 10: 159.
80. Scalapino, K.J. and Daikh, D.I. (2009). Suppression of glomerulonephritis in NZB/NZW lupus prone mice by adoptive transfer of ex vivo expanded regulatory T cells. *PLoS One* 4 (6): e6031.
81. Dall'Era, M., Pauli, M.L., Remedios, K. et al. (2019). Adoptive Treg cell therapy in a patient with systemic lupus erythematosus. *Arthritis Rheumatol* 71 (3): 431–440.
82. Doglio, M., Ugolini, A., Bercher-Brayer, C. et al. (2024). Regulatory T cells expressing CD19-targeted chimeric antigen receptor restore homeostasis in systemic lupus erythematosus. *Nat Commun* 15 (1): 2542.
83. Mackensen, A., Muller, F., Mougiakakos, D. et al. (2022). Anti-CD19 CAR T cell therapy for refractory systemic lupus erythematosus. *Nat Med* 28 (10): 2124–2132.
84. Wang, X., Zhang, Y., Wang, H. et al. (2025). Allogeneic CD19-targeting T cells for treatment-refractory systemic lupus erythematosus: a phase 1 trial. *Nat Med* 31: 3713–3724.
85. Uhlig, H.H., Coombes, J., Mottet, C. et al. (2006). Characterization of Foxp3+CD4+CD25+ and IL-10-secreting CD4+CD25+ T cells during cure of colitis. *J Immunol* 177 (9): 5852–5860.
86. Voskens, C., Stoica, D., Rosenberg, M. et al. (2023). Autologous regulatory T-cell transfer in refractory ulcerative colitis with concomitant primary sclerosing cholangitis. *Gut* 72 (1): 49–53.
87. Canavan, J.B., Scotta, C., Vossenkamper, A. et al. (2016). Developing *in vitro* expanded CD45RA+ regulatory T cells as an adoptive cell therapy for Crohn's disease. *Gut* 65 (4): 584–594.

88. Roncarolo, M.G., Yssel, H., Touraine, J.L. et al. (1988). Autoreactive T cell clones specific for class I and class II HLA antigens isolated from a human chimera. *J Exp Med* 167 (5): 1523–1534.
89. Roncarolo, M.G., Gregori, S., Bacchetta, R. et al. (2018). The biology of T regulatory type 1 cells and their therapeutic application in immune-mediated diseases. *Immunity* 49 (6): 1004–1019.
90. Cui Y, David M, Bouchareychas L, et al. IL23R-specific CAR Tregs for the treatment of Crohn's disease. *J Crohns Colitis* 2025;19(3): jjae135. https://doi.org/10.1093/ecco-jcc/jjae135.
91. Boardman, D.A., Wong, M.Q., Rees, W.D. et al. (2023). Flagellin-specific human CAR Tregs for immune regulation in IBD. *J Autoimmun* 134: 102961.
92. Morita, T., Shima, Y., Wing, J.B. et al. (2016). The proportion of regulatory T cells in patients with rheumatoid arthritis: a meta-analysis. *PLoS One* 11 (9): e0162306.
93. Jiang, Q., Yang, G., Liu, Q. et al. (2021). Function and role of regulatory T cells in rheumatoid arthritis. *Front Immunol* 12: 626193.
94. Morgan, M.E., Flierman, R., van Duivenvoorde, L.M. et al. (2005). Effective treatment of collagen-induced arthritis by adoptive transfer of CD25+ regulatory T cells. *Arthritis Rheum* 52 (7): 2212–2221.
95. Raffin, C., Zhou, Y., Piccoli, L. et al. (2018). Development of citrullinated-vimentin-specific CAR for targeting Tregs to treat autoimmune rheumatoid arthritis. *J Immunol* 200: 176.17.
96. Verreycken, J., Baeten, P., and Broux, B. (2022). Regulatory T cell therapy for multiple sclerosis: breaching (blood-brain) barriers. *Hum Vaccin Immunother* 18 (7): 2153534.
97. Dominguez-Villar, M., Baecher-Allan, C.M., and Hafler, D.A. (2011). Identification of T helper type 1-like, Foxp3+ regulatory T cells in human autoimmune disease. *Nat Med* 17 (6): 673–675.
98. Stephens, L.A., Malpass, K.H., and Anderton, S.M. (2009). Curing CNS autoimmune disease with myelin-reactive Foxp3+ Treg. *Eur J Immunol* 39 (4): 1108–1117.
99. Chwojnicki, K., Iwaszkiewicz-Grzes, D., Jankowska, A. et al. (2021). Administration of CD4(+)CD25(high)CD127(−)FoxP3(+) regulatory T cells for relapsing-remitting multiple sclerosis: a phase 1 study. *BioDrugs* 35 (1): 47–60.
100. Mekala, D.J. and Geiger, T.L. (2005). Immunotherapy of autoimmune encephalomyelitis with redirected CD4+CD25+ T lymphocytes. *Blood* 105 (5): 2090–2092.
101. Mekala, D.J., Alli, R.S., and Geiger, T.L. (2005). IL-10-dependent infectious tolerance after the treatment of experimental allergic encephalomyelitis with redirected CD4+CD25+ T lymphocytes. *Proc Natl Acad Sci U S A* 102 (33): 11817–11822.
102. Fransson M, Piras E, Burman J, et al. CAR/FoxP3-engineered T regulatory cells target the CNS and suppress EAE upon intranasal delivery. *J Neuroinflammation* 2012;9:112. https://doi.org/10.1186/1742-2094-9-112
103. De Paula Pohl, A., Schmidt, A., Zhang, A.H. et al. (2020). Engineered regulatory T cells expressing myelin-specific chimeric antigen receptors suppress EAE progression. *Cell Immunol* 358: 104222.
104. Kim, Y.C., Zhang, A.H., Yoon, J. et al. (2018). Engineered MBP-specific human Tregs ameliorate MOG-induced EAE through IL-2-triggered inhibition of effector T cells. *J Autoimmun* 92: 77–86.
105. Frikeche, J., David, M., Mouska, X. et al. (2024). MOG-specific CAR Tregs: a novel approach to treat multiple sclerosis. *J Neuroinflammation* 21 (1): 268.
106. Chung, J.B., Brudno, J.N., Borie, D., and Kochenderfer, J.N. (2024). Chimeric antigen receptor T cell therapy for autoimmune disease. *Nat Rev Immunol* 24 (11): 830–845.
107. Rezvani, K. (2019). Adoptive cell therapy using engineered natural killer cells. *Bone Marrow Transplant* 54 (Suppl 2): 785–788.
108. Daher, M. and Rezvani, K. (2025). iPSC-derived CAR-NK cells: off-the-shelf cellular therapy for systemic sclerosis. *Cell* 188 (16): 4173–4174.

109. Wang, X., Zhang, Y., Jin, Y. et al. (2025). An iPSC-derived CD19/BCMA CAR-NK therapy in a patient with systemic sclerosis. *Cell* 188 (16): 4225–4238.e12.
110. Rampotas, A., Richter, J., Isenberg, D., and Roddie, C. (2025). CAR-T cell therapy embarks on autoimmune disease. *Bone Marrow Transplant* 60 (1): 6–9.
111. Sasaki, K., Kubo, M., Wang, Y.C. et al. (2024). Multiple infusions of ex vivo-expanded regulatory T cells promote CD163(+) myeloid cells and kidney allograft survival in non-lymphodepleted non-human primates. *Kidney Int* 105 (1): 84–98.
112. Brunstein, C.G., Miller, J.S., McKenna, D.H. et al. (2016). Umbilical cord blood-derived T regulatory cells to prevent GVHD: kinetics, toxicity profile, and clinical effect. *Blood* 127 (8): 1044–1051.
113. Cuadrado, E., van den Biggelaar, M., de Kivit, S. et al. (2018). Proteomic analyses of human regulatory T cells reveal adaptations in signaling pathways that protect cellular identity. *Immunity* 48 (5): 1046–1059.e6.
114. Dawson NAJ, Rosado-Sanchez I, Novakovsky GE, et al. Functional effects of chimeric antigen receptor co-receptor signaling domains in human regulatory T cells. *Sci Transl Med* 2020;12(557): eaaz3866. https://doi.org/10.1126/scitranslmed.aaz3866.
115. Brehm, M.A., Kenney, L.L., Wiles, M.V. et al. (2019). Lack of acute xenogeneic graft-versus-host disease, but retention of T-cell function following engraftment of human peripheral blood mononuclear cells in NSG mice deficient in MHC class I and II expression. *FASEB J* 33 (3): 3137–3151.
116. Shultz, L.D., Saito, Y., Najima, Y. et al. (2010). Generation of functional human T-cell subsets with HLA-restricted immune responses in HLA class I expressing NOD/SCID/IL2r gamma(null) humanized mice. *Proc Natl Acad Sci USA* 107 (29): 13022–13027.
117. Khosravi-Maharlooei, M., Madley, R., Borsotti, C. et al. (2022). Modeling human T1D-associated autoimmune processes. *Mol Metab* 56: 101417.
118. Trinschek, B., Luessi, F., Gross, C.C. et al. (2015). Interferon-beta therapy of multiple sclerosis patients improves the responsiveness of T cells for immune suppression by regulatory T cells. *Int J Mol Sci* 16 (7): 16330–16346.
119. Boardman, D.A., Philippeos, C., Fruhwirth, G.O. et al. (2017). Expression of a chimeric antigen receptor specific for donor HLA class I enhances the potency of human regulatory T cells in preventing human skin transplant rejection. *Am J Transplant* 17 (4): 931–943.
120. Noyan, F., Zimmermann, K., Hardtke-Wolenski, M. et al. (2017). Prevention of allograft rejection by use of regulatory T cells with an MHC-specific chimeric antigen receptor. *Am J Transplant* 17 (4): 917–930.
121. Rana, J., Perry, D.J., Kumar, S.R.P. et al. (2021). CAR- and TRuC-redirected regulatory T cells differ in capacity to control adaptive immunity to FVIII. *Mol Ther* 29 (9): 2660–2676.
122. Henschel, P., Landwehr-Kenzel, S., Engels, N. et al. (2023). Supraphysiological FOXP3 expression in human CAR-Tregs results in improved stability, efficacy, and safety of CAR-Treg products for clinical application. *J Autoimmun* 138: 103057.
123. Cochrane, R.W., Allen, E., and Ferreira, L.M.R. (2025). Expanding the engineered Treg multiverse. *Mol Ther* 33 (3): 833–836.
124. Valentin-Quiroga, J., Zarauza-Santovena, A., Lopez-Collazo, E., and Ferreira, L.M.R. (2025). Chimeric anti-HLA antibody receptor-engineered human regulatory T cells suppress alloantigen-specific B cells from pre-sensitized transplant recipients. *Front Immunol* 16: 1601385.
125. Du, W., Noyan, F., McCallion, O. et al. (2025). Gene editing of CD3 epsilon to redirect regulatory T cells for adoptive T cell transfer. *Mol Ther* 33 (3): 997–1013.
126. Zhang, A.H., Yoon, J., Kim, Y.C., and Scott, D.W. (2018). Targeting antigen-specific B cells using antigen-expressing transduced regulatory T cells. *J Immunol* 201 (5): 1434–1441.
127. Boardman, D.A., Mangat, S., Gillies, J.K. et al. (2025). Armored human CAR T(reg) cells with PD1 promoter-driven IL-10 have enhanced suppressive function. *Sci Adv* 11 (24): eadx7845.

128. Mohseni, Y.R., Saleem, A., Tung, S.L. et al. (2021). Chimeric antigen receptor-modified human regulatory T cells that constitutively express IL-10 maintain their phenotype and are potently suppressive. *Eur J Immunol* 51 (10): 2522–2530.
129. Rui, X., Alvarez Calderon, F., Wobma, H. et al. (2024). Human OX40L-CAR-T(regs) target activated antigen-presenting cells and control T cell alloreactivity. *Sci Transl Med* 16 (769): eadj9331.
130. Tripathi, S.K., Grimm, A., Dahl, N.P. et al. (2025). HLA-A2 CAR/IL-2-CISC engineered Treg display robust in vitro and in vivo antigen-specific regulatory function. *Mol Ther Methods Clin Dev* 33 (3): 101561.
131. McGovern, J., Holler, A., Thomas, S., and Stauss, H.J. (2022). Forced Fox-P3 expression can improve the safety and antigen-specific function of engineered regulatory T cells. *J Autoimmun* 132: 102888.
132. MacDonald, K.G., Hoeppli, R.E., Huang, Q. et al. (2016). Alloantigen-specific regulatory T cells generated with a chimeric antigen receptor. *J Clin Invest* 126 (4): 1413–1424.
133. Yoon, J., Schmidt, A., Zhang, A.H. et al. (2017). FVIII-specific human chimeric antigen receptor T-regulatory cells suppress T- and B-cell responses to FVIII. *Blood* 129 (2): 238–245.
134. Wright, G.P., Notley, C.A., Xue, S.A. et al. (2009). Adoptive therapy with redirected primary regulatory T cells results in antigen-specific suppression of arthritis. *Proc Natl Acad Sci U S A* 106 (45): 19078–19083.
135. Bittner, S., Ruhland, B., Hofmann, V. et al. (2022). Biosensors for inflammation as a strategy to engineer regulatory T cells for cell therapy. *Proc Natl Acad Sci U S A* 119 (40): e2208436119.
136. Hombach, A.A., Kofler, D., Rappl, G., and Abken, H. (2009). Redirecting human CD4+CD25+ regulatory T cells from the peripheral blood with pre-defined target specificity. *Gene Ther* 16 (9): 1088–1096.
137. Porret R, Alcaraz-Serna A, Peter B, et al. T cell receptor precision editing of regulatory T cells for celiac disease. *Sci Transl Med* 2025;17(790):eadr8941.https://doi.org/10.1126/scitranslmed.adr8941.
138. Indart A, Lyu H, Nguyen VQ, et al. Receptor-tethered orthogonal IL-2 enhances regulatory T cell therapy. *bioRxiv* 2025. https://doi.org/10.1101/2025.07.19.665688
139. Doglio, M., Rana, J., Stucchi, A. et al. (2025). CXCR5 engineered human and murine Tregs for targeted suppression in secondary and tertiary lymphoid organs. *Front Immunol* 16: 1513009.
140. Sanchez-Fueyo, A., Taylor, A., Martinez-Llordella, M. et al. (2025). FRI-511 QEL-001 LIBERATE study expansion cohort, CAR (chimeric antigen receptor) T regulatory (Treg) cells engraftment and expansion following rATG (rabbit anti-thymocyte globulin) conditioning in post liver transplantation. *J Hepatol* 82: S394–S395.

12

Immunotherapy in Transplantation Settings

JAMES W. WELLS[1,2]

[1] Faculty of Health, Medicine and Behavioural Sciences, Frazer Institute, The University of Queensland, Brisbane, Queensland, Australia

[2] Faculty of Health, Medicine and Behavioural Sciences, Dermatology Research Centre, The University of Queensland, Brisbane, Queensland, Australia

LEARNING OBJECTIVES

After reading this chapter, the reader should be able to:

- Explain the mechanisms of action of major immunosuppressive drugs and how they are used in the clinic.
- Compare and contrast acute GVHD and chronic GVHD and first-line management strategies.
- Describe early, intermediate, and late post-transplant infectious complications and associated prophylactic and treatment strategies.
- Distinguish between the divergent risks of ICI therapy in solid organ versus haematopoietic stem cell transplant recipients.
- Evaluate emerging strategies to manage transplant-associated complications, including the rationale for local immunotherapy approaches and the potential of genetically modified pig xenotransplantation to address organ shortages.

12.1 INTRODUCTION

The transplantation of tissues and cells between individuals represents one of the most remarkable achievements in modern healthcare. Often lifesaving, the field encompasses diverse procedures from solid organ transplants like pancreas, heart, lung, liver, and kidney to cellular therapies like islet cells, bone marrow, and stem cells (see Figure 12.1). In addition to the challenge of sourcing viable organs and cells, a fundamental challenge facing successful transplantation is overcoming the destruction of donor tissues by the host's immune system.

The immune system has evolved to protect the body against pathogens and abnormal cells, such as cancer. However, it is just as effective at eliminating beneficial transplanted material. This can occur through three main pathways: the direct pathway, the indirect pathway, and the semi-direct pathway. In the direct pathway,

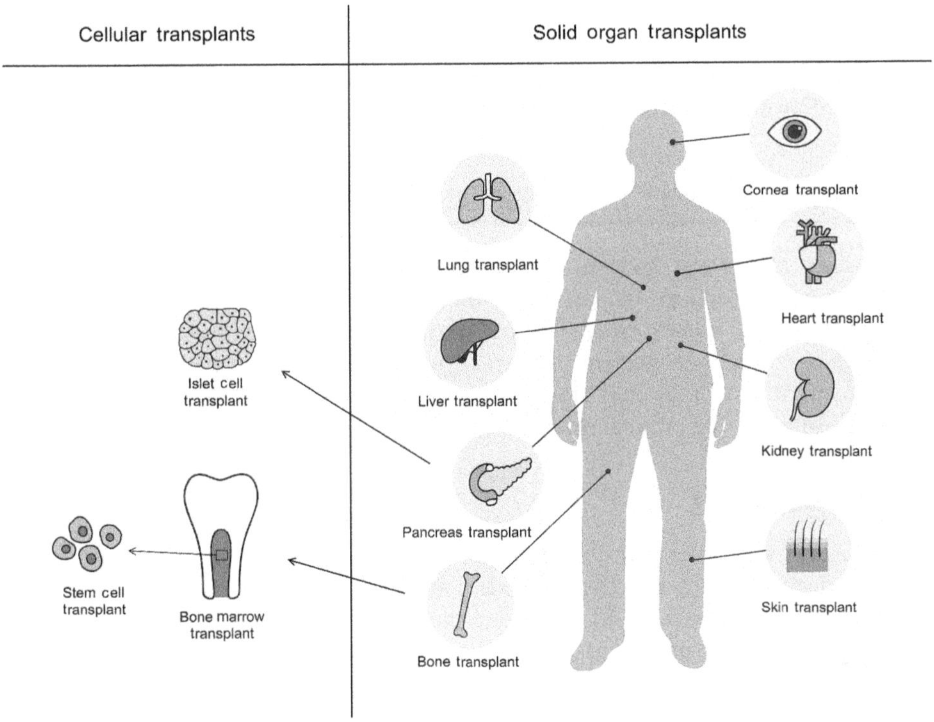

FIGURE 12.1 Types of clinical transplantation. Transplantation encompasses both cellular transplants (left) and solid organ transplants (right). Cellular transplants include islet cells, stem cells, and bone marrow transplants for treating metabolic, haematologic, and immunological disorders. Solid organ transplants include vascularized organs (heart, lungs, liver, pancreas, kidney) and non-vascularized tissues (cornea, skin, bone) for replacing failed or damaged organs.

host T cells recognise donor major histocompatibility complex (MHC) molecules on donor antigen-presenting cells (APCs) [1]. In the indirect pathway, host APCs process donor MHC antigens and present them as peptides to host T cells [2]. Finally, in the semi-direct pathway, donor MHC molecules are transferred to host antigen-presenting cells through a process known as cross-dressing [3].

To prevent the rejection of transplanted material by the host immune system, transplant recipients receive broad immunosuppressive medication before or during surgery and continue to take these drugs daily for the rest of their lives. These medications typically suppress the activation and/or function of host T cells. Amongst the most successful drugs are the calcineurin inhibitors tacrolimus and cyclosporine and the mammalian target of rapamycin (mTOR) inhibitors sirolimus and everolimus. To lower the doses of these drugs used and reduce their kidney-damaging effects, these drugs are frequently given in combination with corticosteroids like prednisone and antimetabolites such as mycophenolate mofetil [4].

While the use of immunosuppressive drugs has dramatically improved short-term transplant survival, they carry significant long-term risks, including increased susceptibility to infections, malignancies (particularly skin cancers), cardiovascular disease, and nephrotoxicity. Furthermore, despite optimal immunosuppressive therapy, chronic transplant rejection and graft dysfunction remain major challenges [5, 6].

This chapter explores mechanisms of immunosuppressive drug action, discusses the challenges associated with treating post-transplant malignancies, graft-versus-host disease (GVHD), and infectious complications, and outlines future directions for the field, from skin cancer preventative strategies to xenotransplantation.

12.2 KEY MILESTONES IN TRANSPLANT SUCCESS

Modern-day transplant success relies on pharmacological immunosuppression to prevent graft rejection. In particular, the discovery of the calcineurin inhibitors cyclosporin A and tacrolimus, the mTOR inhibitor rapamycin, and the inosine monophosphate dehydrogenase inhibitor mycophenolate mofetil have revolutionised transplant outcomes and transformed transplantation from an experimental procedure into routine clinical practice.

12.2.1 Cyclosporin A

Cyclosporin A specifically and reversibly inhibits lymphocyte function, prolonging allograft survival in both preclinical models and clinical transplantation (e.g. kidney, pancreas, liver, and heart) [7, 8]. Early clinical trials produced concerning outcomes, including high lymphoma incidence and mortality, nephrotoxicity and hepatotoxicity [8]. A breakthrough came when cyclosporin A was combined with steroids at lower doses, substantially improving survival, reducing nephrotoxicity, and minimising lymphoproliferative tumours (predominantly Epstein–Barr virus driven) [9, 10].

12.2.2 Tacrolimus

Tacrolimus inhibits calcineurin with approximately 100-fold greater potency than cyclosporin A [11]. Clinical trials demonstrated reduced acute allograft rejection episodes by 31% and reduced graft loss by 44% at 6 months post-transplantation [12]. Tacrolimus offers an improved cardiovascular risk profile and fewer cosmetic side effects (e.g. gingival hyperplasia and hirsutism), substantially improving patient tolerability [13–15].

12.2.3 Rapamycin

Rapamycin targets mTOR, blocking interleukin-2-driven T cell proliferation [16]. Clinical trials demonstrated dramatic reductions in acute rejection rates when rapamycin was combined with cyclosporin A and steroids [17, 18]. However, rapamycin causes substantial adverse effects, including impaired wound healing, metabolic disturbances (dyslipidaemia and hyperglycaemia), haematologic toxicities, and pulmonary complications, resulting in discontinuation rates of up to 49% [19]. Everolimus, a rapamycin derivative with improved pharmacokinetics and tissue penetration, a shorter half-life and a superior tolerability profile, is the preferred mTOR inhibitor in modern transplant regimens [20, 21].

12.2.4 Mycophenolate Mofetil

Mycophenolate mofetil is a potent and reversible inhibitor of inosine monophosphate dehydrogenase, the rate-limiting enzyme in *de novo* purine synthesis. This selectively depletes guanine nucleotides in T and B cells, inhibiting deoxyribonucleic acid (DNA) synthesis and proliferation [22]. A landmark 1995 kidney transplant trial demonstrated that mycophenolate mofetil with cyclosporine and corticosteroids reduced first biopsy-proven acute rejection to 19.8% compared to 38.0% of patients receiving azathioprine-based regimens [23]. However, mycophenolate mofetil cannot be used as a monotherapy, as evidenced by a liver transplant trial that was terminated when three of five patients developed severe organ rejection [24]. Adverse effects include gastrointestinal complications like diarrhoea and colitis and haematologic side effects like anaemia, leukopenia, and neutropenia [25, 26]. Despite these limitations, mycophenolate mofetil remains a cornerstone of current immunosuppressant combination regimens.

12.3 CLINICAL APPLICATIONS

Success in transplantation medicine requires the sophisticated manipulation of the immune system. This section explores three pivotal clinical domains where immunological principles directly translate to clinical outcomes for patients: optimising immunosuppressive regimens to prevent graft rejection whilst minimising toxicity, managing GVHD in haematopoietic transplantation, and harnessing graft-versus-leukaemia (GVL) effects to treat malignancy.

12.3.1 Immunosuppressive Regimens in Contemporary Transplant Care

Current multidrug treatment regimens are dominated by calcineurin inhibitors, tailored to organ type, immunological risk, and comorbidity profile. Tacrolimus combined with mycophenolate and variably with corticosteroids remains the benchmark, reliably preventing acute rejection while permitting dose modulation to minimise toxicity.

12.3.1.1 Kidney Transplantation

Tacrolimus and mycophenolate with early or late steroid withdrawal are now standard for low-to-moderate-risk recipients. The SAILOR trial showed that complete steroid avoidance versus steroid maintenance resulted in comparable acute rejection rates, graft loss, and renal function at two years post-transplant, indicating that steroids may not be necessary in selected patients [27].

A significant advancement is the introduction of mTOR inhibitors to minimise tacrolimus exposure. In *de novo* low-to-moderate risk recipients, the use of rabbit anti-thymocyte globulin to deplete T cells, followed by everolimus with reduced tacrolimus, achieved similar efficacy to standard tacrolimus/mycophenolate therapy while attenuating tacrolimus-associated nephrotoxicity [28]. This strategy is increasingly used, particularly in patients with early renal dysfunction or malignancy risk.

12.3.1.2 Liver Transplantation

In liver transplantation, tacrolimus-based regimens also predominate, but balancing rejection prevention with renal preservation is challenging due to high posttransplant kidney injury rates. Randomised trials demonstrated that everolimus with reduced tacrolimus provides comparable rejection protection to standard tacrolimus while significantly improving renal function [29]. The five-year CERTITUDE observational study found everolimus-based regimens were associated with fewer cardiovascular events, though adverse events and treatment discontinuation rates were higher [30].

12.3.1.3 Heart Transplantation

Triple therapy with calcineurin inhibitors, mycophenolate, and corticosteroids is standard. The SCHEDULE trial showed everolimus with early cyclosporin A withdrawal significantly reduced cardiac allograft vasculopathy progression and improved renal function, although it was associated with a higher incidence of early rejection [31]. Long-term follow-up confirmed sustained renal benefits [32], and recent retrospective registry data validate the clinical utility of tacrolimus combined with everolimus as an effective alternative, offering vascular benefits in adult heart transplant recipients [33].

Across organs, therefore, contemporary regimens are converging on tacrolimus-based combinations integrating mycophenolate, steroids, and everolimus in organ- and risk-specific ways, providing complementary mechanisms for robust immunosuppression with reduced long-term toxicity.

12.3.2 Graft-Versus-Host Disease

Haematopoietic stem cell transplantation (HSCT), which encompasses bone marrow, peripheral blood stem cell, and cord blood transplants, is often used to treat leukaemia/lymphoma, bone marrow failure, and genetic and hereditary disorders [34]. GVHD is a major complication of allogeneic HSCT, occurring when donor T cells recognise recipient major and/or minor histocompatibility molecules as foreign, damaging host tissues and causing severe complications and death [35, 36].

HSCT is often preceded by a conditioning regimen, such as chemotherapy or irradiation, designed to suppress the recipient's immune system to prevent graft rejection and make space for donor cells to engraft. Conditioning regimens, however, can induce tissue damage, releasing danger signals and proinflammatory cytokines that enhance antigen presentation and T cell recruitment to target organs [37]. Chronic GVHD involves additional pathogenic mechanisms, including follicular helper T-cell-driven germinal centre formation, pathogenic B cell activation with autoantibody production, and fibrotic remodelling [36]. This leads to sicca syndrome of the eyes and mouth, bronchiolitis obliterans in the lungs, genital involvement, and joint/fascia restriction [38, 39].

Acute GVHD typically presents within the first 100 days post-transplant, affecting skin (maculopapular rash), the gastrointestinal tract (diarrhoea, nausea, and anorexia), and the liver (cholestatic hyperbilirubinaemia) [40], driven by alloreactive T-cell-mediated epithelial injury and cytokine storm [35].

Management centres on prophylaxis and treatment. Standard prophylaxis includes calcineurin inhibitors (cyclosporine A or tacrolimus) combined with the antimetabolite methotrexate, with anti-thymocyte globulin or post-transplant cyclophosphamide recommended for unrelated donor transplants [41]. First-line treatment for established GVHD is corticosteroids. For steroid-refractory disease, drugs that target and inhibit intracellular signalling pathways involved in immune and inflammatory responses, like ruxolitinib (a Janus kinase (JAK)1/2 inhibitor), are now standard of care for both acute and chronic GVHD, with pivotal data demonstrating superior response rates [42, 43]. Additional options for refractory chronic GVHD include belumosudil (a rho-associated coiled-coil-containing protein kinase 2 (ROCK2) inhibitor) and ibrutinib [a Bruton's tyrosine kinase (BTK) inhibitor] [44–46].

12.3.3 Graft-Versus-Leukaemia

Allogeneic HSCT undertaken to treat leukaemia and other haematological malignancies can induce a GVL effect. GVL is mediated predominantly by donor-derived T cells that recognise residual leukaemia cells through T cell receptor engagement with recipient MHC molecules presenting tumour-associated antigens or minor histocompatibility antigens [47]. $CD8^+$ cytotoxic T lymphocytes are the primary effectors, though $CD4^+$ helper T cells provide critical help for sustained responses [48]. Natural killer cells contribute independently, particularly when donor–recipient killer immunoglobulin-like receptor ligand mismatches permit natural killer cell alloreactivity against leukaemia cells [49]. B cell responses generating antibodies against specific minor histocompatibility antigens may further augment anti-leukaemic immunity [50].

Clinically, patients who develop GVHD tend to have lower cancer relapse rates, indicating that GVL is taking place [51]. Moreover, patients who are at a high risk of disease relapse but who currently show no active GVHD may receive a donor lymphocyte infusion to deliberately induce a controlled GVL effect, improving overall survival [52]. Disease susceptibility to GVL, however, varies substantially. For example, chronic myeloid leukaemia is highly GVL-sensitive, with complete response rates up to 80% following donor lymphocyte infusion. In contrast, acute myeloid leukaemia and acute lymphoblastic leukaemia demonstrate more modest responses, up to 40% [53]. Relapse may occur through immune escape mechanisms, including genomic loss of MHC heterozygosity, preventing presentation of critical alloantigens [54].

Current consensus recommends initiating donor lymphocyte infusion at 1×10^7 $CD3^+$ T-cells/kg with dose escalation at 4-week intervals, carefully balancing anti-leukaemic efficacy against GVHD risk [55]. Novel approaches under investigation to boost the anti-leukaemia effect of donor T cells while reducing GVHD include: adoptive regulatory T cell therapy to selectively suppress GVHD while preserving GVL, metabolic modulation of donor T cells to make them more resilient and effective and genetically engineering donor lymphocytes to enhance tumour specificity while minimising alloreactivity.

12.4 CHALLENGES AND CONTROVERSIES

The immunosuppressive environment necessary for transplant acceptance simultaneously heightens susceptibility to opportunistic infections and complicates cancer immunotherapy. This section examines these two critical clinical dilemmas where immunological management conflicts directly challenge clinical decision-making in solid organ transplant recipients.

12.4.1 Post-transplant Infectious Complications

Transplant patients are highly vulnerable to infectious complications due to immunosuppression required to prevent allograft rejection. Infections represent a leading cause of morbidity and mortality and follow a predictable timeline: the pre-engraftment/early period (0–30 days), the intermediate immunosuppression period (1–6 months), and the late post-engraftment period (>6 months) [56].

12.4.1.1 Early Period (0–30 Days)

During the pre-engraftment/early period, patients often experience severe immunosuppression and mucosal barrier damage. In HSCT recipients, the loss of neutrophils (neutropenia) combined with chemotherapy-induced inflammation of the mucous membranes lining the digestive tract (mucositis) leads to bacterial bloodstream infections in 20–30% of patients [57, 58]. Solid organ transplant recipients face nosocomial (hospital-related), surgical site, bloodstream, and organ-specific infections, particularly in liver transplant recipients (59–68% of patients) [59]. Early *Candida* fungal infections occur in both populations but are also most common in liver transplantation (5–42% of patients) [60]. Prophylactic antimicrobials prevent most early infections, while established infections require broad-spectrum antibiotics and antifungal therapy.

12.4.1.2 Intermediate Period (1–6 Months)

This period carries the highest opportunistic infection risk. Cytomegalovirus (CMV) is the most significant viral pathogen, causing direct end-organ disease (pneumonitis, hepatitis, colitis, and retinitis) and indirect immunomodulatory effects that increase susceptibility to further infections, rejection, and mortality [61]. In HSCT recipients (particularly allogeneic), latent CMV reactivation occurs in 40–60% of seropositive recipients without prophylaxis [62]. Solid organ transplant recipients have lower but organ-specific disease rates (8–32% in kidney, 9–23% in heart, 22–29% in liver, and 50–75% in lung [61, 63]). CMV-seronegative recipients of seropositive organs (Donor$^+$/Recipient$^-$) face the highest risk of severe primary infection. Prophylaxis with valganciclovir or letermovir (preferred due to lower haematologic toxicity) reduces disease substantially [64]. Active CMV disease requires intravenous ganciclovir or valganciclovir. Resistant infection necessitates the use of foscarnet or cidofovir despite significant toxicity [65–67].

HSCT recipients also face severe opportunistic infections, including Pneumocystis jirovecii pneumonia, invasive *Aspergillus* and *Candida*, Epstein–Barr virus, herpes simplex virus, and community-acquired respiratory viruses, with invasive fungal infection mortality rates exceeding 70% [68, 69]. Solid organ transplant recipients experience lower rates of these pathogens.

12.4.1.3 Late Post-engraftment Period (>6 Months)

In HSCT recipients, varicella zoster virus reactivation occurs in approximately 25% within the first year [70], and late CMV disease can emerge after prophylactic antiviral cessation [71]. Encapsulated bacterial infections (e.g. *Streptococcus pneumoniae* and *Haemophilus influenzae*) predominate in patients with active chronic GVHD [72], often requiring revaccination with pneumococcal conjugate, *H. influenzae* type b, and meningococcal vaccines [73]. Solid organ transplant recipients with chronic rejection or higher-dose immunosuppression remain at ongoing infection risk, with lung and pancreas transplantation carrying the highest late infection rates [74].

12.4.2 Cancer Immunotherapy in Transplant Recipients

Solid organ transplant recipients and HSCT recipients face an increased malignancy risk due to impaired T cell surveillance, but their cancer profiles differ substantially.

12.4.2.1 Cancer Epidemiology

In solid organ transplant recipients, keratinocyte skin cancers [squamous cell carcinoma (SCC) and basal cell carcinoma] predominate (>90% of all posttransplant cancers in Caucasian recipients), with 10-year cumulative incidence ranging from 10% in Southern Europe to 45% in Northern Europe and 70–82% at 20 years in Australia [75]. One in twenty solid organ transplant recipients develops a highly morbid or fatal cutaneous SCC after transplantation [76]. HSCT recipients experience a different malignancy spectrum: therapy-related myelodysplastic syndrome/acute myeloid leukaemia, posttransplant lymphoproliferative disorders, and solid tumours (particularly oropharyngeal and lung cancers associated with chronic GVHD).

12.4.2.2 Immune Checkpoint Inhibitors in Solid Organ Transplant Recipients

Immune checkpoint inhibitors (ICIs) targeting programmed cell death protein 1 (PD-1), programmed death-ligand 1 (PD-L1), and cytotoxic T-lymphocyte–associated protein 4 (CTLA-4) have revolutionised cancer treatment, yet transplant recipients have been systematically excluded from pivotal clinical trials because of the risk of organ rejection (see Figure 12.2) [77]. Case series and retrospective analyses confirm that ICIs demonstrate objective response rates of 31–41%, with particularly favourable responses in cutaneous SCC (61–64%) and melanoma (31–48.5%) [78, 79]. However, acute graft rejection occurs in 26–42% of patients, with a median onset at 24–52 days after treatment initiation, and more than half progress to irreversible graft failure [78]. PD-1 inhibitors carry the highest rejection rate, and combination CTLA-4/PD-1 therapy produces rejection rates up to 80% [78].

Management requires multidisciplinary coordination between transplant physicians and oncologists. A Phase I trial demonstrated that maintaining baseline immunosuppression during ICI therapy achieved beneficial responses with no allograft losses, suggesting that baseline immunosuppression need not be sacrificed for antitumour efficacy [80]. Conversion to mTOR inhibitors (everolimus, sirolimus) may offer a dual benefit through intrinsic antitumour properties and lower rejection rates [81].

12.4.2.3 Immune Checkpoint Inhibitors in HSCT Recipients

In HSCT recipients, relapsed leukaemia represents a dire clinical scenario with an extremely poor prognosis. ICIs are being investigated to reverse immune dysfunction by blocking the PD-1/PD-L1 axis, which causes T-cell exhaustion. However, a comprehensive review of 176 HSCT recipients found that 25% developed GVHD,

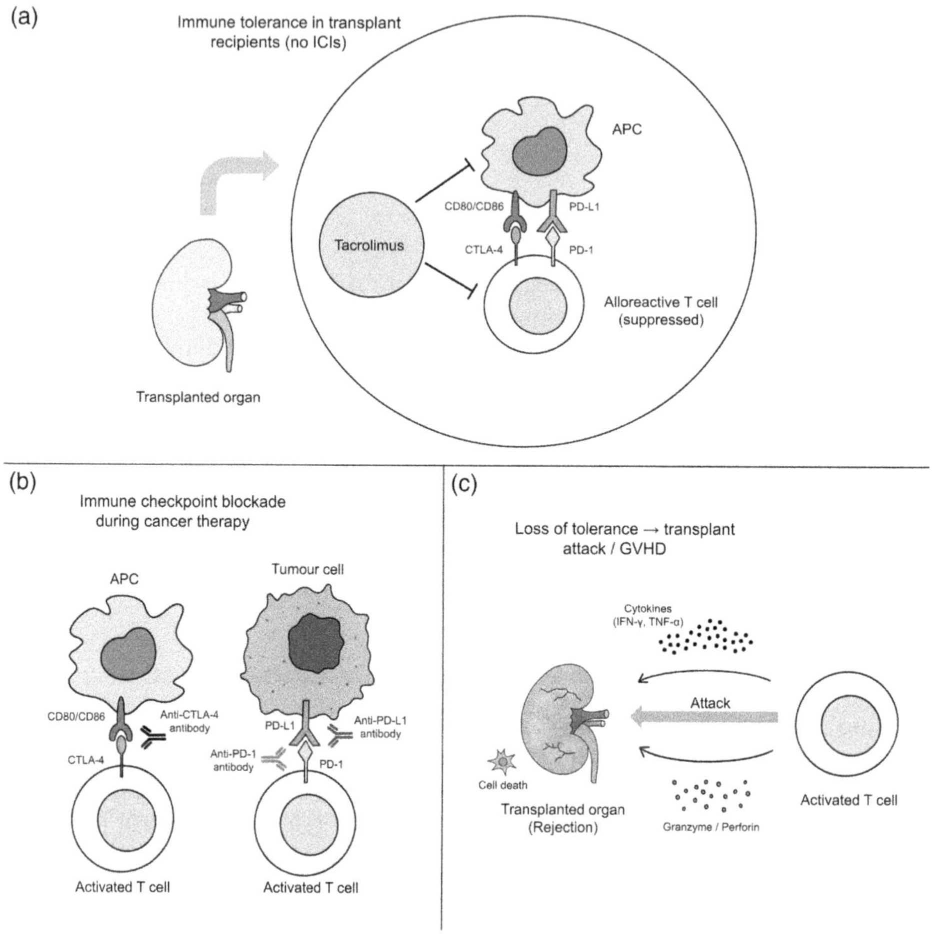

FIGURE 12.2 The paradox of immunosuppression and immune checkpoint inhibition in transplant recipients. (a) Under standard immunosuppression with tacrolimus, immune tolerance is maintained through suppression of costimulatory molecules (CD80/CD86, CTLA-4, PD-1/PD-L1) on antigen-presenting cells (APCs) and T cells, preventing alloreactive T cell activation and transplant rejection. (b) Immune checkpoint inhibitor (ICI) therapy targeting CTLA-4 and PD-1/PD-L1 pathways reactivates T cells for anti-tumour immunity by blocking inhibitory signals on both APCs and tumour cells. (c) Paradoxically, restoration of T cell costimulation during ICI therapy can break transplant tolerance, leading to loss of allograft protection. Activated T cells recognise transplant alloantigens and mediate organ attack through cytokine release (IFN-γ, TNF-α) and cytotoxic granule delivery (granzyme/perforin), resulting in transplant rejection or graft-versus-host disease (GVHD).

leading to 11 deaths [82]. In patients with a history of prior GVHD, the acute GVHD incidence reached 63% [83]. The GVHD risk can be partially mitigated through post-transplantation cyclophosphamide prophylaxis (90% reduced acute risk) [84] and delayed ICI initiation (≥180 days posttransplant) [85].

12.5 FUTURE DIRECTIONS

Emerging technologies are poised to reshape transplant outcomes, from skin cancer management and local immune checkpoint therapy to xenotransplantation approaches. This section examines cutting-edge strategies that promise to expand therapeutic options, enable personalised immune interventions, and address persistent challenges in organ transplantation.

12.5.1 Emerging Approaches for the Treatment of Transplant-Associated Skin Cancer

12.5.1.1 Locally Counteracting the Impact of Immunosuppression in the Skin

Reduction or withdrawal of systemic immunosuppression can induce spontaneous regression of established skin cancers in transplant recipients. Case reports demonstrate remarkable tumour regression following immunosuppression reduction; for example, 2 patients with metastatic melanoma experienced complete regression of advanced disease after discontinuing azathioprine, with one remaining melanoma-free for 10 years [86]. Similarly, reduction of immunosuppression in renal transplant recipients with aggressive SCC has been shown to prolong metastatic disease-free survival and, in select cases, induce tumour regression, suggesting immune reconstitution can re-establish antitumour surveillance [87]. However, this approach is rarely implemented clinically because it precipitates rapid and severe allograft rejection [88].

Q-2361 is a first-in-class small molecule that antagonises tacrolimus, sirolimus, and everolimus binding to FK506-binding protein (FKBP12) [89] (see Figure 12.3). In tacrolimus-suppressed mouse models of cutaneous SCC, the local delivery of Q-2361 drives CD8-dependent tumour regression, with negligible systemic exposure and no intrinsic immunosuppressive activity. Pharmacokinetic studies demonstrate high and sustained skin concentrations with minimal blood levels, supporting a therapeutic window for local immune surveillance restoration while maintaining systemic allograft tolerance [89]. Preliminary data suggest Q-2361 also reduces ultraviolet (UV)-damaged skin cell transformation into skin tumours (unpublished). This mechanistically distinct, local immunotherapy approach offers a promising strategy to prevent or treat transplant-associated skin cancer while preserving conventional tacrolimus/sirolimus/everolimus-based immunosuppression.

12.5.1.2 Local Immune Checkpoint Therapy

As discussed in Section 12.5.2.2, ICIs delivered systemically offer transformative efficacy against advanced malignancies but carry substantial risk of allograft rejection in transplant recipients. Intratumoural or intralesional delivery of ICIs represents an emerging strategy to concentrate immunomodulatory activity within the tumour microenvironment while limiting systemic immune activation [90]. Preclinical data demonstrate that intratumoural, but not systemic, anti-PD-1 combined with toll-like

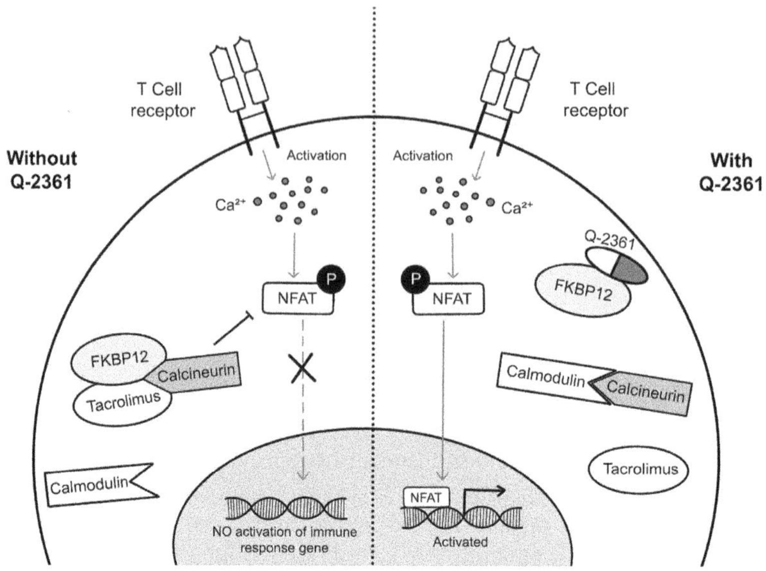

FIGURE 12.3 Mechanism of action of Q-2361 for local immunotherapy in transplant recipients. Q-2361 is a small-molecule antagonist that selectively blocks the binding of tacrolimus to FKBP12. Left panel (without Q-2361): Tacrolimus binds FKBP12 and complexes with calcineurin, inhibiting its phosphatase activity. This prevents calcineurin-mediated dephosphorylation of NFAT, blocking T cell receptor (TCR)-driven nuclear translocation of phosphorylated NFAT and suppressing activation of immune response genes. Right panel (with Q-2361): Q-2361 occupies FKBP12, preventing tacrolimus binding and complexing with calcineurin. Calcineurin remains active and can dephosphorylate NFAT, permitting NFAT nuclear entry and activation of immune response genes, thereby restoring local antitumour T cell immunity. This selective local antagonism of tacrolimus allows immune reconstitution in skin tumours while systemic immunosuppression is maintained through continued tacrolimus exposure in other tissues.

receptor 9 agonism promotes potent antitumour responses without accelerating cardiac allograft rejection in immunosuppressed mice, provided the tumour and graft do not share MHC antigens [91]. Similarly, peritumoural delivery of low-dose anti-CTLA-4 and other ICIs in immunocompetent murine models triggers systemic antitumour immunity while avoiding the autoimmune toxicity observed with systemic high-dose administration [90]. Clinical studies are now evaluating intratumoural oncolytic and immune-modulating agents in transplant recipients with locally advanced or metastatic cutaneous SCC [92, 93]. These localised approaches may ultimately enable immune function at the tumour site while preserving the immunosuppressive balance required for graft survival.

12.5.2 Xenotransplantation

Xenotransplantation offers a transformative solution to organ shortage by using genetically modified pigs as organ donors (see Figure 12.4), providing an essentially unlimited organ supply and eliminating transplant waitlists.

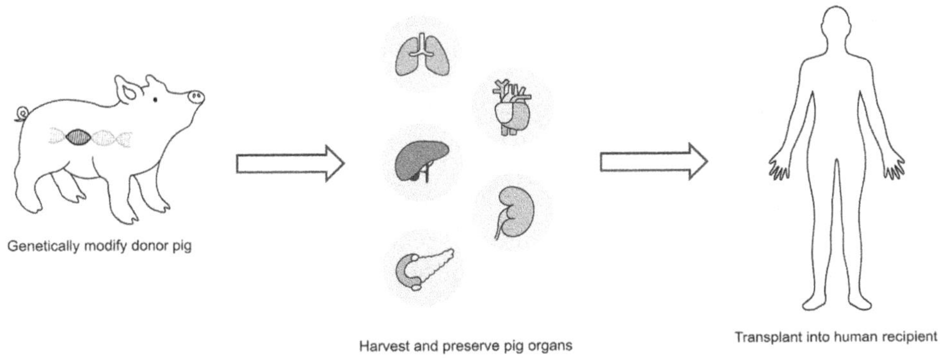

FIGURE 12.4 Xenotransplantation workflow: from genetic engineering to clinical transplantation. The xenotransplantation pathway comprises three key steps. First, donor pigs are genetically modified to eliminate or reduce xenoantigens (e.g. α-Gal, Neu5Gc, and Sda) through knockout of xenoantigen genes (GGTA1, CMAH, β4GalNT2, and GHR) and insertion of human transgenes encoding complement regulatory proteins (CD46, CD55), coagulation factors (thrombomodulin, endothelial protein C receptor), and immunomodulatory molecules (CD47, haem oxygenase-1). Second, organs are harvested from genetically modified pigs and preserved for transplantation. Third, the xenograft is transplanted into a human recipient, where it provides replacement function for failed organs, including lungs, heart, liver, pancreas, and kidneys.

However, significant immunological and safety challenges remain. Hyperacute rejection, driven by preformed antibodies against porcine carbohydrate antigens (e.g. α-Gal, Neu5Gc, and Sda), historically caused immediate graft failure [94]. Beyond antibody-mediated injury, innate immune responses from natural killer cells, macrophages, and complement activation contribute substantially to xenograft rejection [95]. Coagulation dysregulation from molecular incompatibilities between porcine and human coagulation cascades poses additional risk [96]. Furthermore, zoonotic pathogens, including porcine endogenous retroviruses, require rigorous screening and surveillance.

Successful clinical cases employ multigene-edited pigs combining knockout of xenoantigen genes (e.g. alpha-1,3-galactosyltransferase 1 (GGTA1), cytidine 5′-monophosphate N-acetylneuraminic acid hydroxylase (CMAH), beta-1,4-N-acetylgalactosaminyltransferase 2 (β4GalNT2), and growth hormone receptor (GHR)) with insertion of human complement regulatory proteins (e.g. CD46, CD55), thrombomodulin and endothelial protein C receptor (coagulation factors), CD47 (to inhibit macrophage phagocytosis), and haem oxygenase-1 (to reduce reactive oxygen species and inflammatory cell inflammation) [97].

In January 2022, a 10-gene-edited pig heart functioned for approximately 2 months in a living patient before failing due to porcine CMV reactivation and antibody-mediated rejection [97, 98]. Subsequent pig heart transplants into brain-dead recipients demonstrated excellent early function without hyperacute rejection or detectable zoonotic transmission [99].

In kidney xenotransplantation, 10-gene-edited pig kidneys maintained creatinine clearance for 7 days in a decedent model [100]. Recently, patient survival well past six months with functioning pig kidneys has been reported [101, 102]. In early

2025, the first formal clinical trials of genetically edited pig kidney transplants into living humans received approval, using kidneys with 69 gene edits (including 59 viral inactivations) [103].

In 2024, a six-gene-edited pig liver maintained auxiliary function for 10 days in a brain-dead recipient [104]. In 2025, the world's first genetically modified pig auxiliary liver transplant in a living human remained functional for 38 days with a 10-gene-edited organ [105].

Ongoing research focuses on optimising gene-editing combinations, developing CD40–CD154 costimulatory blockade to control T cell and antibody responses, eliminating latent porcine viruses from donor herds, and tailoring immunosuppression to xenograft-specific rejection pathways [106, 107]. Single-cell transcriptomic analyses are revealing cellular dynamics to inform future genetic modifications [108].

KEY TERMS & DEFINITIONS SIDEBAR

Immunosuppression Pharmacological or biological suppression of the adaptive immune system (T cells and B cells) to prevent rejection of transplanted organs or tissues while accepting the trade-off of increased infection and malignancy risk.

Graft rejection Destruction of transplanted tissue by the host immune system, occurring through direct recognition of donor MHC molecules, indirect recognition via processed donor antigens, or semi-direct pathways involving cross-dressed host APCs.

Calcineurin inhibitors A class of immunosuppressive drugs (tacrolimus and cyclosporine) that block the phosphatase calcineurin, preventing T-cell activation and cytokine production by inhibiting nuclear factor of activated T cells (NFAT) signalling.

mTOR inhibitors Immunosuppressive agents (sirolimus and everolimus) that block mTOR, a key regulator of cell growth and proliferation, thereby inhibiting interleukin-2-driven T-cell proliferation and cell cycle progression.

Graft-versus-host disease (GVHD) A serious complication of allogeneic HSCT in which immunocompetent donor T cells recognise recipient MHC and minor histocompatibility antigens as foreign, triggering an immune attack on host tissues (skin, gastrointestinal tract, liver, and lungs).

Graft-versus-leukaemia (GVL) The beneficial antitumour effect mediated by donor-derived T cells (primarily CD8+ cytotoxic T lymphocytes) that recognise and eliminate residual leukaemia cells through T cell receptor engagement with recipient MHC presenting tumour-associated or minor histocompatibility antigens.

Donor lymphocyte infusion A therapeutic strategy in which donor T lymphocytes are deliberately infused into transplant recipients at risk of disease relapse but without active GVHD, administered at escalating doses (starting at 1×10^7 CD3+ T cells/kg at 4-week intervals) to induce a controlled GVL effect.

Immune checkpoint inhibitors (ICIs) Monoclonal antibodies or small molecules (targeting PD-1, PD-L1, or CTLA-4) that block inhibitory signals on T cells, thereby releasing T cell exhaustion and restoring antitumour immunity – but with paradoxical complications in transplant recipients (allograft rejection in solid organ recipients and GVHD in HSCT recipients).

Xenotransplantation The transplantation of organs, tissues, or cells from one species (typically genetically modified pigs) into recipients of a different species (humans), offering a potential solution to organ shortage through on-demand production of physiologically compatible donor organs.

Donor-derived cell-free DNA (dd-cfDNA) Circulating DNA fragments released from transplanted tissue into the bloodstream, serving as a non-invasive biomarker for graft injury and rejection that can provide 10–15 days of early warning before clinically apparent allograft dysfunction.

LIST OF ABBREVIATIONS

β4GalNT2	beta-1,4-N-acetylgalactosaminyltransferase 2
BTK	Bruton's tyrosine kinase
CD	cluster of differentiation
CMAH	cytidine 5′-monophosphate N-acetylneuraminic acid hydroxylase
CMV	cytomegalovirus
CTLA-4	cytotoxic T-lymphocyte-associated protein 4
CXCL	C-X-C motif chemokine ligand
DNA	deoxyribonucleic acid
FKBP	FK506-binding protein
GGTA1	alpha-1,3-galactosyltransferase 1
GHR	growth hormone receptor
GVHD	graft-versus-host disease
GVL	graft-versus-leukaemia
HSCT	haematopoietic stem cell transplantation
ICIs	immune checkpoint inhibitors
JAK	Janus kinase
MHC	major histocompatibility complex
mTOR	mammalian target of rapamycin
PD-1	programmed cell death protein 1
PD-L1	programmed death-ligand 1
ROCK2	rho-associated coiled-coil-containing protein kinase 2
SCC	squamous cell carcinoma
UV	ultraviolet

CASE STUDY: LETERMOVIR PROPHYLAXIS FOR CMV IN HAEMATOPOIETIC-CELL TRANSPLANTATION

BACKGROUND

CMV infection represents a major complication following allogeneic haematopoietic-cell transplantation (HCT), contributing significantly to morbidity and mortality in CMV-seropositive recipients.

STUDY DESIGN

A Phase III, double-blind, randomised controlled trial enrolled 565 adult CMV-seropositive transplant recipients. Patients were randomised 2:1 to receive letermovir (a CMV terminase-complex inhibitor) or placebo, administered orally or intravenously through week 14 post-transplantation [1].

PRIMARY ENDPOINT

The primary efficacy endpoint was clinically significant CMV infection through week 24 after transplantation.

KEY RESULTS

Among 495 patients with undetectable CMV DNA at randomisation, significantly fewer patients receiving letermovir developed clinically significant CMV infection compared to placebo (37.5 versus 60.6%; $P < 0.001$). During the prophylaxis period (through week 14), only 19.1% of letermovir recipients developed infection versus 50.0% of placebo recipients. All-cause mortality at 48 weeks was lower with letermovir (20.9 vs. 25.5%). Adverse events were predominantly low-grade, with similar rates of myelotoxic and nephrotoxic events between groups.

SIGNIFICANCE

This trial established letermovir as an effective and well-tolerated prophylactic agent for CMV infection in high-risk transplant recipients, subsequently leading to FDA approval for this indication.

Marty et al. [109].

REVIEW QUESTIONS

1. Contemporary immunosuppressive regimens now commonly employ 'triple therapy', combining drugs with complementary mechanisms of action (e.g. calcineurin inhibitors, antimetabolites, and corticosteroids). Why is combination therapy superior to monotherapy for preventing graft rejection? What are the trade-offs between achieving robust immunosuppression and minimising long-term toxicities like nephrotoxicity, infections, and malignancy?
2. In HSCT, GVHD and GVL represent two sides of the same immunological phenomenon – donor T cell recognition of host tissues. Yet one is harmful (GVHD), and one is beneficial (GVL). How can the same donor immune response produce such different clinical outcomes? What strategies might allow clinicians to enhance GVL while minimising GVHD?

3. ICIs restore anti-tumour immunity by releasing T cell exhaustion. Yet in transplant recipients, they pose opposite risks: allograft rejection in solid organ recipients versus GVHD in haematopoietic stem cell recipients. Explain why the same mechanism of immune activation creates divergent complications in these two transplant populations, and discuss how this reflects fundamental differences in transplant immunobiology.

REFERENCES

1. Sherman, L.A. and Chattopadhyay, S. (1993). The molecular basis of allorecognition. *Annu Rev Immunol* 11: 385–402.
2. Benichou, G., Takizawa, P.A., Olson, C.A. et al. (1992). Donor major histocompatibility complex (MHC) peptides are presented by recipient MHC molecules during graft rejection. *J Exp Med* 175 (1): 305–308.
3. Liu, Q., Rojas-Canales, D.M., Divito, S.J. et al. (2016). Donor dendritic cell-derived exosomes promote allograft-targeting immune response. *J Clin Invest* 126 (8): 2805–2820.
4. Jung, J.W., Overgaard, N.H., Burke, M.T. et al. (2016). Does the nature of residual immune function explain the differential risk of non-melanoma skin cancer development in immunosuppressed organ transplant recipients? *Int J Cancer* 138 (2): 281–292.
5. Sun, H., Deng, M., Chen, W. et al. (2022). Graft dysfunction and rejection of lung transplant, a review on diagnosis and management. *Clin Respir J* 16 (1): 5–12.
6. Lai, X., Zheng, X., Mathew, J.M. et al. (2021). Tackling chronic kidney transplant rejection: challenges and promises. *Front Immunol* 12: 661643.
7. Calne, R.Y., White, D.J., Rolles, K. et al. (1978). Prolonged survival of pig orthotopic heart grafts treated with cyclosporin A. *Lancet* 1 (8075): 1183–1185.
8. Calne, R.Y., Rolles, K., White, D.J. et al. (1979). Cyclosporin A initially as the only immunosuppressant in 34 recipients of cadaveric organs: 32 kidneys, 2 pancreases, and 2 livers. *Lancet* 2 (8151): 1033–1036.
9. Starzl, T.E., Nalesnik, M.A., Porter, K.A. et al. (1984). Reversibility of lymphomas and lymphoproliferative lesions developing under cyclosporin-steroid therapy. *Lancet* 1 (8377): 583–587.
10. Starzl, T.E., Weil, R. III, Iwatsuki, S. et al. (1980). The use of cyclosporin A and prednisone in cadaver kidney transplantation. *Surg Gynecol Obstet* 151 (1): 17–26.
11. Kino, T., Hatanaka, H., Miyata, S. et al. (1987). FK-506, a novel immunosuppressant isolated from a *Streptomyces*. II. Immunosuppressive effect of FK-506 *in vitro*. *J Antibiot (Tokyo)* 40 (9): 1256–1265.
12. Webster, A.C., Woodroffe, R.C., Taylor, R.S. et al. (2005). Tacrolimus versus ciclosporin as primary immunosuppression for kidney transplant recipients: meta-analysis and meta-regression of randomised trial data. *BMJ* 331 (7520): 810.
13. Zadrazil, J., Horak, P., Zahalkova, J. et al. (2009). Improvement of cardiovascular risk factors and cosmetic side effects in kidney transplant recipients after conversion to tacrolimus. *Biomed Pap Med Fac Univ Palacky Olomouc Czech Repub* 153 (1): 67–73.
14. Penninga, L., Moller, C.H., Gustafsson, F. et al. (2010). Tacrolimus versus cyclosporine as primary immunosuppression after heart transplantation: systematic review with meta-analyses and trial sequential analyses of randomised trials. *Eur J Clin Pharmacol* 66 (12): 1177–1187.
15. Lucey, M.R., Abdelmalek, M.F., Gagliardi, R. et al. (2005). A comparison of tacrolimus and cyclosporine in liver transplantation: effects on renal function and cardiovascular risk status. *Am J Transplant* 5 (5): 1111–1119.

16. Kuo, C.J., Chung, J., Fiorentino, D.F. et al. (1992). Rapamycin selectively inhibits interleukin-2 activation of p70 S6 kinase. *Nature* 358 (6381): 70–73.
17. MacDonald, A.S. and Group RGS (2001). A worldwide, phase III, randomized, controlled, safety and efficacy study of a sirolimus/cyclosporine regimen for prevention of acute rejection in recipients of primary mismatched renal allografts. *Transplantation* 71 (2): 271–280.
18. Kahan, B.D., Julian, B.A., Pescovitz, M.D. et al. (1999). Sirolimus reduces the incidence of acute rejection episodes despite lower cyclosporine doses in Caucasian recipients of mismatched primary renal allografts: a phase II trial. Rapamune Study Group. *Transplantation* 68 (10): 1526–1532.
19. Schmucki, K., Gaisl, T., Hofmann, P. et al. (2024). mTOR inhibitors after lung transplantation: a real-life experience. *J Thorac Dis* 16 (5): 3007–3018.
20. Klawitter, J., Nashan, B., and Christians, U. (2015). Everolimus and sirolimus in transplantation-related but different. *Expert Opin Drug Saf* 14 (7): 1055–1070.
21. Tenderich, G., Fuchs, U., Zittermann, A. et al. (2007). Comparison of sirolimus and everolimus in their effects on blood lipid profiles and haematological parameters in heart transplant recipients. *Clin Transplant* 21 (4): 536–543.
22. Allison, A.C. (2005). Mechanisms of action of mycophenolate mofetil. *Lupus* 14 (Suppl 1): S2–S8.
23. Sollinger, H.W. (1995). Mycophenolate mofetil for the prevention of acute rejection in primary cadaveric renal allograft recipients. U.S. Renal Transplant Mycophenolate Mofetil Study Group. *Transplantation* 60 (3): 225–232.
24. Stewart, S.F., Hudson, M., Talbot, D. et al. (2001). Mycophenolate mofetil monotherapy in liver transplantation. *Lancet* 357 (9256): 609–610.
25. Kaye, A.D., Shah, S.S., Johnson, C.D. et al. (2025). Tacrolimus- and mycophenolate-mediated toxicity: clinical considerations and options in management of post-transplant patients. *Curr Issues Mol Biol* 47 (1): 2.
26. Ferrer-Machin, A., Vera-Cabrera, M., Plasencia-Garcia, I. et al. (2021). Evaluation of neutropenia secondary to mycophenolate mofetil associated with valganciclovir in liver transplant patients. *Farm Hosp* 45 (2): 77–81.
27. Ekberg, J., Baid-Agrawal, S., Jespersen, B. et al. (2022). A randomized controlled trial on safety of steroid avoidance in immunologically low-risk kidney transplant recipients. *Kidney Int Rep* 7 (2): 259–269.
28. Nunes Ficher, K., Dreige, Y., Gessolo Lins, P.R. et al. (2022). Long-term efficacy and safety of everolimus versus mycophenolate in kidney transplant recipients receiving tacrolimus. *Transplantation* 106 (2): 381–390.
29. Lee, S.G., Jeng, L.B., Saliba, F. et al. (2021). Efficacy and safety of everolimus with reduced tacrolimus in liver transplant recipients: 24-month results from the pooled analysis of 2 randomized controlled trials. *Transplantation* 105 (7): 1564–1575.
30. Saliba, F., Duvoux, C., Dharancy, S. et al. (2022). Five-year outcomes in liver transplant patients receiving everolimus with or without a calcineurin inhibitor: results from the CERTITUDE study. *Liver Int* 42 (11): 2513–2523.
31. Andreassen, A.K., Andersson, B., Gustafsson, F. et al. (2014). Everolimus initiation and early calcineurin inhibitor withdrawal in heart transplant recipients: a randomized trial. *Am J Transplant* 14 (8): 1828–1838.
32. Bollano, E., Andreassen, A.K., Eiskjaer, H. et al. (2024). Long-term follow-up of the randomized, prospective Scandinavian heart transplant everolimus de novo study with early calcineurin inhibitors avoidance (SCHEDULE) trial. *J Heart Lung Transplant* 43 (12): 1948–1959.
33. Vigil-Escalera, M., Catala, P., Alonso, V. et al. (2025). Maintenance immunosuppression with tacrolimus and everolimus in heart transplantation compared with the usual tacrolimus and micophenolate protocol: results from a retrospective registry. *Transplant Proc* 57 (1): 59–66.

34. Snowden, J.A., Sanchez-Ortega, I., Corbacioglu, S. et al. (2022). Indications for haematopoietic cell transplantation for haematological diseases, solid tumours and immune disorders: current practice in Europe, 2022. *Bone Marrow Transplant* 57 (8): 1217–1239.
35. Ghimire, S., Weber, D., Mavin, E. et al. (2017). Pathophysiology of GvHD and other HSCT-related major complications. *Front Immunol* 8: 79.
36. Hill, G.R., Betts, B.C., Tkachev, V. et al. (2021). Current concepts and advances in graft-versus-host disease immunology. *Annu Rev Immunol* 39: 19–49.
37. Ramadan, A. and Paczesny, S. (2015). Various forms of tissue damage and danger signals following hematopoietic stem-cell transplantation. *Front Immunol* 6: 14.
38. Jagasia, M.H., Greinix, H.T., Arora, M. et al. (2015). National Institutes of Health Consensus Development Project on criteria for clinical trials in chronic graft-versus-host disease: I. The 2014 diagnosis and staging working group report. *Biol Blood Marrow Transplant* 21 (3): 389–401.e1.
39. Duque-Afonso, J., Rassner, P., Walther, K. et al. (2024). Evaluation of risk for bronchiolitis obliterans syndrome after allogeneic hematopoietic cell transplantation with myeloablative conditioning regimens. *Bone Marrow Transplant* 59 (12): 1744–1753.
40. Kujawska, J., Zeiser, R., and Gil, L. (2025). Recent advances in acute gastrointestinal graft versus host disease (aGvHD): aspects of steroid-resistant disease. *Ann Hematol* 104 (2): 855–865.
41. Penack, O., Marchetti, M., Aljurf, M. et al. (2024). Prophylaxis and management of graft-versus-host disease after stem-cell transplantation for haematological malignancies: updated consensus recommendations of the European Society for Blood and Marrow Transplantation. *Lancet Haematol* 11 (2): e147–e159.
42. Zeiser, R., von Bubnoff, N., Butler, J. et al. (2020). Ruxolitinib for glucocorticoid-refractory acute graft-versus-host disease. *N Engl J Med* 382 (19): 1800–1810.
43. Zeiser, R., Polverelli, N., Ram, R. et al. (2021). Ruxolitinib for glucocorticoid-refractory chronic graft-versus-host disease. *N Engl J Med* 385 (3): 228–238.
44. Cutler, C., Lee, S.J., Arai, S. et al. (2021). Belumosudil for chronic graft-versus-host disease after 2 or more prior lines of therapy: the ROCKstar study. *Blood* 138 (22): 2278–2289.
45. Miklos, D., Cutler, C.S., Arora, M. et al. (2017). Ibrutinib for chronic graft-versus-host disease after failure of prior therapy. *Blood* 130 (21): 2243–2250.
46. Pidala, J., Kim, J., Kalos, D. et al. (2025). Ibrutinib for therapy of steroid-refractory chronic graft-versus-host disease: a multicenter real-world analysis. *Blood Adv* 9 (5): 1040–1048.
47. Dickinson, A.M., Norden, J., Li, S. et al. (2017). Graft-versus-leukemia effect following hematopoietic stem cell transplantation for leukemia. *Front Immunol* 8: 496.
48. Zheng, H., Matte-Martone, C., Li, H. et al. (2008). Effector memory CD4+ T cells mediate graft-versus-leukemia without inducing graft-versus-host disease. *Blood* 111 (4): 2476–2484.
49. Cooley, S., Weisdorf, D.J., Guethlein, L.A. et al. (2014). Donor killer cell Ig-like receptor B haplotypes, recipient HLA-C1, and HLA-C mismatch enhance the clinical benefit of unrelated transplantation for acute myelogenous leukemia. *J Immunol* 192 (10): 4592–4600.
50. Miklos, D.B., Kim, H.T., Miller, K.H. et al. (2005). Antibody responses to H-Y minor histocompatibility antigens correlate with chronic graft-versus-host disease and disease remission. *Blood* 105 (7): 2973–2978.
51. Kim, H.T., Soiffer, R.J., Cutler, C. et al. (2025). Reduced incidence of relapse and graft-versus-host disease in acute myeloid leukemia after allogeneic hematopoietic cell transplantation. *Haematologica* 110 (9): 1998–2008.
52. Wu, N., Yan, C.H., Kong, J. et al. (2025). Prophylactic versus preemptive donor lymphocyte infusion in refractory/relapsed AML post-allogeneic transplant: a retrospective comparative study. *Transplant Cell Ther* https://doi.org/10.1016/j.jtct.2025.10.029.
53. Maurer, K. and Antin, J.H. (2024). The graft versus leukemia effect: donor lymphocyte infusions and cellular therapy. *Front Immunol* 15: 1328858.

54. Pagliuca, S., Gurnari, C., Hercus, C. et al. (2023). Leukemia relapse via genetic immune escape after allogeneic hematopoietic cell transplantation. *Nat Commun* 14 (1): 3153.
55. Pagliuca, S., Schmid, C., Santoro, N. et al. (2024). Practice harmonization and guidelines committee and the cellular therapy and immunobiology working party of the European Society for Blood and Marrow Transplantation (EBMT) donor lymphocyte infusion after allogeneic haematopoietic cell transplantation for haematological malignancies: basic considerations and best practice recommendations from the EBMT. *Lancet Haematol* 11 (6): e448–e458.
56. van Delden, C., Stampf, S., Hirsch, H.H. et al. (2020). Burden and timeline of infectious diseases in the first year after solid organ transplantation in the Swiss transplant cohort study. *Clin Infect Dis* 71 (7): e159–e169.
57. Balletto, E. and Mikulska, M. (2015). Bacterial infections in hematopoietic stem cell transplant recipients. *Mediterr J Hematol Infect Dis* 7 (1): e2015045.
58. Gustinetti, G. and Mikulska, M. (2016). Bloodstream infections in neutropenic cancer patients: a practical update. *Virulence* 7 (3): 280–297.
59. Singh, N., Wagener, M.M., Obman, A. et al. (2004). Bacteremias in liver transplant recipients: shift toward gram-negative bacteria as predominant pathogens. *Liver Transpl* 10 (7): 844–849.
60. Senoner, T., Breitkopf, R., Treml, B., and Rajsic, S. (2023). Invasive fungal infections after liver transplantation. *J Clin Med* 12 (9): 3238.
61. Azevedo, L.S., Pierrotti, L.C., Abdala, E. et al. (2015). Cytomegalovirus infection in transplant recipients. *Clinics (Sao Paulo)* 70 (7): 515–523.
62. Kaito, S., Nakajima, Y., Hara, K. et al. (2020). Heterogeneous impact of cytomegalovirus reactivation on nonrelapse mortality in hematopoietic stem cell transplantation. *Blood Adv* 4 (6): 1051–1061.
63. Cukuranovic, J., Ugrenovic, S., Jovanovic, I. et al. (2012). Viral infection in renal transplant recipients. *Sci. World J.* 2012: 820621.
64. Limaye, A.P., Budde, K., Humar, A. et al. (2023). Letermovir vs valganciclovir for prophylaxis of cytomegalovirus in high-risk kidney transplant recipients: a randomized clinical trial. *JAMA* 330 (1): 33–42.
65. Kotton, C.N., Kumar, D., Manuel, O. et al. (2025). The fourth international consensus guidelines on the management of cytomegalovirus in solid organ transplantation. *Transplantation* 109 (7): 1066–1110.
66. Avery, R.K., Arav-Boger, R., Marr, K.A. et al. (2016). Outcomes in transplant recipients treated with foscarnet for ganciclovir-resistant or refractory cytomegalovirus infection. *Transplantation* 100 (10): e74–e80.
67. Mehta Steinke, S.A., Alfares, M., Valsamakis, A. et al. (2021). Outcomes of transplant recipients treated with cidofovir for resistant or refractory cytomegalovirus infection. *Transpl Infect Dis* 23 (3): e13521.
68. Pereira, M.R., Pouch, S.M., and Scully, B. (2019). Infections in allogeneic stem cell transplantation. In: *Principles and Practice of Transplant Infectious Diseases* (ed. A. Safdar), 209–226. Springer.
69. Rahi, M.S., Jindal, V., Pednekar, P. et al. (2021). Fungal infections in hematopoietic stem-cell transplant patients: a review of epidemiology, diagnosis, and management. *Ther Adv Infect Dis* 8: 20499361211039050.
70. Gea-Banacloche, J. (2016). Risks and epidemiology of infections after hematopoietic stem cell transplantation. In: *Transplant Infections* (ed. P. Ljungman, D. Snydman, and M. Boeckh), 81–99. Springer.
71. Einsele, H., Ljungman, P., and Boeckh, M. (2020). How I treat CMV reactivation after allogeneic hematopoietic stem cell transplantation. *Blood* 135 (19): 1619–1629.
72. Chaaban, S., Zimmer, A., Bhatt, V.R. et al. (2023). Bacterial pathogens causing pneumonia post hematopoietic stem cell transplant: the chronic GVHD population. *Pathogens* 12 (5): 726.

73. Singh, N. and Limaye, A.P. (2015). Infections in solid-organ transplant recipients. In: *Mandell, Douglas, and Bennett's Principles and Practice of Infectious Diseases* (ed. J.E. Bennett, R. Dolin, and M.J. Blaser), 3440–3452. Elsevier.
74. San Juan, R., Aguado, J.M., Lumbreras, C. et al. (2007). Incidence, clinical characteristics and risk factors of late infection in solid organ transplant recipients: data from the RESITRA study group. *Am J Transplant* 7 (4): 964–971.
75. Granata, S., Tessari, G., Stallone, G., and Zaza, G. (2023). Skin cancer in solid organ transplant recipients: still an open problem. *Front Med (Lausanne)* 10: 1189680.
76. Bibee, K., Swartz, A., Sridharan, S. et al. (2020). Cutaneous squamous cell carcinoma in the organ transplant recipient. *Oral Oncol* 103: 104562.
77. Van Meerhaeghe, T., Murakami, N., Le Moine, A. et al. (2024). Fine-tuning tumor- and allo-immunity: advances in the use of immune checkpoint inhibitors in kidney transplant recipients. *Clin Kidney J* 17 (4): sfae061.
78. Ji, S., Liu, H., Pachella, L. et al. (2023). Use of immune checkpoint inhibitors in solid organ transplant recipients with advanced cutaneous malignancies. *Front Transplant* 2: 1284740.
79. Saleem, N., Wang, J., Rejuso, A. et al. (2025). Outcomes of solid organ transplant recipients with advanced cancers receiving immune checkpoint inhibitors: a systematic review and individual participant data meta-analysis. *JAMA Oncol* 11 (10): 1150–1159.
80. Carroll, R.P., Boyer, M., Gebski, V. et al. (2022). Immune checkpoint inhibitors in kidney transplant recipients: a multicentre, single-arm, phase 1 study. *Lancet Oncol* 23 (8): 1078–1086.
81. Murakami, N., Mulvaney, P., Danesh, M. et al. (2021). A multi-center study on safety and efficacy of immune checkpoint inhibitors in cancer patients with kidney transplant. *Kidney Int* 100 (1): 196–205.
82. Ijaz, A., Khan, A.Y., Malik, S.U. et al. (2019). Significant risk of graft-versus-host disease with exposure to checkpoint inhibitors before and after allogeneic transplantation. *Biol Blood Marrow Transplant* 25 (1): 94–99.
83. Haverkos, B.M., Abbott, D., Hamadani, M. et al. (2017). PD-1 blockade for relapsed lymphoma post-allogeneic hematopoietic cell transplant: high response rate but frequent GVHD. *Blood* 130 (2): 221–228.
84. Saberian, C., Abdel-Wahab, N., Abudayyeh, A. et al. (2021). Post-transplantation cyclophosphamide reduces the incidence of acute graft-versus-host disease in patients with acute myeloid leukemia/myelodysplastic syndromes who receive immune checkpoint inhibitors after allogeneic hematopoietic stem cell transplantation. *J Immunother Cancer* 9 (2): e001818.
85. Herbaux, C., Merryman, R., Devine, S. et al. (2018). Recommendations for managing PD-1 blockade in the context of allogeneic HCT in Hodgkin lymphoma: taming a necessary evil. *Blood* 132 (1): 9–16.
86. Dillon, P., Thomas, N., Sharpless, N., and Collichio, F. (2010). Regression of advanced melanoma upon withdrawal of immunosuppression: case series and literature review. *Med Oncol* 27 (4): 1127–1132.
87. Moloney, F.J., Kelly, P.O., Kay, E.W. et al. (2004). Maintenance versus reduction of immunosuppression in renal transplant recipients with aggressive squamous cell carcinoma. *Dermatol Surg* 30 (4 Pt 2): 674–678.
88. Pisano, C., Leitenberger, J.J., Pugliano-Mauro, M., and Carroll, B.T. (2024). Updates in skin cancer in transplant recipients and immunosuppressed patients: review of the 2022-2023 scientific symposium of the International Immunosuppression and Transplant Skin Cancer Collaborative. *Transpl Int* 37: 12387.
89. Veitch, M., Beaumont, K., Pouwer, R. et al. (2023). Local blockade of tacrolimus promotes T-cell-mediated tumor regression in systemically immunosuppressed hosts. *J Immunother Cancer* 11 (9): e006783.
90. Wright, Q.G., Sinha, D., Wells, J.W. et al. (2024). Peritumoral administration of immunomodulatory antibodies as a triple combination suppresses skin tumor growth without systemic toxicity. *J Immunother Cancer* 12 (1): e007960.

91. Dang, N., Waer, M., Sprangers, B., and Lin, Y. (2021). Intratumoral immunotherapy with anti-PD-1 and TLR9 agonist induces systemic antitumor immunity without accelerating rejection of cardiac allografts. *Am J Transplant* 21 (1): 60–72.
92. Joo, V., Abdelhamid, K., Noto, A. et al. (2024). Primary prophylaxis with mTOR inhibitor enhances T cell effector function and prevents heart transplant rejection during talimogene laherparepvec therapy of squamous cell carcinoma. *Nat Commun* 15 (1): 3664.
93. Vidovic, D., Simms, G.A., Pasternak, S. et al. (2021). Case report: combined intra-lesional IL-2 and topical imiquimod safely and effectively clears multifocal, high-grade cutaneous squamous cell cancer in a combined liver and kidney transplant patient. *Front Immunol* 12: 678028.
94. Ko, J., Lee, G., Kim, H.W. et al. (2025). Current status of xenotransplantation from an immunobiological standpoint. *Clin Transplant Res* 39 (2): 97–115.
95. Maeda, A., Kogata, S., Toyama, C. et al. (2022). The innate cellular immune response in xenotransplantation. *Front Immunol* 13: 858604.
96. Ali, A., Kurome, M., Kessler, B. et al. (2024). What genetic modifications of source pigs are essential and sufficient for cell, tissue, and organ xenotransplantation? *Transpl Int* 37: 13681.
97. Griffith, B.P., Goerlich, C.E., Singh, A.K. et al. (2022). Genetically modified porcine-to-human cardiac xenotransplantation. *N Engl J Med* 387 (1): 35–44.
98. Mohiuddin, M.M., Singh, A.K., Scobie, L. et al. (2023). Graft dysfunction in compassionate use of genetically engineered pig-to-human cardiac xenotransplantation: a case report. *Lancet* 402 (10399): 397–410.
99. Moazami, N., Stern, J.M., Khalil, K. et al. (2023). Pig-to-human heart xenotransplantation in two recently deceased human recipients. *Nat Med* 29 (8): 1989–1997.
100. Judd, E., Kumar, V., Porrett, P.M. et al. (2024). Physiologic homeostasis after pig-to-human kidney xenotransplantation. *Kidney Int* 105 (5): 971–979.
101. Fieldhouse, R. (2025). 'Amazing feat': US man still alive six months after pig kidney transplant. *Nature* 645 (8081): 571–572.
102. Qin, F. (2025). Gene-edited pig kidney functions for over 200 days [Press release]. China Daily. https://www.chinadaily.com.cn/a/202509/25/WS68d53397a3108622abca2f7d.html. (Accessed 25 November 2025).
103. Deeley, M. (2025). FDA greenlights first clinical trials for genetically modified pig kidney transplants in humans. American Kidney Fund. https://www.kidneyfund.org/article/fda-greenlights-first-clinical-trials-genetically-modified-pig-kidney-transplants-humans.
104. Tao, K.S., Yang, Z.X., Zhang, X. et al. (2025). Gene-modified pig-to-human liver xenotransplantation. *Nature* 641 (8064): 1029–1036.
105. Zhang, W., Xu, Q., Xu, K. et al. (2025). Genetically engineered pig-to-human liver xenotransplantation. *J Hepatol* 84 (3): 587–598.
106. Cooper, D.K.C. and Pierson, R.N. III (2023). Milestones on the path to clinical pig organ xenotransplantation. *Am J Transplant* 23 (3): 326–335.
107. Alobaidi, S. and Alobaidi, S. (2025). Xenotransplantation of solid organs: revolutionizing transplantation through innovation, ethics, and global solutions. *Med Princ Pract* 34 (5): 418–431.
108. Cheung, M.D., Asiimwe, R., Erman, E.N. et al. (2024). Spatiotemporal immune atlas of a clinical-grade gene-edited pig-to-human kidney xenotransplant. *Nat Commun* 15 (1): 3140.
109. Marty, F.M., Ljungman, P., Chemaly, R.F. et al. (2017). Letermovir prophylaxis for cytomegalovirus in hematopoietic-cell transplantation. *N Engl J Med* 377 (25): 2433–2444.

CHAPTER 13

Immunotherapy for the Global Prevention of Haemolytic Disease of the Foetus and Newborn

BEHNAZ HEYDARCHI[1,2] AND IAN P. WICKS[1,2]
[1] Walter and Eliza Hall Institute of Medical Research, Parkville, Victoria, Australia
[2] Department of Medical Biology, The University of Melbourne, Melbourne, Victoria, Australia

LEARNING OBJECTIVES

- Understand the immunological basis of HDFN, clinical needs, and current treatment in a global context.
- Review the challenges in maintaining a sustainable supply of RhD-pIgG.
- Discuss the key features that define an effective mAb therapy as a viable alternative to RhD-pIgG.
- Explain antibody engineering approaches to enhance mAb effector function.

13.1 INTRODUCTION

Haemolytic disease of the foetus and newborn (HDFN) is a major cause of foetal anaemia, jaundice, recurrent miscarriage, and stillbirth worldwide [1]. The most common cause of HDFN is maternal antibodies to Rhesus D (RhD), a blood group antigen only found on human red blood cells (RBCs) [2]. When an RhD negative (RhD ^{neg}) mother carries an RhD positive (RhD ^{pos}) baby, foetal RBCs can enter the maternal circulation during pregnancy and after delivery, inducing an Ab response to the paternally derived RhD molecule that can destroy foetal RBCs [3] (see Figure 13.1). This alloimmune response increases with each at-risk pregnancy [3, 4].

When HDFN develops, it requires intensive prenatal management for the baby to survive [5]. Intrauterine transfusions (IUTs) can treat foetal anaemia but are only available in specialised centres and carry risks such as further alloimmunisation, infection, and miscarriage. Intravenous immunoglobulin (IVIG) can reduce foetal anaemia and the need for IUTs in some cases. However, it has variable efficacy, is costly, and the supply of IVIG is also limited [6]. Postnatally, HDFN requires phototherapy or exchange transfusions, often resulting in extended stays in a neonatal

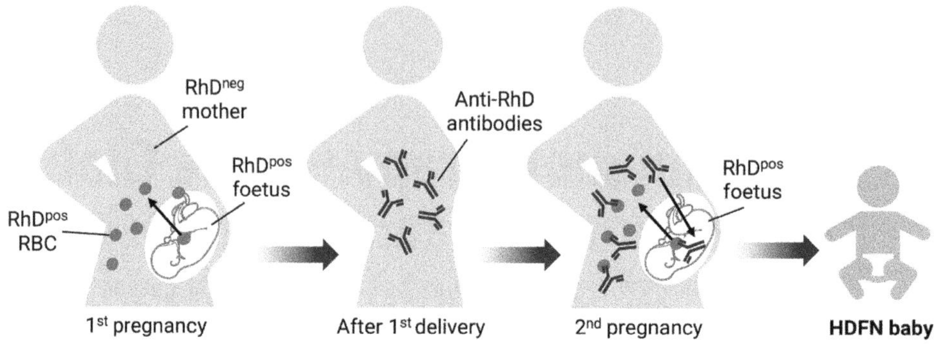

FIGURE 13.1 Schematic representation of HDFN. During a first pregnancy, an RhD ^{neg} mother carrying an RhD ^{pos} foetus may become immunised and produce anti-RhD antibodies, particularly after delivery-associated transplacental haemorrhage. In subsequent pregnancies, maternal anti-RhD antibodies can cross the placenta and destroy foetal RhD ^{pos} RBCs, resulting in HDFN.

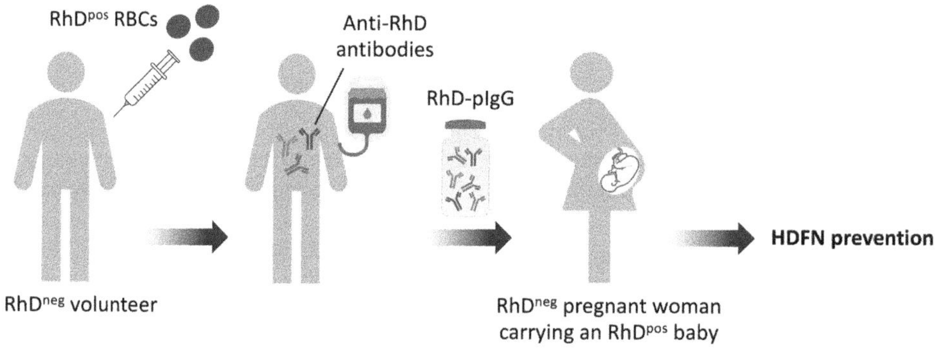

FIGURE 13.2 HDFN prevention mediated by donor-derived RhD-pIgG. RhD ^{neg} volunteers receive repeated injections of RhD ^{pos} RBCs to stimulate the production of anti-RhD antibodies. Once antibodies are generated, blood samples are collected, and the polyclonal IgG fraction is purified, which contains anti-RhD IgG (RhD-pIgG). Administration of RhD-pIgG to RhD ^{neg} pregnant women prevents HDFN.

intensive care unit (NICU). Maternal anti-RhD Abs can persist in the baby for up to 6 months, requiring prolonged monitoring. The complexities of managing HDFN emphasise the critical need for effective prevention strategies [5, 7].

In a remarkable example of applied immunology, researchers suggested administering polyclonal anti-RhD immunoglobulin G (RhD-pIgG) might prevent HDFN in RhD ^{neg} pregnant women (see Figure 13.2) [8]. This approach proved highly effective, reducing perinatal deaths from HDFN by over 98% in those countries where it was made available. Despite its success, many countries still have inadequate anti-RhD prophylaxis programmes due to cost and insufficient healthcare resources [7, 9]. The supply of RhD-pIgG is expensive and resource intensive to maintain, and, in some jurisdictions, it has been discontinued due to ethical concerns [10]. As a result, many countries now rely on imports from the United States, where plasma is sourced from paid donors. Outside of the USA, deriving anti-RhD plasma depends on altruistic blood donors, who sometimes become unwell after immunisation with 'foreign' RBCs. There are also risks of immunisation against other alloantigens on RBCs [11]. The COVID-19 pandemic exposed significant vulnerabilities in global blood and plasma supply chains [12], which are likely to increase in the future [13].

There is growing scientific and clinical interest in developing recombinant anti-RhD monoclonal antibodies (mAbs) as a more standardised, sustainable, and ethically preferable alternative to RhD-pIgG. This chapter reviews previous efforts to develop anti-RhD mAbs and highlights how advances in antibody engineering might facilitate the generation of recombinant anti-RhD mAbs with defined specificity, enhanced effector functions, and scalable manufacturing potential. We begin by outlining the immunological mechanisms underpinning alloimmunisation in HDFN and antibody-mediated clearance of RhD ^{pos} RBCs. We then describe technological platforms that have enabled the identification and optimisation of human anti-RhD mAbs. We examine the current state of clinical translation, comparing recombinant mAbs with RhD-pIgG and outlining challenges and future directions. Importantly, we believe mAb therapy offers a path towards equitable and scalable prevention of RhD-mediated HDFN worldwide.

13.2 MOLECULAR FEATURES OF RHD

13.2.1 Structure and Function

RhD and RhCE proteins comprise the Rhesus blood group system (now known as RH), expressed on human RBCs. Both RhD and RhCE are polymorphic proteins that can be antigenic, but antibodies to the highly variable RhD antigens are a major cause of alloimmune reactions [14]. The RhD molecule is a transmembrane protein with six extracellular loops. It has homology to ammonia transporters, although there may be other cationic substrates [15, 16]. Unlike the ABO blood groups, expression of RhD is restricted to the surface of RBCs, where two RhD or RhCE proteins and two Rh-associated glycoproteins (RhAG) form a 'core complex'. This complex is associated with a group of accessory proteins that have functional and structural roles and is linked to the spectrin-actin RBC cytoskeleton through interaction with ankyrin [17].

13.2.2 Genetic Variation

Rh proteins derive from homologous RhD and RhCE genes on chromosome 1, in a complex locus characterised by multiple allelic variants [18, 19]. More than 720 RhD alleles have been reported [20]. Genetic variation in RhD gives rise to quantitative and qualitative effects on expression, including the absence of RhD protein (RhD null or markedly reduced in the DEL phenotype), 'weak RhD' and 'partial RhD' phenotypes [19]. The weak RhD phenotype is characterised by reduced expression of the RhD antigen, typically due to mutations in intracellular or transmembrane regions that affect antigen density. Despite lower antigen density, the RhD epitopes remain intact, and individuals with weak D are generally considered RhD ^{pos} [21]. In contrast, the partial RhD phenotype involves structural alterations in the RhD antigen due to specific point mutations in the extracellular region. These changes can lead to the absence of one or more epitopes, making individuals with partial RhD at risk of producing anti-RhD antibodies if exposed to RhD ^{pos} RBCs [22].

13.2.3 Geographical Distribution of RhD Variants

RhD variants produce conformation-dependent epitopes that can be detected serologically and have been divided into categories [20, 23]. Genetic diversity in the Rh complex has not been fully defined in many parts of the world, particularly in low- and middle-income countries [24]. The frequency of RhD 'weak' expression phenotypes is up to 15% in Caucasians with European ancestry but is lower in Nigeria and India (~5%) and China (~1%) [25, 26]. In Europe [27] and Australia [28], the most prevalent variants are weak RhD types 1–3, generally considered RhD ^{pos} for clinical purposes. The predominant partial RhD phenotypes in Europe are DNB, DVI, and DVII, whereas in the United States, partial RhD phenotypes are frequently observed in individuals of African ancestry [29, 30]. In East Asia, particularly China, DEL/Asia-type variants are more common [31]. In sub-Saharan Africa, a high diversity of RhD alleles is observed, including the DAU cluster and multiple partial-RhD alleles, which frequently alter epitope expression and complicate serologic typing [32, 33].

13.3 EVOLUTION OF THERAPY FOR THE PREVENTION OF HDFN

13.3.1 Early Clinical Trials of RhD-pIgG

Following the recognition of the Rh complex as separate from the major ABO blood groups on human RBCs [34], it was observed that ABO incompatibility conferred a degree of protection against maternal sensitisation to RhD [8]. This led to the concept that feto-maternal incompatibility for RhD might be the basis for HDFN [35] and, furthermore, that immune-mediated removal of foetal RBCs might prevent HDFN [36]. Dr. John Gorman, an Australian physician, and his colleagues Freda and Pollack, also hypothesised that passive administration of anti-RhD antibodies would actively suppress the maternal immune response to RhD. Subsequent challenge studies of RhD ^{neg} males showed protection against sensitisation with anti-RhD coated RBCs and against RhD ^{pos} RBCs with co-administration of plasma containing anti-RhD polyclonal immunoglobulin (RhD-pIgG), or with a concentrated preparation of RhD-pIgG [37–40]. In landmark studies, it was then shown that 'passive immunisation' with RhD-pIgG conferred almost complete maternal protection against the immunological challenge of an RhD incompatible pregnancy [41–45]. Importantly, protection against maternal sensitisation continued in subsequent RhD-mismatched pregnancies. The 1980 Lasker Prize was awarded to Cyril Clarke and William Pollack, for 'illuminating the genetics of Rh factor', and to Vincent Freda, John Gorman, and Ronald Finn, for 'developing an anti-Rh vaccine, leading to the conquest of HDFN'.

13.3.2 Mechanism of Action of RhD-pIgG

Prevention of HDFN by RhD-pIgG clearly occurs via antibody-mediated immune suppression (AMIS). Although the precise mechanisms underlying AMIS remain incompletely understood, clearance of foetal RhD pos RBCs, epitope masking, antigen modulation, and suppression of maternal B cells are considered the major factors. As summarised in Figure 13.3:

- Removal of foetal RhD pos RBCs from the maternal circulation is mediated primarily by splenic macrophages expressing activating Fcγ receptors (FcγRI, FcγRII, and FcγRIII) [46]. Opsonised RBCs might therefore be phagocytosed by splenic macrophages before they can be recognised by the maternal immune system [46, 47].

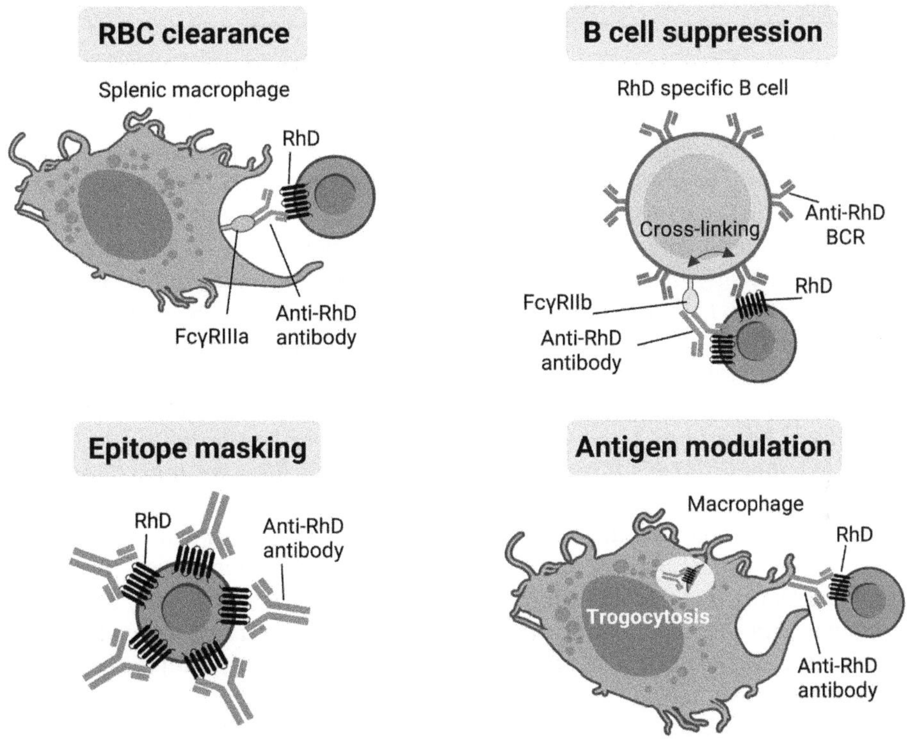

FIGURE 13.3 Proposed mechanisms of antibody-mediated immune suppression by RhD-pIgG. Splenic macrophages remove anti-RhD opsonised foetal RhD pos RBCs from the maternal circulation via FcγRIIIa-mediated phagocytosis (RBC clearance). Crosslinking of the B cell receptor (BCR) with the inhibitory FcγRIIB receptor in the presence of anti-RhD antibody suppresses B-cell activation and antibody production (B cell suppression). Binding of anti-RhD antibodies to RhD epitopes on foetal RBCs sterically hinders recognition by maternal B-cell receptors, preventing the initiation of an alloimmune response (epitope masking). Interaction of anti-RhD antibodies with RhD on foetal RBCs induces internalisation or modulation of the antigen, reducing RhD density and limiting immunogenicity (antigen modulation).

- RhD-pIgG could also mask RhD antigens on the foetal RBC surface, preventing recognition by B cell receptors [48].
- Trogocytosis, in which immune cells acquire fragments of RBC membranes, might further reduce antigen availability and limit B cell activation [49, 50].
- Finally, RhD-pIgG bound to foetal RBCs may also form immune complexes that engage the inhibitory FcγRIIB receptor on maternal RhD-specific B cells, suppressing antigen-specific B cell activation [51, 52].

Notably, anti-RhD IgG1 antibodies in alloimmunised patients [53–55], as well as the anti-RhD fraction of RhD-pIgG preparations [56, 57], display low fucosylation and increased galactosylation. These features are known to enhance FcγRIII engagement and antibody-dependent effector functions [57, 58] and are also likely contribute to efficient clearance of foetal RhD ^{pos} RBCs.

13.4 THE IMPACT OF HDFN

13.4.1 Personal Perspectives From High-Income Countries

Katie Shanahan – *As a parent of a child severely affected by HDFN due to anti-RhD maternal alloimmunisation, our family faced the complex clinical and emotional challenges of this condition first-hand. I developed anti-RhD antibodies after not being offered RhD-pIgG when I should have been, so I deeply understand the critical importance of prevention. Managing high-risk pregnancies with HDFN often involves intensive monitoring, including frequent specialised ultrasounds, and in some cases, invasive procedures to treat foetal anaemia. While these interventions are lifesaving, they can be physically and emotionally demanding, with a profound impact on families.*

Our own alloimmunised pregnancy required four intrauterine blood transfusions to keep our son alive before birth, and each procedure carried risk and uncertainty. After delivery, he required neonatal intensive care and four post-birth transfusions over the first five months of his life. The early months of his life were marked by weekly laboratory tests, hospital visits, and intensive monitoring; an experience that shaped our understanding of how isolating and overwhelming this diagnosis can be for families. Navigating these challenges led me to connect with and ultimately work for the Allo Hope Foundation, a global non-profit that provides education, advocacy, and support for patients and providers managing HDFN (allohopefoundation.org). Through our journey, I became deeply committed to ensuring that no other family faces the same preventable risks.

Even in well-resourced healthcare systems, HDFN places a heavy emotional burden on parents. Recent studies highlight the mental health burden of this condition, with patients reporting increased levels of anxiety, stress, and post-traumatic stress disorder related to the demands of navigating this rare and high-risk condition [59]. *The mother is the only constant in an otherwise siloed care pathway of multiple specialists: obstetrics, maternal-foetal medicine, neonatology, paediatrics, and haematology, leading to a high degree of advocacy burden. Through our work with Allo Hope, we have seen that this burden is even greater in low- and middle-income countries, where access to RhD-pIgG, specialised prenatal monitoring, and neonatal care is limited or non-existent. In these settings, preventable foetal and neonatal losses are devastatingly common, further emphasising the urgent need for equitable access to prevention globally.*

Lyndsay Pastega (Australia) – *After the birth of our first daughter in 2014, my bloodwork indicated RhD antibodies, which would affect my ability to have babies in the future. As a mother, it was traumatic. Our first son was born at 37 weeks, after having received an intrauterine blood transfusion at 32 weeks. He required a three-week stay in the NICU. In 2019, I fell pregnant with our daughter, who was treated with IVIG and monitored weekly for anti-RhD antibody levels and with middle cerebral artery scans. She went to 37 weeks but was born anaemic with heart failure and died in my arms at 2 days old. Our second son had 5 IUT's from 25 weeks and spent 8 weeks in the NICU. Navigating this condition will stay with me for a lifetime.*

13.4.2 HDFN in Low- and Middle-Income Countries (LMICs)

Despite proven efficacy, the global demand for RhD-pIgG has never been met in LMICs [25]. While the frequency of RhD negativity in LMICs is lower compared to countries with a predominantly Caucasian population, HDFN is still a significant cause of neonatal morbidity and mortality [60], because access to RhD-pIgG is limited. Lack of effective anti-RhD prophylaxis leads to stillbirth in up to 14% of affected babies and long-term neurological damage in up to 60% of those who survive neonatal jaundice (kernicterus) [7]. In India and China, where the prevalence of RhD ^{neg} is relatively low (around 5% and 1%, respectively), millions of pregnancies are still at risk, simply due to population size [26]. In 2010, it was estimated that sensitisation of RhD ^{neg} mothers to paternally derived RhD resulted in 373,300 live births affected by HDFN, with many children incurring lifelong neurological disabilities from neonatal jaundice and 114,100 avoidable neonatal deaths [7]. A global modelling study estimated that approximately 2.5 million doses of RhD-pIgG are required annually to meet the antenatal and post-partum demand of sub-Saharan Africa alone. However, only ~110,000 doses were administered, representing less than 5% coverage of the population in need [25].

The persistent shortage of RhD-pIgG in LMIC has prompted efforts to develop alternatives. For example, Rhoclone was developed by Bharat Serums and Vaccines Limited and is currently the only available anti-RhD mAb in India and some countries in Asia and Africa. To date, clinical validation of Rhoclone has been limited to small, non-inferiority trials [61–63], without reporting of key inclusion criteria, such as parity and ABO incompatibility [64]. In addition, Rhoclone lacked efficacy in an antibody-dependent cellular cytotoxicity (ADCC) assay, which is the key *in vitro* predictor of the efficacy of anti-RhD antibodies in human clinical trials [65].

13.5 MAINTAINING THE SUPPLY OF RhD-pIgG

Production of RhD-pIgG is costly, resource-intensive, and has been discontinued in Europe due to ethical concerns [10]. Many countries now rely on imports from the United States, where plasma is sourced from paid donors. Maintaining volunteer donors for RhD-pIgG production is proving difficult for blood collection agencies such as Australian Red Cross Lifeblood, and this challenge is likely to grow in the future [13]. RhD-pIgG has also been used as an alternative to IVIG to treat immune thrombocytopenia, further straining limited supplies.

CASE STUDY: AUSTRALIA'S MOST PROLIFIC ANTI-RhD BLOOD DONOR

Australian Red Cross Lifeblood (ARCL): Australia remains the only country in the world to have a voluntary, non-remunerated anti-RhD donor programme, which has been managed by Lifeblood since 1967 [66]. Australia's RhD-pIgG supply comes from a pool of fewer than 180 altruistic donors, most of whom need periodic 'boosting' with RhD ^{pos} RBCs to maintain high levels of anti-RhD antibodies. However, only about 50% of those boosted produce enough anti-RhD for their plasma to be suitable for RhD-pIgG manufacturing. Some notable Lifeblood donors, such as James Harrison OAM, developed anti-RhD antibodies without boosting. For James, this occurred at age 14 following multiple blood transfusions after lung surgery, including at least one suspected RhD ^{pos} transfusion. James was committed to giving back after those transfusions saved his life. He became a lifelong plasma donor, donating 1,173 times between 1968 and his retirement in 2018, as part of ARCL's anti-D donor programme, helping to protect over two million pregnancies. Over the course of his donor career, the rate of deaths due to HDFN in Australia dropped 100-fold to around 0.01 per 1,000 births. James Harrison died in 2025 and was eulogised in the New York Times.

In summary, while RhD-pIgG has been used successfully for decades, its dependence on a small pool of donors and hyperimmunisation with foreign RBCs, pose major challenges for long-term sustainability. Recombinant anti-RhD mAbs would provide a safer, more consistent, and ethically preferable alternative to traditional RhD-pIgG (Table 13.1).

TABLE 13.1 Comparison of RhD-pIgG and recombinant anti-RhD mAbs.

	RhD-pIgG	**Recombinant anti-RhD mAbs**
Supply	■ Derived from plasma of RhD ^{neg} donors sensitised with RhD ^{pos} RBCs	■ Sequences of mAbs identified from *in vitro* screening, or from sensitised donors ■ Produced recombinantly in mammalian cell lines
Clonality	■ Polyclonal	■ Monoclonal (single or cocktail formulation)
Mechanism of action	■ Induces antibody-mediated immune suppression (AMIS)	■ Designed to replicate AMIS
Advantages	■ Long-established clinical efficacy and safety record ■ Naturally polyclonal, providing broad RhD epitope coverage	■ RhD specific ■ Fully defined composition with minimal batch variability ■ Donor-independent and reduces pathogen-transmission risk ■ Amenable to Fc and glycoengineering to enhance effector function and reduce the required dosage ■ Scalable and sustainable recombinant protein production

TABLE 13.1 (Continued)

	RhD-pIgG	Recombinant anti-RhD mAbs
Limitations	▪ Donor-dependent ▪ Ethically and logistically constrained ▪ Limited and unsustainable supply (does not meet the global demand) ▪ Batch to batch variability ▪ Potential risk of transmitting blood-borne pathogens ▪ Mixture of RhD and non-RhD antibodies ▪ Potential for alloimmunisation against other RBC antigens	▪ May not fully reproduce the broad epitope recognition of polyclonal IgG ▪ Subject to formulation, manufacturing costs might be high ▪ Limited clinical data currently available
Clinical efficacy	▪ Approved globally	▪ Several candidates have demonstrated promising preclinical and early clinical trial success but have yet to achieve regulatory approval
Safety profile	▪ Excellent long-term record ▪ Only rare mild reactions	▪ Favourable safety in early trials ▪ Lower risk of infection or donor-derived contaminants ▪ Immunogenicity requires monitoring
Overall assessment	Clinically proven but donor-dependent and unsustainable in the long-term	Promising alternative, offering standardised, scalable, and sustainable supply, pending demonstration of clinical equivalence

13.6 CASE STUDIES OF ALTERNATIVES TO RhD-pIgG

13.6.1 Rozrolimupab: An Anti-RhD mAb Cocktail

One of the earliest efforts to find an alternative to plasma-derived RhD-pIgG was Rozrolimupab (SYM-001), developed by Symphogen. Rozrolimupab is a cocktail of 25 distinct IgG1 mAbs isolated from 8 RhD ^{neg} female donors with high-titre anti-RhD Abs. It was produced in CHO cells using the Flp-In system, with different batches showing similar RhD binding and high purity [67, 68]. Rozrolimupab demonstrated binding to a broad spectrum of RhD variants, with potency comparable to plasma-derived RhD-pIgG products [69].

In vitro functional assays revealed that Rozrolimupab facilitated phagocytosis and ADCC against RhD ^{pos} RBCs, using human effector cells [70]. Clinical trials demonstrated promising safety and efficacy profiles for Rozrolimupab in males with immune thrombocytopenia [70]. However, the efficacy of Rozrolimumab in preventing HDFN in pregnant women has not been reported, and it seems the inherent complexity and high costs of manufacturing a cocktail of 25 mAbs ultimately led to a commercial decision to discontinue this programme.

13.6.2 BRAD-3: An Anti-RhD IgG3 mAb

BRAD-3 is a human IgG3 anti-RhD mAb generated through the fusion of Epstein–Barr virus transformed human B lymphocytes (isolated from a sensitised RhD ^{neg} donor) with a human myeloma cell line, resulting in a heterohybridoma [71]. Functional studies demonstrated that BRAD-3 effectively mediated ADCC, leading to the clearance of RhD ^{pos} RBCs [72]. Early-phase clinical trials indicated that BRAD-3 could suppress the primary immune response to RhD ^{pos} RBCs, with some subjects remaining non-sensitised even after subsequent exposures [72]. BRAD-3 produced in CHO cells exhibited relatively low ADCC activity. However, in later studies using Fc engineering (by targeted mutagenesis or afucosylation), we found its ADCC could be significantly enhanced, to levels exceeding those of RhD-pIgG [58]. However, clinical development of BRAD-3 has not been pursued, and further studies are required to fully assess its efficacy and safety profile.

13.6.3 FOG-1: An Anti-RhD IgG1 mAb

FOG-1 is a recombinant human IgG1 anti-RhD mAb from an immunised RhD ^{neg} donor and was originally produced from a human–mouse heterohybridoma [73]. In early studies, FOG-1 was less effective than RhD-pIgG in mediating RBC clearance [74]. However, subsequent work demonstrated that FOG-1 produced in the rat myeloma cell line (YB2/0) mediated more rapid clearance of autologous RBCs compared with its heterohybridoma-derived counterpart [75]. Enhanced clearance was attributed to altered Fc glycosylation associated with production in YB2/0 cells, leading to increased binding to low-affinity Fcγ receptors, particularly FcγRIII, and thereby augmenting ADCC [57, 75]. We subsequently showed that FOG-1 produced in CHO cells had reduced ADCC, but afucosylation or Fc mutagenesis enhanced ADCC to levels surpassing those of RhD-pIgG [58]. These findings underscore the role of the antibody Fc region in determining the efficacy of anti-RhD mAbs and the importance of Fc optimisation when developing therapeutic mAbs to prevent HDFN.

13.6.4 Roledumab: An Anti-RhD IgG1 mAb

Roledumab (LFB-R593) was developed by LFB Biotechnologies and is a human IgG1 mAb. It was produced in YB2/0 cells, generating low Fc fucosylation and enhanced ADCC activity [76].

Clinical evaluation of Roledumab demonstrated low immunogenicity, favourable pharmacokinetic properties, and effective RBC clearance. Evaluation in healthy individuals confirmed safety and the apparent lack of alloimmune reactions [77, 78]. Pharmacokinetic and safety data from a trial in RhD ^{neg} pregnant women carrying RhD ^{pos} foetuses were made available, and no serious adverse events were reported. However, the data from five participants were incomplete, and outcomes related to alloimmunisation were not disclosed [79]. Roledumab is believed to target epitope 13.1, which is absent in several RhD variants. Additionally, Roledumab failed to bind to weak RhD variants 10, 11, 18, 38, and 58 (ClinicalTrials.gov protocol NCT02287896). To our knowledge, Roledumab is no longer in clinical development.

13.6.5 Nipocalimab: An Anti-FcRn mAb to Reduce Maternal IgG Transfer

Nipocalimab is a fully human IgG1 mAb that targets the human neonatal Fc receptor (FcRn) and thus inhibits IgG recycling, reducing the transplacental transfer of maternal IgG antibodies (including anti-RhD antibodies) [80]. Unlike traditional anti-RhD mAbs that specifically bind RhD ^{pos} foetal RBCs, Nipocalimab non-specifically inhibits placental IgG transport, reducing the harmful effects of existing maternal alloantibodies on the foetus. In the Phase 2 UNITY trial, Nipocalimab demonstrated promising efficacy, with 54% of high-risk pregnancies resulting in live births at or beyond 32 weeks, without the need for IUTs [81]. Nipocalimab may serve as a valuable therapeutic option for the management of HDFN in women who have already developed alloantibodies. However, its mechanism of action does not replicate the AMIS induced by RhD-specific IgG, and it cannot prevent maternal B cell activation or replace preventative anti-RhD prophylaxis.

13.7 CHALLENGES IN DEVELOPING A NEW IMMUNOTHERAPY FOR HDFN

13.7.1 Epitope Coverage

One of the major challenges in developing a mAb-based immunotherapy for RhD-pIgG is achieving sufficiently broad epitope coverage. It is thought that donor-derived RhD-pIgG response targets multiple, non-overlapping epitopes on the RhD protein [82], and this broad reactivity is believed to be critical for preventing maternal alloimmunisation. In contrast, single mAbs generally recognise only one epitope, which may be insufficient to replicate the protective effects of RhD-pIgG against polymorphic RhD antigens [83].

To address this limitation, candidate mAbs must either recognise a conserved epitope expressed by RhD variants or be combined into cocktails targeting non-overlapping epitopes. However, as demonstrated by Rozrolimupab, production of mAb cocktails poses both technical and regulatory challenges, including manufacturing complexity, quality control, and cost. Recent technological innovations, such as continuous or hybrid production modes [84], antibody modification [57, 58], and cell line engineering [85], can be used to optimise upstream/downstream mAb production processes [86] and could make mAb therapies more economically feasible, particularly for LMIC.

13.7.2 Limitations of *In Vitro* Assays to Predict mAb Efficacy in Clinical Trials

The spleen is most likely the key site for RBC clearance *in vivo* [46, 47], and it is suggested that RhD-pIgG opsonised RBCs are phagocytosed and destroyed intracellularly [87] via splenic macrophages, which express FcγRIIIa [75, 88]. As human splenic macrophages aren't routinely accessible, *in vitro* ADCC assays often utilise peripheral blood mononuclear cells (PBMCs, expressing all human FcγRs) or natural killer (NK) cells (expressing FcγRIIIa) [57, 58, 89] as surrogates for splenic macrophages [87]. However, the complexity of the *in vivo* environment, including immune cell interactions and cytokine networks, cannot be fully captured by *in vitro* assays, which only measure FcγR-mediated interactions [87]. As discussed, Fc glycosylation of anti-RhD mAbs also affects binding to FcγRs, impacting RBC clearance kinetics [57]. Therefore, while *in vitro* assays provide valuable insights, ideally, these should be complemented with *in vivo* evaluation to help predict the efficacy and safety of anti-RhD mAbs.

13.7.3 Lack of an Appropriate Animal Model of HDFN

Current animal models do not fully recapitulate the features of HDFN or the protective role of anti-RhD antibodies. In xenogeneic systems, AMIS tends to be transient, dose-dependent, and mainly restricted to primary immune responses, which differs from the robust and enduring protection reported with RhD prophylaxis in humans. Immunocompetent mice challenged with human RBC xenografts mount innate and inflammatory responses, but those reactions do not accurately reflect the *in vivo* dynamics of allogeneic human RBCs and anti-RhD antibodies [89]. Humanised NOD-SCID mice allow comparison of the relative clearance rates of human RhD ^{pos} RBCs between anti-RhD and non-specific antibodies, but do not reproduce the effects of antibody isotype, Fc glycosylation, or other effector mechanisms observed in humans [90]. Likewise, rabbits challenged with defined blood groups capture certain aspects of anti-RhD responses, but don't fully replicate the complex interactions involved in human RhD immunisation and prevention [91].

Chimpanzees are physiologically closer to humans and share some Rh genetic architecture, such as conservation of exon 7 [92] and characteristic intron polymorphisms [93]. However, binding profiles of human anti-RhD antibodies to chimpanzee RBCs [94] suggest differences in accessibility to key epitopes. In addition, human RBCs undergo rapid, antibody-independent RBC clearance in chimpanzees [95]. Ethical concerns and high costs further restrict the use of non-human primates for research on HDFN.

In summary, experimental models that accurately reflect the pathophysiology of HDFN and the operation of AMIS *in vivo* remain elusive, highlighting the translational challenges in developing mAb therapies to prevent HDFN.

13.7.4 mAb Safety in Pregnancy

The safety and efficacy of anti-RhD mAbs must be rigorously validated before administration to pregnant or post-partum women. However, clinical trials in non-pregnant adults do not replicate the unique immunological environment of gestation. Alloimmune responses to RhD are generally slow and low-titre, arising after foetal–maternal haemorrhage, which leads to prolonged splenic phagocytosis of foetal RBCs [96, 97]. In an inflammatory context, splenic macrophages can adopt dendritic-like properties, causing activation of T helper cells and promotion of maternal alloantibody production [47]. Haemolysis underlies the pathology of HDFN, and the extracellular release of haemoglobin breakdown products may contribute to local or systemic inflammation. Pregnancy itself induces mild systemic immune activation via syncytiotrophoblast microparticles and is biased towards Th2 responses, facilitating alloimmunisation even with minimal exposure to foetal RBCs [98–100]. These considerations underscore the need to balance efficient RBC clearance with the avoidance of excessive immune activation when developing therapeutic anti-RhD antibodies.

IgG is the only antibody class able to cross the placental barrier, and anti-RhD responses are predominantly of the IgG1 subclass, with IgG3 contributing to a lesser extent [101]. Anti-RhD mAbs will thus require careful Fc modifications to enhance RBC clearance in the mother, while avoiding/minimising haemolysis and inflammatory activation in the foetus. Glycosylation plays a critical role in the efficacy of anti-RhD mAb [57], and Fc engineering (e.g. the GASDALIE mutation in Fc) can enhance FcγR-mediated effector functions and RBC clearance [58]. However, overactivation of splenic macrophages could inadvertently augment maternal immune responses. Engineered anti-RhD mAbs must ensure maternal and foetal safety while allowing robust clearance of foetal RBCs from the maternal circulation.

13.8 FUTURE DIRECTIONS

13.8.1 Integration of AI and Machine Learning in Anti-RhD mAb Discovery

Despite decades of research, the precise structure of the RhD protein remains unresolved, due to its hydrophobic, multi-pass transmembrane nature and an obligatory interaction with RhAG in the RBC cell surface, which complicates crystallisation and structural resolution. This knowledge gap has hindered rational, structure-guided engineering of anti-RhD mAbs. Recent advances in artificial intelligence (AI) [102, 103] and machine learning (ML) [104] now offer alternative strategies, enabling high-accuracy prediction of mAb structures (e.g. AlphaFold [105, 106] and Rosetta-Antibody [107]) and antigen recognition features, even in the absence of experimentally determined structures. AI/ML approaches hold promise for designing anti-RhD mAbs with enhanced RBC binding and effector functions.

13.8.2 Development of Improved Preclinical Models of HDFN

A critical obstacle to the development of anti-RhD mAbs is the limited predictive value of traditional animal models, as discussed above. To address this, *ex vivo* human organ perfusion models may be more physiologically relevant. Human spleens perfused for short periods *ex vivo* maintain structure, vascular flow, and metabolic activity, allowing investigation of splenic macrophage-mediated clearance of altered or infected erythrocytes in a manner not possible in rodent or xenogeneic models [108]. Increased RBC rigidity correlated strongly with rapid splenic retention and clearance in an isolated perfused human spleen [109]. An *ex vivo* spleen model could allow testing of RBC opsonisation and Fc-mediated clearance mechanisms in HDFN, under conditions more closely resembling normal human splenic architecture and function.

Ex vivo human placental perfusion could also provide insight into maternal-to-foetal transfer of IgG, including anti-RhD mAbs, and the role of FcRn and other placental IgG transport regulators. In one study, engineered variants of anti-RhD IgG1 and IgG3 were compared, and modifications in the IgG hinge regions were found to influence placental transfer [110]. Placental perfusion literature demonstrates consistent findings: variability in transfer depends on IgG subclass, FcRn binding, and Fc glycosylation [111].

These *ex vivo* organ perfusion models may help bridge the gap between *in vitro* functional assays and *in vivo* human responses, offering a more translationally predictive platform for evaluating both the efficacy and safety of candidate anti-RhD mAbs.

13.8.3 Potential for Collaboration and Equitable Distribution of a Validated mAb Therapy for Global Prevention of HDFN

Immunotherapy for HDFN was introduced in a very different ethical and regulatory era. Modern standards mandate stringent safety and efficacy studies, and clinical trials in the context of pregnancy are, understandably, even more demanding. It is vital for all stakeholders to realistically address the consequences of continued reliance on RhD-pIgG. Women from all countries, especially LMIC, need to be included in the design of innovative and ethically acceptable clinical trials for the prevention of HDFN, so that new approaches can be developed. The COVAX initiative was a global attempt to accelerate vaccine development and ensure fair access to COVID-19 vaccines. COVAX provides an inspiring model for development and distribution of a mAb therapeutic alternative to prevent HDFN, including expertise in scaled manufacturing, cold-chain logistics, and equitable allocation, combined with World Health Organisation support and guidance.

Putting this vision into practice for HDFN will require close alignment with existing patient and health care networks. The Allo Hope Foundation (https://allohopefoundation.org) provides education for patients and providers and clinical guidelines for managing HDFN, along with global advocacy efforts. WIRhE (Worldwide Initiative for Rh Disease Eradication; https://wirhe.org) brings together healthcare professionals, researchers, and patient advocates to promote universal access to anti-RhD prophylaxis. AFRICARhE (African Initiative for Rh Eradication, https://wirhe.org/partners-africarhe/) leads field studies in sub-Saharan Africa (partnering with institutions in Ethiopia, Malawi, and Tanzania) that aim to quantify the burden of HDFN and help embed local implementation and capacity-building for the prevention of HDFN. It will also be essential to partner with biotechnology to generate an alternative to RhD pIgG that is practical and cost-effective. Such a partnership will have to address the financial realities of mAb development, manufacturing, and distribution. However, it will be just as important to weigh these economic considerations against the true societal costs of HDFN around the globe, including the management of lifelong disabilities and the continuing toll of human suffering inflicted by HDFN on women and their families.

KEY TERMS & DEFINITIONS SIDEBAR

ADCC (Antibody-Dependent Cellular Cytotoxicity) An immune mechanism in which effector cells, such as natural killer (NK) cells, recognise and kill target cells that are coated with antibodies. ADCC is critical for the therapeutic activity of many monoclonal antibodies and is predictive of anti-RhD antibody success in clinical trials.

Alloimmunisation The immune response against foreign RBC antigens, which can occur following transfusion or pregnancy and may cause HDFN.

Antibody Immune Repertoire The complete collection of distinct antibodies produced by an individual's B cells at a given time, reflecting the immune system's capacity to recognise and respond to a wide variety of antigens. This repertoire includes antibodies of different classes, specificities, and affinities and can change dynamically in response to infections, vaccination, or therapeutic interventions.

COVAX A worldwide initiative aimed at equitable access to COVID-19 vaccines.

DEL Phenotype A variant characterised by extremely low RhD antigen density, often missed by routine serologic testing but detectable by molecular methods.

Epitope The specific region of an antigen recognised by an antibody. Changes in RhD epitopes can affect serologic detection and immune responses.

Haemolytic Disease of the Foetus and Newborn (HDFN) A pregnancy-associated condition in which maternal antibodies cross the placenta and target foetal RBCs, leading to their destruction (haemolysis). HDFN can cause anaemia, jaundice (kernicterus), miscarriage, and perinatal mortality and is most commonly associated with RhD incompatibility between mother and child.

Monoclonal Antibody (mAb) An antibody derived from a single B-cell clone that recognises a specific epitope on an antigen. Monoclonal antibodies are now widely used in therapy, diagnostics, and research.

Partial RhD Variants in which one or more RhD epitopes are missing, potentially leading to alloimmunisation if exposed to the complete RhD antigen through transfusion or pregnancy.

RhD Antigen A highly polymorphic protein expressed on the surface of human RBCs, encoded by the RHD gene, responsible for the Rh blood group system. Its presence or absence determines RhD ^{pos} or RhD ^{neg} status, but genetic variation at the Rh locus gives rise to multiple RhD variants.

RhD-pIgG Anti-RhD immunoglobulin derived from RhD ^{neg} male donors, repeatedly immunised with RhD ^{pos} RBCs, or from women who have suffered HDFN. RhD-pIgG prevents alloimmunisation during pregnancy or after exposure to RhD ^{pos} RBCs.

Weak RhD RhD variants with reduced antigen expression on human RBCs typically result from point mutations in the RHD gene. Most weak D types are considered RhD ^{pos} for transfusion purposes.

LIST OF ABBREVIATIONS

ADCC	antibody-dependent cellular cytotoxicity
AFRICARhE	African Initiative for Rh Eradication
AI	artificial intelligence
AMIS	antibody-mediated immune suppression
HDFN	Haemolytic Disease of the Foetus and Newborn
Fc	fragment crystallisable
FcRn:	neonatal Fc receptor
Fcγ	Fc gamma receptors
IgG	immunoglobulin G
IUTs	intrauterine transfusions
IVIG	intravenous immunoglobulin
LMICs	low- and middle-income countries

MAb	monoclonal antibody
ML	machine learning
NK	natural killer
PBMCs	peripheral blood mononuclear cells
RBC	red blood cell
RhAG	Rh-associated glycoproteins
RhD	Rhesus D
RhD ^{neg}	RhD negative
RhD ^{pos}	RhD positive
RhD-pIgG	Polyclonal anti-RhD immunoglobulin G
WHO	World Health Organisation
WIRhE	Worldwide Initiative for Rh Disease Eradication

REVIEW QUESTIONS

1. What is the immunological basis for HDFN?
2. How does current prophylaxis prevent HDFN?
3. Describe previous attempts to generate alternatives to current treatment for HDFN.
4. What factors must be considered in optimising an anti-RhD mAb?

REFERENCES

1. Bowman, J.M. (1998). RhD hemolytic disease of the newborn. *N Engl J Med* 339 (24): 1775–1777.
2. Urbaniak, S.J. and Greiss, M.A. (2000). RhD haemolytic disease of the fetus and the newborn. *Blood Rev* 14 (1): 44–61.
3. de Haas, M., Thurik, F.F., Koelewijn, J.M., and van der Schoot, C.E. (2015). Haemolytic disease of the fetus and newborn. *Vox Sang* 109 (2): 99–113.
4. Christensen, R.D., Bahr, T.M., Wong, R.J. et al. (2023). A "Gold Standard" test for diagnosing and quantifying hemolysis in neonates and infants. *J Perinatol* 43 (12): 1541–1547.
5. Andrews, J. and Grace, M.R. (2024). Time to optimise management of haemolytic disease of the fetus and newborn. *Lancet Haematol* 11 (12): e884–e885.
6. Legler, T.J. (2020). RhIg for the prevention Rh immunization and IVIg for the treatment of affected neonates. *Transfus Apher Sci* 59 (5): 102950.
7. Bhutani, V.K., Zipursky, A., Blencowe, H. et al. (2013). Neonatal hyperbilirubinemia and rhesus disease of the newborn: incidence and impairment estimates for 2010 at regional and global levels. *Pediatr Res* 74: 86–100.
8. Clarke, C.A. (ed.) (1975). *Rhesus Haemolytic Disease*. Lancaster, England. Medical and Technical Publishing Co. Ltd.
9. Visser, G.H.A., Di Renzo, G.C., Spitalnik, S.L., and FIGO Committee Safe Motherhood and Newborn Health (2019). The continuing burden of Rh disease 50 years after the introduction of anti-Rh(D) immunoglobin prophylaxis: call to action. *Am J Obstet Gynecol* 221 (3): 227.e1–227.e4.
10. Farrugia, A. and Robert, P. (2006). Plasma protein therapies: current and future perspectives. *Best Pract Res Clin Haematol* 19 (1): 243–258.

11. Viayna, E., Gehrie, E.A., Blanchette, C. et al. (2022). Red cell alloimmunization is associated with increased health care costs, longer hospitalizations, and higher mortality. *Blood Adv* 6 (20): 5655–5658.
12. Saillant, N.N., Kornblith, L.Z., Moore, H. et al. (2022). The national blood shortage—an impetus for change. *Ann Surg* 275 (4): 641–643.
13. Viennet, E., Dean, M.M., Kircher, J. et al. (2025). Blood under pressure: how climate change threatens blood safety and supply chains. *Lancet Planet Health* 9 (4): e304–e313.
14. Avent, N.D. and Reid, M.E. (2000). The Rh blood group system: a review. *Blood* 95 (2): 375–387.
15. Hemker, M.B., Cheroutre, G., van Zwieten, R. et al. (2003). The Rh complex exports ammonium from human red blood cells. *Br J Haematol* 122 (2): 333–340.
16. Westhoff, C.M., Ferreri-Jacobia, M., Mak, D.O., and Foskett, J.K. (2002). Identification of the erythrocyte Rh blood group glycoprotein as a mammalian ammonium transporter. *J Biol Chem* 277 (15): 12499–12502.
17. Vallese, F., Kim, K., Yen, L.Y. et al. (2022). Architecture of the human erythrocyte ankyrin-1 complex. *Nat Struct Mol Biol* 29 (7): 706–718.
18. Avent, N.D., Madgett, T.E., Lee, Z.E. et al. (2006). Molecular biology of Rh proteins and relevance to molecular medicine. *Expert Rev Mol Med* 8 (13): 1–20.
19. Flegel, W.A. (2007). The genetics of the rhesus blood group system. *Blood Transfus* 5 (2): 50–57.
20. Floch, A., Teletchea, S., Tournamille, C. et al. (2021). A review of the literature organized into a new database: reference. *Transfus Med Rev* 35 (2): 70–77.
21. Wagner, F.F., Gassner, C., Müller, T.H. et al. (1999). Molecular basis of weak D phenotype. *Blood* 93 (1): 385–393.
22. Wagner, F.F. and Flegel, W.A. (2000). RHD gene deletion occurred in the rhesus box. *Blood* 95 (12): 3662–3668.
23. Denomme, G.A., Wagner, F.F., Fernandes, B.J. et al. (2005). Partial D, weak D types, and novel RHD alleles among 33,864 multiethnic patients: implications for anti-D alloimmunization and prevention. *Transfusion* 45 (10): 1554–1560.
24. Wheeler, M.M., Lannert, K.W., Huston, H. et al., NHLBI trans-omics for precision medicine (TOPMed) consortium. (2019). Genomic characterization of the RH locus detects complex and novel structural variation in multi-ethnic cohorts. *Genet Med* 21 (2): 477–486.
25. Pegoraro, V., Urbinati, D., Visser, G.H.A. et al. (2020). Hemolytic disease of the fetus and newborn due to Rh(D) incompatibility: A preventable disease that still produces significant morbidity and mortality in children. *PLoS One* 15 (7): e0235807.
26. Zipursky, A., Bhutani, V.K., and Odame, I. (2018). Rhesus disease: a global prevention strategy. *Lancet Child Adolesc Health* 2 (7): 536–542.
27. Barriteau, C.M., Lindholm, P.F., Hartman, K. et al. (2022). RHD genotyping to resolve weak and discrepant RhD patient phenotypes. *Transfusion* 62 (11): 2194–2199.
28. McGowan, E.C., Lopez, G.H., Knauth, C.M. et al. (2017). Diverse and novel RHD variants in Australian blood donors with a weak D phenotype: implication for transfusion management. *Vox Sang* 112 (3): 279–287.
29. Sandler, S.G., Flegel, W.A., Westhoff, C.M. et al. (2015). It's time to phase in RHD genotyping for patients with a serologic weak D phenotype. College of American Pathologists Transfusion Medicine Resource Committee Work Group. *Transfusion* 55 (3): 680–689.
30. von Zabern, I., Wagner, F.F., and Moulds, J.M. (2013). D category IV: a group of clinically relevant and phylogenetically diverse partial D. *Transfusion* 53 (11 Suppl 2): 2960–2973.
31. Yin, Q. and Flegel, W.A. (2021). DEL in China: the D antigen among serologic RhD-negative individuals. *J Transl Med* 19 (1): 439.
32. Wagner, F.F., Ladewig, B., Angert, K.S. et al. (2002). The DAU allele cluster of the RHD gene. *Blood* 100 (1): 306–311.

33. Wagner, F.F., Moulds, J.M., Tounkara, A. et al. (2003). RHD allele distribution in Africans of Mali. *BMC Genet* 4: 14.
34. Landsteiner, K. and Wiener, A.S. (1941). Studies on an agglutinogen (Rh) in human blood reacting with anti-rhesus sera and with human isoantibodies. *J Exp Med* 74 (4): 309–320.
35. Levine, P.B.L., Katzin, E.M., and Vogel, P. (1941). The role of iso-immunization in the pathogenesis of erythroblastosis fetalis. *Am J Obstet Gynecol* 42: 925–937.
36. Finn, R., Clarke, C.A., Donohoe, W.T. et al. (1961). Experimental studies on the prevention of Rh haemolytic disease. *Br Med J* 1 (5238): 1486–1490.
37. Freda, V.J., Gorman, J.G., and Pollack, W. (1964). Successful prevention of experimental Rh sensitization in man with an anti-Rh Gamma2-globulin antibody preparation: a preliminary report. *Transfusion* 4: 26–32.
38. Stern, K., Goodman, H.S., and Berger, M. (1961). Experimental isoimmunization to hemoantigens in man. *J Immunol* 87 (2): 189–198.
39. Mollison, P.L., Hughes-Jones, N.C., Lindsay, M., and Wessely, J. (1969). Suppression of primary RH immunization by passively-administered antibody. Experiments in volunteers. *Vox Sang* 16 (4): 421–439.
40. Clarke, C.A., Donohoe, W.T., Mc, C.R. et al. (1963). Further experimental studies on the prevention of Rh haemolytic disease. *Br Med J* 1 (5336): 979–984.
41. Freda, V.J., Gorman, J.G., and Pollack, W. (1966). Rh factor: prevention of isoimmunization and clinical trial on mothers. *Science* 151 (3712): 828–830.
42. BMJ (1971). Prevention of Rh-haemolytic disease: final results of the "high-risk" clinical trial. A combined study from centres in England and Baltimore. *Br Med J* 2 (5762): 607–609.
43. Bowman, J.M., Chown, B., Lewis, M., and Pollock, J.M. (1978). Rh isoimmunization during pregnancy: antenatal prophylaxis. *Can Med Assoc J* 118 (6): 623–627.
44. Tovey, L.A., Townley, A., Stevenson, B.J., and Taverner, J. (1983). The Yorkshire antenatal anti-D immunoglobulin trial in primigravidae. *Lancet* 2 (8344): 244–246.
45. Woodrow, J.C., Clarke, C.A., McConnell, R.B. et al. (1971). Prevention of Rh-haemolytic disease: results of the Liverpool "low-risk" clinical trial. *Br Med J* 2 (5762): 610–612.
46. Nagelkerke, S.Q., Bruggeman, C.W., den Haan, J.M.M. et al. (2018). Red pulp macrophages in the human spleen are a distinct cell population with a unique expression of Fc-gamma receptors. *Blood Adv* 2 (8): 941–953.
47. Kumpel, B.M. (2006). On the immunologic basis of Rh immune globulin (anti-D) prophylaxis. *Transfusion* 46 (9): 1652–1656.
48. Hjelm, F., Carlsson, F., Getahun, A., and Heyman, B. (2006). Antibody-mediated regulation of the immune response. *Scand J Immunol* 64 (3): 177–184.
49. Cruz-Leal, Y., Marjoram, D., and Lazarus, A.H. (2018). Erythrocyte saturation with IgG is required for inducing antibody-mediated immune suppression and impacts both erythrocyte clearance and antigen-modulation mechanisms. *J Immunol* 200 (4): 1295–1305.
50. Cruz-Leal, Y., Norris, P.A.A., Gil Gonzalez, L. et al. (2024). Trogocytosis drives red blood cell antigen loss in association with antibody-mediated immune suppression. *Blood* 143 (9): 807–821.
51. Sinclair, N.R. and Chan, P. (1971). Regulation of the immune response. IV. The role of the Fc-fragment in feedback inhibition by antibody. *Adv Exp Med Biol* 12: 609–615.
52. Sinclair, N.R. (2001). Fc-signalling in the modulation of immune responses by passive antibody. *Scand J Immunol* 53 (4): 322–330.
53. Kapur, R., Della Valle, L., Sonneveld, M. et al. (2014). Low anti-RhD IgG-Fc-fucosylation in pregnancy: a new variable predicting severity in haemolytic disease of the fetus and newborn. *Br J Haematol* 166 (6): 936–945.
54. Sonneveld, M.E., Koelewijn, J., de Haas, M. et al. (2017). Antigen specificity determines anti-red blood cell IgG-Fc alloantibody glycosylation and thereby severity of haemolytic disease of the fetus and newborn. *Br J Haematol* 176 (4): 651–660.

55. de Graaf, E.L., Larsen, M.D., van der Bolt, N. et al. (2024). Assessment of IgG-Fc glycosylation from individual RhD-specific B cell clones reveals regulation at clonal rather than clonotypic level. *Immunology* 171 (3): 428–439.
56. Kapur, R., Della Valle, L., Verhagen, O.J. et al. (2015). Prophylactic anti-D preparations display variable decreases in Fc-fucosylation of anti-D. *Transfusion* 55 (3): 553–562.
57. Kumpel, B.M., Saldova, R., Koeleman, C.A.M. et al. (2020). Anti-D monoclonal antibodies from 23 human and rodent cell lines display diverse IgG Fc-glycosylation profiles that determine their clinical efficacy. *Sci Rep* 10 (1): 1464.
58. Heydarchi, B., D'Silva, D.B., Wong, H. et al. (2025). Fc mutagenesis enhances the functionality of anti-RhD monoclonal antibodies. *Blood Adv* 9 (7): 1522–1533.
59. Sherwood, M.R., Weathersby, B.M., Granger, M.E. et al. (2025). Alloimmunization in pregnancy: patient-reported quality of care, mental health effects, and impact upon daily life. *AJP Rep* 15 (3): e146–e153.
60. Visser, G.H.A., Thommesen, T., Di Renzo, G.C. et al. (2021). FIGO/ICM guidelines for preventing rhesus disease: a call to action. *Int J Gynaecol Obstet* 152 (2): 144–147.
61. Chauhan, A.R., Bhattacharyya, M.S., Turakhia, N., and Daftary, G.V. (2002). Efficacy and safety of monoclonal anti-D immunoglobulin in comparison with polyclonal anti-D immunoglobulin in prevention of rho isoimmunization. *J Assoc Physicians India* 50: 1341–1342.
62. Chauhan, A.R., Nandanwar, Y.S., Ramaiah, A. et al. (2019). A multicenter, randomized, open-label trial comparing the efficacy and safety of monoclonal anti-Rh (D) immunoglobulin with polyclonal anti-Rh (D) immunoglobulin for the prevention of maternal Rh-isoimmunization. *J Obstet Gynaecol India* 69 (5): 420–425.
63. Mayekar, R.V., Paradkar, G.V., Bhosale, A.A. et al. (2020). Recombinant anti-D for prevention of maternal-foetal Rh(D) alloimmunization: a randomized multi-centre clinical trial. *Obstet Gynecol Sci* 63 (3): 315–322.
64. Verweij, E., Tura, A.K., Gure, T. et al. (2024). Monoclonal RhD prophylaxis: high time to evaluate efficacy. *Lancet* 403 (10429): 806–807.
65. Contreras, M., Kumpel, B., and Olovnikova, N. (2024). Anti-D prophylaxis should protect all newborns from haemolytic disease, regardless of their country of residence. *Vox Sang* 119 (12): 1221–1222.
66. Thyer, J., Wong, J., Thomson, A. et al. (2018). Fifty years of RhD immunoglobulin (anti-D) therapy in Australia: celebrating a public health success story. *Med J Aust* 209 (8): 336–339.
67. Frandsen, T.P., Naested, H., Rasmussen, S.K. et al. (2011). Consistent manufacturing and quality control of a highly complex recombinant polyclonal antibody product for human therapeutic use. *Biotechnol Bioeng* 108 (9): 2171–2181.
68. Wiberg, F.C., Rasmussen, S.K., Frandsen, T.P. et al. (2006). Production of target-specific recombinant human polyclonal antibodies in mammalian cells. *Biotechnol Bioeng* 94 (2): 396–405.
69. Stasi, R. (2010). Rozrolimupab, symphobodies against rhesus D, for the potential prevention of hemolytic disease of the newborn and the treatment of idiopathic thrombocytopenic purpura. *Curr Opin Mol Ther* 12 (6): 734–740.
70. Robak, T., Windyga, J., Trelinski, J. et al. (2012). Rozrolimupab, a mixture of 25 recombinant human monoclonal RhD antibodies, in the treatment of primary immune thrombocytopenia. *Blood* 120 (18): 3670–3676.
71. Thomson, A., Contreras, M., Gorick, B. et al. (1990). Clearance of Rh D-positive red cells with monoclonal anti-D. *Lancet* 336 (8724): 1147–1150.
72. Kumpel, B.M., Goodrick, M.J., Pamphilon, D.H. et al. (1995). Human Rh D monoclonal antibodies (BRAD-3 and BRAD-5) cause accelerated clearance of Rh D+ red blood cells and suppression of Rh D immunization in Rh D- volunteers. *Blood* 86 (5): 1701–1709.
73. Bye, J.M., Carter, C., Cui, Y. et al. (1992). Germline variable region gene segment derivation of human monoclonal anti-Rh(D) antibodies. Evidence for affinity maturation by somatic hypermutation and repertoire shift. *J Clin Invest* 90 (6): 2481–2490.

74. Beliard, R. (2006). Monoclonal anti-D antibodies to prevent alloimmunization: lessons from clinical trials. *Transfus Clin Biol* 13 (1–2): 58–64.
75. Armour, K.L., Smith, C.S., Ip, N.C. et al. (2014). Clearance of human IgG1-sensitised red blood cells in vivo in humans relates to the in vitro properties of antibodies from alternative cell lines. *PLoS One* 9 (10): e109463.
76. Beck, A. and Reichert, J.M. (2012). Marketing approval of mogamulizumab: a triumph for glyco-engineering. *MAbs* 4 (4): 419–425.
77. Yver, A., Homery, M.C., Fuseau, E. et al. (2012). Pharmacokinetics and safety of roledumab, a novel human recombinant monoclonal anti-RhD antibody with an optimized Fc for improved engagement of FCgammaRIII, in healthy volunteers. *Vox Sang* 103 (3): 213–222.
78. Laboratoire français de Fractionnement et de Biotechnologies (LFB) (2009). Dose-finding study of LFB-R593, A monoclonal anti-RhD antibody, in healthy RhD negative volunteers. NCT00952575. https://clinicaltrials.gov/study/NCT00952575 (accessed 6 October 2025).
79. Laboratoire Français de Fractionnement et de Biotechnologies (2014). Pharmacokinetics and safety of Roledumab, in RhD-negative pregnant women carrying an RhD-positive foetus. NCT02287896. https://clinicaltrials.gov/study/NCT02287896 (accessed 6 October 2025)
80. Ling, L.E., Hillson, J.L., Tiessen, R.G. et al. (2019). M281, an anti-FcRn antibody: pharmacodynamics, pharmacokinetics, and safety across the full range of IgG reduction in a first-in-human study. *Clin Pharmacol Ther* 105 (4): 1031–1039.
81. Moise, K.J. Jr., Ling, L.E., Oepkes, D. et al. (2024). Nipocalimab in early-onset severe hemolytic disease of the fetus and newborn. *N Engl J Med* 391 (6): 526–537.
82. Chang, T.Y. and Siegel, D.L. (1998). Genetic and immunological properties of phage-displayed human anti-Rh(D) antibodies: implications for Rh(D) epitope topology. *Blood* 91 (8): 3066–3078.
83. Westhoff, C.M. (2004). The Rh blood group system in review: a new face for the next decade. *Transfusion* 44 (11): 1663–1673.
84. Partopour, B. and Pollard, D. (2025). Advancing biopharmaceutical manufacturing: economic and sustainability assessment of end-to-end continuous production of monoclonal antibodies. *Trends Biotechnol* 43 (2): 462–475.
85. Majumdar, S., Desai, R., Hans, A. et al. (2025). From efficiency to yield: exploring recent advances in CHO cell line development for monoclonal antibodies. *Mol Biotechnol* 67 (2): 369–392.
86. Gronemeyer, P., Ditz, R., and Strube, J. (2014). Trends in upstream and downstream process development for antibody manufacturing. *Bioengineering (Basel)* 1 (4): 188 212.
87. Kumpel, B.M. (2007). Efficacy of RhD monoclonal antibodies in clinical trials as replacement therapy for prophylactic anti-D immunoglobulin: more questions than answers. *Vox Sang* 93 (2): 99–111.
88. Engelfriet, C.P. (1992). The immune destruction of red cells. *Transfus Med* 2 (1): 1–6.
89. Kumpel, B.M. and Elson, C.J. (2001). Mechanism of anti-D-mediated immune suppression—a paradox awaiting resolution? *Trends Immunol* 22 (1): 26–31.
90. Bazin, R., Aubin, É., Boyer, L. et al. (2002). Functional in vivo characterization of human monoclonal anti-D in NOD-scid mice. *Blood* 99 (4): 1267–1272.
91. Mage, R.G., Esteves, P.J., and Rader, C. (2019). Rabbit models of human diseases for diagnostics and therapeutics development. *Dev Comp Immunol* 92: 99–104.
92. Westhoff, C.M. and Wylie, D.E. (1996). Investigation of the RH locus in gorillas and chimpanzees. *J Mol Evol* 42 (6): 658–668.
93. Apoil, P.A. and Blancher, A. (2000). Rh gene evolution in primates: study of intron sequences. *Mol Biol Evol* 17 (1): 127–136.
94. Owens, N.A., Hui, H.L., and Green, F.A. (1982). The binding characteristics of anti-Rho(D)-positive human and chimpanzee erythrocytes measured with ^{14}C protein A. *J Immunol* 129 (4): 1471–1473.

95. Blancher, A., Socha, W.W., Roubinet, F. et al. (1993). Human monoclonal anti-D-induced clearance of human D-positive red cells in a chimpanzee model. *Vox Sang* 65 (1): 47–54.
96. BMJ (1966). Prevention of Rh-haemolytic disease: results of the clinical trial. A combined study from centres in England and Baltimore. *Br Med J* 2 (5519): 907–914.
97. Gunson, H.H., Stratton, F., Cooper, D.G., and Rawlinson, V.I. (1970). Primary immunization of Rh-negative volunteers. *Br Med J* 1 (5696): 593–595.
98. Germain, S.J., Sacks, G.P., Sooranna, S.R. et al. (2007). Systemic inflammatory priming in normal pregnancy and preeclampsia: the role of circulating syncytiotrophoblast microparticles. *J Immunol* 178 (9): 5949–5956.
99. Göhner, C., Plösch, T., and Faas, M.M. (2017). Immune-modulatory effects of syncytiotrophoblast extracellular vesicles in pregnancy and preeclampsia. *Placenta* 60 (Suppl 1): S41–S51.
100. Kumpel, B.M. and Manoussaka, M.S. (2012). Placental immunology and maternal alloimmune responses. *Vox Sang* 102 (1): 2–12.
101. Proulx, C., Filion, M., Goldman, M. et al. (1994). Analysis of immunoglobulin class, IgG subclass and titre of HPA-1a antibodies in alloimmunized mothers giving birth to babies with or without neonatal alloimmune thrombocytopenia. *Br J Haematol* 87 (4): 813–817.
102. Cheng, J., Liang, T., Xie, X.Q. et al. (2024). A new era of antibody discovery: an in-depth review of AI-driven approaches. *Drug Discov Today* 29 (6): 103984.
103. Gaudreault, F., Sulea, T., and Corbeil, C.R. (2025). AI-augmented physics-based docking for antibody-antigen complex prediction. *Bioinformatics* 41 (4): btaf129.
104. Wossnig, L., Furtmann, N., Buchanan, A. et al. (2024). Best practices for machine learning in antibody discovery and development. *Drug Discov Today* 29 (7): 104025.
105. Jumper, J., Evans, R., Pritzel, A. et al. (2021). Highly accurate protein structure prediction with AlphaFold. *Nature* 596 (7873): 583–589.
106. Tunyasuvunakool, K., Adler, J., Wu, Z. et al. (2021). Highly accurate protein structure prediction for the human proteome. *Nature* 596 (7873): 590–596.
107. Weitzner, B.D., Jeliazkov, J.R., Lyskov, S. et al. (2017). Modeling and docking of antibody structures with Rosetta. *Nat Protoc* 12 (2): 401–416
108. Buffet, P.A., Milon, G., Brousse, V. et al. (2006). Ex vivo perfusion of human spleens maintains clearing and processing functions. *Blood* 107 (9): 3745–3752.
109. Safeukui, I., Buffet, P.A., Deplaine, G. et al. (2018). Sensing of red blood cells with decreased membrane deformability by the human spleen. *Blood Adv* 2 (20): 2581–2587.
110. Mathiesen, L., Nielsen, L.K., Andersen, J.T. et al. (2013). Maternofetal transplacental transport of recombinant IgG antibodies lacking effector functions. *Blood* 122 (7): 1174–1181.
111. Sand, K.M.K., Gruber, M.M., Sandlie, I. et al. (2022). Contribution of the ex vivo placental perfusion model in understanding transplacental immunoglobulin G transfer. *Placenta* 127: 77–87.

14

Advances in Engineered Immune Cells

Latest Advancements in CRISPR, CAR-T, and Other Immune Cell Engineering Techniques

LAMBERTO TORRALBA-RAGA[1,2] AND KARL-JOHAN MALMBERG[1,2,3]

[1] Department of Cancer Immunology, Institute for Cancer Research, Oslo University Hospital, Oslo, Norway

[2] Precision Immunotherapy Alliance, Institute for Clinical Medicine, The University of Oslo, Oslo, Norway

[3] Center for Infectious Medicine, Department of Medicine Huddinge, Karolinska Institutet, Stockholm, Sweden

LEARNING OBJECTIVES

- Distinguish autologous versus allogeneic/iPSC-derived immune-cell products and how gene editing addresses their key limitations.
- Compare CARs, TCRs, and synthetic circuits (logic-gated, SynNotch/SNIPR, switch receptors) for tumour recognition and safety.
- Summarise the main delivery platforms (viral and non-viral, including EV-based) and their pros and cons for clinical translation.
- Explain how CRISPR and next-generation gene-writing tools enable multiplex, stealth, and functional template editing of immune cells.

14.1 INTRODUCTION

T cells engineered with chimeric antigen receptors (CAR-T cells) have transformed the treatment of B cell malignancies, resulting in several Food and Drug Administration (FDA)- and European Medicines Agency (EMA)-approved therapies [1–3]. Yet their broader application to non-B-cell haematologic cancers and solid tumours is limited by major logistic and scientific hurdles [4–6]. Building on the preceding discussion of CAR-T and CAR-NK therapies (Chapter 6), this chapter focuses on the gene-editing and synthetic engineering strategies that enable their next generation of function, precision, and scalability (Figures 14.1 and 14.2).

Current CAR T manufacturing is labour-intensive: patient cells must be harvested, shipped to centralised facilities for genetic engineering and expansion, and then

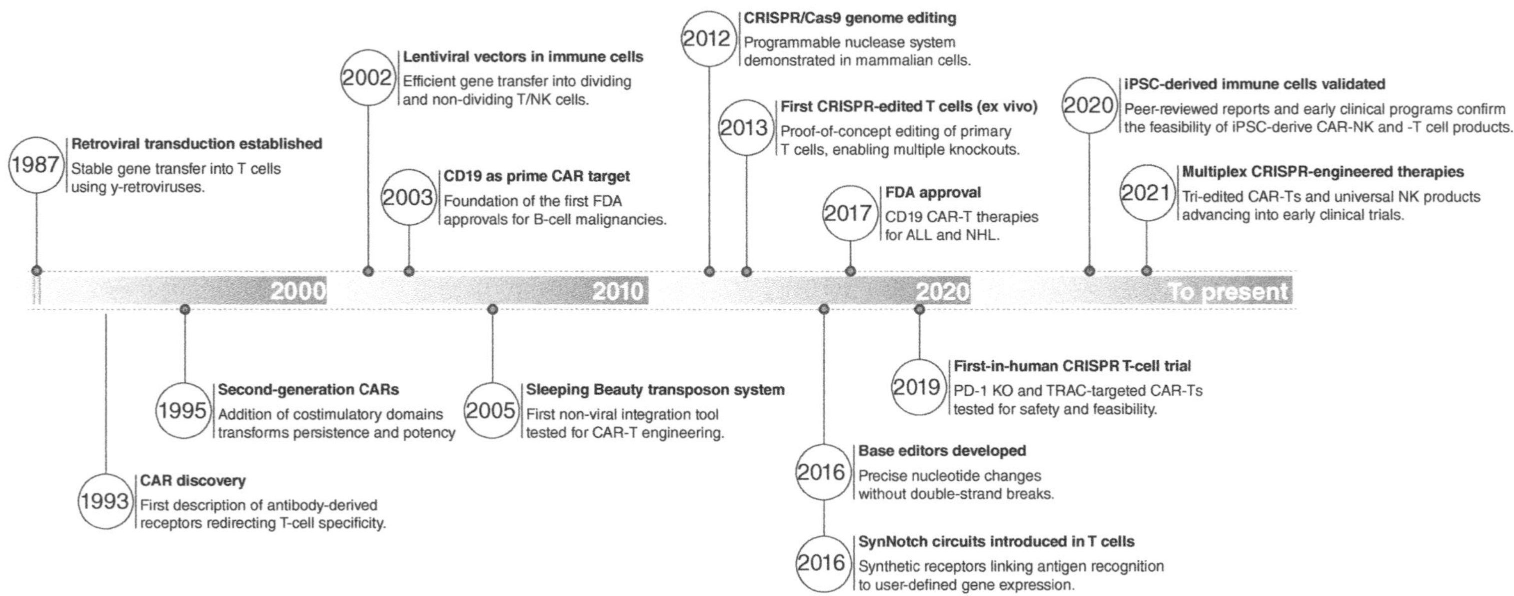

FIGURE 14.1 Milestones in immune-cell engineering.

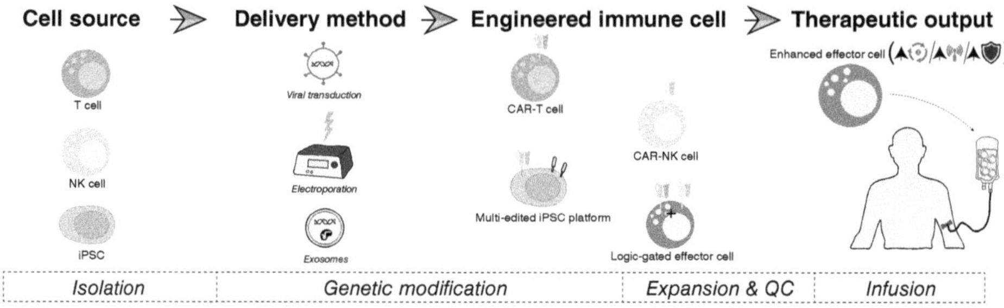

FIGURE 14.2 Overview of the immune-cell engineering workflow.

cryopreserved for return to the clinic. Each dose is patient-specific, increasing costs and risking failure when patient-derived T cells are functionally compromised by disease or prior therapy [7–9]. Moreover, the number of feasible edits per dose is limited, since each additional modification reduces yield and consistency. These bottlenecks can be alleviated by editing allogeneic immune cells, where a single round of engineering can generate hundreds of off-the-shelf doses. Induced pluripotent stem cells (iPSCs) are especially promising, as multiplex editing can be performed at the pluripotent stem cell stage to establish master cell banks capable of producing virtually unlimited therapeutic doses [10, 11].

The main strength of autologous CAR-T strategies is their persistence, often lasting months to years with robust antigen-driven *in vivo* expansion. In contrast, allogeneic CAR-T and -NK cells are typically cleared within two to three weeks by host immunity [12, 13]. Extending the persistence of allogeneic products through immune evasion edits is thus a central challenge [1, 14, 15]. Future gene-editing technologies are likely to streamline autologous manufacturing, potentially even enabling rapid, robust decentralised editing at a fast pace, and at the same time enhance persistence and potency of allogeneic therapies.

Whether autologous or allogeneic cells represent the optimal platform will likely depend on disease context: durable engraftment may be critical in some settings, whereas repeated short-course dosing of highly specialised multi-plex edited off-the-shelf cells may be the better choice for other indications. Shared priorities across both approaches include expanding the range of targetable antigens, improving tumour homing, overcoming the tumour microenvironment, and reprogramming metabolic and regulatory circuits to sustain function. In particular, edits that intelligently tune key transcriptional and signalling circuits to optimise the 'functional template' of immune cells represent one of the most exciting future directions [16–21]. In this chapter, we outline the categories of edits aimed at improving specificity, function, and persistence, and review the current tools that enable precision engineering of immune cells.

14.2 ENGINEERING SPECIFICITY AND FUNCTIONAL MODALITIES

14.2.1 Antigen Targeting Through CARs and TCRs

The genetic reprogramming of lymphocytes with synthetic receptors has transformed the field of cancer immunotherapy. The best-established approach is the use of CARs, in which an antibody-derived single-chain variable fragment (scFv) is fused to intracellular signalling modules derived from the T-cell receptor (TCR) complex (see Chapter 6) [22–25]. CARs confer the ability to recognise surface antigens independently of HLA presentation, enabling robust tumour cell killing. Clinical successes in B-cell malignancies, notably with CD19- and BCMA-directed CAR T cells, have established this principle and led to multiple approved therapies. However, the scarcity of tumour-specific surface molecules and the risk of on-target/off-tumour toxicities remain major barriers to extending CAR therapy to other haematological malignancies and solid tumours [1].

By contrast, TCRs expand the targetable antigen space. TCRs recognise short peptides derived from intracellular or extracellular proteins when presented on the cell surface by HLA molecules [26]. This provides access to a much larger repertoire of potential tumour antigens, including neoantigens generated by somatic mutations, post-translational modifications, or metabolic dysregulation [26–28]. TCR-based therapies can therefore target intracellular oncogenic drivers that are inaccessible to conventional CARs. The challenge lies in ensuring sufficient affinity and specificity, given that most patient-derived TCRs are of low avidity due to central and peripheral tolerance. Strategies to overcome this include isolating high-affinity TCRs from healthy donor repertoires or engineering affinity-enhanced variants [29].

A growing area of innovation lies in combinatorial and synthetic receptor designs. Switch receptors can rewire inhibitory pathways into activating signals, thereby expanding the range of contexts in which engineered cells respond to tumours. Gated or logic-based receptors, such as synNotch constructs [30], allow engineered lymphocytes to integrate multiple signals before activation, reducing the risk of off-target toxicity. These designs, discussed in more detail in Section 14.3, can be layered on top of conventional CAR or TCR architectures to provide context-aware antigen recognition.

Together, CARs and TCRs represent complementary antigen-targeting strategies: CARs provide rapid, HLA-independent recognition of cell-surface molecules, while TCRs open access to the intracellular proteome. Their integration into multiplex engineering frameworks, particularly in stem-cell-derived or allogeneic immune cells, is poised to broaden the scope and safety of engineered cell therapies.

14.2.2 Functional Edits Through Modulation of Regulatory Pathways

Beyond receptor targeting, the long-term success of engineered lymphocytes depends on their ability to maintain activity in hostile environments. A promising strategy is to reprogram the regulatory circuits that define cell identity, differentiation, and stress responses. Recent advances in functional genomics have enabled systematic mapping of such regulatory networks. Tools such as genome-wide CRISPR perturbations, pooled knockout/activation libraries, and single-cell multi-omics readouts now allow unbiased identification of transcriptional regulators that dictate effector function under specific conditions [16, 17, 31–33]. For example, by coupling CRISPR-based perturbation with high-dimensional phenotyping, one can resolve which TFs control responsiveness to cytokines, cytotoxic granule dynamics, or adaptation to tumour-derived stressors.

The goal of functional template editing is to programme therapeutic cells into states that maximise their performance. This can be achieved by locking cells into an effector-competent fate, strengthening transcriptional circuits that support metabolic

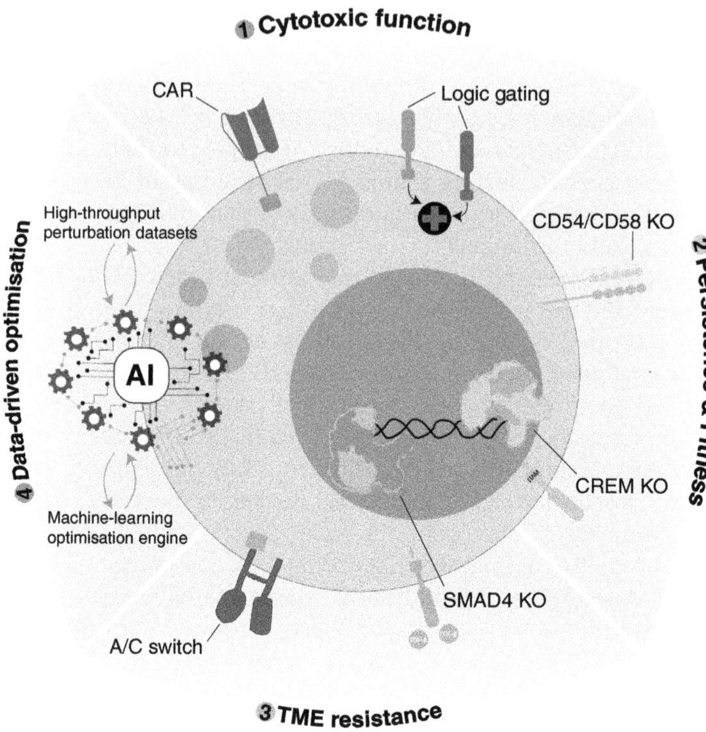

FIGURE 14.3 Functional template editing framework for engineered immune cells.

fitness, or removing repressors that drive exhaustion. Editing the regulatory architecture of immune cells offers a path to therapies that are not only antigen-specific but also intrinsically equipped to withstand suppression and maintain activity over time (Figure 14.3).

14.2.3 Stealth Editing to Enhance Persistence

A central challenge for allogeneic immune cell therapies is their rapid elimination by the host immune system. Allogeneic lymphocytes are typically rejected within one to two weeks through recognition by host T cells, NK cells, macrophages, and preformed antibodies. This short therapeutic window limits efficacy and complicates multi-dosing strategies [34]. Extending the persistence of transferred cells, therefore, requires strategies that minimise their immunogenicity while preserving antitumour activity.

Stealth editing refers to the genetic modification of immune cells to reduce visibility to host immune surveillance. Viruses and tumours provide blueprints for immune evasion, highlighting pathways that can be co-opted in therapeutic design [35]. A common strategy, already in clinical testing, is disruption of HLA class I and II molecules to reduce recognition by recipient T cells, for example through knockout of β2-microglobulin (B2M) or CIITA [36–38]. However, global HLA loss provokes NK cell 'missing-self' responses [39, 40]. More refined designs preserve or reintroduce non-polymorphic HLA molecules such as HLA-E or HLA-G to deliver inhibitory signals, or selectively delete subsets of HLA alleles while maintaining others (e.g. HLA-C), thereby balancing evasion of both T and NK cells [41, 42]. Another strategy that has already reached clinical testing is based on overexpression of the 'don't eat me signal' CD47, which protect cells from macrophages but also reduces NK cell-mediated recognition [43–45].

Stable immune synapse formation is essential for cytotoxic rejection. Deletion of adhesion ligands such as CD54 (ICAM-1) and CD58 (LFA-3) impairs conjugate formation between therapeutic and host effector cells. Combined knockout of CD54/CD58 has been shown to markedly reduce NK-cell-mediated clearance across diverse NK subsets without impairing tumour cytotoxicity and may complement T cell stealth strategies in future clinical trials [46].

Stealth strategies must balance immune invisibility with retained effector function. Excessive deletion of recognition molecules may impair trafficking, conjugate formation, or cytotoxic synapse stability. For this reason, systematic mapping of host-cell interactions and iterative testing in rejection assays are essential to identify edits that achieve the desired immune-evasive phenotype without compromising tumour killing.

Because rejection involves adaptive and innate immune arms as well as humoral responses, single edits are rarely sufficient. Multiplexed strategies, integrating HLA disruption, inhibitory ligand expression, adhesion molecule knockout, and novel circuits that directly eliminate activated alloreactive lymphocytes, are emerging as promising solutions. By selectively targeting recognition pathways, it is possible to extend the lifespan of engineered cells *in vivo*, enabling repeated dosing or durable engraftment, and ultimately broadening the clinical applicability of off-the-shelf cellular immunotherapies [14].

14.3 ENGINEERING 'SMARTER' CELLS

14.3.1 Logic-Gated Circuits for Safer and Smarter Immune Cells

As engineered cell therapies moved from proof-of-concept into routine clinical use, it became clear that single-receptor designs were not sufficient for the challenges ahead. The first waves of CAR-T cells demonstrated the transformative power of redirecting lymphocytes against malignant cells [23, 25, 47], but they also exposed the limitations of a single-axis design: off-tumour toxicity against healthy tissues [48], severe cytokine release syndromes [49], and limited homing to and persistence in solid tumours [50, 51]. In this context, future therapies will therefore need to be context-aware, that is with cells able to integrate multiple inputs from the environment and become activated only under the right conditions and discriminating between malignant and healthy cells with greater precision.

One promising strategy is the design of logic-gated circuits, which borrows principles from digital computing and applies them to immune-cell receptors. In these designs, the recognition of tumour-associated antigens (TAAs) and the resulting signalling are arranged according to Boolean logic rules such as 'AND', 'OR', and 'NOT', ensuring that therapeutic cells only act when the appropriate decision criteria are met [52] (Figure 14.3). By integrating these principles, engineered lymphocytes can function more like biological computers rather than simple on–off switches, adding critical layers of safety and specificity. These benefits are especially valuable in solid tumours, where healthy and malignant tissues often share antigens and the microenvironment promotes immune escape. In this setting, logic gating helps limit toxicity while supporting multiplex strategies that make immune-cell therapies more precise and resilient.

In an **AND gate**, activation strictly occurs when two independent receptors are engaged simultaneously, greatly reducing the likelihood of attacking healthy tissues that may express one but not both TAAs. This can be achieved, for example, with split-CAR designs [53, 54], where one receptor binds antigen A and provides the activation signal, while a second receptor binds antigen B and delivers co-stimulation. Such designs are particularly valuable in solid tumours, where malignant cells often co-express a tumour-restricted antigen alongside another marker that is also found on normal tissue. In an **OR gate**, activation occurs if either of two TAA is detected, a strategy well-suited to heterogeneous tumours or those prone to antigen loss, with dual CARs or tandem CARs (TanCARs) serving as practical examples that broaden target coverage and limit relapse [55, 56]. A **NOT gate** works in the opposite way, using an inhibitory receptor that halts activation when a 'safe' antigen associated with healthy tissue is encountered, thereby protecting vital organs even when they share markers with tumour cells [57]. Importantly, while these systems add important safeguards, they are not without challenges: AND gates can be limited by variable antigen co-expression, OR gates may increase the risk of on-target/off-tumour toxicity risks, and NOT gates require exquisitely specific inhibitory antigens to avoid silencing therapeutic activity. Preclinical studies have shown that AND-gated circuits can prevent off-tumour toxicity in solid tumour models such as glioblastoma and mesothelioma [58]. OR-gated designs have been tested in B-cell malignancies, where they reduce relapse by limiting antigen escape [56]. Approaches using logic-gated circuits in NK cells are now progressing towards early-phase clinical evaluation [57].

14.3.2 SynNotch Receptors for Controlled Activation

The advent of synthetic Notch (SynNotch) receptors represents one of the most innovative applications of synthetic biology to immune-cell engineering [30]. Inspired by the natural Notch family, which plays central roles in embryonic development and cell-fate decisions [59], SynNotch receptors convert surface-ligand recognition into transcriptional outputs. Mechanistically, when a SynNotch receptor binds its target antigen, a conformational change exposes a cleavage site, releasing an intracellular transcription factor that translocates to the nucleus and activates any gene under its defined promoter. This basic mechanism can be reprogrammed for therapy by modular engineering of both domains. The extracellular region can be replaced with an scFv or ligand-binding domain to define the antigen sensed, while the intracellular portion is tailored to release a chosen transcription factor upon activation. Unlike CARs, which directly trigger activation, SynNotch functions as a programmable switch that only induces the expression of a secondary, downstream component, such as CARs, cytokines, costimulatory molecules, or other synthetic modules, once the receptor has been engaged. By separating sensing from acting, and offering plug-and-play flexibility, SynNotch receptors represent a powerful backbone for building context-aware cell therapies, particularly when combined with the previously described logic-gating strategies.

Preclinical studies have shown that SynNotch circuits enhance tumour specificity by requiring dual antigen recognition, for instance, using a broadly expressed antigen such as EGFR to trigger CAR expression against a more tumour-restricted antigen like EphA2, thereby reducing off-tumour effects [30, 58]. Beyond such antigen gating, SynNotch designs have been used to programme T cells to secrete checkpoint inhibitors, activate sequential signalling cascades, or remodel the tumour microenvironment. This versatility has already reached the clinic, with a first-in-human study in glioblastoma demonstrating both feasibility and safety, marking an important milestone for synthetic biology in immunotherapy [60].

Despite its promise, SynNotch-based synthetic circuits have some practical limitations. Because its activation relies on mechanical pulling forces, it can only recognise membrane-bound ligands, making it ineffective for soluble cues such as cytokines [58]. In addition, some degree of signal leakage has been observed, where basal transcription occurs even without ligand engagement, potentially reducing specificity [58]. Researchers are actively refining the system by adjusting receptor expression, optimising cleavage domains, and adding feedback loops to tighten control. These challenges, however, also motivated the development of next-generation platforms such as synthetic intramembrane proteolysis receptors (SNIPRs [61, 62]). Building on the SynNotch concept, SNIPRs incorporate design improvements that reduce leakage, broaden the types of inputs that can be sensed, and provide more precise transcriptional control. Together, these innovations reflect the field's trajectory towards immune cells acting as 'living computers', capable of integrating multiple signals and adapting dynamically to the tumour microenvironment.

14.3.3 Switch Receptors, Converting Suppression to Activation

While CARs are designed as a direct 'on switch', giving effector cells the ability to recognise a chosen tumour antigen and immediately trigger activation and killing, **switch receptors** function more like 'signal inverters', re-wiring the meaning of an existing signal [63, 64]. Instead of providing the primary activation like a CAR does, a switch receptor reprograms how the cell interprets its environment: the extracellular portion detects an inhibitory cue such as PD-L1 or TGF-β or HLA-E, while the intracellular tail is replaced with an activating domain like CD3ζ, CD28, or 4-1BB. As a result, what would normally silence or suppress the immune cell is converted into a stimulatory signal, effectively turning a tumour's 'stop' message into a 'go' signal. This inversion helps engineered lymphocytes resist immunosuppression and sustain their activity, often complementing the function of a CAR or other naturally encoded activating receptor. For example HLA-E is highly expressed in most solid tumours [65] and engages the inhibitory receptor NKG2A on NK cells, dampening their cytotoxicity [66]. To overcome this, researchers have engineered an A/C switch receptor, where the extracellular domain of NKG2A is fused to an activating signalling tail. In this configuration, binding of tumour HLA-E no longer transmits an inhibitory 'stop' signal but instead delivers an activating cue, thereby converting a common immune evasion mechanism into a trigger for NK-cell activation [67]. This illustrates the power of switch receptor design to invert tumour-driven suppression into productive anti-tumour responses.

14.4 PRECISION ENGINEERING TOOLS

Implementation of edits that enhance immune-cell function requires precise delivery of new genetic material or modification of existing loci. This section covers the field's progression from viral transduction, the backbone of today's approved cell therapies, to precision genome editing, including CRISPR ribonucleoproteins (RNPs), base and prime editors, and emerging non-viral carriers (electroporation, lipid nanoparticles (LNPs), and extracellular vesicles (EVs)). In this section, we discuss efficiency, control, and limitations of the different methods (Table 14.1). Some cell-type-specific considerations of gene editing approaches in terms of clinical use and specific limitations are summarised in Table 14.2.

TABLE 14.1 Comparative overview of delivery and genome-editing platforms for immune-cell engineering.

Category	Tool/Method	Efficiency	Precision	Limitations
Delivery system	Retroviral/ lentiviral vectors	★★★★	★★☆☆	Random/semi-random integration; insertional mutagenesis risk; costly GMP manufacturing
	Electroporation (*ex vivo*)	★★★★	★★★☆	DNA toxicity in NK cells; requires optimisation; transient unless combined with template
	Exosome- or EV-mediated delivery	★★☆☆	★★☆☆	Scale-up, reproducibility, and cargo loading remain major hurdles
	Lipid nanoparticles	★★☆☆	★★★☆	Suboptimal delivery to lymphocytes vs hepatocytes; potential immunogenicity
Editing system	Transposons (SB, PB)	★★★☆	★★☆☆	Semi-random integration; variable expression; lower clinical maturity
	CRISPR/Cas9	★★★★	★★★☆	Off-target risk; DSBs can cause rearrangements or p53 activation
	Cas12a (Cpf1)	★★★☆	★★★☆	PAM restrictions; less validated clinically
	Base editors	★★★☆	★★★★	Limited to C→T or A→G edits; risk of off-target deamination
	Prime editors	★★☆☆	★★★★	Large/complex machinery; low efficiency in primary lymphocytes
	FiCAT and CRISPR integrases	★★☆☆	★★★☆	Still experimental; efficiency in human immune cells unproven

TABLE 14.2 Cell sources for engineered immune therapies.

Cell source	Clinical use	Persistence	Advantages	Limitations
Primary T cells	Current products are autologous; allogeneic use requires TCR/HLA editing	High (memory subsets)	Clinically validated; robust expansion protocols; strong cytotoxic activity; physiological relevance	Donor variability; limited proliferative capacity; risk of GvHD (allogeneic use); cryopreservation can impair function
Primary NK cells	Allogeneic, off-the-shelf	Low, need cytokine support	Natural antitumour activity; safer inflammatory profile; allogeneic use feasible; lower CRS/neurotoxicity risk	Difficult to transduce/edit (DNA sensitivity, antiviral sensors); heterogeneity across donors; limited persistence
γδ T cells	Primarily allogeneic; early trials ongoing	Limited, can form memory subsets	MHC-independent recognition; potential "off-the-shelf" use; reduced GvHD risk	Lower expansion efficiency; fewer established protocols; clinical experience still limited
iPSCs	Allogeneic, off-the-shelf	Can be differentiated into memory-like T or NK cells	Unlimited renewable source; clonal editing possible at stem-cell stage; standardised, homogeneous starting material; enables "off-the-shelf" universal products	Complex differentiation protocols; high cost and regulatory hurdles; genomic/epigenetic stability concerns
Immortalised cell lines (e.g., NK-92)	Universal (cell line, requires irradiation)	None (irradiated)	Easy to culture and expand; high transduction efficiency; homogeneous populations; scalable manufacturing	Require irradiation before infusion (no *in vivo* persistence); limited clinical use; potential tumorigenicity

14.4.1 Viral Vectors

Viral vectors are gene-delivery vehicles built from modified viral backbones that retain their ability to enter eukaryotic cells but lack the capacity to replicate. They mediate efficient transfer of engineered nucleic acid payloads through a controlled transduction process. The current FDA-approved engineered cell therapies, most notably CAR-T cells, have almost exclusively relied on viral transduction as the delivery method [68–70]. This approach allows the delivery and stable insertion of recombinant DNA encoding a CAR or other synthetic receptor, giving T cells or NK cells the capacity to recognise targets beyond their natural repertoire. Viral vectors achieve this by packaging engineered genetic material into particles that enter the target cell, where the transgene is then incorporated into the host genome or maintained episomally, depending on the vector type. The result is a durable expression of the introduced genetic payload, although in integrating systems, this occurs at largely random genomic sites.

The earliest clinical studies with CAR T cells employed **γ-retroviral vectors**, which stably integrate their cargo into dividing T cells, and with a practical packaging capacity of ~8 to 9 kb (Figure 14.1). While efficient, retroviruses cannot transduce non-dividing cells, and their integration profile has raised safety concerns [71]. Nevertheless, they enabled the first generation of CAR-T trials that proved the principle of adoptive transfer of genetically modified lymphocytes [72]. **Lentiviruses** (LVs), derived from HIV-1, were developed to overcome this limitation. LVs can transduce both dividing and quiescent cells, making them especially well-suited for *ex vivo* modification of T cells, NK cells, and iPSC-derived progenitors. Lentiviruses support cargo sizes up to ~8 kb and have relatively predictable integration patterns, although they still integrate semi-randomly into the host genome. In fact, most FDA-approved CAR-T products today, including tisagenlecleucel and axicabtagene ciloleucel [73, 74], rely on lentiviral transduction for CAR delivery. **Adenoviruses** provide very high transduction efficiency and a large packaging capacity (~36 kb), which permits delivery of multiple or large payloads. Unlike retro- and lentiviruses, adenoviral genomes remain episomal, leading to strong but transient expression. However, their high innate immunogenicity has limited their use in *ex vivo* T and NK engineering, but they remain valuable in vaccine development and oncolytic virotherapy [75]. **Adeno-associated viruses** (AAV) vectors are derived from non-pathogenic parvoviruses and offer a different profile: very low immunogenicity, primarily episomal persistence, and efficient transduction of both dividing and non-dividing cells [76]. The major limitation is their small packaging capacity (~4.7 kb), which can restrict inclusion of large CAR constructs or multi-gene circuits. Of note, AAVs are particularly useful in precise gene knock-in strategies, where CRISPR nucleases create double-strand breaks, and AAV provides the homology template for targeted repair.

However, viral integration remains only partially controllable, carrying a rare but real risk of insertional mutagenesis [71] despite improvements such as self-inactivating designs [77]. At the same time, the high cost and regulatory burden of GMP-grade vector production make viral manufacturing one of the most resource-intensive steps in cell therapy development. [78] In summary, while viral vectors remain the clinical standard for their efficiency and proven track record, their drawbacks, including random integration, cost, and limited suitability for multiplex engineering, have encouraged the development of alternative strategies.

14.4.2 Non-viral Approaches

While viral vectors remain the clinical standard for engineering T and NK cells, their reliance on semi-random integration, restricted cargo capacity, and the expense of GMP-grade production have motivated the search for alternatives. Non-viral approaches aim to provide more precise, flexible, and cost-effective editing, often without the need for stable integration (Table 14.1). These methods range from direct delivery of nucleic acids or protein–RNA complexes to more innovative vesicle-based carriers. Among them, electroporation is now the mainstay for *ex vivo* cell engineering: a physical method that transiently permeabilises the plasma membrane, allowing plasmid DNA, mRNA, or pre-assembled CRISPR RNPs to enter immune cells with high efficiency.

14.4.3 Electroporation

Electroporation works by using brief electrical pulses to temporarily disrupt the plasma membrane of cells. When a strong but carefully calibrated electric field is applied, it causes the lipid bilayer to reorganise and form transient nanopores. These pores increase membrane permeability, allowing charged molecules such as plasmid DNA, mRNA, or protein–RNA complexes (e.g. Cas9 RNPs) to pass into the cytoplasm [79]. After the pulse ends, the cell membrane reseals within seconds to minutes, ideally trapping the delivered cargo inside while maintaining cell viability. The cargo can then follow its natural intracellular routes: DNA migrates to the nucleus for transcription, mRNA is translated in the cytoplasm, and proteins like Cas9 can access the nucleus to edit genomic DNA. In immune-cell engineering, electroporation is widely used because it can efficiently deliver large and complex cargos into primary lymphocytes, which are otherwise difficult to transfect. However, its success depends on careful optimisation. Pulse strength and duration must be tuned to avoid cell death or impaired function, and the choice of cargo is equally important. For instance, NK cells are particularly sensitive to DNA because of their strong antiviral sensors, making protein–RNA complexes such as CRISPR RNPs a more effective option [80].

14.4.4 Transposon Systems

While RNA delivery provides short-lived expression, DNA transposons such as Sleeping Beauty and piggyBac enable stable integration of genetic payloads without using viral vectors [81]. These systems rely on a transposase enzyme that mediates 'cut-and-paste' insertion of DNA into the genome at TA- or TTAA-rich sites, allowing long-term expression of CARs, cytokines, or synthetic circuits [82]. Both platforms have been adapted for electroporation into T and NK cells and have progressed into early clinical trials, where piggyBac-modified CAR-T cells achieved sustained engraftment and durable responses [83]. Newer variants improve efficiency and reduce insertional bias, while ongoing engineering efforts aim to combine them with CRISPR guidance for targeted integration. Owing to their simplicity, scalability, and GMP compatibility, transposon systems remain attractive non-viral alternatives for large-scale immune-cell manufacturing.

14.4.5 Transient RNA Programming: mRNA and circRNA

mRNA electroporation enables transient expression of CARs, cytokines, or genome editors without genomic integration, offering a rapid, flexible, and highly safe way to test receptor designs or add short-lived 'arming' functions during manufacturing [84]. Expression typically lasts hours to a few days, which reduces long-term risk but may require re-dosing or repeated stimulation to sustain activity. To extend the window without sacrificing non-integration, circular RNAs (circRNAs) have emerged as a next-generation format. Their covalently closed structure resists exonuclease degradation, supporting multi-day protein production while maintaining a similar safety profile to linear mRNA [85]. In practice, mRNA is well suited for quick prototyping, transient CAR or cytokine boosts, or one-time delivery of genome editors (e.g. Cas9 or base editors), whereas circRNA is attractive when longer, still-transient expression is desired (e.g. IL-15 support, inducible switches, or staged circuit components).

14.4.6 Lipid and Polymeric Nanoparticles

LNPs have become a leading non-viral delivery platform, validated at a global scale through their use in COVID-19 mRNA vaccines [86]. Their basic principle is to encapsulate nucleic acids such as mRNA, sgRNA, or even Cas9 protein within lipid bilayer structures that protect the cargo from degradation and facilitate uptake by endocytosis. Once inside the cell, the lipid formulation helps release the nucleic acid into the cytoplasm for translation or editing. For immune-cell engineering, LNPs offer several advantages: they are fully synthetic, relatively straightforward to manufacture under GMP conditions, and can be chemically tuned to influence stability, biodistribution, and tropism [87]. Emerging formulations have been designed to preferentially target lymphocytes or haematopoietic cells, although transfection efficiency remains lower than electroporation in *ex vivo* settings. Their real promise lies in *in vivo* delivery, where they could bypass labour-intensive *ex vivo* manipulation altogether and edit or reprogram circulating immune cells directly inside the patient. Polymeric nanoparticles provide an alternative synthetic vehicle with broader chemical flexibility [88]. While polymeric nanoparticles can deliver DNA, RNA, or RNPs with tunable charge, degradability, and release, concerns over toxicity, stability, and reproducibility have limited their clinical translation compared to LNPs.

14.4.7 Exosomes and Extracellular Vesicles

Exosomes and other EVs are nanoscale, membrane-bound particles (30–150 nm) naturally secreted by most cell types as part of intercellular communication [89]. They carry proteins, lipids, and nucleic acids, and their biological role in antigen presentation and immune modulation has made them attractive candidates for therapeutic delivery vehicles [89]. For cell engineering, exosomes can be loaded with mRNA, proteins, or CRISPR RNPs, thereby offering a means to transfer editing machinery without the need for viral vectors or harsh physical methods [90]. A major advantage of exosomes is their low immunogenicity and ability to evade rapid clearance by the immune system. Unlike synthetic nanoparticles, they are naturally stable in circulation and can cross biological barriers, such as the blood–brain barrier. While exosome secretion is generally non-polarised and non-specific [91], surface engineering can enhance their tropism by decorating vesicles with targeting ligands or antibodies, thereby directing them more selectively to tumours, lymphoid tissues, or defined immune subsets [92].

Despite this promise, significant technical hurdles remain. Current methods for exosome isolation and cargo loading, especially for larger Cas9 nucleases, vary widely and are often inefficient, making scale-up and reproducibility difficult. In summary, exosomes and other EVs represent a biologically inspired, potentially transformative delivery system for immune-cell engineering. Their ability to combine stealth, tropism, and modularity positions them as promising alternatives to viral or synthetic carriers, particularly for *in vivo* applications. However, improvements in manufacturing, loading technologies, and regulatory harmonisation will be essential before exosome-based approaches can become mainstream in clinical immunotherapy.

14.4.8 CRISPR Editing

The discovery of the CRISPR/Cas genome-editing system has transformed the field of immune-cell engineering, offering a level of accuracy and control that was previously unattainable. Functioning as a molecular scalpel, the CRISPR system uses a Cas nuclease guided by a short RNA sequence to recognise complementary DNA, which is then cleaved at the target site [93]. Depending on how the cell repairs the DNA break, two main outcomes are possible. Most often, the lesion is resolved by non-homologous end joining (NHEJ), an error-prone pathway that introduces insertions or deletions, leading to gene disruption and a functional knockout (KO). Alternatively, if a DNA repair template is supplied, the cell can use homology-directed repair (HDR) to precisely insert or replace sequences at the break site, enabling a targeted knock-in (KI). Together, these capabilities allow scientists to move beyond random viral integration and instead rewrite the genome of T cells, NK cells, or stem-cell-derived progenitors with unprecedented precision and predictability [94].

Beyond KOs, one of the most powerful applications of CRISPR is the KI of therapeutic cassettes into defined genomic sites. Following a targeted CRISPR-induced double-strand break, synthetic modules such as CARs, cytokines, or safety switches can be integrated into well-characterised 'safe-harbour' loci, where they rely on an exogenous promoter, or directly under the control of endogenous regulatory loci, where they are expressed under natural transcriptional control. The latter approach ensures both uniform expression and avoids issues like tonic signalling. Today, the CRISPR toolbox extends well beyond Cas9, with nucleases like Cas12a broadening targeting options and base or prime editors enabling precise nucleotide changes without double-strand breaks, lowering the risk of genomic instability [95, 96].

The most transformative feature of CRISPR is multiplex genome editing: the possibility of reshaping immune cells through several coordinated modifications. This matters because cancer is not a single-target disease: tumours deploy multiple defences at once, from inhibitory ligands to immunosuppressive cytokines and metabolic barriers [97]. Relying on a single CAR insertion gives therapeutic cells a strong weapon, but not the versatility they need to withstand these combined pressures. Multiplex editing changes this equation. In T cells, this can include checkpoint disruption (e.g. PDCD1 knockout to reduce exhaustion [98]), removal of the endogenous TCR or HLA molecules (e.g. TRAC knockout to prevent graft-versus-host disease [99]), and targeted knock-ins that place CARs under physiological control or add cytokine support modules such as IL-15. In NK cells, edits like CISH knockout enhance IL-15 responsiveness [100], while NKG2A deletion counteracts HLA-E-mediated inhibition [101]. By combining such edits in the same cell, CRISPR enables the design of multiplex, 'armoured' lymphocytes that are safer for allogeneic use, more resistant to suppression, and endowed with enhanced persistence in the tumour microenvironment. Several of these multi-edited products, including tri-edited CAR-T and CAR-NK cells, are already advancing into early-phase clinical trials.

Such advances, however, come with safety and reproducibility challenges. Every additional edit increases the risk of undesirable outcomes. Off-target cuts can introduce accidental mutations [102]; multiple double-strand breaks may cause chromosomal translocations [103] or trigger p53 pathways [104], impairing cell viability. To address this, the field is moving towards DSB-free editors, improved delivery platforms such as LNPs and engineered exosomes, and the use of multi-omic CRISPR screens to rationally guide design. Together, these advances aim to make CRISPR-engineered immune cells safer and more versatile, bringing the vision of programmable 'living drugs' closer to reality.

Immunogenicity is also a concern, since the Cas9 nuclease is of bacterial origin, patients may mount responses against Cas proteins or residual delivery components [105]. Finally, the reproducibility of manufacturing is a critical logistical barrier. Ensuring that each batch of this complex, living therapeutic meets stringent release criteria for editing efficiency, safety, and potency is a formidable bioprocessing and regulatory challenge that must be solved for widespread clinical translation. Overcoming these obstacles is the central focus of current research, paving the way for a future of precisely programmed immunotherapies.

14.4.9 Future-Facing Platforms

The field of immune-cell engineering is expanding beyond traditional nuclease-based editing towards a diverse toolbox of gene-writing platforms. The Find, Cut and Transfer (FiCAT) system exemplifies this shift, enabling precise insertion of large payloads in both dividing and non-dividing lymphocytes, thereby bypassing the constraints of HDR [106]. In parallel, advances in AI-guided protein design are accelerating the development of next-generation genome engineering tools, from optimised nucleases and base editors to synthetic transposases and integrases with programmable specificity and improved safety [107]. At the RNA level, editing strategies harness endogenous ADAR enzymes to introduce precise base changes directly into transcripts, providing reversible modulation of immune functions without permanent genomic alteration [108]. These approaches, combined with multiplex CRISPR designs and integration with synthetic circuits, point towards a future where lymphocytes can not only resist exhaustion and rejection but also dynamically adapt to the tumour microenvironment. Together, these innovations signal the transition from single-gene modifications to programmable, context-aware 'living drugs'.

14.5 CONCLUSION

The advent of programmable living drugs capable of replacing damaged tissues, correcting genetic abnormalities, or executing complex therapeutic tasks marks a true biomedical revolution. We are only beginning to see the impact such therapies will have across all fields of medicine. As illustrated in this chapter, the toolbox for precise, multiplexed genome engineering is expanding rapidly, now complemented by computational frameworks that can predict how genomic perturbations influence cell fate. Lab-in-the-loop designs, where machine learning integrates experimental data in real time, are accelerating the rational design of engineered immune cells.

Realising this potential will require continued research investments in basic biology. Understanding the regulatory elements that govern differentiation, effector function, and persistence is essential for editing strategies to achieve context-dependent functional responses. Equally critical is translating these insights into scalable and safe manufacturing processes that meet the demands of clinical application. Looking ahead, several frontiers are emerging, including (i) universal cell sources such as iPSCs that allow unlimited production and multiplex engineering; (ii) synthetic circuits that enable context-aware responses and improve safety in solid tumours; (iii) functional template editing, where regulatory programmes are tuned to sustain metabolic fitness and resist exhaustion; (iv) stealth and immune-evasive designs that extend persistence of allogeneic products; and (v) computational immunoengineering, where AI models and multi-omics integration guide the choice of edits and predict their outcomes (Figure 14.3).

Together, these innovations are moving engineered lymphocytes from simple antigen-targeting tools towards programmable biological platforms that can sense, decide, and act with increasing sophistication. However, bringing such products to the clinic entails substantial regulatory and GMP demands. Multi-edited cell therapies require exhaustive characterisation of each modification and their combined effects, including integration-site mapping, off-target profiling, and long-term genomic stability, supported by clonally traceable manufacturing and reproducible release testing. The next generation of therapies will not only treat cancer but also address autoimmunity, infectious disease, and regenerative medicine, placing engineered immune cells at the centre of future precision therapies.

KEY POINTS

- Engineered immune cells are shifting from single-gene modifications to programmable, multiplex-edited 'living drugs' capable of sensing, integrating, and responding to complex cues.
- CARs, TCRs, logic-gated circuits, SynNotch/SNIPR systems, and switch receptors enable increasingly precise and context-aware tumour recognition.
- Functional template editing reprograms transcriptional and metabolic circuits to sustain effector function, resist exhaustion, and improve persistence in hostile microenvironments.
- Stealth and immune-evasive designs are essential for durable allogeneic therapies, requiring coordinated edits across HLA, NK-ligand, and adhesion pathways.
- Delivery platforms, from viral vectors to CRISPR RNPs, transposons, mRNA/circRNA, nanoparticles, and exosomes, define feasibility, safety, and scalability of clinical manufacturing.
- Regulatory and GMP frameworks must evolve to accommodate multi-edited products, including rigorous off-target assessment, integration-site mapping, clonality, and reproducible large-scale production.

LIST OF ABBREVIATIONS

AAV	Adeno-associated virus
ADAR	Adenosine deaminase acting on RNA
ATMP	Advanced therapy medicinal product
CAR	Chimeric antigen receptor
CRISPR	Clustered regularly interspaced short palindromic repeats
DSB	Double-strand break
EV	Extracellular vesicle
FiCAT	Find, Cut and Transfer
GMP	Good manufacturing practice
HDR	Homology-directed repair
HLA	Human leukocyte antigen
iPSC	Induced pluripotent stem cell
LNP	Lipid nanoparticle
LV	Lentiviral vector
NHEJ	Non-homologous end joining
PAM	Protospacer adjacent motif
scFv	Single-chain variable fragment
SNIPR	Synthetic intramembrane proteolysis receptor
SynNotch	Synthetic Notch receptor
TAA	Tumour-associated antigen
TCR	T-cell receptor

REVIEW QUESTIONS

1. Compare and contrast the mechanisms and therapeutic implications of CAR and TCR-based immune cell therapies. How do their antigen recognition properties define their respective strengths and limitations in treating haematologic versus solid tumours?
2. Explain the rationale behind stealth editing in allogeneic immune-cell therapies. Which gene targets and molecular strategies are employed to evade host immune rejection while maintaining cytotoxic function?
3. Describe the concept of functional template editing. How can modulation of transcriptional and metabolic circuits enhance persistence and resistance to exhaustion in engineered lymphocytes?
4. Discuss the advantages and drawbacks of viral versus non-viral delivery systems for introducing genetic modifications into immune cells. In what contexts might each be preferable?
5. Outline the emerging role of next-generation gene-writing tools such as FiCAT and base/prime editors in advancing precision immunotherapy. How do these differ from conventional CRISPR approaches in terms of mechanism, efficiency, and clinical potential?

REFERENCES

1. Labanieh, L. and Mackall, C.L. (2023). CAR immune cells: design principles, resistance and the next generation. *Nature* 614 (7949): 635–648.
2. Feucht, J. and Sadelain, M. (2020). Function and evolution of the prototypic CD28zeta and 4-1BBzeta chimeric antigen receptors. *Immunooncol Technol* 8: 2–11.
3. June, C.H. and Sadelain, M. (2018). Chimeric antigen receptor therapy. *N Engl J Med* 379 (1): 64–73.
4. Uslu, U. and June, C.H. (2025). Beyond the blood: expanding CAR T cell therapy to solid tumors. *Nat Biotechnol* 43 (4): 506–515.
5. Biederstadt, A., Basar, R., Park, J.M. et al. (2025). Genome-wide CRISPR screens identify critical targets to enhance CAR-NK cell antitumor potency. *Cancer Cell* 43: 2069–2088.e11.
6. Peng, L., Sferruzza, G., Yang, L. et al. (2024). CAR-T and CAR-NK as cellular cancer immunotherapy for solid tumors. *Cell Mol Immunol* 21 (10): 1089–1108.
7. Chen, A.J., Zhang, J., Agarwal, A., and Lakdawalla, D.N. (2022). Value of reducing wait times for chimeric antigen receptor T-cell treatment: evidence from randomized controlled trial data on tisagenlecleucel for diffuse large B-cell lymphoma. *Value Health* 25 (8): 1344–1351.
8. Westin, J.R., Kersten, M.J., Salles, G. et al. (2021). Efficacy and safety of CD19-directed CAR-T cell therapies in patients with relapsed/refractory aggressive B-cell lymphomas: observations from the JULIET, ZUMA-1, and TRANSCEND trials. *Am J Hematol* 96 (10): 1295–1312.
9. Geethakumari, P.R., Ramasamy, D.P., Dholaria, B. et al. (2021). Balancing quality, cost, and access during delivery of newer cellular and immunotherapy treatments. *Curr Hematol Malig Rep* 16 (4): 345–356.
10. Saetersmoen, M.L., Hammer, Q., Valamehr, B. et al. (2019). Off-the-shelf cell therapy with induced pluripotent stem cell-derived natural killer cells. *Semin Immunopathol* 41 (1): 59–68.
11. Zhu, H. and Kaufman, D.S. (2019). Engineered human pluripotent stem cell-derived natural killer cells: the next frontier for cancer immunotherapy. *Blood Sci* 1 (1): 4–11.
12. Bjorklund, A.T., Carlsten, M., Sohlberg, E. et al. (2018). Complete remission with reduction of high-risk clones following haploidentical NK-cell therapy against MDS and AML. *Clin Cancer Res* 24 (8): 1834–1844.
13. Lamb, M.G., Rangarajan, H.G., Tullius, B.P., and Lee, D.A. (2021). Natural killer cell therapy for hematologic malignancies: successes, challenges, and the future. *Stem Cell Res Ther* 12 (1): 211.
14. Martin, K.E., Hammer, Q., Perica, K. et al. (2024). Engineering immune-evasive allogeneic cellular immunotherapies. *Nat Rev Immunol* 24: 680–693.
15. Jo, S., Das, S., Williams, A. et al. (2022). Endowing universal CAR T-cell with immune-evasive properties using TALEN-gene editing. *Nat Commun* 13 (1): 3453.
16. Yu, H., Qian, W., Song, Y., and Welch, J.D. (2025). PerturbNet predicts single-cell responses to unseen chemical and genetic perturbations. *Mol Syst Biol* 21 (8): 960–982.
17. Wang, G., Liu, T., Zhao, J. et al. (2024). Modeling and predicting single-cell multi-gene perturbation responses with scLAMBDA. *bioRxiv* https://doi.org/10.1101/2024.12.04.626878.
18. Roohani, Y., Huang, K., and Leskovec, J. (2024). Predicting transcriptional outcomes of novel multigene perturbations with GEARS. *Nat Biotechnol* 42 (6): 927–935.
19. Cui, H., Wang, C., Maan, H. et al. (2024). scGPT: toward building a foundation model for single-cell multi-omics using generative AI. *Nat Methods* 21 (8): 1470–1480.
20. Bunne, C., Roohani, Y., and Rosen, Y. (2024). How to build the virtual cell with artificial intelligence: priorities and opportunities. *Cell* 187 (25): 7045–7063.
21. Kamimoto, K., Stringa, B., Hoffmann, C.M. et al. (2023). Dissecting cell identity via network inference and in silico gene perturbation. *Nature* 614 (7949): 742–751.

22. Brentjens, R.J., Latouche, J.B., Santos, E. et al. (2003). Eradication of systemic B-cell tumors by genetically targeted human T lymphocytes co-stimulated by CD80 and interleukin-15. *Nat Med* 9 (3): 279–286.
23. Maher, J., Brentjens, R.J., Gunset, G. et al. (2002). Human T-lymphocyte cytotoxicity and proliferation directed by a single chimeric TCRzeta /CD28 receptor. *Nat Biotechnol* 20 (1): 70–75.
24. Krause, A., Guo, H.F., Latouche, J.B. et al. (1998). Antigen-dependent CD28 signaling selectively enhances survival and proliferation in genetically modified activated human primary T lymphocytes. *J Exp Med* 188 (4): 619–626.
25. Eshhar, Z., Waks, T., Gross, G., and Schindler, D.G. (1993). Specific activation and targeting of cytotoxic lymphocytes through chimeric single chains consisting of antibody-binding domains and the gamma or zeta subunits of the immunoglobulin and T-cell receptors. *Proc Natl Acad Sci USA* 90 (2): 720–724.
26. Foldvari, Z., Brennan, M.S., Titov, A. et al. (2025). Targeting the roots of myeloid malignancies with T cell receptors. *Nat Rev Cancer* 25: 965–985.
27. Weller, C., Bartok, O., McGinnis, C.S. et al. (2025). Translation dysregulation in cancer as a source for targetable antigens. *Cancer Cell* 43 (5): 823–840.e18.
28. Champagne, J., Nielsen, M.M., Feng, X. et al. (2025). Adoptive T cell therapy targeting an inducible and broadly shared product of aberrant mRNA translation. *Immunity* 58 (1): 247–262.e9.
29. Karpanen, T. and Olweus, J. (2017). The potential of donor T-cell repertoires in neoantigen-targeted cancer immunotherapy. *Front Immunol* 8: 1718.
30. Morsut, L., Roybal, K.T., Xiong, X. et al. (2016). Engineering customized cell sensing and response behaviors using synthetic notch receptors. *Cell* 164 (4): 780–791.
31. Dufva, O., Gandolfi, S., Huuhtanen, J. et al. (2023). Single-cell functional genomics reveals determinants of sensitivity and resistance to natural killer cells in blood cancers. *Immunity* 56 (12): 2816–2835.e13.
32. Dubrot, J., Du, P.P., Lane-Reticker, S.K. et al. (2022). In vivo CRISPR screens reveal the landscape of immune evasion pathways across cancer. *Nat Immunol* 23 (10): 1495–1506.
33. Sheffer, M., Lowry, E., Beelen, N. et al. (2021). Genome-scale screens identify factors regulating tumor cell responses to natural killer cells. *Nat Genet* 53 (8): 1196–1206.
34. Benjamin, R., Graham, C., Yallop, D. et al. (2020). Genome-edited, donor-derived allogeneic anti-CD19 chimeric antigen receptor T cells in paediatric and adult B-cell acute lymphoblastic leukaemia: results of two phase 1 studies. *Lancet* 396 (10266): 1885–1894.
35. Momayyezi, P., Bilev, E., Ljunggren, H.G., Hammer, Q. (2023). Viral escape from NK-cell-mediated immunosurveillance: A lesson for cancer immunotherapy? *Eur J Immunol* 53 (11): e2350465. doi:10.1002/eji.202350465. Epub 2023 Aug. 12.PMID: 37526136
36. Riolobos, L., Hirata, R.K., Turtle, C.J. et al. (2013). HLA engineering of human pluripotent stem cells. *Mol Ther* 21 (6): 1232–1241.
37. Cui, D., Wang, J., Zeng, Y. et al. (2016). Generating hESCs with reduced immunogenicity by disrupting TAP1 or TAPBP. *Biosci Biotechnol Biochem* 80 (8): 1484–1491.
38. Abrahimi, P., Chang, W.G., Kluger, M.S. et al. (2015). Efficient Gene Disruption in Cultured Primary Human Endothelial Cells by CRISPR/Cas9. *Circ Res* 117 (2): 121–128.
39. Ljunggren, H.G. and Karre, K. (1990). In search of the 'missing self': MHC molecules and NK cell recognition. *Immunol Today* 11 (7): 237–244.
40. Ljunggren, H.G. and Karre, K. (1985). Host resistance directed selectively against H-2-deficient lymphoma variants. Analysis of the mechanism. *J Exp Med* 162 (6): 1745–1759.
41. Braud, V.M., Allan, D.S.J., O'Callaghan, C.A. et al. (1998). HLA-E binds to natural killer cell receptors CD94/NKG2A, B and C. *Nature* 391 (6669): 795–799.
42. Shiroishi, M., Tsumoto, K., Amano, K. et al. (2003). Human inhibitory receptors Ig-like transcript 2 (ILT2) and ILT4 compete with CD8 for MHC class I binding and bind preferentially to HLA-G. *Proc Natl Acad Sci USA* 100 (15): 8856–8861.

43. Deuse, T., Hu, X., Gravina, A. et al. (2019). Hypoimmunogenic derivatives of induced pluripotent stem cells evade immune rejection in fully immunocompetent allogeneic recipients. *Nat Biotechnol* 37 (3): 252–258.
44. Hu, X., White, K., Olroyd, A.G. et al. (2024). Hypoimmune induced pluripotent stem cells survive long term in fully immunocompetent, allogeneic rhesus macaques. *Nat Biotechnol* 42: 413–423.
45. Carlsson, P.O., Hu, X., Scholz, H. et al. (2025). Survival of transplanted allogeneic beta cells with no immunosuppression. *N Engl J Med* 393 (9): 887–894.
46. Hammer, Q., Perica, K., Mbofung, R.M. et al. (2024). Genetic ablation of adhesion ligands mitigates rejection of allogeneic cellular immunotherapies. *Cell Stem Cell* 31: 1376–1386.e8.
47. Porter, D.L., Levine, B.L., Kalos, M. et al. (2011). Chimeric antigen receptor-modified T cells in chronic lymphoid leukemia. *N Engl J Med* 365 (8): 725–733.
48. Morgan, R.A., Yang, J.C., Kitano, M. et al. (2010). Case report of a serious adverse event following the administration of T cells transduced with a chimeric antigen receptor recognizing ERBB2. *Mol Ther* 18 (4): 843–851.
49. Lee, D.W., Gardner, R., Porter, D.L. et al. (2014). Current concepts in the diagnosis and management of cytokine release syndrome. *Blood* 124 (2): 188–195.
50. Newick, K., O'Brien, S., Moon, E., and Albelda, S.M. (2017). CAR T cell therapy for solid tumors. *Annu Rev Med* 68: 139–152.
51. Sadelain, M., Riviere, I., and Riddell, S. (2017). Therapeutic T cell engineering. *Nature* 545 (7655): 423–431.
52. Roybal, K.T. and Lim, W.A. (2017). Synthetic immunology: hacking immune cells to expand their therapeutic capabilities. *Annu Rev Immunol* 35: 229–253.
53. Kloss, C.C., Condomines, M., Cartellieri, M. et al. (2013). Combinatorial antigen recognition with balanced signaling promotes selective tumor eradication by engineered T cells. *Nat Biotechnol* 31 (1): 71–75.
54. Lanitis, E., Poussin, M., Klattenhoff, A.W. et al. (2013). Chimeric antigen receptor T Cells with dissociated signaling domains exhibit focused antitumor activity with reduced potential for toxicity in vivo. *Cancer Immunol Res* 1 (1): 43–53.
55. Grada, Z., Hegde, M., Byrd, T. et al. (2013). TanCAR: a novel bispecific chimeric antigen receptor for cancer immunotherapy. *Mol Ther Nucleic Acids* 2 (7): e105.
56. Hegde, M., Mukherjee, M., Grada, Z. et al. (2016). Tandem CAR T cells targeting HER2 and IL13Ralpha2 mitigate tumor antigen escape. *J Clin Invest* 126 (8): 3036–3052.
57. Frankel, N.W., Deng, H., Yucel, G. et al. (2024). Precision off-the-shelf natural killer cell therapies for oncology with logic-gated gene circuits. *Cell Rep* 43 (5): 114145.
58. Roybal, K.T., Rupp, L.J., Morsut, L. et al. (2016). Precision tumor recognition by T cells with combinatorial antigen-sensing circuits. *Cell* 164 (4): 770–779.
59. Artavanis-Tsakonas, S., Rand, M.D., and Lake, R.J. (1999). Notch signaling: cell fate control and signal integration in development. *Science* 284 (5415): 770–776.
60. Choe, J.H., Watchmaker, P.B., Simic, M.S. et al. (2021). SynNotch-CAR T cells overcome challenges of specificity, heterogeneity, and persistence in treating glioblastoma. *Sci Transl Med* 13 (591): eabe7378.
61. Piraner, D.I., Abedi, M.H., Duran Gonzalez, M.J. et al. (2025). Engineered receptors for soluble cellular communication and disease sensing. *Nature* 638 (8051): 805–813.
62. Zhu, I., Liu, R., Garcia, J.M. et al. (2022). Modular design of synthetic receptors for programmed gene regulation in cell therapies. *Cell* 185 (8): 1431–1443.e16.
63. Fedorov, V.D., Themeli, M., and Sadelain, M. (2013). PD-1- and CTLA-4-based inhibitory chimeric antigen receptors (iCARs) divert off-target immunotherapy responses. *Sci Transl Med* 5 (215): 215ra172.
64. Liu, X., Ranganathan, R., Jiang, S. et al. (2016). A chimeric switch-receptor targeting PD1 augments the efficacy of second-generation CAR T cells in advanced solid tumors. *Cancer Res* 76 (6): 1578–1590.

65. Thelen, M., Wennhold, K., Lehmann, J. et al. (2021). Cancer-specific immune evasion and substantial heterogeneity within cancer types provide evidence for personalized immunotherapy. *NPJ Precis Oncol* 5 (1): 52.
66. Andre, P., Denis, C., Soulas, C. et al. (2018). Anti-NKG2A mAb is a checkpoint inhibitor that promotes anti-tumor immunity by unleashing both T and NK cells. *Cell* 175 (7): 1731–1743.e13.
67. Saetersmoen, M., Kotchetkov, I.S., Torralba-Raga, L. et al. (2025). Targeting HLA-E-overexpressing cancers with a NKG2A/C switch receptor. *Med* 6 (2): 100521.
68. Maude, S.L., Frey, N., Shaw, P.A. et al. (2014). Chimeric antigen receptor T cells for sustained remissions in leukemia. *N Engl J Med* 371 (16): 1507–1517.
69. Milone, M.C., Fish, J.D., Carpenito, C. et al. (2009). Chimeric receptors containing CD137 signal transduction domains mediate enhanced survival of T cells and increased antileukemic efficacy in vivo. *Mol Ther* 17 (8): 1453–1464.
70. Milone, M.C. and O'Doherty, U. (2018). Clinical use of lentiviral vectors. *Leukemia* 32 (7): 1529–1541.
71. Hacein-Bey-Abina, S., Garrigue, A., Wang, G.P. et al. (2008). Insertional oncogenesis in 4 patients after retrovirus-mediated gene therapy of SCID-X1. *J Clin Invest* 118 (9): 3132–3142.
72. Brentjens, R.J., Riviere, I., Park, J.H. et al. (2011). Safety and persistence of adoptively transferred autologous CD19-targeted T cells in patients with relapsed or chemotherapy refractory B-cell leukemias. *Blood* 118 (18): 4817–4828.
73. Maude, S.L., Laetsch, T.W., Buechner, J. et al. (2018). Tisagenlecleucel in children and young adults with B-cell lymphoblastic leukemia. *N Engl J Med* 378 (5): 439–448.
74. Locke, F.L., Neelapu, S.S., Bartlett, N.L. et al. (2017). Phase 1 results of ZUMA-1: a multicenter study of KTE-C19 anti-CD19 CAR T cell therapy in refractory aggressive lymphoma. *Mol Ther* 25 (1): 285–295.
75. Crystal, R.G. (2014). Adenovirus: the first effective in vivo gene delivery vector. *Hum Gene Ther* 25 (1): 3–11.
76. Wang, D., Tai, P.W.L., and Gao, G. (2019). Adeno-associated virus vector as a platform for gene therapy delivery. *Nat Rev Drug Discov* 18 (5): 358–378.
77. Miyoshi, H., Blomer, U., Takahashi, M. et al. (1998). Development of a self-inactivating lentivirus vector. *J Virol* 72 (10): 8150–8157.
78. Ayala Ceja, M., Khericha, M., Harris, C.M. et al. (2024). CAR-T cell manufacturing: major process parameters and next-generation strategies. *J Exp Med* 221 (2): e20230903.
79. Neumann, E., Schaefer-Ridder, M., Wang, Y., and Hofschneider, P.H. (1982). Gene transfer into mouse lyoma cells by electroporation in high electric fields. *EMBO J* 1 (7): 841–845.
80. Pomeroy, E.J., Hunzeker, J.T., Kluesner, M.G. et al. (2020). A genetically engineered primary human natural killer cell platform for cancer immunotherapy. *Mol Ther* 28 (1): 52–63.
81. Sandoval-Villegas, N., Nurieva, W., Amberger, M., and Ivics, Z. (2021). Contemporary transposon tools: a review and guide through mechanisms and applications of sleeping beauty, piggyBac and Tol2 for genome engineering. *Int J Mol Sci* 22 (10): 5084.
82. Ivics, Z., Hackett, P.B., Plasterk, R.H., and Izsvak, Z. (1997). Molecular reconstruction of sleeping beauty, a Tc1-like transposon from fish, and its transposition in human cells. *Cell* 91 (4): 501–510.
83. Kebriaei, P., Singh, H., Huls, M.H. et al. (2016). Phase I trials using Sleeping Beauty to generate CD19-specific CAR T cells. *J Clin Invest* 126 (9): 3363–3376.
84. Foster, J.B., Barrett, D.M., and Kariko, K. (2019). The emerging role of in vitro-transcribed mRNA in adoptive T cell immunotherapy. *Mol Ther* 27 (4): 747–756.
85. Wesselhoeft, R.A., Kowalski, P.S., and Anderson, D.G. (2018). Engineering circular RNA for potent and stable translation in eukaryotic cells. *Nat Commun* 9 (1): 2629.
86. Baden LR, El Sahly HM, Essink B. et al. Efficacy and safety of the mRNA-1273 SARS-CoV-2 vaccine. *N Engl J Med* 2021;384(5):403–416.

87. Hou, X., Zaks, T., Langer, R., and Dong, Y. (2021). Lipid nanoparticles for mRNA delivery. *Nat Rev Mater* 6 (12): 1078–1094.
88. Smith, T.T., Stephan, S.B., Moffett, H.F. et al. (2017). In situ programming of leukaemia-specific T cells using synthetic DNA nanocarriers. *Nat Nanotechnol* 12 (8): 813–820.
89. van Niel, G., D'Angelo, G., and Raposo, G. (2018). Shedding light on the cell biology of extracellular vesicles. *Nat Rev Mol Cell Biol* 19 (4): 213–228.
90. Kalluri, R. and LeBleu, V.S. (2020). The biology, function, and biomedical applications of exosomes. *Science* 367 (6478): eaau6977.
91. Mathieu, M., Martin-Jaular, L., Lavieu, G., and Thery, C. (2019). Specificities of secretion and uptake of exosomes and other extracellular vesicles for cell-to-cell communication. *Nat Cell Biol* 21 (1): 9–17.
92. Xu, Q., Zhang, Z., Zhao, L. et al. (2020). Tropism-facilitated delivery of CRISPR/Cas9 system with chimeric antigen receptor-extracellular vesicles against B-cell malignancies. *J Control Release* 326: 455–467.
93. Jinek, M., Chylinski, K., Fonfara, I. et al. (2012). A programmable dual-RNA-guided DNA endonuclease in adaptive bacterial immunity. *Science* 337 (6096): 816–821.
94. Doudna, J.A. and Charpentier, E. (2014). Genome editing. The new frontier of genome engineering with CRISPR-Cas9. *Science* 346 (6213): 1258096.
95. Zetsche, B., Gootenberg, J.S., Abudayyeh, O.O. et al. (2015). Cpf1 is a single RNA-guided endonuclease of a class 2 CRISPR-Cas system. *Cell* 163 (3): 759–771.
96. Anzalone, A.V., Koblan, L.W., and Liu, D.R. (2020). Genome editing with CRISPR-Cas nucleases, base editors, transposases and prime editors. *Nat Biotechnol* 38 (7): 824–844.
97. Binnewies, M., Roberts, E.W., Kersten, K. et al. (2018). Understanding the tumor immune microenvironment (TIME) for effective therapy. *Nat Med* 24 (5): 541–550.
98. Su, S., Zou, Z., Chen, F. et al. (2017). CRISPR-Cas9-mediated disruption of PD-1 on human T cells for adoptive cellular therapies of EBV positive gastric cancer. *Oncoimmunology* 6 (1): e1249558.
99. Eyquem, J., Mansilla-Soto, J., Giavridis, T. et al. (2017). Targeting a CAR to the TRAC locus with CRISPR/Cas9 enhances tumour rejection. *Nature* 543 (7643): 113–117.
100. Delconte, R.B., Kolesnik, T.B., Dagley, L.F. et al. (2016). CIS is a potent checkpoint in NK cell-mediated tumor immunity. *Nat Immunol* 17 (7): 816–824.
101. Bexte, T., Alzubi, J., Reindl, L.M. et al. (2022). CRISPR-Cas9 based gene editing of the immune checkpoint NKG2A enhances NK cell mediated cytotoxicity against multiple myeloma. *Oncoimmunology* 11 (1): 2081415.
102. Tsai, S.Q. and Joung, J.K. (2016). Defining and improving the genome-wide specificities of CRISPR-Cas9 nucleases. *Nat Rev Genet* 17 (5): 300–312.
103. Smith, C., Gore, A., Yan, W. et al. (2014). Whole-genome sequencing analysis reveals high specificity of CRISPR/Cas9 and TALEN-based genome editing in human iPSCs. *Cell Stem Cell* 15 (1): 12–13.
104. Haapaniemi, E., Botla, S., Persson, J. et al. (2018). CRISPR-Cas9 genome editing induces a p53-mediated DNA damage response. *Nat Med* 24 (7): 927–930.
105. Charlesworth, C.T., Deshpande, P.S., Dever, D.P. et al. (2019). Identification of preexisting adaptive immunity to Cas9 proteins in humans. *Nat Med* 25 (2): 249–254.
106. Pallares-Masmitja, M., Ivancic, D., Mir-Pedrol, J. et al. (2021). Find and cut-and-transfer (FiCAT) mammalian genome engineering. *Nat Commun* 12 (1): 7071.
107. Jumper, J., Evans, R., Pritzel, A. et al. (2021). Highly accurate protein structure prediction with AlphaFold. *Nature* 596 (7873): 583–589.
108. Weng, S., Yang, X., Yu, N. et al. (2024). Harnessing ADAR-mediated site-specific RNA editing in immune-related disease: prediction and therapeutic implications. *Int J Mol Sci* 25 (1): 351.

PART

V

Advanced Immunotherapy Techniques and Applications

15

Personalised Immunotherapy and Biomarker-Driven Approaches

NAOMI BERRELL[1,2], DENISE GOH[3], CLARA LAWLER[2], MEG L. DONOVAN[1,2], JOE YEONG[3,4,5,6], AND ARUTHA KULASINGHE[1,2]

[1] Queensland Spatial Biology Centre, Wesley Research Institute, The Wesley Hospital, Brisbane, Queensland, Australia

[2] Faculty of Health, Medicine and Behavioural Sciences, Frazer Institute, The University of Queensland, Brisbane, Queensland, Australia

[3] Institute of Molecular and Cell Biology (IMCB), Agency for Science, Technology and Research (A*STAR), Singapore, Singapore

[4] Department of Anatomical Pathology, Singapore General Hospital, Singapore, Singapore

[5] Department of Microbiology, Singapore General Hospital, Singapore, Singapore

[6] Duke-NUS Medical School, Singapore, Singapore

LEARNING OBJECTIVES

- Tumour microenvironment profiling and biomarkers.
- Established and emerging spatial technologies and their applications.
- Current challenges of working with spatial data.
- How multi-omic integration and deep learning will contribute to biomarker discovery.

15.1 INTRODUCTION

Modern medical research advancements have seen the standardisation of whole genome sequencing in clinical and non-clinical settings and have evolved from bulk sequencing, measuring the average analyte expression across a sample, to single cell sequencing, measuring the analyte expression of each cell in a sample, to now spatial sequencing technologies. To gain deeper insights into effective cancer therapeutics, we need a comprehensive understanding of the underlying tumour microenvironment (TME). The TME consists of a dynamic milieu of structural and immune cells interacting to maintain the tumour and associated stromal tissue. Single-cell technologies have enabled valuable insights into disease states, but the loss of key cellular interactions through tissue dissociation has been recovered by spatial technologies. Modern methods are capable of capturing hundreds to thousands of molecular readouts while simultaneously maintaining their tissue location (Figure 15.1).

These spatial profiling tools, paired with deep learning and artificial intelligence (AI) approaches, are rapidly changing the way researchers are able to understand the TME. This chapter will explore the evolution and current landscape of spatial biology techniques and their applications for immunotherapy and biomarker profiling. Specifically, this chapter will focus on spatial transcriptomics (ST), proteomics, metabolomics, epigenomics, and 'multi-omic' integration.

The location of cells within the context of tissue or disease is important in understanding the function or effect that these cells have. For example, within the TME, identifying whether certain immune cells have infiltrated the tumour, and to what

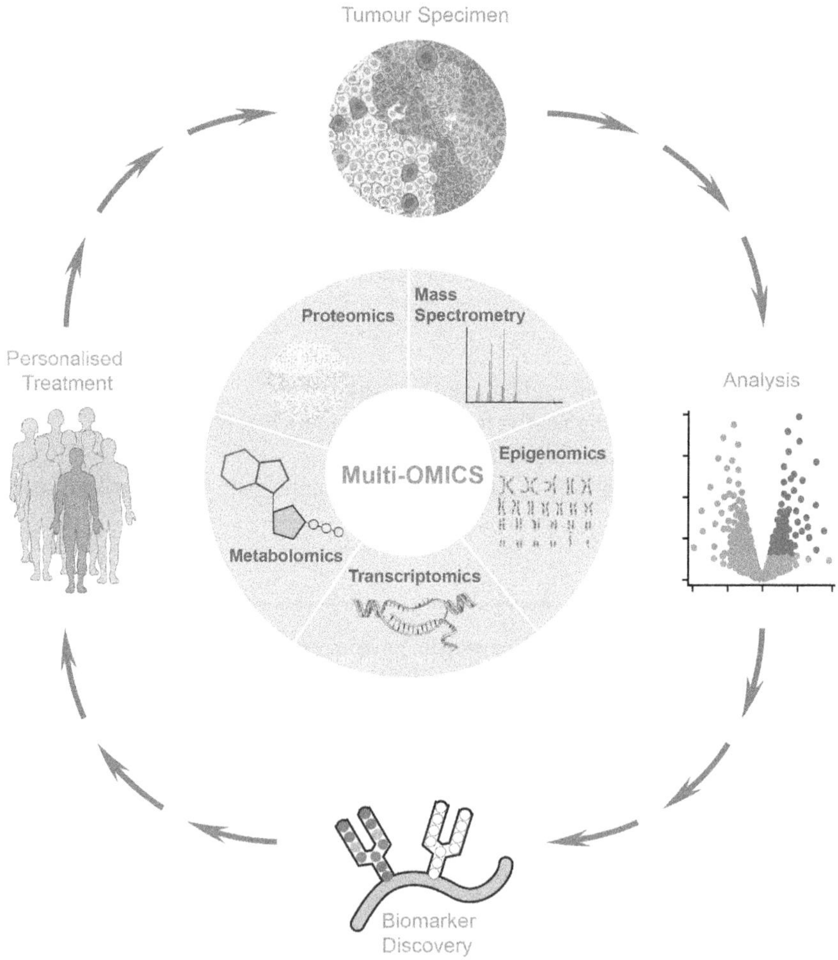

FIGURE 15.1 High plex multi-omic profiling and integration are driving biomarker discovery and enabling advancements in personalised treatment. Development of omic technologies is enabling scientists to better understand the complexities of biology and decipher the driving factors that are contributing disease outcomes. In particular, integrating different modalities provides a more comprehensive insight into basic biology and immune activity.

extent, could have significant implications for therapy response and disease outcomes. This is important due to tissue heterogeneity, where one region may experience tumour infiltration while another region could display immune exclusion, leading to partial responses throughout the tumour. These clinical insights would not be identifiable or might be misinterpreted by looking exclusively at cellular counts or readouts and not their location. Spatial profiling methods include investigating the spatial distribution of RNA, proteins, metabolites, and epigenomic readouts. Systems biology and AI undoubtedly enable more streamlined biomarker discovery. This chapter will explore prominent omic techniques, how they can be integrated to accelerate biomarker discovery and personalise therapies, and the current challenges that come with large and complex datasets. The convergence of omic technologies into multi-omic integration promises to capture the complexities in genotype, phenotype, and overall environment of disease states that might dictate the most appropriate intervention.

15.2 SPATIAL TRANSCRIPTOMICS

ST was named the 'Method of the Year' in 2020 by Nature Methods, and provides an unbiased overview of the mRNA composition of intact tissue sections, demonstrating potential in identifying tumour-immune interactions and in the generation of tissue/disease-specific molecular maps [1]. It has evolved through technological breakthroughs, enabling the readout of mRNA using sequencing or imaging-based modalities [2].

Whole-transcriptome profiling of tissue samples using sequencing-based readouts can be achieved using the GeoMx Digital Spatial Profiler (Bruker Spatial Biology), Visium and Visium HD (10x Genomics, USA), Curio Seeker (Curio Biosciences), and SpaTial Enhanced Resolution Omics-sequencing (Stereo-seq; BGI, China). Each device has a different core technology, resolution, tissue preparation requirement, and mRNA coverage, described in Table 15.1. Visium and Stereo-seq integrate spatially barcoded arrays with next-generation sequencing to map the location and expression levels of transcripts within tissues. Visium uses RNA-binding probes attached to an array of approximately 5000 barcoded spots that are spaced 100 μm apart. Stereo-seq uses DNA nanoball technology for in situ RNA capture, achieving near sub-cellular resolution with spot sizes of 0.22 μm spaced 0.5 μm apart. Both techniques have advanced cancer research: Visium revealed spatial archetypes of triple-negative breast cancer (TNBC) with distinct molecular profiles that impact immunotherapy response [3], and identified a novel T-cell state that drives immunotherapy resistance [4]. With increased barcoding density, Visium HD enabled spatial mapping of distinct macrophage subpopulations in different tumour niches and the identification of a clonally expanded T-cell population within an anti-tumour macrophage-rich niche [5]. Stereo-seq identified invasive zones in liver cancer that promote immune suppression and tumour progression [6], and developed a spatial transcriptome atlas of colorectal cancer in immunotherapy-treated patients, revealing an association between the spatial organisation of tumour-stroma boundary and treatment responsiveness [7]. The SpaTial Enhanced Resolution single-cell sequencing (Stereo-cell) pipeline evolved from Stereo-seq technology, seeing high-throughput profiling, improved cell segmentation and doublet exclusion, cell type

TABLE 15.1 Overview of spatial transcriptomics and current capabilities of technologies.

Platform	Technology	Resolution	Tissue Types	mRNA Coverage
GeoMx DSP	Barcoding with UV-cleavable oligos (Sequencing)	Region/area specific up to 660 μm	FF and FFPE	Targeted (cancer transcriptome atlas), whole transcriptome (WTA), and 1,200 proteins (DPA)
Visium	Spot-based detection (Sequencing)	55 μm	FF and FFPE	Whole transcriptome
Visium HD	Spot-based detection (Sequencing)	5 μm	FF and FFPE	Whole transcriptome
Stereo-seq	DNA nanoball arrays (Sequencing)	1 μm	FF	Whole transcriptome (v2)
Curio Seeker	Slide-seq technology	10 μm	FF	Whole transcriptome
MERSCOPE	Error-robust barcoding (Imaging)	100 nm/pixel	FF and FFPE	Up to 1,000 custom genes
CosMx SMI	Single-molecule imaging (Imaging)	Sub-cellular	FF and FFPE	1,000, 6,000, whole transcriptome
Xenium	ISH and ISS (Imaging)	0.2 μm/pixel	FF and FFPE	Up to 5,000 genes

identification, and rare cell detection [8]. GeoMx, Visium, and Stereo-seq technologies are widely adopted, and analytical tools are readily available, including Space Ranger for Visium data and StandR for GeoMx [9].

Recently developed imaging-based ST enables sequencing-free detection and visualisation of RNA molecules directly from intact tissues using transcript detection in situ through fluorescently labelled probes that bind to unique RNA sequences. Technologies that leverage fluorescent in situ hybridisation (FISH) or in situ sequencing (ISS) as their core foundation include CosMx SMI (Bruker Spatial Biology, USA), MERSCOPE (Vizgen, UK), and Xenium (10× Genomics, USA). The barcodes are decoded computationally, providing *x*, *y*, and *z* coordinates for transcripts. These datasets are often quite large (gigabytes to terabytes per slide) and require extensive computational resources for storage and analysis. Combination with single-molecule fluorescence imaging (smFISH) provides quantitative insights into the spatial localisation of RNA within individual cells [10]. Xenium combines ISH and ISS to first hybridize the padlock probe to an RNA transcript, followed by signal amplification, detection, and imaging [11]. The application of ST techniques on clinical samples is enabling a deeper understanding of the TME and identifying novel biomarkers. In a hepatocellular carcinoma study, mature dendritic cells preferentially localised within immune niches, closely interacting with other immune cell types [12]. In breast cancer, CosMx Whole Transcriptome identified two distinct tumour regions, each subdivided into subregions with unique and shared gene expression profiles [13]. The integration of a Xenium dataset with H&E and immunofluorescence (IF) staining found region-specific stromal compositions linked to immune response, tumour progression, and tumour-suppressive properties [14]. Assessing the TME of NSCLC, Xenium revealed anti-tumoral $CXCL9^+$ and $CXCL13^+$ cells that localise around tumour cells after combination treatment of anti-PD-L1 and radiotherapy [15].

Although ST can provide critical insights into gene expression patterns and cellular organisation, it captures only one layer of biological regulation. Proteins, as the direct targets of most therapies, offer a complementary dimension that cannot be inferred solely from RNA.

15.3 SPATIAL PROTEOMICS

Spatial proteomics was named 'Method of the Year' in 2024 by Nature Methods, and underscores its potential for addressing key gaps left by traditional methods, primarily by preserving spatial information [16]. It refers to a collection of methodologies and technologies that can detect a multitude of proteins expressed in the same fixed tissue section, either by sequential immunofluorescence or by mass spectrometry. This method offers an unprecedented level of spatial resolution, revealing intricate details of tissue architecture, cell–cell communication, immune signalling pathways, and tumour-specific antigen presentation. Spatial proteomics is distinct from traditional technologies such as immunohistochemistry (IHC) and immunofluorescence (IF), which have limited multiplexing capabilities, enabling the investigation of many cell types and processes simultaneously.

Conventional IHC remains the gold standard for diagnosis of tissue pathology despite having high inter-observer variability as a single-marker technique. Various PD-L1 IHC assays have been approved as a companion diagnostic to predict immune checkpoint blockade responsiveness. However, as demonstrated in gastric cancer, different PD-L1 assays can influence the eligibility for immunotherapy [17]. In identifying other biomarkers with predictive value, IHC scoring of CD38 in the TME predicts immune checkpoint inhibitor (ICI) responsiveness with superior overall survival in liver cancer [18]. Combined with multiplex IHC (mIHC), CD38 expression was observed to co-localise with CD68, a macrophage lineage marker [19]. While IHC demonstrated that prognostic and predictive value of CD38, mIHC further revealed that CD38 was predictive only in patients with viral hepatitis, while LAG-3 and CD8 expression correlated with ICI responsiveness regardless of viral status [20]. Enabling the investigation of multiplex biomarkers (up to 100) on a single slide, mIHC can be used to explore the TME comprehensively [21]. With moderate-to-strong correlations in PD-L1 positivity between results obtained through mIHC and IHC, mIHC also represents a promising tool in cancer immunotherapy [22]. Additional spatial analysis, including localisation, structure-based, distance, ligand-receptor, and neighbourhood analysis, can further inform cellular localisation, interaction, and spatial signatures predictive of therapeutic response [23]. Platforms, including COMET (Lunaphore Technologies, Switzerland), PhenoCycler (Akoya Biosciences, USA), and MICS (Miltenyi Biotec, Germany), have also been developed to facilitate comprehensive immune characterisation by offering ultra-high plex (>300) capabilities [24]. For instance, COMET leverages an automated sequential workflow to stain and image 40 markers on a single tissue, under 24 hours, to visualise the TME with spatial information between tissue structure and cellular distribution [25, 26].

Other multiplex approaches are based on the use of metal-tagged antibodies; regardless of how the metals are extracted, both imaging mass cytometry (IMC) and multiplexed ion beam imaging (MIBI) allow simultaneous, spatially resolved, and highly multiplexed protein measurement directly in intact tissue [24]. IMC quantification of 35 proteins in pre-treated melanoma showed that CD45RO + Ki67 + CD8+ T-cell abundance and its proximity to melanoma cells were positively associated with ICI response [27], whereas MIBI profiling of 36 proteins in TNBC revealed distinct tumour–immune archetypes defined by cellular composition, spatial organisation, and regulatory protein expression, which correlated with overall survival [28]. MIBI also demonstrated similar robustness, sensitivity, and reproducibility when compared to IHC stains [29]. Furthermore, advanced mass spectrometry (MS)-based techniques leverage laser capture microdissection (LCM) to isolate defined cell populations from conventionally stained (i.e. H&E and IHC) tissues for region-specific tissue analysis using high-sensitivity MS [30]. This process allows identification of proteins that can be mapped back to their original spatial context. Comparable to PD-L1 IHC assays, LCM-based workflow was also used to quantify PD-L1 expression in various micro-dissected tumours, showcasing its unique ability to capture immune checkpoint molecules on a continuous quantitative scale [31].

Although the development of SP came after ST, its rapid progression underscores its value in capturing the functional state of cells. Its integration with transcriptomic data represents the next frontier in decoding tumour heterogeneity.

15.4 METABOLOMICS

Dysregulated metabolic behaviour of malignant cells can impact both malignant and host immune cells, alter the TME to be inhospitable for immune cells through excreting harmful metabolites and depleting the TME of essential nutrients. This leads to an arms race between tumour and non-tumour cells to survive in these harsh environments. Understanding how specific metabolic and drug patterns influence immune cell activity could assist in predicting the success of immunotherapies [32, 33].

Typically, spatial metabolic profiling uses adaptations of MS techniques or is inferred through transcriptomic and/or proteomic profiles. MS is capable of profiling the metabolic activity of tissues, cells, organs, and exogenous metabolites, such as drugs and pathogenic molecules (Table 15.2). These techniques are particularly powerful when paired with other omic techniques. Compared to bulk protocols, these methods face challenges with coverage depth and amplification due to the decrease in signal that occurs when increasing resolution. Due to volatile nature of metabolome, successful experiments should process samples synchronously with a minimum of 100–1,000 cells each. Other challenges include minimising background noise and sample-to-sample variability, as differences in sample preparation and storage can drastically impact the metabolic profile. Automation of sample preparation and continued development of laser and ion beam technologies should help to minimise these challenges [34].

TABLE 15.2 Characteristics, applications, and considerations of prominent spatial metabolomic techniques.

Technique	Concept	Resolution	Coverage	Considerations
MALDI-MSI (Matrix-assisted desorption ionisation)	Laser rastered across sample after matrix has been applied to tissue surface.	Single cell (if optimised for resolution). 5 μm	Unbiased characterisation of lipids, small metabolites, and protein	Complicated tissue preparation. Resolution can be optimised but may reduce the coverage depth. Tissue non-destructive
DESI-MSI (Desorption electro spray ionisation. Ambient liquid-extraction)	Spray of charged solvents	10 μm	lipids, steroids, metabolites, glycans, proteoforms, proteins, drugs, and drug metabolites	Non-tissue destructive and no sample pre-treatment. Ambient technique
SIMS-TOF (Time-of-flight mass spectrometry. Profiling of secondary ions released from tissue)	Ion beam rastered across sample – secondary ions measured by MS	10–100 nm (~10 nm^3)	Cholesterol, lipids, metals, and non-metals. (Dependent on the primary ion used)	Results can only be interpreted in a semi-quantitative way. Relatively soft ionisation means tissue is less damaged. Cholesterol measurement. Can achieve 3D profiling

Matrix-assisted laser desorption ionisation mass spectrometry imaging (MALDIMSI) involves the application of a matrix on top of the tissue that is used to extract molecules from the tissue [35]. To create a spatial readout, the laser is rastered across the matrix layer where a mass spectrometry read out is generated for each 'spot', allowing the tissue to remain intact for additional assays or histological assessment. The resolution is determined by protocol and instrument optimisation, and while this typically ranges between 20 and 200 μm, newer approaches have been able to achieve readouts to 5–10 μm [35, 36]. Depending on the protocol stage that is optimised, there is a trade-off between resolution and number of captured analytes. Primary limitations of MALDI-MSI approaches arise due to the length and complexity of workflow, introducing delocalisation. In 2024, an updated approach included laser-induced post-ionisation (MALDI-2), which aims to improve the yield of analytes retrieved from small pixel sizes [36].

Desorption electrospray ionisation mass spectrometry imaging (DESI-MSI) creates mass spectrometry readouts by, under ambient conditions, rastering charged solvent droplets that are carried by nebulising gas across the surface of the tissue, causing desorption and ionisation of molecules present on the tissue surface [37, 38]. Because DESI-MSI does not require sample pre-treatment and is non-destructive, it offers a more accessible spatial metabolomic profiling solution and allows same-slide integration of other assays [37]. These molecules are then processed by a mass spectrometer through an atmospheric pressure inlet and registered to the spot's location [37]. Advancements of this technique include nanospray DESI (nano-DESI), which uses ambient liquid-extraction-based ionisation and can capture metabolic readout down to a resolution of 10 μm [38].

Imaging time-of-flight secondary ion mass spectrometry (ToF-SIMS) can capture sub-micron spatial-metabolic information, can detect a lateral resolution of ~100 nm, and has the capability to capture 3D readout information. A beam of primary ions is concentrated onto one spot at a time, and secondary ions in the samples are released and profiled by MS [39, 40]. The primary ions can be elemental, but polyatomic primary ions have been shown to improve organic compound profiling and reduce sample destruction [41]. One benefit of ToF-SIMS is that, due to the relatively soft ionisation beam, fragmentation of the sample is reduced. TOF-SIMS has been reported to be particularly effective in measuring cholesterol expression, a molecule that is notoriously difficult to screen with other techniques [42]. Users should consider that results are limited by being only semi-quantitative in nature and that analytes, especially large molecules, may become fragmented, potentially complicating the interpretation of results [41].

15.5 EPIGENOMICS

Modifications to DNA, without altering the DNA sequence itself, and to associated histones, have emerged as a crucial branch in cancer research [43]. Environmental factors, such as aging and disease progression, trigger epigenetic modifications that have significant contributions to oncogenesis and are recognised as a hallmark of cancer. DNA methylation can silence tumour suppressor genes, permitting uncontrolled cellular proliferation. Histone post-translational modifications alter accessible chromatin and thus gene transcription. Epitranscriptomics moves beyond chromatin alterations, adding a further layer of control over gene expression through RNA methylation and altered expression of non-coding RNAs, which disrupt normal gene regulation to promote cancer cell proliferation, invasion, and metastasis. The reversibility of epigenetic changes presents unique therapeutic opportunities, targeting the source of dysregulation to overcome treatment resistance in combination with therapeutic approaches. DNA methyltransferase inhibitors were pioneer epigenetic drugs (azacitidine and decitabine); however, high toxicity (thrombocytopenia and neutropenia) makes these nucleotide analogues biologically unsuitable. Histone deacetylase inhibitors (vorinostat, romidepsin) have limited value when used alone but have shown benefit in combination therapy (tucidinostat) [44]. The most recent targetable proteins, born from better understanding of epigenetics, are histone methyltransferase inhibitors, lysine demethylase inhibitors, and bromodomain inhibitors, demonstrating synergy between immunotherapy and epigenetic therapy [45, 46].

The convergence of epigenomics and spatial biology offers new opportunities for using dynamic gene regulation pathways to inform treatment outcomes. Spatial profiling of immune cell fate using spatial epigenomics has been possible through recent advancements in technology, allowing genome-wide mapping of chromatin states within specific tissue microenvironments in specific disease states. Taking T cells as an example, their differentiation is highly dependent on chromatin remodelling to dictate lineage and effector function. The $CD8^+$ T-cell exhaustion phenotype, suggested to be mediated by de novo DNA methylation, greatly hinders ICI response. Resistance to ICI is poorly understood and might be explained by 'epigenetic scars' at immune checkpoint loci, where chronic tumour antigen presentation results in synchronised histone methylation and acetylation, which persist despite checkpoint blockade.

Single-cell studies afford insights into profiling of epigenetic modification, but cell dissociation required for these techniques leads to loss of spatial context. Adopting key concepts into FFPE tissue conserves these interactions; the resulting transcriptional plasticity can be mapped to cells within a tissue sample in situ to better understand changes in gene expression. These changes can be localised to specific cell types within the TME to define a cell type-specific gene expression profile. By mapping the coordinates of each defined cell, computational analysis of tumour samples captures a snapshot of the epigenomic landscape, providing an opportunity for new therapeutic targets.

FISH provides gene expression profiles at single-cell resolution using sequential rounds of probe hybridisation. Multiplexed error-robust fluorescence *in situ* hybridisation (MERFISH) was developed to overcome the limitations of FISH. Extensive cross-linking through formalin fixation in FFPE tissue can obstruct chromatin accessibility necessary for epigenetic probing. The spatial assay for transposase-accessible chromatin and RNA using sequencing (ATAC-RNA-seq), which introduces key optimisation to facilitate access [47], and the spatial assay of cleavage under targets and tagmentation and RNA using sequencing (CUT&Tag-RNA-seq) [48] are dual omics approaches allowing correlation of open chromatin regions and transcriptional activity. Epigenetic proximity hybridisation reaction (Epi-PHR) has allowed single-cell three-dimensional organisation of the epigenome to be profiled [49].

Cancer cells coordinate epigenetic reprogramming to facilitate immune evasion. ICIs such as PD-1 are upregulated through DNA methylation. Cancer cells can silence intracellular antigen processing machinery, thus reducing tumour immunogenicity, as well as suppressing MHC-I expression to reduce T-cell recognition and cytotoxicity by gene promoter hypermethylation. Chromatin accessibility patterns vary across tumour neighbourhoods and immune infiltration zones. Tailoring individual therapeutic approaches to maximise treatment efficacy and minimise treatment toxicity remains the overall aim of precision medicine. Patients may share the same gene variant but exhibit significant differences in treatment response, highlighting a shift towards comprehensive genetic and epigenetic diagnostic profiling.

15.6 CHALLENGES AND CONTROVERSIES

Multi-omic technologies allow large amounts of information to be captured from a single sample, enabling rapid gains in biological understanding. Big data, however, comes with inherent limitations, including accessibility of computing resources to allow for storage of large datasets and power required to perform data analysis, development of statistically robust analysis approaches. The high cost-per-slide is another hindrance, contributing to studies with small sample sizes that are not large enough to overcome the statistical implications introduced by large feature-sets during false-discovery-rate correction.

Integrating technologies, such as ST with spatial proteomics, enables workflows that can provide insights into cellular function, heterogeneity, and interaction mechanisms within native tissue contexts [50, 51]. Metabolomic techniques lack cell-type-specific identifiers, meaning that interpreting cell-specific metabolic correlations is difficult, but multi-omic integration offers an approach to overcome this limitation. Based on the current speed of computational, AI, and bioinformatic advancement, the integration and interpretation of these complex datasets will likely soon become streamlined [52], with researchers developing their own multi-omic workflows. Spatial CITE-seq, an extension of CITE-seq, includes spatial resolution by using barcoded surface-capture approach to simultaneously profile protein and whole transcriptomes on a single tissue slide [53]. In human tissue, spatial CITE-seq revealed spatially distinct germinal centre reactions in the tonsil and early immune activation in the skin at mRNA vaccination site. By combining single-cell CITE-seq with single-nuclei sequencing, ST, and SP, Guilliams et al. presented a spatial proteogenomic atlas of healthy and obese human and murine liver, uncovering evolutionarily conserved and spatially restricted signals driving distinct hepatic macrophage phenotypes [54].

To fully leverage multi-omics integration, AI-driven analyses are emerging to align and dissect complex datasets for comprehensive TME overview that enables the discovery of clinically actionable insights. Further description of AI-driven TME analyses is discussed below.

15.7 FUTURE DIRECTIONS

By comparing disease and control groups, researchers can understand mechanisms of disease that can be further stratified into response groups. These detailed insights could inform future directions for novel therapeutics and screening tests. While the direct application of these techniques in the clinic may be currently unfeasible, their role in discovery realigns existing clinical workflow and diagnostic tests. AI integration in analytic pipelines has helped overcome the complexity of interpreting multi-omics datasets by reducing inter- and intra-observer variability while providing a holistic view of disease pathophysiology and supporting cancer precision medicine through automated cell/tissue segmentation, cell/biomarker detection and prediction, and prognostic analysis [55, 56].

Applications of AI integration have been shown to assist with more sensitive identification of cancerous regions and prediction of tumour progression [57–59]. Other applications include the ‘H&E 2.0’ concept that leverages AI to extract molecular and cellular information from routinely acquired H&E images to generate virtual stains trained on multiplexed IHC data [60]. This approach demonstrated success in identifying tumour-specific $CD39^{+}CD8^{+}$ T cells in marker-free images to predict immunotherapy response [61]. H&E 2.0 has extended to transcriptome prediction through RNA sequencing and/or ST data [62, 63]. At the protein level, AI has also enabled cell type-resolved proteomics through approaches such as deep visual proteomics. By integrating high-resolution imaging, AI-guided cell segmentation, laser microdissection, and ultra-high sensitive mass spectrometry, enabling spatially informed and cell type-specific comparison of proteomic profiles [64–66].

15.8 CASE STUDIES AND REAL-WORLD EXAMPLES

Translating spatial technologies into the clinic is restricted by experimental and analytic complexities, as well as by cost. Recent years have seen rapid method and technology development in the field, with most effort focused on data generation as opposed to translation into the clinic. But with many new studies revealing potential novel biomarkers, we may begin seeing more translation into clinical settings. For example, an AI-powered spatial immune scoring system was developed using five biomarkers identified through spatial proteogenomic approaches to predict liver cancer recurrence [56]. Using standard pathological images, the scoring system generates a personalised recurrence risk score for each patient and was able to predict anti-PD-1 treatment response in a group of patients. This flavour of research has the power to stratify patients based on their TME profile, into appropriate clinical recruitment, predict therapeutic outcomes, and highlight novel drug targets. A recent example of spatial multi-omic translation is the development of an FDA-approved predictive signature for drug sensitivity in ovarian cancer. This panel was developed for use in the clinical trial of the CHK1/2 inhibitor therapy, ACR-368, to predict patients who are likely to respond to the treatment [67].

KEY TERMS & DEFINITIONS SIDEBAR

Transcriptomics The study of all RNA within a cell or sample (dependent on technologies resolution capability).

Proteomics The study of all protein species within a cell or sample (dependent on technologies resolution capability).

Metabolomics The study of the collection of small molecules or metabolites found in a cell or system.

Epigenomics The study of DNA modifications, these alter gene expression and cellular behaviour.

Raster The process of scanning across a sample to create a grid of pixels.

Mass spectrometry An analytical process that measures the mass-to-charge ratio of molecules collected from a sample.

Haematoxylin and eosin (H&E) A widely used histological stain used to visualise cells and tissue structures and assist with diagnosis of some diseases. Two dyes, haematoxylin (blue – staining the nucleus and nucleic acids) and eosin (pink – cytoplasm and proteins), stain different cellular compartments enabling the inspection of important histology.

Immunohistochemistry (IHC) Laboratory technique that uses antibodies to detect specific proteins (antigens) present in cells.

Immunofluorescence (IF) Laboratory technique that uses antibodies joined with fluorescent dye to detect proteins present on cells.

LIST OF ABBREVIATIONS

3D	three dimensional
AI	artificial intelligence
ATAC-RNA-seq	transposase-accessible chromatin and RNA using sequencing
CDx	cluster differentiation x
CITE-seq	cellular indexing of transcriptomes and epitopes by sequencing
CUT&Tag-RNA-seq	cleavage under targets and tagmentation and RNA using sequencing
CXCL	chemokine ligand
DESI	desorption electrospray ionisation
DNA	deoxyribonucleic acid
DSP	digital spatial profiler
Epi-PHR	epigenetic proximity hybridisation reaction
FDA	food and drug administration
FF	fresh frozen
FFPE	formalin fixed paraffin embedded
FISH	fluorescent in situ hybridisation
H&E	haematoxylin & eosin
ICI	immune checkpoint inhibitor
IF	immunofluorescence
IHC	immunohistochemistry
IMC	imaging mass cytometry
ISH	in situ hybridisation
ISS	in situ sequencing
LAG3	lymphocyte activation gene −3
LCM	laser capture microdissection
MALDI	matrix-assisted laser desorption ionisation
MERFISH	multiplexed error-robust fluorescence in situ hybridisation
MHC-I	major histocompatibility complex
MIBI	multiplexed ion beam imaging
mRNA	messenger ribonucleic acid
MS	mass spectrometry
MSI	mass spectrometry imaging
NSCLC	non-small cell lung cancer
PD-L1	programmed death ligand 1
RNA	ribonucleic acid
smFISH	single-molecule fluorescence in situ hybridisation
ST	spatial transcriptomics
TIM3	T-cell immunoglobulin and mucin domain-containing protein 3
TME	tumour microenvironment
TOF-SIMS	time of flight–secondary ion mass spectrometry
TNBC	triple-negative breast cancer

REVIEW QUESTIONS

1. Explain the main differences between spatial proteomics and spatial transcriptomics.
2. How is spatial proteomics different from traditional IHC?
3. What is metabolomics, and what is a potential application of this approach?
4. Does epigenomics examine heritable or non-heritable changes in the transcriptome? What are the main proteins targeted for this technique?
5. What spatial biology approach would you choose to implement and why?

REFERENCES

1. Method of the Year (2020). spatially resolved transcriptomics. *Nat Methods* 2021 (18): 1.
2. Lee, R.Y., Ng, C.W., Rajapakse, M.P. et al. (2023). The promise and challenge of spatial omics in dissecting tumour microenvironment and the role of AI. *Front Oncol* 13: 1172314.
3. Wang, X., Venet, D., Lifrange, F. et al. (2024). Spatial transcriptomics reveals substantial heterogeneity in triple-negative breast cancer with potential clinical implications. *Nat Commun* 15 (1): 10232.
4. Chu, Y., Dai, E., Li, Y. et al. (2023). Pan-cancer T cell atlas links a cellular stress response state to immunotherapy resistance. *Nat Med* 29 (6): 1550–1562.
5. Oliveira, M.F., Romero, J.P., Chung, M. et al. (2025). High-definition spatial transcriptomic profiling of immune cell populations in colorectal cancer. *Nat Genet* 57 (6): 1512–1523.
6. Wu, L., Yan, J., Bai, Y. et al. (2023). An invasive zone in human liver cancer identified by Stereo-seq promotes hepatocyte-tumor cell crosstalk, local immunosuppression and tumor progression. *Cell Res* 33 (8): 585–603.
7. Feng, Y., Ma, W., Zang, Y. et al. (2024). Spatially organized tumor-stroma boundary determines the efficacy of immunotherapy in colorectal cancer patients. *Nat Commun* 15 (1): 10259.
8. Zhao, Y., Li, Y., He, Y. et al. (2025). Stereo-seq V2: spatial mapping of total RNA on FFPE sections with high resolution. *Cell* 188: 6554–6571.e21.
9. Liu, N., Bhuva, D.D., Mohamed, A. et al. (2024). standR: spatial transcriptomic analysis for GeoMx DSP data. *Nucleic Acids Res* 52 (1): e2.
10. Jin, Y., Zuo, Y., Li, G. et al. (2024). Advances in spatial transcriptomics and its applications in cancer research. *Mol Cancer* 23 (1): 129.
11. Lim, H.J., Wang, Y., Buzdin, A., and Li, X. (2025). A practical guide for choosing an optimal spatial transcriptomics technology from seven major commercially available options. *BMC Genomics* 26 (1): 47.
12. Magen, A., Hamon, P., Fiaschi, N. et al. (2023). Intratumoral dendritic cell-CD4(+) T helper cell niches enable CD8(+) T cell differentiation following PD-1 blockade in hepatocellular carcinoma. *Nat Med* 29 (6): 1389–1399.
13. Patrick, M., He, S., Ilcisin, S. et al. (2024). Abstract 3644: uncover spatial signatures of tumor microenvironment and oncogenic pathways using 6,000-plex single-cell spatial molecular imaging on FFPE skin squamous cell carcinoma. *Cancer Res* 84 (6_Supplement): 3644.
14. Janesick, A., Shelansky, R., Gottscho, A.D. et al. (2023). High resolution mapping of the tumor microenvironment using integrated single-cell, spatial and in situ analysis. *Nat Commun* 14 (1): 8353.
15. Sakai, S.A., Oyoshi, H., Nakamura, M. et al. (2025). Single-cell spatial analysis with Xenium reveals anti-tumour responses of CXCL13 + T and CXCL9+ cells after radiotherapy combined with anti-PD-L1 therapy. *Br J Cancer* 133 (6): 795–808.
16. (2024). Method of the Year 2024: spatial proteomics. *Nat Methods* 21 (12): 2195–2196.

17. Yeong, J., Lum, H.Y.J., Teo, C.B. et al. (2022). Choice of PD-L1 immunohistochemistry assay influences clinical eligibility for gastric cancer immunotherapy. *Gastric Cancer* 25 (4): 741–750.
18. Ng, H.H.M., Lee, R.Y., Goh, S. et al. (2020). Immunohistochemical scoring of CD38 in the tumor microenvironment predicts responsiveness to anti-PD-1/PD-L1 immunotherapy in hepatocellular carcinoma. *J Immunother Cancer* 8 (2): e000987.
19. Lam, J.H., Ng, H.H.M., Lim, C.J. et al. (2019). Expression of CD38 on macrophages predicts improved prognosis in hepatocellular carcinoma. *Front Immunol* 10: 2093.
20. Cheung, C.C.L., Seah, Y.H.J., Fang, J. et al. (2023). Immunohistochemical scoring of LAG-3 in conjunction with CD8 in the tumor microenvironment predicts response to immunotherapy in hepatocellular carcinoma. *Front Immunol* 14: 1150985.
21. Fincham REA, Bashiri H, Lau MC, Yeong J. Editorial: Multiplex immunohistochemistry/immunofluorescence technique: the potential and promise for clinical application. *Front Mol Biosci* 2022;9 831382.
22. Yeong, J., Tan, T., Chow, Z.L. et al. (2020). Multiplex immunohistochemistry/immunofluorescence (mIHC/IF) for PD-L1 testing in triple-negative breast cancer: a translational assay compared with conventional IHC. *J Clin Pathol* 73 (9): 557–562.
23. Semba, T. and Ishimoto, T. (2024). Spatial analysis by current multiplexed imaging technologies for the molecular characterisation of cancer tissues. *Br J Cancer* 131 (11): 1737–1747.
24. Zhang, Y., Lee, R.Y., Tan, C.W. et al. (2024). Spatial omics techniques and data analysis for cancer immunotherapy applications. *Curr Opin Biotechnol* 87: 103111.
25. Rivest, F., Eroglu, D., Pelz, B. et al. (2023). Fully automated sequential immunofluorescence (seqIF) for hyperplex spatial proteomics. *Sci Rep* 13 (1): 16994.
26. Chong, L.Y., Wee, F., Joseph, C.R. et al. (2024). Automated hyperplex protein staining and imaging system on lung adenocarcinoma tissue using off-the-shelf primary antibodies. *World Sci Ann Rev Cancer Immunol* 01: 2430002.
27. Moldoveanu, D., Ramsay, L., Lajoie, M. et al. (2022). Spatially mapping the immune landscape of melanoma using imaging mass cytometry. *Sci Immunol* 01 (7): eabi5072.
28. Keren, L., Bosse, M., Marquez, D. et al. (2018). A structured tumor-immune microenvironment in triple negative breast cancer revealed by multiplexed ion beam imaging. *Cell* 174 (6): 1373–1387.e19.
29. Angelo, M., Bendall, S.C., Finck, R. et al. (2014). Multiplexed ion beam imaging of human breast tumors. *Nat Med* 20 (4): 436–442.
30. Hu, B., Zhu, J., and Zhao, F. (2024). The evolving landscape of spatial proteomics technologies in the AI age. *Fundam Res* 6 (1): 28–39.
31. Liotta, L.A., Pappalardo, P.A., Carpino, A. et al. (2021). Laser capture proteomics: spatial tissue molecular profiling from the bench to personalized medicine. *Expert Rev Proteomics* 18 (10): 845–861.
32. Xiao, Y., Li, Y., and Zhao, H. (2024). Spatiotemporal metabolomic approaches to the cancer-immunity panorama: a methodological perspective. *Mol Cancer* 23 (1): 202.
33. Alexandrov, T. (2023). Spatial metabolomics: from a niche field towards a driver of innovation. *Nat Metab* 5 (9): 1443–1445.
34. Min, X., Zhao, Y., Yu, M. et al. (2024). Spatially resolved metabolomics: from metabolite mapping to function visualising. *Clin Transl Med* 14 (11): e70031.
35. Aichler, M. and Walch, A. (2015). MALDI imaging mass spectrometry: current frontiers and perspectives in pathology research and practice. *Lab Invest* 95 (4): 422–431.
36. Niehaus, M., Soltwisch, J., Belov, M.E., and Dreisewerd, K. (2019). Transmission-mode MALDI-2 mass spectrometry imaging of cells and tissues at subcellular resolution. *Nat Methods* 16 (9): 925–931.
37. Zickuhr, G.M., Um, I.H., Laird, A. et al. (2024). DESI-MSI-guided exploration of metabolic-phenotypic relationships reveals a correlation between PI 38:3 and proliferating cells in

clear cell renal cell carcinoma via single-section co-registration of multimodal imaging. *Anal Bioanal Chem* 416 (18): 4015–4028.
38. Iqfath, M., Wali, S.N., Amer, S. et al. (2024). Nanospray desorption electrospray ionization mass spectrometry imaging (nano-DESI MSI): a tutorial review. *ACS Meas Sci Au* 4 (5): 475–487.
39. Paudel, B., Dhas, J.A., Zhou, Y. et al. (2024). ToF-SIMS in material research: a view from nanoscale hydrogen detection. *Mater Today* 75: 149–165.
40. Neittaanmäki, N., Zaar, O., Cehajic Kevin, S. et al. (2024). ToF-SIMS imaging reveals changes in tumor cell lipids during metastatic progression of melanoma. *Pigment Cell Melanoma Res* 37 (6): 793–800.
41. Maćkiewicz, E., Rogowski, J., and Szynkowska-Jóźwik, M.I. (2025). Application of time-of-flight secondary ion mass spectrometry (ToF-SIMS) in forensic science – a review. *Forensic Sci Int* 367: 112347.
42. Manaprasertsak, A., Kazi, J.U., Hagerling, C. et al. (2024). Alterations of the chemical profile of cholesterol in cancer tissue as traced with ToF-SIMS. *Analyst* 149 (21): 5344–5352.
43. Ji, Y., Xiao, C., Fan, T. et al. (2025). The epigenetic hallmarks of immune cells in cancer. *Mol Cancer* 24 (1): 66.
44. Zhang, W., Ge, L., Zhang, Y. et al. (2025). Targeted intervention of tumor microenvironment with HDAC inhibitors and their combination therapy strategies. *Eur J Med Res* 30 (1): 69.
45. Seneviratne, J.A., Ravindrarajah, D., Carter, D.R. et al. (2024). Combined inhibition of histone methyltransferases EZH2 and DOT1L is an effective therapy for neuroblastoma. *Cancer Med* 13 (21): e70082.
46. Wang, Z.-Q., Zhang, Z.-C., Wu, Y.-Y. et al. (2023). Bromodomain and extraterminal (BET) proteins: biological functions, diseases and targeted therapy. *Signal Transduct Target Ther* 8 (1): 420.
47. Guo, P., Chen, Y., Mao, L. et al. (2025). Spatial profiling of chromatin accessibility in formalin-fixed paraffin-embedded tissues. *Nat Commun* 16 (1): 5945.
48. Kaya-Okur, H.S., Wu, S.J., Codomo, C.A. et al. (2019). CUT&Tag for efficient epigenomic profiling of small samples and single cells. *Nat Commun* 10 (1): 1930.
49. Chen Y, Radda JSD, Alderman MH, III, et al. (2025). Non-disruptive 3D profiling of combinations of epigenetic marks in single cells. *bioRxiv*. doi: https://doi.org/10.1101/2025.06.13.659535.
50. Fan, R. (2024). Integrative spatial protein profiling with multi-omics. *Nat Methods* 21 (12): 2223–2225.
51. Liu, X., Peng, T., Xu, M. et al. (2024). Spatial multi-omics: deciphering technological landscape of integration of multi-omics and its applications. *J Hematol Oncol* 17 (1): 72.
52. Hu, T., Allam, M., Cai, S. et al. (2023). Single-cell spatial metabolomics with cell-type specific protein profiling for tissue systems biology. *Nat Commun* 14 (1): 8260.
53. Liu, Y., DiStasio, M., Su, G. et al. (2023). High-plex protein and whole transcriptome co-mapping at cellular resolution with spatial CITE-seq. *Nat Biotechnol* 41 (10): 1405–1409.
54. Guilliams, M., Bonnardel, J., Haest, B. et al. (2022). Spatial proteogenomics reveals distinct and evolutionarily conserved hepatic macrophage niches. *Cell* 185 (2): 379–396.e38.
55. Mei, T., Wang, T., and Zhou, Q. (2024). Multi-omics and artificial intelligence predict clinical outcomes of immunotherapy in non-small cell lung cancer patients. *Clin Exp Med* 24 (1): 60.
56. Jia, G., He, P., Dai, T. et al. (2025). Spatial immune scoring system predicts hepatocellular carcinoma recurrence. *Nature* 640 (8060): 1031–1041.
57. Flach, R.N., van Dooijeweert, C., Nguyen, T.Q. et al. (2025). Prospective clinical implementation of Paige prostate detect artificial intelligence assistance in the detection of prostate cancer in prostate biopsies: CONFIDENT P trial implementation of artificial intelligence assistance in prostate cancer detection. *JCO Clin Cancer Inform* 9: e2400193.
58. Perincheri, S., Levi, A.W., Celli, R. et al. (2021). An independent assessment of an artificial intelligence system for prostate cancer detection shows strong diagnostic accuracy. *Mod Pathol* 34 (8): 1588–1595.

59. Schweizer, L., Kenny, H.A., Krishnan, R. et al. (2025). Spatial proteo-transcriptomic profiling reveals the molecular landscape of borderline ovarian tumors and their invasive progression. *Cancer Cell* 43 (8): 1495–1511.e7.
60. Zhang, Y., Lee, R.Y., Joseph, C.R. et al. (2024). H&E2.0—harnessing artificial intelligence to enhance biomarker prediction using hematoxylin and eosin-stained image. *World Sci Ann Rev Cancer Immunol* 01: 2430003.
61. Felicia, W., Willa, Y., Jia, M. et al. (2023). 1311 H&E 2.0: deep learning-enabled identification of tumor-specific CD39+CD8+ T cells in marker-free images for predicting immunotherapy response. *J Immunother Cancer* 11 (Suppl 1): A1459–A1460.
62. Schmauch, B., Romagnoni, A., Pronier, E. et al. (2020). A deep learning model to predict RNA-seq expression of tumours from whole slide images. *Nat Commun* 11 (1): 3877.
63. Wang, C., Chan, A.S., Fu, X. et al. (2025). Benchmarking the translational potential of spatial gene expression prediction from histology. *Nat Commun* 16 (1): 1544.
64. Mund, A., Coscia, F., Kriston, A. et al. (2022). Deep visual proteomics defines single-cell identity and heterogeneity. *Nat Biotechnol* 40 (8): 1231–1240.
65. Nordmann, T.M., Mund, A., and Mann, M. (2024). A new understanding of tissue biology from MS-based proteomics at single-cell resolution. *Nat Methods* 21 (12): 2220–2222.
66. Rosenberger, F.A., Madler, S.C., Thorhauge, K.H. et al. (2025). Deep visual proteomics maps proteotoxicity in a genetic liver disease. *Nature* 642: 1–8.
67. Lee, J.M., MacLaughlan, S., Matei, D. et al. (2024). 744P A phase II study of ACR-368 in patients with ovarian (OvCa) or endometrial carcinoma (EnCa) and prospective validation of OncoSignature patient selection (NCT05548296). *Ann Oncol* 35: S564–S565.

CHAPTER 16

Immunotherapy and the Microbiota: Exploring Microbiota-Immune Interactions and Their Impact on Immunotherapy Efficacy

MERIEM MESSAOUDENE AND MARINE FIDELLE
Inserm UMR1367, Microbiota and Mucosal Immunity for Cancer Immunotherapy, ClinicoBiome, Université Paris-Saclay, Gustave Roussy, Villejuif, France

LEARNING OBJECTIVES

By the end of this chapter, the reader will be able to:

- Define the microbiota and understand its major physiological functions.
- Describe how the microbiota shapes the development and the education of the immune system.
- Understand the mechanisms linking the microbiota and the efficacy of immunotherapies. Identify the opportunities and challenges of microbiota-centred interventions in the therapeutic context of cancer.

16.1 INTRODUCTION

The microbiome has emerged as one of the most influential biological ecosystems in human health. The microbiome is defined as all the microorganisms, including bacteria, archaea, phages, viruses, and fungi that inhabit mucosal and epithelial surfaces, and their genomes [1]. The microbiota represents the microorganisms in the microbiome. Among these ecosystems, the gut microbiota, hosting over 10^{13} microorganisms, represents the most densely populated and the most active one [1, 2]. The role of the gut microbiota extends beyond local gastrointestinal functions, including digestion, nutrient assimilation, and intestinal barrier integrity. Indeed, it is also implicated in neuroendocrine signalling, xenobiotic metabolism [3], and immune education and maturation [4]. Multiple lines of evidence showed that the local and systemic immune system depends profoundly on microbial signals to shape its functions [5, 6]. These observations have established the importance of the microbiota-immunity axis in the shaping of innate and adaptive responses from the earliest stages of development, mainly through the production of a myriad of microbial metabolites that play the role of immunomodulatory messengers, including short-chain fatty acids (SCFAs), tryptophan derivatives, and bile acids [7, 8].

In parallel, immunotherapy has revolutionised the treatment landscape for several diseases, most notably cancer [9]. Immune checkpoint inhibitors (ICIs) [10], cellular therapies such as chimeric antigen receptor T cells (CAR-T cells) [11], cytokine-based treatments [12], and vaccines [13] have transformed the clinical outcomes to multiple malignancies with durable responses. Converging lines of evidence from germ-free animal models, antibiotic-treated mice, human cohort studies, and clinical trials demonstrate that the gut microbiome is a critical regulator of immunotherapy efficacy [14, 15].

This chapter examines these concepts in detail. We begin by defining the microbiome and its biological functions, focusing on its influence on immune development and homeostasis. We then introduce the principles of immunotherapy, before exploring the mechanistic and clinical connections between microbiota composition and therapeutic outcomes. Finally, we discuss current limitations, controversies, and future avenues for microbiota-centred interventions in immunotherapy.

16.2 PHYSIOLOGICAL AND IMMUNOLOGICAL FUNCTIONS OF THE GUT MICROBIOTA

16.2.1 Structure and Organisation of the Gut Microbiota

The gut microbiota contains an abundant microbial community with a remarkable diversity that gathers over 10^{13} microorganisms, composed of archaea, fungi, viruses, phages, and bacteria. The study of its composition relies on complementary techniques, such as the culturomic [16], the sequencing of the small subunit ribosomal ribonucleic acid (RNA) genes (16S rRNA), allowing for taxonomic and phylogenetic analyses [17], and the whole deoxyribonucleic acid (DNA) sequencing (shotgun metagenomic sequencing) based on bioinformatic reconstruction of bacterial genomes [18] and enabling the identification of not yet-cultivated strains [19]. One of the major studies of the human microbiome by high-throughput metagenomics is led by the Human Microbiome Project Consortium and helped to better understand its structure, functions, and diversity [1, 20].

Its bacterial composition is shaped by oxygen and pH gradients [21], nutrient and metabolite availability, and physical architecture of the intestine in the different parts of the gut. The upper small intestine, exposed to bile acids and rapid flow, contains a low density of species enriched in facultative anaerobes, including *Streptococcus* and *Lactobacillus*. In contrast, the colon, anaerobic section of the gut, nutrient-rich, and slow-moving, supports dense species dominated by *Firmicutes* and *Bacteroidetes* [2] prone to digestion of complex carbohydrates and fibre fermentation leading to organic acids production, primarily SCFAs, including acetate, propionate, and butyrate [21]. The composition of the gut microbiota is highly heterogeneous and is influenced by multiple parameters, including genetics, mode of birth (vaginal or C-section), breastfeeding, diet, xenobiotics, medications (especially antibiotics or proton pump inhibitors administration), environment, and aging [3, 22–26]. Given its diversity, richness, and location, the gut microbiome exerts an essential influence on individuals, in maintaining host homeostasis and health, supporting multiple metabolic, structural, endocrine, and immunological functions across the lifespan [20, 27].

16.2.2 Metabolic Roles of the Gut Microbiome

The gut microbiome metabolic activity allows, among others, the breakdown of complex and indigestible dietary fibres and proteins (including complex polysaccharides), synthesis of vitamins (such as K and B-group vitamins), nutrient absorption, glycaemic regulation, lipid metabolism, and the production of SCFAs and secondary bile acids [21, 28]. In addition, through the production of SCFAs such as acetate, propionate, and butyrate, microbial communities nourish colonocytes, maintain epithelial barrier integrity, promote the expression of tight-junction proteins (claudin, occludin), and facilitate tissue repair following mucosal injury [29].

16.2.3 Immunological Functions of the Gut Microbiome

The co-evolution of immune-gut microbiome axis led to a strong bidirectional communication in which multiple microbial functions influence immune maturation, tolerance, regulation, and inflammation [27]. The proof of concept of this cross-talk between gut microbiota and the immune system was demonstrated in germ-free mouse models in which profound structural and immune immaturity, including defective development of Peyer's patches and mesenteric lymph nodes, reduced of total immunoglobulin (Ig)A production, defective T helper 17 cells (Th17) and regulatory T cells (Treg) differentiation, and altered myeloid compartments, highlighting a critical early-life windows for immune shaping that depend on the gut microbiome presence [6, 30].

Furthermore, metabolites of microbial origin are actively integrated into immune regulation. The SCFAs promote Treg differentiation through histone deacetylase inhibition and G-protein-coupled receptor 43 (GPR43)/G-protein-coupled receptor 109A (GPR109A) signalling [31, 32], indole derivatives activate the aryl hydrocarbon receptor (Ahr) to enhance epithelial repair and interleukin (IL)-22 secretion [33], and bile acid metabolites shape the Th17/Treg balance via the farnesoid X receptor (FXR) and the G protein-coupled bile acid receptor 1 (GPBAR1) pathways [34].

In addition to these metabolic and immunomodulatory functions, the microbiome constitutes a first line of defence against invading pathogens through colonisation resistance. Commensal communities occupy ecological niches that restrict pathogen access to nutrients and epithelial attachment sites through the production of bacterial antimicrobial peptides (AMPs) or bacteriocins and the secretion of inhibitory metabolites that directly suppress pathogen growth [35, 36]. In addition, the Paneth cells in the intestine participate in the innate immune response towards pathogens and shape the gut microbiota composition through the secretion of AMPs, such as regenerating family member 3 gamma (Reg3γ) [37]. Commensals and their metabolites can engage pattern recognition receptors (PRRs), including the two major forms of innate immune sensors, Toll-like and NOD-like receptors (TLRs and NLRs), enabling discrimination between harmless and pathogenic signals while preserving mucosal tolerance [38]. For example, Gram-negative bacteria outer membranes are rich in lipopolysaccharide (LPS), a well-characterised microbial-associated molecular pattern (MAMP) that contribute to the initiation of a strong immune response via the TLR4 expressed by macrophages and dendritic cells [39].

Disruption of this organised ecosystem, termed dysbiosis, and characterised by the reduction of microbial and functional diversity, loss of beneficial taxa, and expansion of pathobionts, is associated with chronic inflammation [40] and immune-mediated diseases such as inflammatory bowel disease [41]; rheumatoid arthritis [42]; multiple sclerosis [43]; metabolic disorders, including obesity and type 2 diabetes, through altered butyrate production and bile acid metabolism [44, 45]; and cancer [46], where microbes may promote tumorigenesis via toxins and metabolic by-products leading to oxidative stress, DNA damage, chronic inflammation or immune suppression, as shown in gastric carcinogenesis with *Helicobacter pylori* [47] or the enterotoxigenic *Bacteroides fragilis* in colorectal cancer [48].

Collectively, these findings demonstrate that the microbiome functions not only as a metabolic and protective organ but also as a fundamental educator of the immune system throughout life.

16.3 LINKING THE MICROBIOME TO IMMUNOTHERAPY EFFICACY IN CANCER

16.3.1 Clinical Associations

Over the past decade, converging clinical studies have shown the gut microbiota to be a pivotal determinant of response to ICI. In 2018, three back-to-back publications unravelled the impact of the gut microbiota in modulating ICI activity. By profiling baseline (before ICI initiation) gut microbiota composition of advanced melanoma, non-small cell lung carcinoma (NSCLC), and genitourinary cancer patients amenable to ICI, these studies discerned distinct bacterial signatures enriched in responders compared with non-responder patients [49–51]. Specifically, high gut microbiota diversity and the overrepresentation of health-related species were correlated with a beneficial anti-tumour microenvironment, mostly an increase of interferon gamma (IFN-γ) production and a positive clinical outcome following ICI treatment [49]. In NSCLC, renal cell carcinoma, and hepatocellular carcinoma, enrichment of *Akkermansia muciniphila* has been consistently associated with improved progression-free and overall survival following anti-PD-1 (programmed cell death protein 1) treatment [49, 52, 53]. In metastatic melanoma, a favourable clinical outcome is associated with higher diversity and enrichment in *Ruminococcaceae* and *Lachnospiraceae*, and *Bifidobacterium longum,* correlating with enhanced immune surrogate markers, including tumour-infiltrating $CD8^+$ T cells [50, 51, 54].

In contrast, disruption of the gut microbiome by antibiotic administration 30 days before and up to 42 days after immunotherapy initiation has been largely associated with an unfavourable clinical outcome, showing the causal role of microbial integrity in ICI treatment [49, 55]. By changing the local microbial ecosystem with a decrease of the global gut bacterial richness and specific beneficial taxa, including *Ruminococcaceae, A. muciniphila, Bifidobacterium species* (spp.), *Roseburia* spp., *Faecalibacterium* spp., *Eubacterium* spp., and *Dorea* spp., and, on the other hand, the overrepresentation of immunosuppressive species such as *Enterocloster* spp., *Veillonella* spp., *Proteobacteria* spp., and *Hungatella* spp. [56, 57]. To better characterise the ecological consortia involved in the efficacy or resistance to ICI, a network analysis has been performed on the metagenomic profiles of patients with

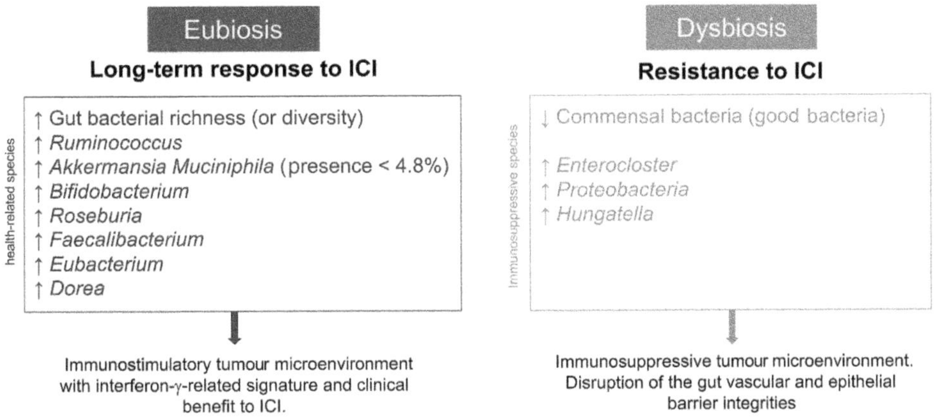

FIGURE 16.1 Impact of gut microbiota profiles on immunotherapy efficacy in cancer. Created by the authors.

NSCLC. This analysis resulted in the identification of two main clusters of bacteria associated with poor (species-interacting groups [SIG]1 cluster) or prolonged (SIG2 cluster) survival in NSCLC patients treated with ICI. The enumeration of each bacterium comprised in each of the clusters gives rise to a score of dysbiosis: the Toposcore, allowing for routine polymerase chain reaction (PCR)-based diagnosis of dysbiosis and validated in different types of cancer [58] (Figure 16.1).

16.3.2 Microbiome-Driven Mechanisms Shaping Immunotherapy Response

Several studies using germ-free and antibiotic-treated mouse models have provided proof of concept for how the composition of the gut microbiota is able to regulate an appropriate antitumor immunity and immunotherapy efficacy. Specific commensals enhance dendritic cell maturation and antigen presentation, promoting effective $CD8^+$ T-cell stimulation and higher effector memory function within the tumours [59, 60]. For example, it was reported that *A. muciniphila* abrogates anti-PD-1 resistance by promoting IL-12-producing dendritic cells and systemic IFN-γ-$CD4^+$ and $CD8^+$ T cells production, and increasing the tumour infiltration of CXC chemokine receptor 3 $(CXCR3)^+$ T cells [49]. Beyond the presence of specific taxa composition, microbial-derived metabolites exert strong immunomodulatory effects. The production of SCFAs, including butyrate and acetate, supports memory T-cell differentiation and mitochondrial fitness [61, 62], while inosine produced by specific bacterial species, including *Bifidobacterium pseudolongum*, enhances T-cell activation and synergises with ICI via A2A adenosine receptor-dependent signalling [63]. In addition, recent works have revealed that specifically antibiotics induce functional and anatomical immune misdirection leading to impaired immunotherapy efficacy. In addition, reports showed that antibiotic exposure affects the local and systemic immune tone by increasing circulating exhausted $CD8^+$ T cells in patients with gastric cancer amenable to ICI [64] and promoting the programmed cell death-ligand 2 (PD-L2) binding to its receptor repulsive guidance molecule b (RGMb) into the tumour [65]. Another study by Fidelle et al. showed that following antibiotic administration, a down-regulation of mucosal addressin cell adhesion molecule 1 (MAdCAM-1) in the ileum, Peyer's patches, and mesenteric lymph nodes is observed, which is associated with gut recolonisation by *Enterocloster* spp. and a disbalance in the bile acids pool, promoting aberrant emigration of enterotropic α4β7⁺ CD4⁺ regulatory Tr17 cells into the tumour [66].

16.4 THERAPEUTIC MODULATION OR PROTECTION OF THE GUT MICROBIOTA TO ENHANCE IMMUNOTHERAPY EFFICACY IN CANCER

The identification of the gut microbiota as a pivotal determinant of immunotherapy efficacy, foregrounding it not only as a static biomarker but also as a therapeutic tool that can be actively manipulated during immunotherapy treatment, with the goal of restoring immune competence. Several strategies, including dietary intervention, prebiotics, probiotics, and faecal microbiota transplantation (FMT), are currently being evaluated in clinical trials to favourably modulate the gut microbiome or to protect him from the deleterious impact of antibiotics (Figure 16.2).

Dietary Interventions Dietary interventions represent a non-invasive and scalable approach to beneficially modulate the gut microbiome. In the literature, among many dietary interventions, high fibre intake has shown positive signals in both preclinical and clinical studies [60]. Indeed, in patients with advanced melanoma treated with ICI, a sufficient dietary fibre intake (>20 g/day) was associated with a better clinical response [60]. In another report, in melanoma patients treated with ICI, similar outcomes were also observed with Mediterranean diet consumption, known to be rich in fibre [67]. Mechanistically, diets enriched in fibre promote the expansion of SCFA-producing taxa, including members of the *Ruminococcaceae* and

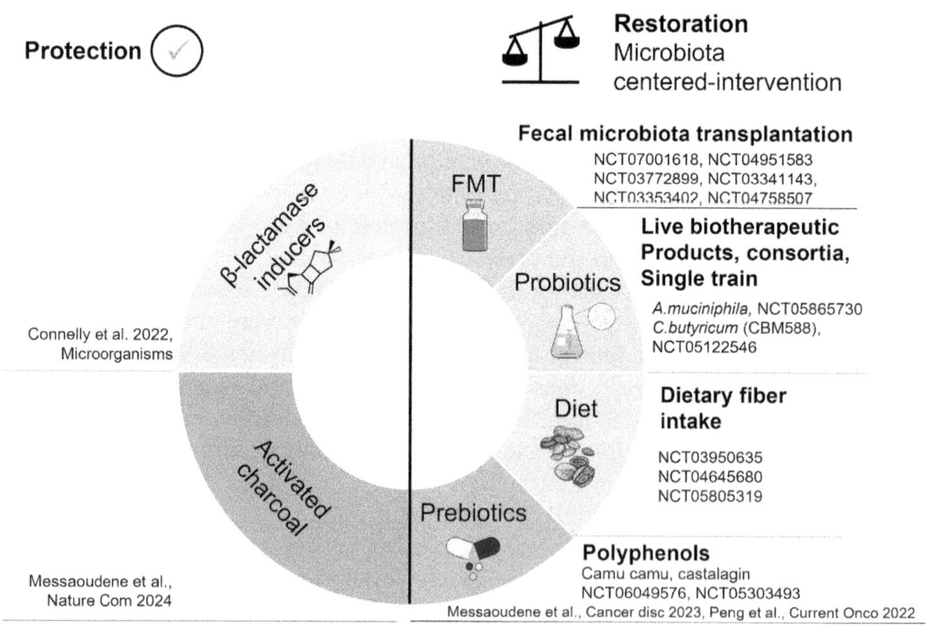

FIGURE 16.2 Microbiome-centred interventions for protection and modulation of the gut microbiota to enhance immunotherapy efficacy in cancer. Adapted from NIAID BioArt [NIH].

Lachnospiraceae families, which are consistently associated with improved anti-tumour immune responses [56], as well as enhanced $CD8^+$ T-cell infiltration, and improved clinical outcomes [60]. Based on these results, the feasibility and a positive signal for a high fibre dietary intervention were shown in a randomised Phase II clinical trial (DIET, NCT04645680). The authors showed that melanoma patients receiving a high fibre diet intervention during ICI treatment exhibited a better clinical response and less toxicity compared to the control group [68].

Prebiotics Supplementation Prebiotics are from different nature and comprise food ingredients that cannot be digested but support the growth of beneficial bacteria in the gut, such as complex prebiotics including fructo-oligosaccharides, inulin, and galacto-oligosaccharides. They are transformed by the gut microbiota into metabolites, including SCFAs, that support epithelial and systemic immune functions. In preclinical models, inulin has been shown to induce favourable modulation of the gut microbiome, leading to an increase in ICI efficacy, particularly through enrichment of *A. muciniphila, Lactobacillus* spp., *and Roseburia* spp., and their SCFA metabolites, which led to exerting potent anti-tumour efficacy, notably through IFN-γ^+ $CD8^+$ T cells, as well as the establishment of stem-like T-cell factor-1 $(Tcf1)^+$ PD-1^+ $CD8^+$ T cells within the tumour [69]. Based on these promising results, inulin is currently under clinical evaluation in patients with metastatic head and neck squamous cell carcinoma (NCT05821751) and metastatic or locally advanced kidney cell cancer (NCT06866262).

Another class of prebiotics, polyphenol-based prebiotics, is mainly derived from secondary plant metabolites found in fruits, vegetables, nuts, and tree heartwood. Their supplementations were mainly correlated with a favourable shift of the microbiome that led to increase and/or overcoming resistance of the immunotherapy responses. In preclinical models, the ellagitannin castalagin, a polyphenol derived from the camu camu berry, has shown a potential to overcome anti-PD-1 resistance by remodelling the gut microbiome composition characterised by an enrichment of *Ruminococcaceae* and *A. muciniphila*, and also by promoting intratumoural increase of $CD8^+$ T cells, PD-$L1^+$ $CD8^+$ T cells, and a high $CD8^+$/Treg cells ratio [70]. These beneficial pleiotropic effects have led to the evaluation of camu camu raw extract in clinical trials in combination with ICI in melanoma [71], NSCLC (NCT05303493), and renal cell carcinoma (NCT06049576).

Faecal Microbiota Transplantation (FMT) FMT has emerged as the most direct strategy to reshape the gut microbiota composition and to restore immunotherapy efficacy. Two initial proof-of-concept studies, in refractory melanoma patients, demonstrated that FMT using faeces from ICI responder patients could overcome the primary resistance to anti-PD-1 treatment with a durable response, translating into pathological tumour regression, and increased activated $CD8^+$ T cells, and a low proportion of IL-8-producing immunosuppressive myeloid cells within the tumour microenvironment [72, 73]. Those studies represented a critical clinical milestone, underscoring that the gut microbiome manipulation can be a causal and actionable lever to overcome immunotherapy resistance rather than a simple associative phenomenon. Building on this success, several FMT trials are currently ongoing in multiple malignancies, and in combination with ICI (Table 16.1).

Probiotics and Live Biotherapeutic Products (LBPs) Among the promising strategies, probiotics and live biotherapeutic products (LBPs) have gained increasing attention, mainly because they represent higher controlled approaches to microbiome manipulation. While traditional probiotics are defined as live microorganisms conferring health benefits when administered at adequate doses, the emergence of defined LBP reflects growing regulatory and mechanistic rigour in this field.

TABLE 16.1 Completed and ongoing clinical trials for FMT-centred interventions.

NCT number	Phase	Cancer type/ population	Study location/ institution
NCT04951583	Phase II	Advanced NSCLC, melanoma, uveal melanoma	CHUM – Montreal, Canada
NCT06623461	Phase II randomised	Melanoma	Canadian Cancer Trials Group – Canada
NCT03341143	Phase II	Melanoma	University of Pittsburgh – USA
NCT04116775	Phase II	Prostate cancer	Portland VA Medical Centre – USA
NCT04758507	Phase II randomised	Advanced renal cell carcinoma	Fondazione Policlinico Univ. Agostino Gemelli IRCCS – Italy
NCT04163289	Phase I	Renal cell carcinoma	Lawson Health Research Institute – Canada
NCT03772899	Phase I	Melanoma	Lawson Health Research Institute – Canada
NCT03353402	Phase I	Melanoma	Sheba Medical Centre – Israel
NCT04988841	Phase II randomised	Melanoma	MaaT Pharma/ AP-HP – France
NCT07001618	Phase II randomised	NSCLC	Gustave Roussy – France/ Europe
NCT03817125	Phase I randomised	Melanoma	Parker Institute for Cancer Immunotherapy – USA
NCT04038619	Phase I	Genitourinary cancers	MD Anderson Cancer Centre – USA
NCT03819296	Phase I	Melanoma or genitourinary cancers	MD Anderson Cancer Centre – USA
NCT04729322	Phase II	Metastatic colorectal cancer	MD Anderson Cancer Centre – USA
NCT06206707	not applicable	Genitourinary cancers or melanoma	University of Aarhus – Denmark
NCT04883762	Phase I	Any malignancy (prevention of ICI-related diarrhoea)	Memorial Sloan Kettering Cancer Centre – USA
NCT05286294	Phase II	Solid tumours	Oslo University Hospital – Norway
NCT05273255	Phase I	Refractory stage IV malignancies	University of Zurich – Switzerland
NCT05502913	Phase II randomised	Lung cancer	Soroka University Medical Centre – Israel
NCT05251389	Phase Ia/IIb	Melanoma	Netherlands Cancer Institute – Netherlands

TABLE 16.1 (Continued)

NCT number	Phase	Cancer type/ population	Study location/ institution
NCT05669846	Phase II	NSCLC	University of Pittsburgh – USA
NCT06030037	Phase II randomised	Advanced melanoma	University of Pittsburgh – USA
NCT06499896	Phase II	Refractory immune-related cutaneous and colitis events	University of Pittsburgh – USA
NCT05008861	Phase I	NSCLC	Shanghai Zhongshan Hospital – China
NCT04577729	Not applicable	Melanoma	Medical University of Graz – Austria
NCT05690048	Phase II randomised	Hepatocellular carcinoma	University Hospital Heidelberg – Germany
NCT04130763	Phase I	Gastrointestinal solid tumours	Peking University – China
NCT05279677	Phase II	Colorectal cancer	Chinese Academy of Medical Sciences – China
NCT06346093	Not specified	Gastric cancer	Changhai Hospital – China
NCT06405113	Phase II	Gastric cancer	Changzhou No. 2 People's Hospital – China
NCT06403111	Phase II	NSCLC	Changzhou No. 2 People's Hospital – China
NCT06613308	Not specified	NSCLC	China–Japan Friendship Hospital – China
NCT05533983	Phase II	Solid tumours	Asan Medical Centre – South Korea
NCT04924374	Not specified	NSCLC	Hospital Univ. Ramón y Cajal – Spain
NCT06643533	Not specified	Hepatocellular carcinoma	Fujian Provincial Hospital – China
NCT06486220	Phase III randomised	Oligometastatic nasopharyngeal carcinoma	Sun Yat-sen University Cancer Centre – China
NCT05750030	Phase II	Hepatocellular carcinoma	Medical University of Vienna – Austria
NCT04056026	Phase I	Mesothelioma	ProgenaBiome – USA
NCT04105270	Phase II randomised	NSCLC	University of Minnesota – USA
NCT04521075	Phase Ib	Melanoma, NSCLC, dMMR gastrointestinal cancers	Ella Therapeutics Ltd. – International

Next-generation probiotics, including defined LBP and minimal microbial consortia such as *A. muciniphila,* and rationally designed multi-species consortia, have been developed to exert specific immunomodulatory functions. Early-phase clinical trials of LBP in combination with ICI have yielded encouraging but heterogeneous results, exemplified by studies using the bifidogenic strain CBM588, which was associated with a better progression-free survival when combined with anti-CTLA-4 and anti-PD-1 [74], as well as by trials evaluating defined consortia such as MET4 [75], underscoring both the promise and the complexity of translating microbiome-centred interventions into clinical benefit. These approaches aim to recapitulate the therapeutic benefits of FMT while improving safety, standardisation, and regulatory compliance. In addition, consortia such as VE800 (NCT04208958) and SER-155 [76] are designed to deliver specific immunostimulatory functions, such as enhanced antigen presentation, T-cell priming, and metabolic support, while avoiding the variability associated with donor-derived material.

Strategies to Overcome Antibiotic-Related Dysbiosis In addition to implementing strict recommendations such as prior confirmation of bacterial infection, use of narrow-spectrum antibiotics, and prescription of the shortest possible duration, it is also important to develop complementary and therapeutic strategies to limit the deleterious impact of antibiotics on the gut microbiota. Among these strategies, an innovative activated charcoal-based product targeting the colon, DAV132, was recently developed to sequester antibiotics in the gut and prevent microbiota destruction. In a randomised Phase I study conducted in healthy volunteers, DAV132 was shown to effectively adsorb several broad-spectrum antibiotics (piperacillin-tazobactam, ceftriaxone, ceftazidime), allowing their systemic absorption while preventing their presence in faeces. This approach preserved microbiota diversity, accelerated its recovery, and protected key beneficial bacteria. Furthermore, DAV132 has also demonstrated, in several preclinical mouse models of cancer, its ability to preserve the efficacy of ICI mainly by protecting important surrogate markers such as $CD8^+$ T cell anti-tumour response [77]. Other strategies are currently being investigated, including the administration of β-lactamase enzymes to hydrolyse β-lactam antibiotics in the colon, in order to reduce their negative impact on the microbiota and decrease the incidence of *Clostridium difficile* infections. However, the protective potential of β-lactamase enzymes on the efficacy of immunotherapies remains unknown [78].

Collectively, these strategies herald a new era in which microbiome modulation becomes an integral component of precision immuno-oncology, with interventions tailored to restore immune competence, optimise therapeutic response, and ultimately extend the benefits of immunotherapy to a broader patient population.

16.5 CHALLENGES AND CONTROVERSIES

Despite the growing body of evidence supporting a role for the gut microbiota in modulating immunotherapy efficacy, several challenges and ongoing controversies complicate the translation into clinical practice. One of the most significant limitations is the lack of reproducibility to identify a specific microbial signature that is associated with ICI response across studies, which underscore inter-individual and inter-cohort variability driven by geography, dietary habits, ethnicity, antibiotic exposure, and lifestyle, as well as technical heterogeneity associated to the microbiome sequencing, bioinformatic pipelines, and sample collection and storage protocols

[79, 80]. This raises the question of whether immunotherapy efficacy is driven by specific immunogenic bacterial species, such as *A. muciniphila or Bifidobacterium* spp., or rather by functions, metabolic pathways, and ecosystem-level interactions that may be conserved despite the gut microbiome differences [15].

In parallel, safety concerns remain a critical barrier to the widespread utilisation of live microbial therapeutics, particularly in immunocompromised cancer patients, where risks of bacteraemia, sepsis, and horizontal gene transfer must be carefully weighed against potential benefits [81]. Despite promising results in FMT trials, the complexity of implementing this type of treatment can be a deterrent. These concerns are compounded by ongoing regulatory complexity, as microbiome-centred interventions span between drugs, biologics, and food supplements, resulting in heterogeneous regulatory frameworks and posing challenges for standardisation, quality control, and large-scale clinical deployment.

16.6 FUTURE DIRECTIONS

Looking ahead, the next decade is poised to transform the microbiome-immunotherapy field from correlative discovery to biomarkers and to precision interventions. Advances in synthetic biology and microbial engineering are expected to enable the rational design of engineered bacterial strains capable of delivering immunomodulatory molecules, enhancing antigen presentation, or selectively reshaping immune cell trafficking within the tumour microenvironment [15, 82, 83]. In parallel, increasing attention is being directed towards microbial metabolites, named 'postbiotics', including SCFAs, bile acids, and nucleosides such as inosine. They can offer the potential to recapitulate key immunomodulatory effects of the microbiome while avoiding the safety and regulatory challenges associated with live organisms [84].

Future clinical strategies are also likely to integrate a specific diet into personalised oncology care, being a scalable and modifiable determinant of microbial and immune functions. Dietary interventions tailored to individual microbial and metabolic profiles may emerge as low-risk adjuncts to immunotherapy [60]. At the same time, the convergence of high-dimensional host and microbial multi-omics – including metagenomics, metabolomics, transcriptomics, and immune profiling, will enable the development of predictive machine learning models capable of stratifying patients, predicting response, and guiding the adequate therapeutic armamentarium [15, 56]. Ultimately, the future of cancer immunotherapy lies in microbiome-centred interventions, that leverage microbial, metabolic, and immune functions to extend durable responses to a broader and more diverse patient population.

BOXED CASE STUDY

Routy et al. conducted a prospective FMT clinical trial using faeces from healthy donors and showed that FMT can durably reshape the gut microbiota, enhance systemic and intratumoural immune activation, and improve the clinical outcomes with an objective response rate of 65% [85] compared to 45% in historical trials treated with anti-PD-1 alone [86, 87]. These positive results have recently been confirmed in three back-to-back publications [88–90].

KEY TERMS & DEFINITIONS SIDEBAR

Dysbiosis A disruption of the gut microbial ecosystem characterised by reduced diversity, loss of beneficial microbes, and expansion of pathological microbes, often associated with inflammation and diseases.

Faecal Microbiota Transplantation (FMT) The transfer of faecal material from a donor to a recipient to restore microbial diversity and functions.

Gut Microbiota The microorganisms inhabiting the gut interact dynamically with the host to regulate metabolism, immunity, and tissue homeostasis.

Live Biotherapeutic Products (LBP) Defined and regulated microbial formulations designed to exert specific therapeutic functions, offering a controlled alternative to conventional probiotics or FMT.

Microbiome The collective microorganisms composed of archaea, fungi, viruses, phages, and bacteria, inhabiting mucosal and epithelial surfaces, and their genomes, such as the gut microbiome.

Microbiota-Centred Interventions Therapeutic approaches aimed at protecting and/or modulating the gut microbiome beneficially, such as diet, prebiotics, probiotics, FMT, or postbiotics.

Prebiotics Substrates that support the growth and activity of beneficial gut microorganisms.

Precision Immuno-oncology An approach that integrates tumour, immune, and microbiome-derived biomarkers to personalise immunotherapy strategies and optimise patient response.

LIST OF ABBREVIATIONS

16S rRNA	16S ribosomal RNA genes
Ahr	aryl hydrocarbon receptor
AMPs	antimicrobial peptides
CAR-T	chimeric antigen receptor T cells
CTLA-4	cytotoxic T-lymphocyte-associated protein 4
CXCR3	CXC chemokine receptor 3
dMMR	deficient MisMatch repair
DNA	deoxyribonucleic acid
FMT	faecal microbiota transplantation
FXR	farnesoid X receptor
GPBAR1	G protein-coupled bile acid receptor 1
GPR43	G-protein-coupled receptor 43
GPR109A	G-protein-coupled receptor 109A
ICIs	immune checkpoint inhibitors
IFN	interferon
IL	interleukin
LBPs	live biotherapeutic products
LPS	lipopolysaccharide
MAdCAM-1	mucosal addressin cell adhesion molecule 1

MAMPs	microbial-associated molecular pattern(s)
NLRs	NOD-like receptors
NSCLC	non-small cell lung carcinoma
PCR	polymerase chain reaction
PD-1	programmed cell death protein 1
PD-L1	programmed death-ligand 1
PD-L2	programmed death-ligand 2
PRRs	pattern recognition receptors
Reg3γ	regenerating family member 3 gamma
RGMb	repulsive guidance molecule b
RNA	ribonucleic acid
SCFAs	short-chain fatty acids
SIG	species-interacting group
Spp	species
Tcf1	T-cell factor-1
Th17	T helper 17 cells
TILs	tumour-infiltrating lymphocytes
TLR	Toll-like receptors
Treg	regulatory T cells

REVIEW QUESTIONS

1. How does the gut microbiota shape immune system development and function?
2. What evidence supports a role for the gut microbiota in immunotherapy efficacy?
3. Which microbial features are associated with better responses to ICI?
4. How do antibiotics affect microbiota-immune interactions and immunotherapy outcomes?
5. What microbiota-centred interventions are being developed to beneficially modulate the gut microbiota to improve cancer immunotherapy?

REFERENCES

1. Gevers, D., Knight, R., Petrosino, J.F. et al. (2012). The human microbiome project: a community resource for the healthy human microbiome. *PLoS Biol* 10 (8): e1001377.
2. Qin, J., Li, R., Raes, J. et al. (2010). A human gut microbial gene catalogue established by metagenomic sequencing. *Nature* 464 (7285): 59–65.
3. Maurice, C.F., Haiser, H.J., and Turnbaugh, P.J. (2013). Xenobiotics shape the physiology and gene expression of the active human gut microbiome. *Cell* 152 (1): 39–50.
4. Tanoue, T., Atarashi, K., and Honda, K. (2016). Development and maintenance of intestinal regulatory T cells. *Nat Rev Immunol* 16 (5): 295–309.
5. Lathrop, S.K., Bloom, S.M., Rao, S.M. et al. (2011). Peripheral education of the immune system by colonic commensal microbiota. *Nature* 478 (7368): 250–254.

6. Round, J.L. and Mazmanian, S.K. (2009). The gut microbiota shapes intestinal immune responses during health and disease. *Nat Rev Immunol* 9 (5): 313–323.
7. Tamburini, S., Shen, N., Wu, H.C., and Clemente, J.C. (2016). The microbiome in early life: implications for health outcomes. *Nat Med* 22 (7): 713–722.
8. Koh, A., De Vadder, F., Kovatcheva-Datchary, P., and Bäckhed, F. (2016). From dietary fiber to host physiology: short-chain fatty acids as key bacterial metabolites. *Cell* 165 (6): 1332–1345.
9. Zhang, M., Liu, C., Tu, J. et al. (2025). Advances in cancer immunotherapy: historical perspectives, current developments, and future directions. *Mol Cancer* 24 (1): 136.
10. Waldman, A.D., Fritz, J.M., and Lenardo, M.J. (2020). A guide to cancer immunotherapy: from T cell basic science to clinical practice. *Nat Rev Immunol* 20 (11): 651–668.
11. Uslu, U. and June, C.H. (2025). Beyond the blood: expanding CAR T cell therapy to solid tumors. *Nat Biotechnol* 43 (4): 506–515.
12. Agliardi, S., Veronese, C., Panzeri, F. et al. (2025). Immunocytokines in cancer treatment: a systematic review. *Cancer Treat Rev* 139: 102978.
13. Pail, O., Lin, M.J., Anagnostou, T. et al. (2025). Cancer vaccines and the future of immunotherapy. *Lancet* 406 (10499): 189–202.
14. Vétizou, M., Pitt, J.M., Daillère, R. et al. (2015). Anticancer immunotherapy by CTLA-4 blockade relies on the gut microbiota. *Science* 350 (6264): 1079–1084.
15. Elkrief, A., Pidgeon, R., Maleki Vareki, S. et al. (2025). The gut microbiome as a target in cancer immunotherapy: opportunities and challenges for drug development. *Nat Rev Drug Discov* 24 (9): 685–704.
16. Lagier, J.C., Dubourg, G., Million, M. et al. (2018). Culturing the human microbiota and culturomics. *Nat Rev Microbiol* 16: 540–550.
17. Hold, G.L., Pryde, S.E., Russell, V.J. et al. (2002). Assessment of microbial diversity in human colonic samples by 16S rDNA sequence analysis. *FEMS Microbiol Ecol* 39 (1): 33–39.
18. Human Microbiome Jumpstart Reference Strains Consortium, Nelson, K.E., Weinstock, G.M. et al. (2010). A catalog of reference genomes from the human microbiome. *Science* 328 (5981): 994–999.
19. Knight, R., Vrbanac, A., Taylor, B.C. et al. (2018). Best practices for analysing microbiomes. *Nat Rev Microbiol* 16 (7): 410–422.
20. Human Microbiome Project Consortium (2012). Structure, function and diversity of the healthy human microbiome. *Nature* 486 (7402): 207–214.
21. Brinck, J.E., Sinha, A.K., Laursen, M.F. et al. (2025). Intestinal pH: a major driver of human gut microbiota composition and metabolism. *Nat Rev Gastroenterol Hepatol* 22 (9): 639 656.
22. Dominguez-Bello, M.G., De Jesus-Laboy, K.M., Shen, N. et al. (2016). Partial restoration of the microbiota of cesarean-born infants via vaginal microbial transfer. *Nat Med* 22 (3): 250–253.
23. Stark, P.L. and Lee, A. (1982). The microbial ecology of the large bowel of breast-fed and formula-fed infants during the first year of life. *J Med Microbiol* 15 (2): 189–203.
24. Maier, L., Pruteanu, M., Kuhn, M. et al. (2018). Extensive impact of non-antibiotic drugs on human gut bacteria. *Nature* 555 (7698): 623–628.
25. Yatsunenko, T., Rey, F.E., Manary, M.J. et al. (2012). Human gut microbiome viewed across age and geography. *Nature* 486 (7402): 222–227.
26. Badal, V.D., Vaccariello, E.D., Murray, E.R. et al. (2020). The gut microbiome, aging, and longevity: a systematic review. *Nutrients* 12: 3759.
27. Iliev, I.D., Blander, J.M., Collins, N. et al. (2025). Microbiota-mediated mechanisms of mucosal immunity across the lifespan. *Nat Immunol* 26 (10): 1645–1659.
28. Collins, S.L., Stine, J.G., Bisanz, J.E. et al. (2023). Bile acids and the gut microbiota: metabolic interactions and impacts on disease. *Nat Rev Microbiol* 21 (4): 236–247.
29. Mukhopadhya, I. and Louis, P. (2025). Gut microbiota-derived short-chain fatty acids and their role in human health and disease. *Nat Rev Microbiol* 23 (10): 635–651.

30. Atarashi, K., Tanoue, T., Oshima, K. et al. (2013). Treg induction by a rationally selected mixture of Clostridia strains from the human microbiota. *Nature* 500 (7461): 232–236.
31. Furusawa, Y., Obata, Y., Fukuda, S. et al. (2013). Commensal microbe-derived butyrate induces the differentiation of colonic regulatory T cells. *Nature* 504 (7480): 446–450.
32. Smith, P.M., Howitt, M.R., Panikov, N. et al. (2013). The microbial metabolites, short-chain fatty acids, regulate colonic Treg cell homeostasis. *Science* 341 (6145): 569–573.
33. Zelante, T., Iannitti, R.G., Cunha, C. et al. (2013). Tryptophan catabolites from microbiota engage aryl hydrocarbon receptor and balance mucosal reactivity via interleukin-22. *Immunity* 39 (2): 372–385.
34. Hang, S., Paik, D., Yao, L. et al. (2019). Bile acid metabolites control TH17 and Treg cell differentiation. *Nature* 576 (7785): 143–148.
35. Buffie, C.G. and Pamer, E.G. (2013). Microbiota-mediated colonization resistance against intestinal pathogens. *Nat Rev Immunol* 13 (11): 790–801.
36. Byndloss, M.X. and Bäumler, A.J. (2018). The germ-organ theory of non-communicable diseases. *Nat Rev Microbiol* 16 (2): 103–110.
37. Wallaeys, C., Garcia-Gonzalez, N., and Libert, C. (2022). Paneth cells as the cornerstones of intestinal and organismal health: a primer. *EMBO Mol Med* 15 (2): e16427.
38. Honda, K. and Littman, D.R. (2016). The microbiota in adaptive immune homeostasis and disease. *Nature* 535 (7610): 75–84.
39. Park, B.S. and Lee, J.O. (2013). Recognition of lipopolysaccharide pattern by TLR4 complexes. *Exp Mol Med* 45 (12): e66.
40. Goel, A., Shete, O., Goswami, S. et al. (2025). Toward a health-associated core keystone index for the human gut microbiome. *Cell Rep* 44 (3): 115378.
41. Zhang, J., Mak, J.W.Y., and Ng, S.C. (2025). Gut microbiome in IBD: past, present and the future. https://gut.bmj.com/content/early/2025/11/11/gutjnl-2025-335626.info (accessed 22 December 2025).
42. Kapoor, B. and Gulati, M. (2025). Gut microbiome and rheumatoid arthritis: revisiting the gut-joint axis. *Int Immunopharmacol* 165: 115503.
43. iMSMS Consortium. Gut microbiome of multiple sclerosis patients and paired household healthy controls reveal associations with disease risk and course. *Cell* 185: 3467–3486.
44. Van Hul, M. and Cani, P.D. (2023). The gut microbiota in obesity and weight management: microbes as friends or foe? *Nat Rev Endocrinol* 19 (5): 258–271.
45. Vrieze, A., Van Nood, E., Holleman, F. et al. (2012). Transfer of intestinal microbiota from lean donors increases insulin sensitivity in individuals with metabolic syndrome. *Gastroenterology* 143 (4): 913–916.e7.
46. Nobels, A., van Marcke, C., Jordan, B.F. et al. (2025). The gut microbiome and cancer: from tumorigenesis to therapy. *Nat Metab* 7 (5): 895–917.
47. Parsonnet, J., Friedman, G.D., Vandersteen, D.P. et al. (1991). Helicobacter pylori infection and the risk of gastric carcinoma. *N Engl J Med* 325 (16): 1127–1131.
48. El Tekle, G. and Garrett, W.S. (2023). Bacteria in cancer initiation, promotion and progression. *Nat Rev Cancer* 23 (9): 600–618.
49. Routy, B., Le Chatelier, E., Derosa, L. et al. (2018). Gut microbiome influences efficacy of PD-1–based immunotherapy against epithelial tumors. *Science* 359 (6371): 91–97.
50. Matson, V., Fessler, J., Bao, R. et al. (2018). The commensal microbiome is associated with anti–PD-1 efficacy in metastatic melanoma patients. *Science* 359 (6371): 104–108.
51. Gopalakrishnan, V., Spencer, C.N., Nezi, L. et al. (2018). Gut microbiome modulates response to anti–PD-1 immunotherapy in melanoma patients. *Science* 359 (6371): 97–103.
52. Derosa, L., Routy, B., Fidelle, M. et al. (2020). Gut bacteria composition drives primary resistance to cancer immunotherapy in renal cell carcinoma patients. *Eur Urol* 78 (2): 195–206.
53. Lee, K.A., Thomas, A.M., Bolte, L.A. et al. (2022). Cross-cohort gut microbiome associations with immune checkpoint inhibitor response in advanced melanoma. *Nat Med* 28 (3): 535–544.

54. McCulloch, J.A., Davar, D., Rodrigues, R.R. et al. (2022). Intestinal microbiota signatures of clinical response and immune-related adverse events in melanoma patients treated with anti-PD-1. *Nat Med* 28 (3): 545–556.
55. Derosa, L., Routy, B., Desilets, A. et al. (2021). Microbiota-centered interventions: the next breakthrough in immuno-oncology? *Cancer Discov* 11 (10): 2396–2412.
56. Thomas, A.M., Fidelle, M., Routy, B. et al. (2023). Gut OncoMicrobiome Signatures (GOMS) as next-generation biomarkers for cancer immunotherapy. *Nat Rev Clin Oncol* 20 (9): 583–603.
57. Andrews, M.C., Duong, C.P.M., Gopalakrishnan, V. et al. (2021). Gut microbiota signatures are associated with toxicity to combined CTLA-4 and PD-1 blockade. *Nat Med* 27 (8): 1432–1441.
58. Derosa, L., Iebba, V., Silva, C.A.C. et al. (2024). Custom scoring based on ecological topology of gut microbiota associated with cancer immunotherapy outcome. *Cell* 187 (13): 3373–3389.e16.
59. Sivan, A., Corrales, L., Hubert, N. et al. (2015). Commensal *Bifidobacterium* promotes antitumor immunity and facilitates anti-PD-L1 efficacy. *Science* 350 (6264): 1084–1089.
60. Spencer, C.N., McQuade, J.L., Gopalakrishnan, V. et al. (2021). Dietary fiber and probiotics influence the gut microbiome and melanoma immunotherapy response. *Science* 374 (6575): 1632–1640.
61. Bachem, A., Makhlouf, C., Binger, K.J. et al. (2019). Microbiota-derived short-chain fatty acids promote the memory potential of antigen-activated CD8+ T cells. *Immunity* 51 (2): 285–297.e5.
62. Balmer, M.L., Ma, E.H., Thompson, A.J. et al. (2020). Memory CD8+ T cells balance pro- and anti-inflammatory activity by reprogramming cellular acetate handling at sites of infection. *Cell Metab* 32 (3): 457–467.e5.
63. Mager, L.F., Burkhard, R., Pett, N. et al. (2020). Microbiome-derived inosine modulates response to checkpoint inhibitor immunotherapy. *Science* 369 (6510): 1481–1489.
64. Kim, C.G., Koh, J.Y., Shin, S.J. et al. (2023). Prior antibiotic administration disrupts anti-PD-1 responses in advanced gastric cancer by altering the gut microbiome and systemic immune response. *Cell Rep Med* 4 (11): 101251.
65. Park, J.S., Gazzaniga, F.S., Wu, M. et al. (2023). Targeting PD-L2-RGMb overcomes microbiome-related immunotherapy resistance. *Nature* 617 (7960): 377–385.
66. Fidelle, M., Rauber, C., Alves Costa Silva, C. et al. (2023). A microbiota-modulated checkpoint directs immunosuppressive intestinal T cells into cancers. *Science* 380 (6649): eabo2296.
67. Bolte, L.A., Lee, K.A., Björk, J.R. et al. (2023). Association of a Mediterranean diet with outcomes for patients treated with immune checkpoint blockade for advanced melanoma. *JAMA Oncol* 9 (5): 705–709.
68. Qiu, Y., Dizman, N., Jiang, Y. et al. (2025). Clinical outcomes of the DIET study: A randomized controlled phase 2 trial of a high fiber diet intervention (HFDI) in patients with melanoma receiving immune checkpoint blockade (ICB). *J Clin Oncol* 43 (16_suppl): 9511.
69. Han, K., Nam, J., Xu, J. et al. (2021). Generation of systemic antitumour immunity via the in situ modulation of the gut microbiome by an orally administered inulin gel. *Nat Biomed Eng* 5 (11): 1377–1388.
70. Messaoudene, M., Pidgeon, R., Richard, C. et al. (2022). A natural polyphenol exerts antitumor activity and circumvents anti-PD-1 resistance through effects on the gut microbiota. *Cancer Discov* 12 (4): 1070–1087.
71. Pang, S.A., Elkrief, A., Capella, M.P., and Miller, W.H. (2023). Two cases of durable and deep responses to immune checkpoint inhibition-refractory metastatic melanoma after addition of Camu prebiotic. *Curr Oncol* 30 (9): 7852–7859.
72. Baruch, E.N., Youngster, I., Ben-Betzalel, G. et al. (2021). Fecal microbiota transplant promotes response in immunotherapy-refractory melanoma patients. *Science* 371 (6529): 602–609.

73. Davar, D., Dzutsev, A.K., McCulloch, J.A. et al. (2021). Fecal microbiota transplant overcomes resistance to anti-PD-1 therapy in melanoma patients. *Science* 371 (6529): 595–602.
74. Ebrahimi, H., Dizman, N., Meza, L. et al. (2024). Cabozantinib and nivolumab with or without live bacterial supplementation in metastatic renal cell carcinoma: a randomized phase 1 trial. *Nat Med* 30 (9): 2576–2585.
75. Spreafico, A., Heirali, A.A., Araujo, D.V. et al. (2023). First-in-class Microbial Ecosystem Therapeutic 4 (MET4) in combination with immune checkpoint inhibitors in patients with advanced solid tumors (MET4-IO trial). *Ann Oncol* 34 (6): 520–530.
76. Halvorsen, E., Vulic, M., O'Brien, E.J. et al. (2021). 130. Design and preclinical characterization of SER-155, an investigational cultivated microbiome therapeutic to restore colonization resistance and prevent infection in patients undergoing hematopoietic stem cell transplantation. *Open Forum Infect Dis* 8 (Suppl 1): S79–S80.
77. Messaoudene, M., Ferreira, S., Saint-Lu, N. et al. (2024). The DAV132 colon-targeted adsorbent does not interfere with plasma concentrations of antibiotics but prevents antibiotic-related dysbiosis: a randomized phase I trial in healthy volunteers. *Nat Commun* 15 (1): 8083.
78. Kokai-Kun, J.F., Roberts, T., Coughlin, O. et al. (2019). Use of ribaxamase (SYN-004), a β-lactamase, to prevent Clostridium difficile infection in β-lactam-treated patients: a double-blind, phase 2b, randomised placebo-controlled trial. *Lancet Infect Dis* 19 (5): 487–496.
79. Sinha, R., Abu-Ali, G., Vogtmann, E. et al. (2017). Assessment of variation in microbial community amplicon sequencing by the Microbiome Quality Control (MBQC) project consortium. *Nat Biotechnol* 35 (11): 1077–1086.
80. Falony, G., Joossens, M., Vieira-Silva, S. et al. (2016). Population-level analysis of gut microbiome variation. *Science* 352 (6285): 560–564.
81. DeFilipp, Z., Bloom, P.P., Soto, M.T. et al. (2019). Drug-resistant *E. coli* bacteremia transmitted by fecal microbiota transplant. *N Engl J Med* 381 (21): 2043–2050.
82. Dizman, N., Meza, L., Bergerot, P. et al. (2022). Nivolumab plus ipilimumab with or without live bacterial supplementation in metastatic renal cell carcinoma: a randomized phase 1 trial. *Nat Med* 28 (4): 704–712.
83. Isabella, V.M., Ha, B.N., Castillo, M.J. et al. (2018). Development of a synthetic live bacterial therapeutic for the human metabolic disease phenylketonuria. *Nat Biotechnol* 36 (9): 857–864.
84. Lavelle, A. and Sokol, H. (2020). Gut microbiota-derived metabolites as key actors in inflammatory bowel disease. *Nat Rev Gastroenterol Hepatol* 17 (4): 223–237.
85. Routy, B., Lenehan, J.G., Miller, W.H. et al. (2023). Fecal microbiota transplantation plus anti-PD-1 immunotherapy in advanced melanoma: a phase I trial. *Nat Med* 29 (8): 2121–2132.
86. Wolchok, J.D., Chiarion-Sileni, V., Rutkowski, P. et al. (2025). Final, 10-year outcomes with nivolumab plus ipilimumab in advanced melanoma. *N Engl J Med* 392 (1): 11–22.
87. Robert, C., Schachter, J., Long, G.V. et al. (2015). Pembrolizumab versus ipilimumab in advanced melanoma. *N Engl J Med* 372 (26): 2521–2532.
88. Duttagupta, S., Messaoudene, M., Hunter, S. et al. (2026). Fecal microbiota transplantation plus immunotherapy in non-small cell lung cancer and melanoma: the phase 2 FMT-LUMINate trial. *Nat Med* 32, 1337–1350. https://doi.org/10.1038/s41591-025-04186-5
89. Fernandes, R., Jabbarizadeh, B., Rajeh, A. et al. (2026). Fecal microbiota transplantation plus immunotherapy in metastatic renal cell carcinoma: the phase 1 PERFORM trial. *Nat Med* 32, 1325–1336. https://doi.org/10.1038/s41591-025-04183-8
90. Porcari, S., Ciccarese, C., Heidrich, V. et al. (2026. Fecal microbiota transplantation plus pembrolizumab and axitinib in metastatic renal cell carcinoma: the randomized phase 2 TACITO trial. *Nat Med* 32, 1316–1324. https://doi.org/10.1038/s41591-025-04189-2

17 Veterinary Immunotherapy

ALEXANDRE HUMBERT, MARIE ABITBOL, AND CAROLE PEROZ
VetAgro Sup Campus vétérinaire, Departement Basic Sciences, Université de Lyon, Marcy-l'Etoile, France

LEARNING OBJECTIVES

After the reading of this chapter, the reader should be able to:

- Provide some examples of licensed immunotherapeutic substances available for companion animals (cats, dogs) to cure osteoarthritis or canine allergic dermatitis.
- Explain the molecular mechanisms behind the action of NGF monoclonal antibodies used for osteoarthritis.
- Provide examples of cancer immunotherapy in dogs.
- Identify the limits of using human monoclonal antibodies in animals.
- Identify the advantages of using client-owned pets, and especially dogs as (preclinical) models for some human immunotherapies.

17.1 INTRODUCTION

Dog is man's best friend. This assertion has been true since the domestication of the first wolves, and in the field of comparative pathology, it has proven to be accurate, particularly for oncology. Comparative oncology has long highlighted similarities between canine and human cancers [1]. These similarities were found for genetic predisposition (shared susceptibility loci) and tumour tissue composition. Spontaneous canine cancer models replicate more accurately the oncogenesis and complex, heterogeneous microenvironment of human tumours than laboratory animal models such as rats or mice, in which genome is often engineered and neoplasia is induced. Furthermore, they are immunocompetent hosts, and their immune response is more representative of the human patient [2]. Pet dogs share their living environment with humans and thus many exposure factors and show clear similarities in terms of the molecular, histological, and immune characteristics of their cancers [3]. Thus, pet dogs with spontaneous cancers have been included in several clinical trials (melanoma, glioma, osteosarcoma, urothelial carcinoma) and can help inform human trial designs [4]. A recent study clustered canine and human cancers with respect to their immune checkpoint expression levels, further highlighting the link between species in certain types of tumours, including glioma and osteosarcoma [5].

The search for susceptibility loci in canine cancers has made great strides since the publication of the canine genome sequence in 2005 [6]. The unique structure of the genome of purebred dogs laid ground to search for genomic variants involved in Mendelian hereditary disorders, as well as susceptibility loci for multifactorial/complex disorders, especially cancers [7, 8]. The population of purebred dogs is divided into breeds originating from small founding populations and maintained over generations by a closed gene pool, which allows a high level of genetic homogeneity to be maintained within most breeds (contributing to the maintenance of morphological and temperamental homogeneity within each breed). Conversely, when breeds are compared with each other, they exhibit considerable genetic diversity. This unique genetic structure, characterised by intra-racial homogeneity and inter-racial heterogeneity, facilitates the search for genomic variants associated with desirable or deleterious traits, using Single Nucleotide Polymorphism (SNP)-based genotyping arrays and Genome-Wide Association Studies (GWAS), a strategy often referred to as 'within- and across-breeds studies' [9].

More recently, advances in next-generation sequencing have enabled the genomes of thousands of canids to be sequenced [10], offering the possibility of moving from SNP chips to whole-genome sequencing for the search for susceptibility loci [11, 12]. For example a multi-omics approach was used to confirm that some oncogenes were shared in human and dog osteosarcoma (such as TP53 or PI3K pathway) [13]. The continuous improvement of tools for studying the canine genome [14], combined with the increase in dogs' life expectancy and their growing medicalisation, has made dog a valuable resource for searching cancer genomic-associated loci [15] and somatic events [16, 17]. However, even if several oncogenes are shared in canine and human tumours, some markers might differ between species. For instance, *ATP Binding Cassette Subfamily C Member 3 (ABCC3)* is overexpressed in human breast cancer but appears to be less expressed in feline mammary cancer [18].

The comprehension of how immune systems function in various species, as well as the pathophysiology of diseases, enabled the development and personalisation of treatments. Veterinary medicine, while deeply linked to the history of immunotherapies (as discussed in Chapter 1), flourishes alongside human medicine. Immunotherapies have thus naturally found their way in the treatment of animals. This chapter, without aiming to be exhaustive, will illustrate the diversity of already (or soon-to-be) available immunotherapies in veterinary practice (Figure 17.1). This chapter will provide information on monoclonal antibodies (mAbs) used to tackle inflammatory and allergic disorders, before addressing antitumoural immunotherapies, through examples of marketed treatments and targets that are the focus of intensive research (Table 17.1).

17.2 MONOCLONAL ANTIBODIES IN THE TREATMENT OF OSTEOARTHRITIS

Osteoarthritis is a very common chronic joint disease in aging dogs and cats, with a prevalence estimated to even reach 90% in older cats [19]. It is characterised by cartilage alteration, bone neoformation, inflammatory infiltration of synovial fluid, and, mostly, chronic pain. Osteoarthritis has no curative treatment yet; therapeutic strategies either aim at slowing down the progression or easing the pain.

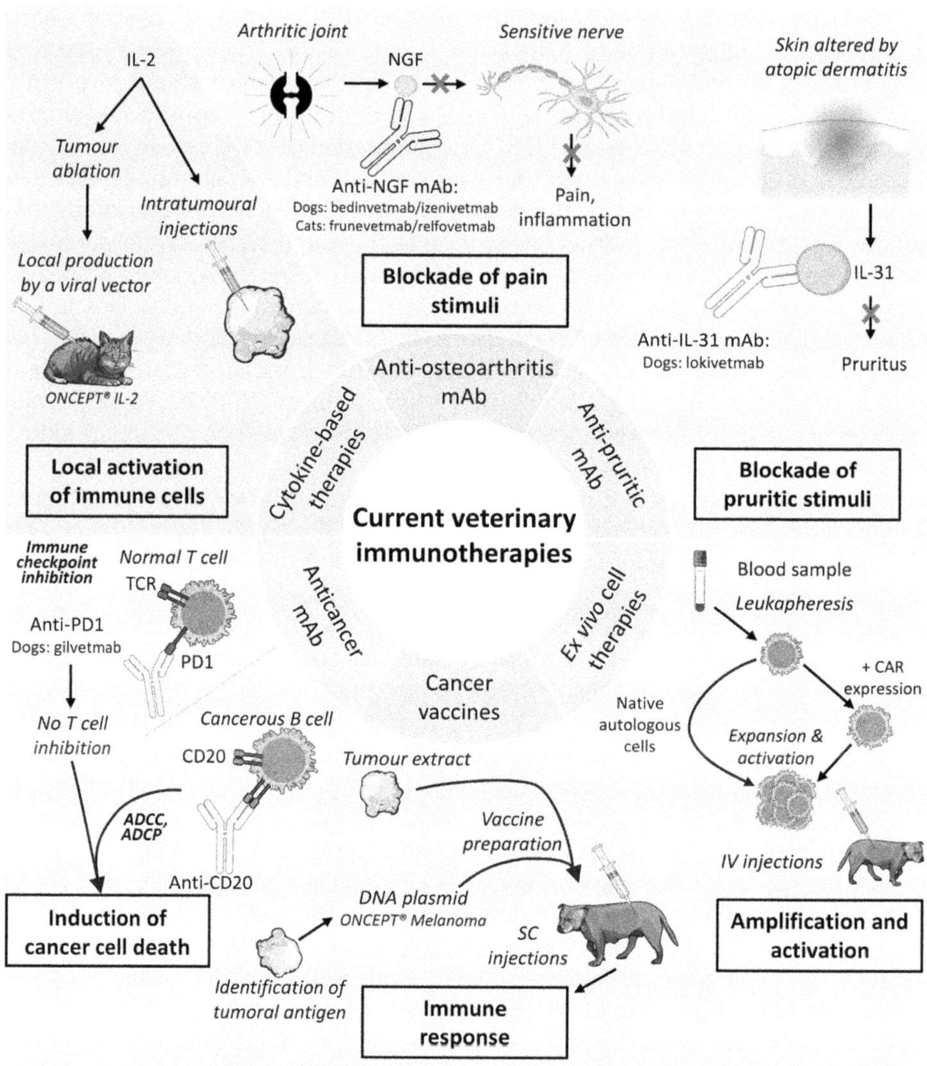

FIGURE 17.1 Current immunotherapy in veterinary medicine. Medications currently on the market, or at the forefront of clinical research, are represented. The reader is advised to keep in mind that monoclonal antibodies presented here heavily differ in their structure. Icons were downloaded from BioArt.
ADCC, antibody-dependent cell cytotoxicity; ADCP, antibody-dependent cell phagocytosis; CAR, chimeric antigen receptor; CD, cluster of differentiation; IL: interleukin; IV, intravenous; NGF: nerve growth factor; mAb: monoclonal antibody; PD-1, programmed cell death protein 1; SC, subcutaneous; TCR, T-cell receptor.

All mAbs (currently bedinvetmab and frunevetmab, newly relfovetmab and izenivetmab) used in companion animals against osteoarthritis target Nerve Growth Factor (NGF), which is highly implicated in pain sensation. Anti-NGF antibodies have been tested in people for at least 15 years. A recent meta-analysis demonstrated

TABLE 17.1 Overview of the monoclonal antibodies with positive opinions or approvals from regulatory agencies (top) or cited in this chapter (bottom).

Antibody (trade name, manufacturer)	Molecular target	Indication, species	Year of authorisation (regulatory agency)	Publications of interest
Bedinvetmab (LIBRELA, Zoetis /BERANSA, Rhodes)	NGF	Osteoarthritis, dogs	2020 (EMA), 2023 (FDA), 2022 (APVMA)	[21, 68]
Frunevetmab (SOLENSIA, Zoetis)	NGF	Osteoarthritis, cats	2021 (EMA), 2022 (FDA), 2022 (APVMA)	[23, 69]
Relfovetmab (PORTELA, Zoetis)	NGF	Osteoarthritis, cats	2025 (EMA, positive opinion only)	*
Izenivetmab (LENIVIA, Zoetis)	NGF	Osteoarthritis, dogs	2025 (EMA, positive opinion only)	[73]
Lokivetmab (CYTOPOINT, Zoetis)	IL-31	Atopic dermatitis, dogs	2017 (EMA), 2016 (USDA), 2018 (APVMA)	[29, 30]
Blontuvetmab (AT-004, BLONTRESS, Aratana Therapeutics) – removed	CD-20	B cell lymphoma, dogs	2015 (USDA)	*
Tamtuvetmab (AT-005, TACTRESS, Aratana Therapeutics) – removed	CD-52	B cell lymphoma, dogs	2016 (USDA)	[52]
Gilvetmab (no trade name Merck/MSD)	PD-1	Mast cell tumours and melanoma, dogs	2023 (USDA, conditional approval)	*
Canine Parvovirus Monoclonal Antibody (CPMA®, Elanco)	Canine Parvovirus viral protein-2	Parvoviral infections, dogs	2025 (USDA, conditional approval)	[70]
4E1–7-B_f (chimeric rat-canine defucosylated)	CD-20	B cell lymphoma, dogs	—	[47]
1E4 (cIgGB = canine IgG B)	CD-20	B cell lymphoma, dogs	—	[51, 71]
6C8	CD-20	B cell lymphoma, dogs	—	[72]
3 N1	CD-20	B cell lymphoma, dogs	—	[49]
NCD1.2 (recombinant, single chain)	CD-20	B cell lymphoma, dogs	—	[50]
c4G12	PD-L1	Oral malignant melanoma, (sarcoma), dogs	—	[54, 55]
NOL226–2-D10	IL-5	Insect bite hypersensitivity, horses	—	[31]

APVMA, Australian Pesticides and Veterinary Medicines Authority; CD, Cluster of Differentiation; EMA, European Medicines Agency; IL: interleukin; NGF: Nerve Growth Factor; PD-1, Programmed Cell Death protein 1; PD-L1, PD1-Ligand 1; USDA, United States Department of Agriculture.

* No peer-reviewed, published data available at the date of writing.

that anti-NGF mAbs are as efficient as standard analgesic drugs, but cause slightly more frequent mild adverse effects [20]. However, some clinical trials concluded that anti-NGF mAbs induced rapidly progressive osteoarthritis (RPOA), leading to premature joint replacement [20]. These potentially dramatic side effects heavily hampered the clinical potential of anti-NGF treatment in people.

To date, only two mAbs have received full authorisation on the veterinary market: bedinvetmab (LIBRELA®, Zoetis or BERANSA®, Rhodes in Australia) and frunevetmab (SOLENSIA®, Zoetis) (Table 17.1). Both are fully, respectively, caninised and felinised using a technology developed by Nexvet, called PETisation [21, 22]. Thus, the immunogenicity of these antibodies was proven to be low [23]. Both drugs are administered subcutaneously once per month and have displayed efficacy greater than or equal to classical treatments (mainly non-steroidal anti-inflammatory drugs).

The European regulatory agency recently released a positive opinion on relfovetmab (PORTELA®, Zoetis) and izenivetmab (LENIVIA®, Zoetis), respectively, designed for cats and dogs with a quarterly injection [24, 25]. Preliminary data even point to a positive effect of relfovetmab for up to 270 days, but the manufacturer remains cautious. However, the results of both clinical trials and the modifications on these antibodies that allow for this longer action time are yet to be disclosed.

A safety concern for bedinvetmab has recently been raised by a group composed of 18 experts, describing 19 cases of dogs presenting musculoskeletal adverse events [26]. Last year, this author had already drawn attention to potential adverse effects following bedinvetmab administration, warranting a response from Zoetis [27]. Briefly, the safety concerns demonstrated the possibility that bedinvetmab administration caused RPOA in treated dogs; the laboratory refuted that claim, stating that RPOA has never been described in dogs. The existence of canine RPOA remains unsolved as several veterinary specialists published contradictory opinions. Given that the medication has only been released for a couple of years, long-term prospective studies assessing the long-term safety of anti-NGF mAb are still to be conducted. Now this debate is up to the regulatory administrations to solve.

17.3 MONOCLONAL ANTIBODIES IN THE TREATMENT OF CANINE ATOPIC DERMATITIS

Canine atopic dermatitis is a hereditary chronic inflammatory skin disease clinically characterised by pruritus that affects 10–15% of dogs [28]. Its causes are multifactorial and incompletely understood, as it is associated with impaired skin barrier, presence of IgE antibodies to environmental allergens, and cutaneous microbiome alterations. Pruritus is not only a symptom but also an aggravating factor, because the constant licking fuels local inflammation and threatens potential secondary infection. Interleukin-31 (IL-31), as one of the main molecular controllers of pruritus, is of utmost therapeutic importance [28].

A caninised mAb targeting IL-31, lokivetmab (CYTOPOINT®, Zoetis), was the first mAb authorised in veterinary medicine close to ten years ago (Table 17.1). Lokivetmab is administered subcutaneously and is recommended to be injected once a month [29]. It is generally assumed to be efficient and safe, rarely generating antidrug antibodies thanks to its caninisation (<2,5% in four different studies) [28–30].

In a similar approach, an equine mAb was recently developed to address insect bite hypersensitivity, a frequent equine allergic condition. Currently available therapies rely on glucocorticoid administration, accompanied by adverse effects, and the avoidance of Culicoides bites by maintaining horses in stables, using rugs, nets, and/or insect repellents. As the implicated allergens have not yet been identified, allergen-specific immunotherapy is not currently available. IL-5, secreted by Th2 cells, is implicated in the activation and regulation of eosinophils and seems implicated in the pathogenesis of this allergic condition. A team recently developed an equine IgG6, an isotype that cannot interact with cellular components of the immune system [31], to target equine IL-5. Additional trials are required to better characterise its safety and usefulness.

17.4 ANTICANCER IMMUNOTHERAPIES

Similar to human medicine, a leading interest of veterinary immunotherapy is directed against cancer. Amongst immunotherapeutic approaches, cytokine administration, cancer vaccines, mAbs targeting either tumour cells or immune checkpoints, adoptive cell transfer (tumour-infiltrating lymphocytes or Chimeric Antigen Receptor [CAR]-T-cell therapy), or immunogene therapies have been tested in companion animals [32–37]. However, only few treatments have been authorised yet, so the bulk of literature consists of preclinical research.

17.4.1 Cytokines-Based Strategies

The prospect of using cytokines to draw the attention of the immune system to cancerous sites has been investigated for more than 20 years. The only treatment that has been authorised relies on a defective canarypox vector used to produce IL-2 locally (ONCEPT® IL-2, Boehringer Ingelheim Animal Health) [38]. It was authorised in the EU in 2013 and conditionally approved by the United States Department of Agriculture (USDA) in 2015 to prevent recurrence of feline fibrosarcoma after surgery and in association with radiotherapy. IL-2 was selected for its stimulatory effect on T cells, and the local production limits adverse effects [38]. It demonstrated satisfactory safety and relatively good efficacy in limiting recurrence, cutting the usually high risk in half after a year [39]. However, feline fibrosarcoma can arise from injections, and ONCEPT IL-2 requires 30 injections (five injections for every one of six administrations). This has heavily limited its use in clinical settings, principally regarding owner compliance.

Given that similar results had been obtained with feline and human IL-2, some teams hypothesised that the feline construct could also work in other animals. Two studies have evaluated its action after intratumoural injections in equine sarcoids [40, 41]. The results were nuanced, with most tumours showing partial regression (in both treated and untreated sarcoids), albeit in only two small cohorts. In cattle, intratumoural IL-2 injections achieved complete regressions of 50–60% of bovine ocular squamous cell carcinomas [42].

These cytokine-based approaches represent a very attractive treatment option in animal cancer patients as they can easily be associated with other therapies, remain affordable, and are well-tolerated.

17.4.2 Vaccination Against Human Tyrosinase in Dog Melanoma

The first authorised cancer vaccine in veterinary medicine was ONCEPT Melanoma (Merial Inc.) in 2009 in the USA [43]. This technology relies on the injection of a DNA plasmid coding for the human tyrosinase, an enzyme necessary for melanin synthesis. Human tyrosinase, while different enough from the canine enzyme to elicit an antibody response, is homologous enough so that antibodies can target canine tyrosinase and thus tumoural melanocytes. However, a recent review concluded that ONCEPT Melanoma lacks efficacy, since median survival time was similar with or without the vaccine [44].

17.4.3 Monoclonal Antibodies Targeting Tumour Antigens

Cluster of Differentiation (CD)20 is a common receptor of B cells of Non-Hodgkin's lymphoma subtypes in people that is also expressed in some canine B cell lymphomas [45]. Rituximab, a human mAb targeting CD20, could not bind canine B cells, probably due to mutations altering specificity [46]. This led to the development of several canine mAbs against canine CD20 (see Table 17.1). The elimination of cancer cells labelled by mAbs depends on the immunogenicity of the antigens and the ability to activate effector functions by the mAbs via interactions with FcR expressed at the surface of immune cells or with effectors like the complement system. The functional properties of some of these anti-canine CD20 mAbs have been studied to describe their biological activities. Some were shown to mediate antibody-dependent cellular cytotoxicity (ADCC) (clones 4E1-7-B_f, maybe 1E4) or antibody-dependent cellular phagocytosis (ADCP) (clones 1E4 and 6C8); however, none were found to induce complement-dependent cytotoxicity (CDC) [47, 48]. The functional abilities of the two remaining clones, NCD1.2, which targets both canine and human CD20, and 3N1, were insufficiently characterised, and information regarding their biological activities is lacking [49, 50]. A caninised anti-CD20 antibody was licenced in 2015 (AT-004, renamed blontuvetmab, BLONTRESS®, Aratana Therapeutics), but its ability to bind to canine CD20 and to induce canine B cell depletion has not been demonstrated. It has been pulled out of the market by the manufacturer due to insufficient specificity and efficacy.

To our knowledge, a single clinical trial using a canine anti-CD20 in dogs suffering from B-cell lymphoma has been published [51]. In this study, 42 owned dogs with diffuse large B-cell lymphoma were treated with the clone AE4-cIgGB in combination with doxorubicin. Despite some adverse effects consistent with doxorubicin administration, a rapid and durable depletion of B cells was observed, which seems promising for clinical use in dogs [51]. However, additional trials are still required to better characterise and demonstrate the benefits of such an approach in canine patients.

Another mAb, tamtuvetmab (TACTRESS®, Aratana Therapeutics), targeting CD52, was licenced in 2016 for the management of T-cell dog lymphoma but was withdrawn from the market along with the already mentioned blontuvetmab. This mAb did not bring sufficient improvement in canine patients in a clinical trial comparing chemotherapy and placebo or chemotherapy and anti-CD52 groups [52].

17.4.4 Immune Checkpoint Inhibition

Tumour cells modulate the immune response through several mechanisms, including regulatory signals via the expression of molecules like Programmed Cell Death protein 1 (PD-1), resulting in inactivation of T lymphocytes. Immune checkpoint inhibition could restore immune recognition and destruction of the cancer cells and is a major point of research in veterinary medicine. The first veterinary immune checkpoint inhibitor available to the public is gilvetmab (no trade name, Merck Animal Health), which received a conditional licence approval for the treatment of dogs suffering from stage I to III mast cell tumours or stage II and III melanoma [53]. Gilvetmab is a caninised mAb derived from a rat mAb through PETisation, as described by Gearing et al. (2013). Preliminary data presented by the manufacturer look promising, with a good tolerability and 60–73% of objective or stable response [53]. Other attempts based on anti-PD1-Ligand-1 (PD-L1) mAb administration were also recently investigated [54, 55].

17.4.5 CAR-T Cells

Cytotoxic T lymphocytes kill the cells they recognise via their TCR when an epitope is presented by the target cell in association with its MHC molecule. An efficient way to improve T lymphocyte effectiveness is based on the engineering of autologous T cells to obtain a chimeric receptor, which can directly recognise targets through the part of the antibody used. The first canine human epidermal growth factor 2 (HER2)-specific [56] and CD20-specific CAR-T cells [57] were developed almost ten years ago in dogs. To overcome immune checkpoint hijacking by the tumour cells, CAR-T cells were generated containing chimeric costimulatory domains, resulting in activation instead of inhibition after PD-1 engagement [58, 59]. More recently, a team also published a protocol to generate feline CAR-T cells [60]. However, clinical use of feline CAR-T cells still requires more immunological tools, like mAbs against feline tumour antigens. Another major limitation to CAR-T cell-based therapies in pet animals is the price, which is currently estimated in people to be around $300–500k [61], not accounting for the fact that few veterinary hospitals have the laboratory equipment yet.

17.4.6 Case-Study: Adoptive Cell Transfer Protocol Against Osteosarcoma (ECI®, Elias Animal Health)

This treatment was fully approved by the USDA in 2025. It consists of a combination of autologous cancer vaccination, adoptive T-cell transfer, and IL-2 administration and was tested in 14 dogs affected by osteosarcoma, after amputation, but in the absence of other treatments [62]. *The vaccine was composed of irradiated tumour cells obtained during amputation. T lymphocytes, obtained by leukapheresis after vaccination, were amplified and activated with a superantigen cocktail before being reinjected. Human recombinant IL-2 was then administered to the dogs five times every other day. Despite no additional chemotherapy, the median overall survival time for these dogs was 415 days, much higher than in untreated dogs* [62]. *This promising pilot study led to a bigger-scale clinical trial which included 86 dogs, whose results, to our knowledge, have not yet been published in a peer-reviewed journal* [63]. *Of note, survival was lower than in the carboplatin-receiving positive control group.*

As already stated, this overview is not exhaustive. Other approaches not developed in this chapter were recently reviewed, such as autologous cancer vaccines in animals [64], immunogene therapy [33], or virotherapy [65].

17.5 PERSPECTIVES

Immunotherapy in companion animals is still in its infancy. Additional studies and trials designed to unveil new therapeutic options will also help better characterise the immune responses in animals. The properties of antibodies (including the effectors they recruit) depend on FcR distribution on immune cells, which might differ between targets (inflammatory, auto-immune, cancer, infectious diseases, etc.) and species. Those differences will have to be taken into account to design a new mAb.

Those serendipitous discoveries can go a long way. For instance, the description of light-chain lacking IgG2 and IgG3 in camels [66] eventually led to the proposal of the combination of an anti-idiotype nanobody with another target-specific nanobody, which results in an 'adaptabody' displaying two different binding sites [67]. The two nanobodies can then be used to easily generate 'new mAb'. Indeed, an adaptabody can recognise the specific target via the first nanobody, and with the other nanobody bind to an already available mAb. With the use of phage display libraries, this technique would make the generation of new mAbs much cheaper in species in which one mAb has already been constructed [67]. This is especially promising in veterinary medicine, where resources to develop new mAb remain limited.

As a concluding remark, the relationship between human and veterinary research is inherently reciprocal. Indeed, veterinary trials can represent preclinical studies to treat people, but human medications also allow for proof-of-concept animal studies. However, this raises an ethical issue: owners likely want their animal to have access to the best therapeutic options, so the benefit/risk balance must always be kept in mind when designing clinical trials in client-owned animals. This requires informed consent, equating to a full awareness of the risks of such preclinical or clinical studies.

KEY TERMS & DEFINITIONS SIDEBAR

ADCC Antibody-dependent cell cytotoxicity designs a process in which a cell coated with antibodies becomes a target for immune cells, like NK cells, expressing Fc receptors. Upon binding of the mAb to the Fc receptor, NK cells become activated, which triggers the release of the cytotoxic content of their granules, resulting in the death of the target cell. The recognition of antibodies by NK cell Fc receptors is restricted to some isotypes.

ADCP Antibody-dependent cellular phagocytosis refers to the process in which the coating of cells with antibodies leads to their recognition via the Fc receptors expressed by phagocytes (like macrophages) and their subsequent engulfment and destruction by phagolysosomal degradation. The recognition of antibodies by phagocytes' Fc receptors is restricted to certain isotypes.

CDC Complement-dependent cytotoxicity arises from activation of the complement system, which leads to the formation of a membrane attack complex on the surface of an antibody-coated cell (like a tumour cell), resulting in its destruction. The ability to activate the complement system differs between the different antibody isotypes.

IL-31 Mainly produced by T cells, IL-31 is considered the main trigger for pruritus in dogs. It is associated with sensory neuronal growth and stimulation (which could participate in sustained pruritus) and negatively impacts skin barrier maintenance (by repressing filaggrin).

NGF NGF is a pro-inflammatory cytokine, secreted by macrophages, mast cells, synoviocytes, and neural cells. It induces neuron proliferation and sensitisation to pain signals in osteoarthritis.

PETisation This process involves identifying the residues within the Fc region of an antibody from a donor species (such as rat) that should be substituted to generate an antibody specific to another species (such as a dog or cat). The recognition domains remain unaltered, while the immunogenicity of the resulting antibody is reduced in the target species.

PD-1 Programmed death-1 is a receptor expressed on activated T cells. Upon engagement with its ligand (PD-L1), it inhibits signalling from the antigen receptor and thus prevents T-cell activation. PD-L1 expression by tumour cells represents an immune escape mechanism.

LIST OF ABBREVIATIONS

ABCC3	ATP binding cassette subfamily C member 3
ADCC	antibody-dependent cell cytotoxicity
ADCP	antibody-dependent cell phagocytosis
CAR	chimeric antigen receptor
CD	cluster of differentiation
CDC	complement dependent cytotoxicity
GWAS	genome-wide association studies
HER2	human epidermal growth factor 2
IL	interleukin
mAb	monoclonal antibody
NGF	nerve growth factor
PD-1	programmed cell death protein 1
PD-L1	PD1-ligand 1
RPOA	rapidly progressive osteoarthritis
SNP	single nucleotide polymorphism
USDA	United States department of agriculture

REVIEW QUESTIONS

1. How do the anti-NGF mAbs used to treat osteoarthritis in cats or dogs function?
2. What is the target of the mAb licenced in dogs to treat (some) allergic dermatitis conditions in dogs?
   - IL-2
   - IL-4
   - IL-5
   - IL-6
   - IL-31
3. Why might mAbs developed in humans not be relevant for animals?
4. For what reasons do dogs represent interesting models to study some immunotherapeutic approaches in preclinical studies (or translational research)?
5. What is the genetic characteristic explaining why the canine species can be useful in identifying cancer (or other disorder) genomic-associated loci?

REFERENCES

1. Schiffman, J.D. and Breen, M. (2015). Comparative oncology: what dogs and other species can teach us about humans with cancer. *Philos Trans R Soc B Biol Sci* 370 (1673): 20140231. https://doi:10.1098/rstb.2014.0231
2. LeBlanc, A.K. and Mazcko, C.N. (2020). Improving human cancer therapy through the evaluation of pet dogs. *Nat Rev Cancer* 20 (12): 727–742. https://doi:10.1038/s41568-020-0297-3
3. Cahill, J.A., Smith, L.A., Gottipati, S. et al. (2024). Bringing the genomic revolution to comparative oncology: human and dog cancers. *Annu Rev Biomed Data Sci* 7 (1): 107–129. https://doi:10.1146/annurev-biodatasci-102423-111936
4. Mendez-Gomez, H.R., DeVries, A., Castillo, P. et al. (2024). RNA aggregates harness the danger response for potent cancer immunotherapy. *Cell* 187 (10): 2521–2535.e21 https://doi:10.1016/j.cell.2024.04.003.
5. Kocikowski, M., Yébenes Mayordomo, M., Alfaro, J., and Parys, M. (2025). Barking up the right tree: immune checkpoint signatures of human and dog cancers. *PLOS Comput Biol* 21 (8): e1013270. https://doi:10.1371/journal.pcbi.1013270
6. Lindblad-Toh, K., Broad Sequencing Platform Members, Wade, C.M. et al. (2005). Genome sequence, comparative analysis and haplotype structure of the domestic dog. *Nature* 438 (7069): 803–819. https://doi:10.1038/nature04338
7. Cadieu, E. and Ostrander, E.A. (2007). Canine genetics offers new mechanisms for the study of human cancer. *Cancer Epidemiol Biomarkers Prev* 16 (11): 2181–2183. https://doi:10.1158/1055-9965.EPI-07-2667
8. Shearin, A.L. and Ostrander, E.A. (2010). Leading the way: canine models of genomics and disease. *Dis Model Mech* 3 (1–2): 27–34. https://doi:10.1242/dmm.004358
9. Boyko, A.R. (2011). The domestic dog: man's best friend in the genomic era. *Genome Biol* 12 (2): 216. https://doi:10.1186/gb-2011-12-2-216
10. Ostrander, E.A., Wang, G.D., Larson, G. et al. (2019). Dog10K: an international sequencing effort to advance studies of canine domestication, phenotypes and health. *Natl Sci Rev* 6 (4): 810–824. https://doi:10.1093/nsr/nwz049
11. Binversie, E.E., Momen, M., Rosa, G.J.M. et al. (2022). Across-breed genetic investigation of canine hip dysplasia, elbow dysplasia, and anterior cruciate ligament rupture using whole-genome sequencing. *Front Genet* 13: 913354. https://doi:10.3389/fgene.2022.913354
12. Meadows, J.R.S., Kidd, J.M., Wang, G.D. et al. (2023). Genome sequencing of 2000 canids by the Dog10K consortium advances the understanding of demography, genome function and architecture. *Genome Biol* 24 (1): 187. https://doi:10.1186/s13059-023-03023-7
13. Gardner, H.L., Sivaprakasam, K., Briones, N. et al. (2019). Canine osteosarcoma genome sequencing identifies recurrent mutations in DMD and the histone methyltransferase gene SETD2. *Commun Biol* 2 (1): 266. https://doi:10.1038/s42003-019-0487-2
14. Zhou, T., Pu, S.Y., Zhang, S.J. et al. (2025). Dog10K: an integrated Dog10K database summarizing canine multi-omics. *Nucleic Acids Res* 53 (D1): D939–D947. https://doi:10.1093/nar/gkae928
15. Cook, S.R., Hugen, S., Hayward, J.J. et al. (2025). Genomic analyses identify 15 risk loci and reveal HDAC2, SOX2-OT, and IGF2BP2 in a naturally occurring canine model of gastric cancer. *Proc Natl Acad Sci USA* 122 (22): e2416723122. https://doi:10.1073/pnas.2416723122
16. Fuller, A.M., DeVine, A., Murazzi, I. et al. (2022). Comparative oncology reveals DNMT3B as a molecular vulnerability in undifferentiated pleomorphic sarcoma. *Cell Oncol* 45 (6): 1277–1295. https://doi:10.1007/s13402-022-00717-1
17. Sarver, A.L., Mills, L.J., Makielski, K.M. et al. (2023). Distinct mechanisms of PTEN inactivation in dogs and humans highlight convergent molecular events that drive cell division in the pathogenesis of osteosarcoma. *Cancer Genet* 276–277: 1–11. https://doi:10.1016/j.cancergen.2023.05.001
18. Aruvornlop, P., Ploypetch, S., Sakcamduang, W. et al. (2025). Phosphoproteomic profiling of feline mammary carcinoma: insights into tumor grading and potential therapeutic targets. *PLOS One* 20 (8): e0330520. https://doi:10.1371/journal.pone.0330520

19. Enomoto, M., Mantyh, P.W., Murrell, J. et al. (2019). Anti-nerve growth factor monoclonal antibodies for the control of pain in dogs and cats. *Vet Rec* 184 (1): 23–23. https://doi:10.1136/vr.104590
20. Gao, Y., Hu, Z., Huang, Y. et al. (2022). Efficacy and safety of anti–nerve growth factor antibody therapy for hip and knee osteoarthritis: a meta-analysis. *Orthop J Sports Med* 10 (4): 23259671221088590. https://doi:10.1177/23259671221088590
21. Gearing, D.P., Virtue, E.R., Gearing, R.P., and Drew, A.C. (2013). A fully caninised anti-NGF monoclonal antibody for pain relief in dogs. *BMC Vet Res* 9 (1): 226. https://doi:10.1186/1746-6148-9-226
22. Gearing, D.P., Huebner, M., Virtue, E.R. et al. (2016). In vitro and in vivo characterization of a fully felinized therapeutic anti-nerve growth factor monoclonal antibody for the treatment of pain in cats. *J Vet Intern Med* 30 (4): 1129–1137. https://doi:10.1111/jvim.13985
23. Walters, R.R., Boucher, J.F., and De Toni, F. (2021). Pharmacokinetics and immunogenicity of frunevetmab in osteoarthritic cats following intravenous and subcutaneous administration. *Front Vet Sci* 8: 687448. https://doi:10.3389/fvets.2021.687448
24. Zoetis. Zoetis receives positive opinion from CVMP for Portela (relfovetmab) to alleviate pain associated with osteoarthritis in cats [Internet] 2025. Available from: https://news.zoetis.com/press-releases/press-release-details/2025/Zoetis-Receives-Positive-Opinion-from-CVMP-for-Portela-relfovetmab-to-Alleviate-Pain-Associated-with-Osteoarthritis-in-Cats/default.aspx
25. Zoetis. Zoetis receives positive opinion from CVMP for Lenivia® (izenivetmab) to reduce pain associated with osteoarthritis (OA) in dogs [Internet]. 2025 [cited 2025 Oct 15]. Available from: https://news.zoetis.com/press-releases/press-release-details/2025/Zoetis-Receives-Positive-Opinion-from-CVMP-for-Lenivia-izenivetmab-to-Reduce-Pain-Associated-with-Osteoarthritis-OA-in-Dogs/default.aspx
26. Farrell, M., Waibel, F.W.A., Carrera, I. et al. (2025). Musculoskeletal adverse events in dogs receiving bedinvetmab (Librela). *Front Vet Sci* 12: 1581490. https://doi:10.3389/fvets.2025.1581490
27. Werts, A., Reece, D., Simon, T., and Cole, P. (2024). Re: Re: Laboratory safety evaluation of bedinvetmab, a canine anti-nerve growth factor monoclonal antibody, in dogs. *Vet J* 306: 106175. https://doi:10.1016/j.tvjl.2024.106175
28. Kasper, B., Zablotski, Y., and Mueller, R.S. (2024). Long-term use of lokivetmab in dogs with atopic dermatitis. *Vet Dermatol* 35 (6): 683–693. https://doi:10.1111/vde.13286
29. Michels, G.M., Ramsey, D.S., Walsh, K.F. et al. (2016). A blinded, randomized, placebo-controlled, dose determination trial of lokivetmab, a caninized, anti-canine IL-31 monoclonal antibody in client owned dogs with atopic dermatitis. *Vet Dermatol* 27 (6): 478–e129. https://doi:10.1111/vde.12376
30. Michels, G.M., Walsh, K.F., Kryda, K.A. et al. (2016). A blinded, randomized, placebo-controlled trial of the safety of lokivetmab, a caninized anti-canine IL-31 monoclonal antibody in client-owned dogs with atopic dermatitis. *Vet Dermatol* 27 (6): 505. https://doi:10.1111/vde.12364
31. Langreder, N., Schäckermann, D., Meier, D. et al. (2023). Development of an inhibiting antibody against equine interleukin 5 to treat insect bite hypersensitivity of horses. *Sci Rep* 13 (1): 4029. https://doi:10.1038/s41598-023-31173-y
32. Bergman, P.J. (2024). Cancer immunotherapy. *Vet Clin North Am Small Anim Pract* 54 (3): 441–468. https://doi:10.1016/j.cvsm.2023.12.002
33. Glikin, G.C. and Finocchiaro, L.M.E. (2025). Clinical trials of cancer immunogene therapies in companion animals: an update (2017–2024). *Vet Sci* 12 (4): 329. https://doi:10.3390/vetsci12040329
34. Hampel, J.M., Cheuk, N., Barbosa, M.M.P., and Fan, T.M. (2024). The promise of immunotherapeutic strategies to advance cancer treatment in pet dogs. *J Am Vet Med Assoc* 262 (12): 1583–1593. https://doi:10.2460/javma.24.08.0532
35. Mestrinho, L.A. and Santos, R.R. (2021). Translational oncotargets for immunotherapy: From pet dogs to humans. *Adv Drug Deliv Rev* 172: 296–313. https://doi:10.1016/j.addr.2021.02.020
36. Regan, D., Guth, A., Coy, J., and Dow, S. (2016). Cancer immunotherapy in veterinary medicine: current options and new developments. *Vet J* 207: 20–28. https://doi:10.1016/j.tvjl.2015.10.008

37. Wang, J., Zhou, X., Elazab, S.T. et al. (2025). Current review of monoclonal antibody therapeutics in small animal medicine. *Animals* 15 (4): 472. https://doi:10.3390/ani15040472
38. Jourdier, T.M., Moste, C., Bonnet, M.C. et al. (2003). Local immunotherapy of spontaneous feline fibrosarcomas using recombinant poxviruses expressing interleukin 2 (IL2). *Gene Ther* 10 (26): 2126–2132. https://doi:10.1038/sj.gt.3302124
39. Jas, D., Soyer, C., De Fornel-Thibaud, P. et al. (2015). Adjuvant immunotherapy of feline injection-site sarcomas with the recombinant canarypox virus expressing feline interleukine-2 evaluated in a controlled monocentric clinical trial when used in association with surgery and brachytherapy. *Trials Vaccinol* 4: 1–8. https://doi:10.1016/j.trivac.2014.11.001
40. Loschelder-Ostrowski, J., Winter, J.C., Merle, R. et al. (2021). Treatment of equine sarcoids using recombinant poxviruses expressing feline interleukin-2. *Vet Dermatol* 32 (3): 283. https://doi:10.1111/vde.12941
41. Saba, C., Eggleston, R., Parks, A. et al. (2022). ALVAC-fIL2, a feline interleukin-2 immunomodulator, as a treatment for sarcoids in horses: a pilot study. *J Vet Intern Med* 36 (3): 1179–1184. https://doi:10.1111/jvim.16425
42. Stewart, R.J.E., Masztalerz, A., John, J.L., and Den Otter, W. (2005). Local interleukin-2 and interleukin-12 therapy of bovine ocular squamous cell carcinomas. *Vet Immunol Immunopathol* 106 (3–4): 277–284. https://doi:10.1016/j.vetimm.2005.03.002
43. Bergman, P.J., Camps-Palau, M.A., McKnight, J.A. et al. (2006). Development of a xenogeneic DNA vaccine program for canine malignant melanoma at the Animal Medical Center. *Vaccine* 24 (21): 4582–4585. https://doi:10.1016/j.vaccine.2005.08.027
44. Pellin, M.A. (2022). The use of Oncept melanoma vaccine in veterinary patients: a review of the literature. *Vet Sci* 9 (11): 597. https://doi:10.3390/vetsci9110597
45. Jubala, C.M., Wojcieszyn, J.W., Valli, V.E.O. et al. (2005). CD20 expression in normal canine B cells and in canine non-Hodgkin lymphoma. *Vet Pathol* 42 (4): 468–476. https://doi:10.1354/vp.42-4-468
46. Impellizeri, J.A., Howell, K., McKeever, K.P., and Crow, S.E. (2006). The role of rituximab in the treatment of canine lymphoma: an ex vivo evaluation. *Vet J* 171 (3): 556–558. https://doi:10.1016/j.tvjl.2005.03.005
47. Mizuno, T., Kato, Y., Kaneko, M.K. et al. (2020). Generation of a canine anti-canine CD20 antibody for canine lymphoma treatment. *Sci Rep* 10 (1): 11476. https://doi:10.1038/s41598-020-68470-9
48. Mizuno, T., Kato, Y., Tsukui, T., and Igase, M. (2025). Characterization of anti-canine CD20 antibody 4E1-7-B_f and comparison with commercially available anti-human CD20 antibodies. *PLOS One* 20 (6): e0325526. https://doi:10.1371/journal.pone.0325526
49. Dias, J.N.R., Almeida, A., André, A.S. et al. (2022). Characterization of the canine CD20 as a therapeutic target for comparative passive immunotherapy. *Sci Rep* 12 (1): 2678. https://doi:10.1038/s41598-022-06549-1
50. Jain, S., Aresu, L., Comazzi, S. et al. (2016). The development of a recombinant scFv monoclonal antibody targeting canine CD20 for use in comparative medicine. *PLOS One* 11 (2): e0148366. https://doi:10.1371/journal.pone.0148366
51. McLinden, G.P., Avery, A.C., Gardner, H.L. et al. (2024). Safety and biologic activity of a canine anti-CD20 monoclonal antibody in dogs with diffuse large B-cell lymphoma. *J Vet Intern Med* 38 (3): 1666–1674. https://doi:10.1111/jvim.17080
52. Musser, M.L., Clifford, C.A., Bergman, P.J. et al. (2022). Randomised trial evaluating chemotherapy alone or chemotherapy and a novel monoclonal antibody for canine T-cell lymphoma: a multicentre US study. *Vet Rec Open* 9 (1): e49. https://doi:10.1002/vro2.49
53. Madison N, Merck Animal Health. Gilvetmab – product insert [Internet]. 2022 [cited 2025 Oct 3]. Available from: https://merckusa.cvpservice.com/product/basic/view/1047586
54. Maekawa, N., Konnai, S., Takagi, S. et al. (2017). A canine chimeric monoclonal antibody targeting PD-L1 and its clinical efficacy in canine oral malignant melanoma or undifferentiated sarcoma. *Sci Rep* 7 (1): 8951. https://doi:10.1038/s41598-017-09444-2
55. Deguchi, T., Maekawa, N., Konnai, S. et al. (2023). Enhanced systemic antitumour immunity by hypofractionated radiotherapy and anti-PD-L1 therapy in dogs with pulmonary metastatic oral malignant melanoma. *Cancers* 15 (11): 3013. https://doi:10.3390/cancers15113013

56. Mata, M., Vera, J.F., Gerken, C. et al. (2014). Toward immunotherapy with redirected T cells in a large animal model: ex vivo activation, expansion, and genetic modification of canine T cells. *J Immunother* 37 (8): 407–415. https://doi:10.1097/CJI.0000000000000052
57. Panjwani, M.K., Smith, J.B., Schutsky, K. et al. (2016). Feasibility and safety of RNA-transfected CD20-specific chimeric antigen receptor T cells in dogs with spontaneous B cell lymphoma. *Mol Ther* 24 (9): 1602–1614. https://doi:10.1038/mt.2016.146
58. Sakai, O., Igase, M., and Mizuno, T. (2020). Optimization of canine CD20 chimeric antigen receptor T cell manufacturing and in vitro cytotoxic activity against B-cell lymphoma. *Vet Comp Oncol* 18 (4): 739–752. https://doi:10.1111/vco.12602
59. Yoshimoto, S., Kudo, A., Rotolo, A. et al. (2024). Validation of a PD-1/CD28 chimeric switch receptor to augment CAR-T function in dogs with spontaneous B cell lymphoma. *iScience* 27 (9): 110863. https://doi:10.1016/j.isci.2024.110863
60. Cockey, J.R., Zhou, G.M., Kulp, E.N. et al. (2025). Generation of primary feline chimeric antigen receptor T cells. *Am J Vet Res* 86 (1): ajvr.24.08.0247. https://doi:10.2460/ajvr.24.08.0247
61. Choi, G., Shin, G., and Bae, S. (2022). Price and prejudice? The value of chimeric antigen receptor (CAR) T-cell therapy. *Int J Environ Res Public Health* 19 (19): 12366. https://doi:10.3390/ijerph191912366
62. Flesner, B.K., Wood, G.W., Gayheart-Walsten, P. et al. (2020). Autologous cancer cell vaccination, adoptive T-cell transfer, and interleukin-2 administration results in long-term survival for companion dogs with osteosarcoma. *J Vet Intern Med* 34 (5): 2056–2067. https://doi:10.1111/jvim.15852
63. ELIAS Animal Health. ELIAS cancer immunotherapy – autologous prescription product [Internet]. 2024 [cited 2025 Oct 13]. Available from: https://eliasanimalhealth.com/wp-content/uploads/2025/08/ECI-Product-Insert.pdf
64. Greenberg, C.B., Suckow, M.A., Clauson, R.M. et al. (2025). Autologous cancer vaccines: a precision immunotherapy strategy for veterinary cancer patients. *Anticancer Res* 45 (10): 4115–4130. https://doi:10.21873/anticanres.17766
65. Sánchez, D., Cesarman-Maus, G., Amador-Molina, A., and Lizano, M. (2018). Oncolytic viruses for canine cancer treatment. *Cancers* 10 (11): 404. https://doi:10.3390/cancers10110404
66. Hamers-Casterman, C., Atarhouch, T., Muyldermans, S. et al. (1993). Naturally occurring antibodies devoid of light chains. *Nature* 363 (6428): 446–448. https://doi:10.1038/363446a0
67. González-Techera, A., Lassabe, G., Chabalgoity, J.A. et al. (2025). Adaptabodies: retargeting a predefined monoclonal antibody with bispecific nanobodies for antibody therapy. *Biotechnol J* 20 (8): e70089. https://doi:10.1002/biot.70089
68. Corral, M.J., Moyaert, H., Fernandes, T. et al. (2021). A prospective, randomized, blinded, placebo-controlled multisite clinical study of bedinvetmab, a canine monoclonal antibody targeting nerve growth factor, in dogs with osteoarthritis. *Vet Anaesth Analg* 48 (6): 943--955. https://doi:10.1016/j.vaa.2021.08.001
69. Gruen, M.E., Myers, J.A.E., and Lascelles, B.D.X. (2021). Efficacy and safety of an anti-nerve growth factor antibody (Frunevetmab) for the treatment of degenerative joint disease-associated chronic pain in cats: a multisite pilot field study. *Front Vet Sci* 8: 610028. https://doi:10.3389/fvets.2021.610028
70. Larson, L., Miller, L., Margiasso, M. et al. (2024). Early administration of canine parvovirus monoclonal antibody prevented mortality after experimental challenge. *J Am Vet Med Assoc* 262 (4): 506–512. https://doi:10.2460/javma.23.09.0541
71. Rue, S.M., Eckelman, B.P., Efe, J.A. et al. (2015). Identification of a candidate therapeutic antibody for treatment of canine B-cell lymphoma. *Vet Immunol Immunopathol* 164 (3–4): 148–159. https://doi:10.1016/j.vetimm.2015.02.004
72. Ito, D., Brewer, S., Modiano, J.F., and Beall, M.J. (2015). Development of a novel anti-canine CD20 monoclonal antibody with diagnostic and therapeutic potential. *Leuk Lymphoma* 56 (1): 219–225. https://doi:10.3109/10428194.2014.914193
73. Werts, A., Saad, K., Hummel, B., Mangus, L., Green, E., Guillot, M., Carlson, C., Bedard, A., Boyce, R., Knauer, C. S., Roode, S., & Cole, P.(2026). Laboratory safety evaluations of izenivetmab, a caninized anti-nerve growth factor monoclonal antibody, for three-month alleviation of osteoarthritic pain in dogs. *Vet J* 317, 106635. https://doi.org/10.1016/j.tvjl.2026.106635

CHAPTER 18

Emerging Immunotherapies and Future Horizons

JINGCHEN ZHOU[1], JIYA JOSE[1], MATT VANBROCKLIN[2], JOHN D. HOOPER[3], BRETT M. PATERSON[4], AND FERNANDO SOUZA-FONSECA-GUIMARAES[1]

[1] Frazer Institute, Faculty of Health, Medicine and Behavioural Sciences, The University of Queensland, Woolloongabba, QLD, Australia

[2] Department of Surgery, Huntsman Cancer Institute, University of Utah, Salt Lake City, UT, USA

[3] Mater Research Institute, The University of Queensland, Woolloongabba, QLD, Australia

[4] Centre for Advancing Imaging, Australian Institute for Bioengineering and Nanotechnology, The University of Queensland, Brisbane, QLD, Australia

LEARNING OBJECTIVES

- Understand how multispecific antibodies are designed, and how they work in targeting cancer cells.
- Evaluate principles of antibody–drug conjugates (ADCs), including formulation, payload, and linkage.
- Explain how oncolytic viruses (OVs) target and kill cancer cells.
- Discuss the main challenges facing these therapies, safety concerns, and manufacturing challenges.
- Identify where the field is heading next, including new platforms like mRNA-based immunotherapy.

18.1 INTRODUCTION

The landscape of cancer immunotherapy has undergone a remarkable transformation since the landmark US Food and Drug Administration (FDA) approval of the first checkpoint inhibitor antibody anti-CTLA-4 (ipilimumab) for metastatic melanoma treatment in 2011 [1]. What began as a nascent field has become a cornerstone of oncology, with over 150 FDA approvals by 2024 and real-world usage increasing more than 20-fold since 2011 [2]. However, the initial wave of immune checkpoint inhibitors (ICIs), although revolutionary, marks only the beginning of immunotherapy's full potential. ICIs have transformed oncology and now represent the most widely approved class of cancer immunotherapies by the FDA. However, despite their clinical success, limitations remain. For instance, a substantial proportion of patients do not respond to therapy, others develop resistance over time, and several tumour types remain largely refractory to therapy [3, 4]. These challenges have driven a wave of innovation towards next-generation immunotherapies that extend beyond traditional monoclonal antibodies (mAbs), embracing multi-modal targeting strategies and novel immune activation mechanisms.

Modern antibody engineering exemplifies how the field has progressed beyond the classical full-length immunoglobulin to multifunctional platforms. Figure 18.1 illustrates the evolution of antibody formats, from conventional antibodies and fragments such as fragment antigen-binding (Fab), Fab′, $F(ab')_2$, and single-chain variable fragments (scFv), to alternative formats like heavy-chain antibodies (HcAbs) and their derived nanobodies. More complex constructs include bispecific and trispecific antibodies (TsAbs) as well as antibody–drug conjugates (ADCs). scFvs have also been extensively exploited for applications employing the cancer antigen recognition domains of chimeric antigen receptors (CARs), explored in *Chapter 6 – 'CAR T cell and CAR NK cell therapies'* of this book. Beyond conventional CAR designs, emerging innovations such as SynNotch CAR circuits, fourth-generation armoured CAR constructs, and in vivo CAR delivery approaches represent the next frontier in engineered cellular immunotherapy [5–7]. These diverse formats enable tailored functional enhancements for specific therapeutic objectives.

Bispecific and TsAbs represent a major advancement, enabling simultaneous engagement of multiple antigens [8]. These engineered molecules can redirect immune effector cells to tumour cells, inhibit multiple immune checkpoints concurrently, or condition the tumour microenvironment for improved immune cell infiltration. By integrating the advantages of combination therapy into a single off-the-shelf agent, they offer simplified manufacturing, therapeutic synergy, and potentially reduced systemic toxicity. In parallel, ADCs have redefined the function of antibodies by transforming them into precision delivery vehicles for cytotoxic agents [9]. These constructs combine tumour-specific binding with the potent cell-killing capacity of chemotherapeutic or radiotherapeutic payloads. Advances in linker stability, payload potency, and target selection have significantly improved the safety and efficacy of ADCs, enabling the clinical use of agents that would be otherwise intolerable in unmodified form [10]. This therapeutic modality exploits tumour-enriched surface antigens to deliver lethal agents selectively to malignant cells, sparing healthy tissues.

Oncolytic viruses (OVs) are a class of therapeutics that selectively infect and destroy tumour cells, while also stimulating anti-cancer immune responses, offering a dual mechanism of action distinct from other therapeutic approaches [11]. Although OVs are mechanistically distinct from antibody-based therapies, both approaches share a common aim: to enhance therapeutic precision, overcome resistance, and reshape the tumour microenvironment. However, unlike antibody-based therapies, OVs offer a fundamentally different therapeutic approach. These viruses, either naturally occurring or genetically engineered, selectively infect, replicate in, and lyse cancer cells. Their therapeutic activity involves both direct oncolysis and indirect activation of host immune responses [12]. Contemporary OV platforms are increasingly versatile, capable of expressing immunostimulatory payloads such as cytokines, ICIs, or pro-apoptotic proteins [13]. These engineered viruses can convert immunologically 'cold' tumours into inflamed, immune-responsive environments.

Another immune-modulating advancement in recent years has been the emergence of mRNA-based immunotherapies. Accelerated by the clinical success of mRNA vaccines during the COVID-19 pandemic, this platform enables in vivo immune programming without the need for complex ex vivo cell manufacturing and is now being heavily investigated in the immunotherapy field [14]. As a recent example,

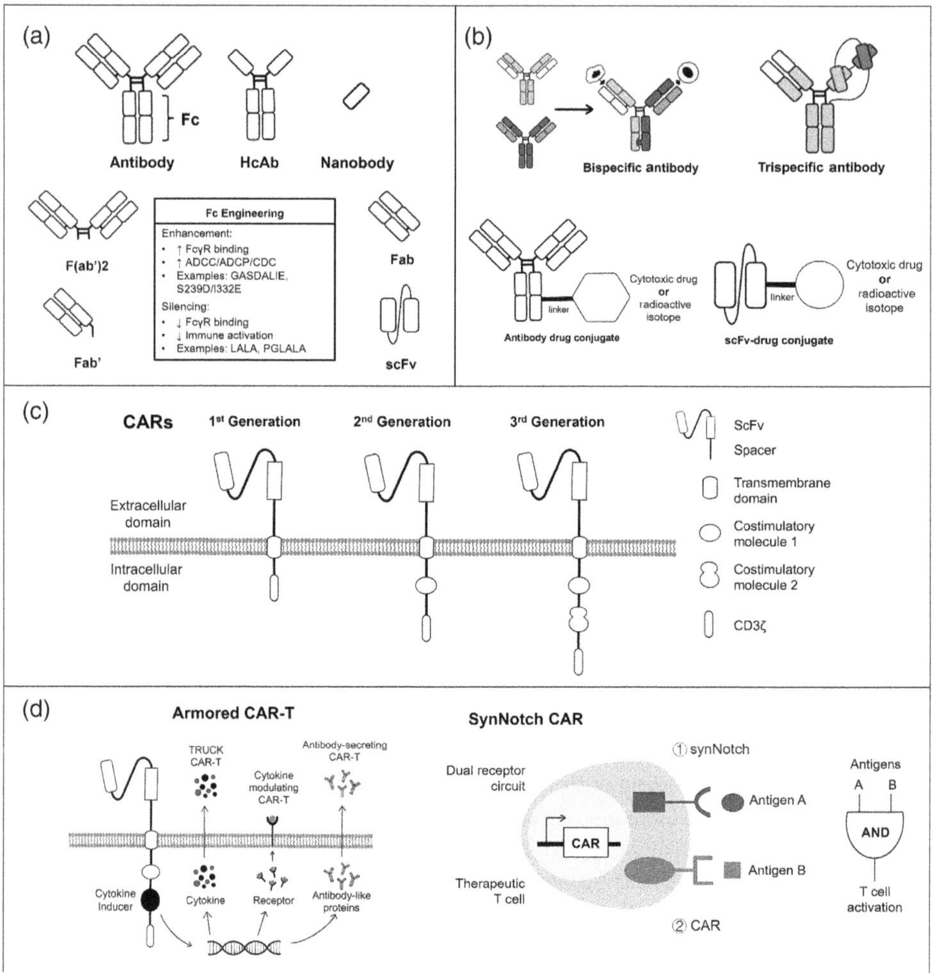

FIGURE 18.1 Engineered antibody formats and CAR design platforms. (a) Antibody formats and Fc engineering. Antibodies can be fragmented into F(ab′)$_2$, Fab′, Fab, or scFv formats, or engineered as heavy-chain antibodies (HcAbs) or nanobodies. Fc engineering can enhance or silence effector functions. Enhancement mutations (e.g. GASDALIE and S239D/I332E) increase FcγR binding and immune activity, while silencing mutations (e.g. LALA and PGLALA) reduce immune activation. (b) Multispecific antibodies and drug conjugates. Bispecific and trispecific antibodies target multiple antigens for enhanced specificity or immune engagement. ADCs or scFv-drug conjugates deliver cytotoxins or radioisotopes via linkers. (c) CAR generations. First-generation CARs feature a transmembrane domain fused to CD3ζ with limited in vivo proliferation. Second-generation CARs incorporate one costimulatory domain, while third-generation CARs contain two costimulatory domains (commonly CD28 or CD137/4-1BB) for improved T cell activation and persistence. (d) Advanced CAR-T strategies. Armoured CAR-T cells are engineered to secrete cytokines, modulate receptors, or produce antibody-like proteins. SynNotch CAR-T systems use a dual-receptor circuit to trigger CAR expression only upon recognition of a specific antigen, enabling logic-gated T cell responses.

lipid nanoparticle (LNP)-mediated delivery of mRNA encoding CAR has been shown to generate functional CAR-T cells directly *in vivo*, potentially circumventing the logistical and technical challenges associated with *ex vivo* formulation of the current adoptive cell therapies for allogeneic reinfusion [15]. This approach provides a flexible, scalable, and potentially more accessible strategy for immunotherapeutic intervention.

The convergence of advances in protein engineering, viral vector design, and a deeper understanding of tumour–immune system interactions has opened unprecedented avenues for therapeutic innovation. As the field enters its next phase, these novel immunotherapies aim not only to overcome existing barriers but also to redefine the future of cancer treatment. This final chapter explores emerging modalities at the forefront of therapeutic antibody evolution, alongside recent progress in OV-based strategies for tumour targeting.

18.2 CORE CONTENT SECTIONS

18.2.1 Bispecific/Trispecific Antibodies

mAbs are therapeutic proteins comprising antigen-binding sites formed by the variable domains of heavy and light chains, paired with an Fc region that can mediate immune effector functions [16]. Bispecific antibodies (BsAbs) are an advancement in antibody engineering, designed to bind two different epitopes either on the same antigen or on distinct antigens. BsAb development began in the 1960s with re-association of antigen-binding fragments (Fabs) from polyclonal sera into bispecific $F(ab')_2$ molecules [17]. The advent of hybridoma technology in 1975 enabled mAb production and laid the foundation for BsAb generation [18]. A major advancement occurred in 1996 with the introduction of the knobs-into-holes technology, which significantly improved BsAb engineering [19]. This technological progress eventually led to the first FDA approval of a BsAb, blinatumomab, in 2014 for the treatment of acute lymphoblastic leukaemia (ALL) [20], marking a pivotal milestone in translating decades of research into clinical practice.

BsAbs can function through two primary mechanisms: through combinatorial or obligate activity [21]. In combinatorial activity (in-trans binding), the antibody's two binding sites engage targets on different cells, for example, in T cell engagers (TCEs) that bridge a tumour cell with a cytotoxic T cell [22]. TCEs represent an important category of BsAbs, with at least 12 TCEs now approved for clinical use, out of more than 20 BsAbs overall [23]. In obligate activity (in-cis binding), both binding sites target distinct epitopes on the same cell, enabling effects such as dual signalling blockade or receptor clustering and enhanced signalling. These mechanisms support a wide range of therapeutic applications, including immune effector cell recruitment (T cells, NK cells, macrophages) [24], checkpoint inhibition (e.g. PD-1, CTLA-4, and LAG-3) [25], and suppression of inflammatory mediators (e.g. TNF and IL-17) [26].

Building on these advances, TsAbs represent the latest generation of multi-targeting antibody-based therapeutics. By incorporating three distinct binding sites, TsAbs are designed to address limitations of bispecific formats such as antigen escape and suboptimal immune activation [8]. Common designs include two tumour-associated antigens (TAAs) and one immune effector target, such as CD3 or CD16, allowing for enhanced selectivity and immune cell engagement. Dual TAA targeting can reduce off-tumour toxicity and improve tumour specificity by requiring co-expression of both antigens on the same cell. In addition, some formats combine checkpoint blockades and co-stimulatory signals within a single molecule to enhance T cell activity. Trispecific constructs can also be engineered for improved pharmacokinetics, such as extended serum half-life via albumin-binding domains or Fc modifications, offering potential dosing and cost advantages over combination antibody therapies [27].

Optimising therapeutic efficacy across all multispecific antibody formats requires careful engineering of both antigen-binding domains and the Fc region. The Fc region is frequently modified to enhance or suppress immune effector functions, including antibody-dependent cellular cytotoxicity (ADCC), complement-dependent cytotoxicity (CDC), and antibody-dependent cell-mediated phagocytosis (ADCP) [28]. For example, FcγR-silencing mutations (such as N297A) are used to suppress effector functions and mitigate off-target immune activation. In T cell-engaging bispecific immunotherapies, Fc silencing prevents FcγR-driven T cell sequestration and cytokine release, thereby preserving T cell trafficking into tumours and improving antitumour efficacy [29]. Conversely, glycoengineering approaches such as reduction of core fucosylation enhance binding to activating FcγRs, thereby boosting ADCC and ADCP when stronger immune-mediated killing is desired [30]. One example is obinutuzumab, which uses glycoengineering to increase bisecting N-acetylglucosamine on the Fc region and thereby enhance ADCC activity [31]. Additionally, antigen-binding functionalities have been engineered into the Fc region itself, specifically within the CH2 and CH3 constant heavy-chain domains. These domains, located in the lower stem of the antibody's Y-shaped structure below the variable regions, can be modified to create compact 'nanoantibodies' that combine antigen specificity with extended half-life properties [32].

Several BsAbs have advanced into clinical use across diverse indications. For example, blinatumomab (CD19 × CD3) is the first FDA-approved bispecific TCE for the treatment of ALL, with demonstrated efficacy in both relapsed/refractory and minimal residual disease (MRD)-positive settings [33]. In the phase III TOWER trial, it significantly improved overall survival (OS) (7.7 vs. 4.0 months) and achieved higher remission rates (34 vs. 16%) compared to chemotherapy [34]. Teclistamab (BCMA × CD3) was FDA approved in 2022 for relapsed/refractory multiple myeloma previously exposed to immunomodulators, proteasome inhibitors, and anti-CD38 antibodies [35]. In the phase I/II MajesTEC-1 trial, it achieved a 63% overall response rate (ORR), with over 46% complete responses and a median duration of response of 24 months [35]. Building on these advances, ISB 2001 is a novel trispecific TCE that targets CD3 on T cells and both BCMA and CD38 on myeloma cells [36]. In preclinical studies, ISB 2001 demonstrated high cytotoxic potency against various myeloma cell lines, significantly outperforming teclistamab and other BCMA-targeting agents while retaining strong activity in the presence of soluble immunosuppressive factors. Despite enhanced efficacy, cytokine release levels (IL-6, IFN-γ, TNF-α) were comparable to existing treatments. In xenograft models, ISB 2001 induced complete tumour regression in 100% of mice at a dose of 0.1 $mg\,kg^{-1}$, whereas no complete responses were observed in the control group. These results highlight the advantage of simultaneously targeting two tumour antigens to enhance T cell redirection in multiple myeloma while limiting off-tumour activity [36].

Bispecific and TsAbs represent a transformative advancement in immunotherapy, overcoming limitations of traditional mAbs through multi-targeting strategies. Clinical successes like blinatumomab and teclistamab, alongside promising trispecific candidates such as ISB 2001, demonstrate enhanced tumour selectivity, reduced antigen escape, and improved immune activation. Through continued engineering of antigen-binding domains and Fc regions, these multispecific formats are poised to become essential tools in precision oncology, offering more effective and safer cancer treatments.

18.2.2 Antibody–Drug Conjugates

The scientific foundation of ADCs is rooted in Paul Ehrlich's early 20th-century concept of the 'magic bullet', a therapeutic agent capable of selectively targeting disease-causing cells while sparing healthy tissue [37].

Structurally, an ADC consists of three core components: a mAb that targets specific TAAs, a highly potent cytotoxic payload, and a chemical linker that connects the two [38]. Linker chemistry is pivotal as it must ensure systemic stability while enabling controlled intracellular release of the drug [39]. Several classes of linkers are employed based on their cleavage mechanisms: hydrazone linkers, which are cleaved in acidic intracellular environments (e.g. endosomes or lysosomes); enzyme-cleavable linkers (e.g. valine–citrulline) sensitive to lysosomal proteases such as cathepsin B; disulphide linkers, which respond to intracellular reducing conditions; and non-cleavable linkers, which rely on antibody degradation to release the drug [38]. Each linker type contributes differently to drug stability, release kinetics, and therapeutic selectivity. Payload selection requires balancing cytotoxic potency with favourable physicochemical properties: sufficient lipophilicity to cross membranes, aqueous solubility to enable conjugation, chemical stability through circulation and intracellular trafficking, and reactive functional groups for stable conjugation [40]. ADCs mainly employ three classes of cytotoxic payloads: microtubule-disrupting agents such as auristatins and maytansinoids; DNA-damaging compounds, including calicheamicins, duocarmycins, and exatecans; and recent immunomodulatory molecules, notably agonists of Toll-like receptors (TLRs) and stimulator of interferon genes (STINGs) [38]. Drug-to-antibody ratios (DARs) are typically constrained to ≤ 4 to maintain solubility, stability, and consistent pharmacokinetics [41]. Beyond therapy, ADCs also show promise as theranostic platforms; by incorporating fluorescent agents or radiolabels, they can simultaneously diagnose, monitor, and treat malignancies, enabling assessment of antigen expression and therapeutic response through fluorescence imaging and ex vivo analysis [42]. This dual capacity reinforces ADCs as versatile tools in precision oncology.

The principle of the 'magic bullet' became a clinical reality in 2000 with the approval of Mylotarg (gemtuzumab ozogamicin), the first ADC [43], which is an anti-CD33 antibody covalently linked to the highly cytotoxic DNA-damaging antibiotic N-acetyl calicheamicin via a cleavable hydrazone linker [44]. Since then, innovations in molecular design have driven the development of more potent and selective ADCs, from first-generation agents like Mylotarg to advanced third-generation ADCs like Enhertu and Trodelvy [38]. While Mylotarg is effective, its linker is prone to instability, risking premature drug release and off-target toxicity [45]. In contrast, third-generation agents Enhertu and Trodelvy employ more stable peptide linkers.

Enhertu is designed to target the HER2 receptor and delivers deruxtecan, a drug that inhibits the enzyme topoisomerase I, which is essential for DNA replication in cancer cells [46]. Trodelvy targets the Trop-2 antigen and carries SN-38, another topoisomerase I inhibitor that interferes with tumour cell division and survival [47]. While both agents offer improved tumour selectivity and bystander killing effects, their potent payloads can also harm healthy dividing cells, leading to side effects such as neutropenia and gastrointestinal toxicity [46, 48]. The number of approved ADCs, all in oncology to date, has grown rapidly in recent years and now totals 16 [23].

The concept of using an antibody to guide a potent payload directly to tumour cells has also been applied in other therapeutic platforms. Radioimmunotherapy (RIT) applies a comparable strategy, substituting the chemical drug payload with a therapeutic radionuclide [49]. Agents such as Bexxar (^{131}I-tositumomab) and Zevalin (^{90}Y-ibritumomab tiuxetan) target CD20-expressing B-cell lymphomas, delivering cytotoxic radiation directly to malignant cells while limiting exposure to normal tissue [50, 51].

Recent clinical trials have demonstrated the therapeutic potential of ADCs across multiple cancer types. FS-1502, a HER2-targeted ADC with β-glucuronide linker and MMAF payload, was tested in 150 patients with HER2-expressing advanced solid tumours. The phase Ia/Ib trial (NCT03944499) established a recommended phase II dose of 2.3 mg kg^{-1} every 3 weeks and achieved 53.7% ORR in HER2-positive breast cancer patients, with manageable reversible ocular and pulmonary toxicities [52]. DB-1310, a HER3-targeted ADC with a cleavable peptide linker and a topoisomerase I inhibitor payload, demonstrated encouraging antitumour activity in 123 heavily pretreated patients with advanced solid tumours. The Phase I/IIa (NCT05914116) trial showed 35.7% response rate in EGFR-mutated non-small-cell lung cancer (NSCLC) and 25.5% ORR, with manageable safety profile and median progression-free survival of 7.0 months in the EGFR-mutated subset [53]. DB-1311/BNT324, a B7H3-targeted ADC with FDA Fast-Track designation, demonstrated promising activity in 65 heavily pretreated castration-resistant prostate cancer patients. ThePhase I/IIa trial (NCT05914116) showed 27.9% ORR and 95.3% disease control rate, with median radiographic progression-free survival of 8.3 months and manageable safety profile characterised primarily by grade 1–2 nausea and haematological events [54].

ADCs demonstrate the power of rational drug design in oncology, successfully combining targeted delivery with potent cytotoxicity to achieve therapeutic selectivity. The evolution from first-generation agents to sophisticated platforms like FS-1502, DB-1310, and DB-1311 highlights how optimised linker chemistry and payload selection can enhance efficacy while maintaining manageable safety profiles. Beyond traditional cytotoxic applications, the expansion of ADCs into theranostic capabilities illustrates their versatility as both diagnostic and therapeutic tools. This molecular engineering approach establishes ADCs as valuable educational models for understanding targeted therapy principles and their clinical translation.

18.2.3 Oncolytic Virotherapy

Oncolytic virotherapy traces its roots to the early 20th century, with one of the earliest reports of tumour regression following viral infection documented by DePace in 1912 [55]. Although clinical trials during the 1950s and 1960s employed viruses such as adenovirus and West Nile virus, therapeutic outcomes were limited due to safety concerns and poor specificity [12]. The emergence of molecular cloning and genetic engineering in the 1990s revitalised the field by enabling the creation of tumour-targeted viral vectors. This advancement led to the first regulatory approvals of OVs, starting with Rigvir, a picornavirus approved in Latvia in 2004 for melanoma [56], followed by H101, a genetically modified adenovirus approved in China in 2005 for nasopharyngeal carcinoma [12]. Later approvals included talimogene laherparepvec (T-VEC) in the United States and European Union in 2015 for melanoma [57, 58], and teserpaturev (DELYTACT) in Japan in 2021 for malignant glioma [59]. OVs are viruses, either naturally occurring or genetically engineered, that selectively infect and destroy cancer cells while sparing healthy tissue [60]. Their therapeutic activity is mediated by both direct and indirect mechanisms: OVs can replicate within and lyse tumour cells (oncolysis) and also stimulate an antitumour immune response, thereby engaging the broader immune system (Figure 18.2) [13]. Modern OVs are either attenuated strains or genetically modified to preferentially infect, replicate within, and lyse malignant cells while sparing normal tissue. This tumour specificity is achieved through the exploitation of aberrant signalling pathways, such as RAS mutations or p53 deficiencies, or by targeting tumour-overexpressed receptors [11]. For example, poliovirus uses CD155, and herpes simplex virus can exploit EGFR, both of which are more abundant on certain cancer cells, allowing the virus to preferentially infect tumour tissue. Viral vectors, including adenovirus, herpes simplex virus, and vaccinia virus, have become foundational platforms due to their amenability to genetic manipulation and capacity for transgene incorporation. These vectors can be armed with therapeutic payloads, such as cytokines (e.g. GM-CSF), ICIs, or pro-apoptotic factors that enhance oncolysis and stimulate robust antitumour immune responses. Transgene expression is often controlled by tumour-specific promoters or regulatory elements responsive to the tumour microenvironment, ensuring selective activation [11].

Recent studies have explored the potential of OVs in combination immunotherapy for difficult-to-treat cancers. In a phase Ib trial, 30 patients with resectable stage III or IV M1a acral melanoma received neoadjuvant therapy with the OV OrienX010 and the anti-PD-1 antibody toripalimab. Treatment was administered over 12 weeks, followed by surgical resection and 1 year of adjuvant toripalimab. The pathological response rate was 77.8%, including 33.3% major pathological responses, while the radiographic response rate reached 36.7%. The one- and two-year recurrence-free survival rates were 85.2 and 81.5%, respectively. The combination was well tolerated, with mostly grade 1–2 adverse events. These results suggest promising efficacy and safety in acral melanoma, a subtype typically resistant to ICIs [61]. In another study, NDV-GT, a recombinant Newcastle disease virus encoding the porcine α1,3-galactosyltransferase (α1,3GT) gene, was evaluated in an interventional trial involving 23 patients with advanced, treatment-refractory solid tumours. Tumour types included hepatocellular carcinoma (HCC), ovarian, cervical, lung, rectal, breast, oesophageal cancer, and melanoma. NDV-GT was administered intravenously and demonstrated a favourable safety profile, with no severe adverse events or significant induction of neutralising antibodies. Among 20 evaluable patients, the disease control rate was 90%, including 1 complete remission and 6 partial responses. Mechanistically, NDV-GT induced tumour-specific α-Gal expression, triggering hyperacute rejection and enhancing both humoral and cellular immune responses, resulting in significant and durable tumour regression across cancer types [62].

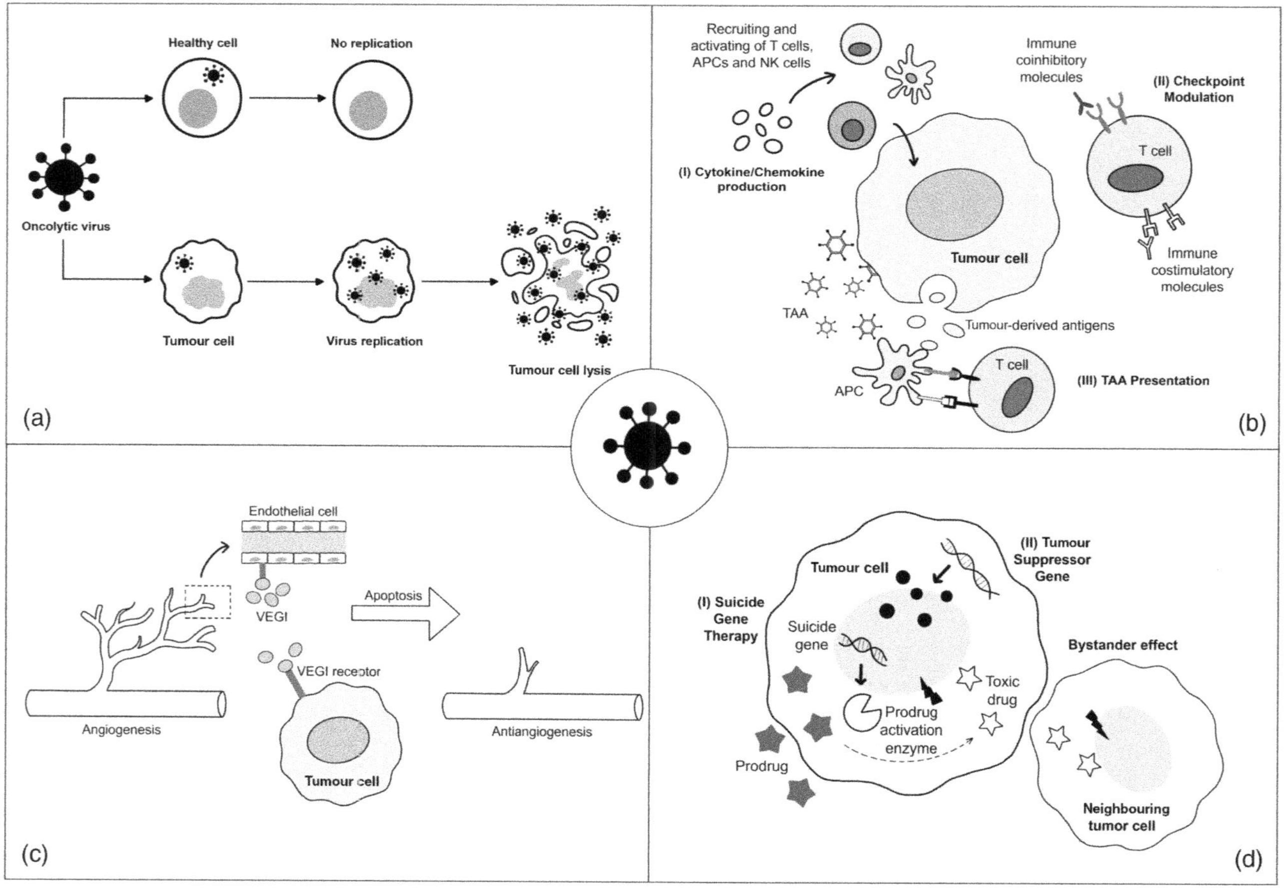

FIGURE 18.2 Mechanisms of oncolytic virotherapy. (a) Selective viral replication: oncolytic viruses preferentially infect and replicate in tumour cells with defective antiviral responses while sparing healthy cells, leading to tumour cell lysis and viral progeny release. (b) Immune modulation: (i) cytokine/chemokine production recruits and activates T cells, APCs, and NK cells; (ii) checkpoint modulation through coinhibitory blockers and costimulatory enhancers overcomes T cell exhaustion; (iii) TAA presentation by APCs primes tumour-specific T cell responses following viral lysis. (c) Microenvironment modification: anti-angiogenic factors (e.g. VEGI) inhibit tumour angiogenesis and promote vessel regression, starving tumours while enhancing viral spread. (d) Direct cytotoxic effects: (i) suicide gene therapy converts prodrugs to toxic metabolites with bystander effects on neighbouring cells; (ii) tumour suppressor gene delivery restores apoptotic pathways and growth control.

Oncolytic virotherapy exemplifies multifaceted cancer treatment through diverse mechanisms, including selective viral replication, immune modulation, microenvironment modification, and direct cytotoxic effects. The evolution from early observations to genetically engineered platforms capable of expressing therapeutic transgenes demonstrates remarkable scientific advancement. Clinical studies with OrienX010 and NDV-GT showcase OVs' ability to achieve substantial response rates across treatment-resistant cancers through combination strategies and novel immune activation pathways. This comprehensive mechanistic approach positions OVs as versatile therapeutic platforms that integrate viral biology with immunotherapy principles, offering valuable educational insights into multi-modal cancer treatment strategies.

18.3 CASE STUDY

To further illustrate advances in emerging immunology in more detail, the following case studies highlight recent clinical trials that exemplify how engineered biologics and immune strategies are being applied in practice.

18.3.1 Phase IIa Study Using Anti-Her2 Bispecific Antibody Delivered as Multimodal Therapy

Among the molecular subtypes of breast cancer, hormone receptor–positive, HER2-positive disease is particularly challenging to treat because crosstalk between the oestrogen receptor and HER2 signalling pathways drives resistance to both endocrine therapy and HER2-targeted agents [63]. Many patients eventually progress despite multiple lines of treatment, leaving few effective options. Zanidatamab represents an important advance in this setting. As a BsAb, it binds two non-overlapping epitopes on HER2, which forces receptor clustering and internalisation, leading to stronger degradation and suppression of downstream signalling. At the same time, dual binding enhances antibody-dependent immune cytotoxicity, giving zanidatamab a mechanistic advantage over single-epitope HER2 antibodies like trastuzumab. This illustrates how careful antibody engineering can directly reshape both tumour signalling and immune responses, offering a strategy to overcome acquired resistance.

To evaluate this approach clinically, a Phase IIa open-label trial tested zanidatamab in combination with palbociclib, a CDK4/6 inhibitor, and fulvestrant, a selective oestrogen receptor degrader. This triple therapy was rationally designed to block three complementary pathways: HER2 signalling, cell cycle progression, and oestrogen receptor activity. The study enrolled 51 patients across 13 centres, all of whom had received multiple prior HER2-targeted therapies, including trastuzumab, trastuzumab emtansine (T-DM1), and pertuzumab. Treatment involved zanidatamab infusions every two weeks, oral palbociclib on a 21-day schedule, and intramuscular fulvestrant at standard intervals. Results were encouraging: 66.7% of patients remained progression-free at 6 months, with a median progression-free survival of 11.7 months and an objective response rate (ORR) of 34.8%, including complete responses [64]. By comparison, fulvestrant monotherapy historically achieved only a 21.5% ORR in treatment-naive patients [65]. The triple combination's superior performance in this heavily pretreated population, typically less responsive due to acquired resistance, suggests it can effectively overcome conventional resistance mechanisms [64]. This case illustrates how BsAbs can serve as backbone agents in rational combination therapies, enabling simultaneous suppression of multiple resistance pathways while maintaining manageable safety profiles.

18.3.2 AFM13-Precomplexed Allogeneic NK Cells in Refractory CD30+ Lymphoma

In CD30-positive lymphomas, resistance to both brentuximab vedotin (BV) and anti-PD-1 inhibitors highlights a critical gap in treatment, with conventional approaches offering limited benefit [66]. To address this challenge, investigators designed a novel therapeutic platform that combines allogeneic natural killer (NK) cells with a bispecific NK cell engager, AFM13, to enhance immune targeting of resistant lymphomas. AFM13 is engineered to bridge NK cells and tumour cells by binding CD16A on NK cells and CD30 on tumour cells, thereby redirecting innate cytotoxicity specifically towards malignant cells. Prior to infusion, cord blood-derived NK cells were expanded, cytokine-activated (IL-12, IL-15, IL-18), and preloaded with AFM13, while patients received lymphodepleting chemotherapy to improve engraftment.

In a Phase I study, 42 heavily pretreated patients underwent 2–4 treatment cycles. Each cycle involved lymphodepleting chemotherapy followed by AFM13-NK cell infusion and three weekly AFM13 antibody doses over approximately 28 days. The regimen demonstrated excellent tolerability, with no cytokine release syndrome, neurotoxicity, or graft-versus-host disease. Remarkably, the ORR reached 92.9%, with 66.7% achieving complete responses, including 73% among Hodgkin lymphoma patients. Durable responses persisted for up to 40 months in some cases, even among patients who had failed CAR-T therapy.

Highlighting AFM13's bispecific function, preclinical studies showed that cytokine-preactivated NK cells loaded with AFM13 had significantly higher antitumour activity than unloaded NK cells, whereas single-agent AFM13 monotherapy achieved only 11.5–16% response rates in similar patient populations [67]. This trial illustrates how BsAbs can effectively redirect innate effectors, supporting their promise as 'off-the-shelf' immunotherapies for refractory cancers.

18.3.3 VG161 Oncolytic Virotherapy for Refractory Hepatocellular Carcinoma

HCC remains one of the most life-threatening cancers globally, with an approximate five-year survival rate of only 18% [68], with limited treatment options beyond second-line therapies. VG161, a genetically engineered oncolytic herpes simplex virus, represents a novel immunotherapeutic approach to this challenge. The virus is designed with a dual mechanism of action: it directly lyses tumour cells while simultaneously stimulating systemic antitumour immunity. Mechanistically, VG161 selectively replicates within cancer cells, causing their destruction and releasing TAAs. At the same time, it expresses multiple immunomodulatory transgenes, including IL-12, IL-15, IL-15Rα, and a PD-1/PD-L1-blocking fusion protein, which remodel the tumour microenvironment. These modifications enhance T cell and NK-cell activity and counteract immune evasion pathways, effectively transforming immunologically 'cold' tumours into 'hot' tumours. This case illustrates how synthetic virotherapy can bridge direct oncolysis with immune activation, reshaping treatment possibilities for refractory cancers.

In a multicentre phase I clinical trial, VG161 was evaluated in 44 heavily pre-treated patients, including 40 with HCC and 4 with intrahepatic cholangiocarcinoma. The treatment was delivered through intratumoural injections with dose escalation from 1.0×10^8 to 5.0×10^8 plaque-forming units (PFUs). The recommended phase II dose was determined as 1.0×10^8 PFU, administered on days 1–3 of each 28-day cycle, with treatment repeated until progression or intolerance; in this phase I trial, patients received between 1 and 9 cycles. Results showed an ORR of 18.9% and a disease control rate of 64.9% among evaluable HCC patients. Median progression-free survival was 2.9 months, and OS reached 12.4 months, with longer benefit observed in patients who had prior checkpoint inhibitor exposure. The trial also confirmed a favourable safety profile, with no dose-limiting toxicities and manageable adverse events [69].

In comparison, the phase III RESORCE trial with regorafenib, a standard second-line therapy, reported an ORR of 10% and an OS of 10.6 months [70]. Together, these findings demonstrate the clinical promise of VG161 as a third-line option and underscore the potential of OVs in advancing cancer immunotherapy by bridging direct oncolysis with immune activation.

18.4 CHALLENGES AND CONTROVERSIES

The development of next-generation cancer therapeutics, bispecific and TsAbs, ADCs, and OVs, faces multifaceted challenges that significantly impact their clinical translation. Safety concerns represent paramount challenges across all four modalities, with bispecific and TsAbs prone to cytokine release syndrome, neurotoxicity and 'on-target off-tumour' toxicity when targeting antigens expressed on normal tissues [71, 72], ADCs producing off-target toxicity in healthy tissue and drug resistance mechanisms [10], and OVs triggering potentially harmful antiviral immune responses [11]. One approach to overcoming this off-target toxicity challenge can be found in pretargeted radioimmunotherapy (PRIT). PRIT addresses similar toxicity challenges by separating tumour targeting from payload delivery. It uses a BsAb for tumour localisation, followed by a radiolabelled small molecule that clears rapidly from healthy tissue. This strategy achieves higher therapeutic indices and may inspire future two-step ADC design [73, 74].

Moreover, delivery efficiency represents another fundamental challenge for antibody-based therapeutics. Clinical studies with radiolabelled antibodies have demonstrated that only $\leq 0.1\%$ of the injected dose per gram reaches tumour tissue, with most being catabolised elsewhere in the body, and this biodistribution limitation is presumed to also affect ADCs [23].

Manufacturing complexities pose substantial hurdles, particularly for BsAbs, where over 100 different molecular formats require specialised production methods to ensure proper heavy-light chain pairing while preventing immunogenicity [75]. ADCs face unique manufacturing challenges in achieving homogeneous conjugation, with current heterogeneous approaches resulting in millions of different ADC species and limited DARs [76]. For OVs, the production of high-quality purified viral stocks requires complex, large-scale cell culture systems coupled with rigorous downstream purification, making the process technically demanding and costly [77]. Regulatory hurdles further complicate development, as these first-in-class therapeutics often lack established approval pathways, require novel companion diagnostics for patient selection, and face uncertainty in regulatory standards.

18.5 FUTURE DIRECTION

The future of these advanced therapeutics lies in pushing beyond current formats towards more sophisticated, integrated designs. While bispecific and TsAbs have already shown proof-of-concept, ongoing efforts focus on next-generation multispecific immune cell engagers that can broaden targeting scope and refine control. NK cell platforms, for example, have progressed from bispecific killer engagers (BiKEs) to trispecific formats (TriKEs), some of which incorporate IL-15 to prolong NK activity. Building on this, tetraspecific designs engage multiple activating receptors such as CD16a, NKG2D, NKp30, and NKp46 [78]. Similarly, TCEs are adopting logic-gated architectures, requiring combinations of antigens or microenvironmental cues before activation. By integrating 'AND' or 'NOT' gate principles, these constructs aim to maximise tumour specificity while reducing off-tumour toxicity, representing a more intelligent layer of immune redirection [79].

Parallel innovations are transforming OVs from purely lytic agents into versatile 'armoured' platforms. These engineered viruses function as both tumour-selective cytolytic agents and local delivery systems for immune-modulatory payloads, including cytokines (e.g. GM-CSF and IL-12), chemokines, costimulatory ligands, or bispecific engagers to enhance immune infiltration and function [80]. By releasing these factors within the tumour microenvironment, armoured viruses can shift it from immune-excluded to inflamed, supporting more robust antitumour responses [81]. Refinements like tumour-selective promoters, microRNA targeting, and synergistic payload combinations further enhance safety and efficacy [81].

Building upon emerging engineering strategies, a future direction lies in systematically combining multiple therapeutic modalities. Recent advances have begun to explore combining adoptive cell therapies with personalised vaccines to enhance antitumour efficacy. For instance, vaccines delivering tumour associated or neoantigen peptides have been shown to expand and sustain infused CAR-T cells in vivo, thereby prolonging their therapeutic activity [82]. Personalised neoantigen-specific T cell therapy, generated from autologous lymphocytes primed against patient-specific mutations, offers a tailored approach capable of addressing tumour heterogeneity [83]. At the same time, interventions that remodel the tumour microenvironment, such as boosting chemokine expression or promoting vascular normalisation, can facilitate T cell infiltration. This allows both transferred cells and vaccine-induced responses to more effectively reach tumour sites [84].

Meanwhile, artificial intelligence (AI) offers another promising avenue for the future of immunotherapy. One area where this has already shown value is vaccine development. For example, machine learning applied to genomic and protein data can predict epitopes and prioritise antigens with strong immunogenic potential. Generative models have been used to design optimised immunogens, while molecular simulations assess stability and interactions [85]. Similarly, AI is being applied to antibody discovery and multi-parameter optimisation, integrating structural, functional, and safety considerations to accelerate therapeutic design [23]. Looking forward, AI applications may extend beyond these examples to support innovation across immunotherapy.

Equally important is ensuring that these advances reach patients worldwide. Expanding global access may involve scaling up manufacturing in low- and middle-income regions through modular, cost-efficient production and technology transfer partnerships. Building local capacity can reduce reliance on centralised facilities, lower costs, and improve the timely availability of these innovative treatments in resource-limited settings. Advances in technology, paired with strategies to expand access, may determine the real-world impact of next-generation immunotherapies.

KEY TERMS & DEFINITIONS SIDEBAR

Bispecific Antibody An engineered antibody designed to recognise and bind simultaneously to two distinct antigens.

Trispecific Antibody An engineered antibody designed to recognise and bind simultaneously to three distinct antigens.

T Cell Engager A type of engineered molecule, often a bispecific antibody, that redirects the patient's own immune T cells to recognise and kill cancer cells.

Antibody–Drug Conjugate A type of biopharmaceutical consisting of a monoclonal antibody covalently attached to a cytotoxic agent through a specialised linker molecule. The antibody selectively binds to target proteins or receptors expressed on specific cell types, including cancer cells. Upon binding and internalisation, the linker facilitates controlled release of the therapeutic payload within target cells, resulting in selective cytotoxicity while minimising damage to non-target cellular populations.

Oncolytic Virus A naturally occurring or engineered virus that selectively infects and kills cancer cells while largely sparing normal tissues.

Radioimmunotherapy A radiotherapeutic approach using radioisotope-conjugated monoclonal antibodies administered systemically. The antibody targets specific cellular antigens, while the attached radionuclide delivers localised ionising radiation to induce selective cytotoxicity.

Pretargeted Radioimmunotherapy A two-step strategy in which tumour targeting is separated from radioactive payload delivery, enhancing both the safety and efficacy of the therapy.

Fragment Antigen-Binding The part of an antibody that binds to antigens, consisting of variable regions from both heavy and light chains.

Single-Chain Variable Fragment A fusion protein containing the variable regions of antibody heavy and light chains connected by a flexible linker.

Heavy-Chain Antibody Naturally occurring antibodies found in certain animals that lack light chains provide the basis for nanobody development.

Chimeric Antigen Receptor A genetically engineered receptor expressed on immune cells, such as T-lymphocytes, that enables specific recognition of antigens on cancer cells. CARs redirect immune cells to selectively target and eliminate tumour cells, effectively reprogramming host lymphocytes into potent, tumour-directed effector cells.

SynNotch CAR Circuit Engineered T cell receptors incorporating a synthetic Notch (SynNotch) system that detects a specific disease-associated antigen and, upon activation, induces expression of a CAR targeting a second antigen.

Immune Checkpoint Inhibitors – drugs that block immune checkpoint proteins, which normally inhibit T cell activation, thereby enhancing the immune system's ability to recognise and attack cancer cells.

Knobs-into-Holes Technology An antibody engineering strategy for bispecific antibody production that promotes correct heavy chain heterodimerisation by introducing a 'knob' on one CH3 domain and a complementary 'hole' on the other, minimising unwanted homodimer formation.

Minimal Residual Disease A small population of cancer cells that persists after treatment and remains below the detection threshold of standard diagnostic methods.

Antibody-dependent cell-mediated cytotoxicity An immune mechanism in which antibodies bind to a target cell, marking it for destruction by effector cells such as NK cells or macrophages. These effector cells recognise the antibody-coated target via Fc receptors and release cytotoxic molecules to eliminate the cell.

Complement-Dependent Cytotoxicity An immune process in which antibodies bind to antigens on target cells, such as cancer cells, activating the complement system to form a membrane attack complex (MAC) that lyses the cell.

Antibody-Dependent Cellular Phagocytosis – an immune process in which a target cell, such as a pathogen or tumour cell, is coated with antibodies (opsonisation). Phagocytic cells, including macrophages, recognise the antibody-coated target via Fc receptors and engulf it for subsequent degradation.

Drug-to-Antibody Ratio The average number of drug molecules attached to each antibody molecule.

Viral Vector A genetically engineered, non-replicating virus used as a delivery vehicle to introduce specific genetic material, such as a gene, into target cells.

Tumour-Associated Antigen Proteins that are overexpressed on cancer cells and serve as targets for immunotherapy are expressed at lower levels on normal tissues.

Logic-Gated Therapies Immunotherapies engineered to require multiple inputs or conditions for activation, enhancing tumour specificity and minimising off-target effects.

Antigen Escape The process by which cancer cells evade immune detection by downregulating or losing expression of target antigens.

Cytokine Release Syndrome A potentially life-threatening inflammatory response triggered by rapid immune cell activation, resulting in excessive cytokine release.

Off-Target Toxicity Harmful effects on healthy tissues that express the same antigens targeted by cancer therapies.

LIST OF ABBREVIATIONS

ADC antibody drug conjugate

ADCC antibody-dependent cellular cytotoxicity

ADPC antibody-dependent cellular mediated phagocytosis

ALL acute lymphoblastic leukaemia

BiKE bispecific killer engager

BsAb bispecific antibody

BV brentuximab vedotin

CAR chimeric antigen receptor

CDC complement-dependent cellular cytotoxicity
DAR drug-to-antibody ratio
Fab fragment antigen-binding
FDA Food and Drug Administration
NK natural killer
HcAb heavy-chain antibody
ICI immune checkpoint inhibitor
mAb monoclonal antibody
MRD minimal residual disease
ORR objective response rate
OS overall survival
OV oncolytic virus
PFU plaque-forming unit
PRIT pretargeted radioimmunotherapy
RIT radioimmunotherapy
scFv single-chain variable fragments
TAA tumour-associated antigen
TCE T cell engager
TLR Toll-like receptor
TriKE trispecific killer engager
TsAb trispecific antibody

REVIEW QUESTIONS

1. Describe the three core components of an ADC and explain how linker type affects drug release and safety.
2. How do oncolytic viruses selectively target cancer cells, and what direct and what indirect and direct mechanisms do they use to kill them?
3. Compare the toxicity challenges associated with bispecific antibodies, ADCs, and oncolytic viruses. In addition, describe one engineering strategy used to reduce off-target effects in these modalities.
4. Using one case study from this chapter, explain how combining immunotherapy modalities can overcome resistance that limits singleagent treatment.

REFERENCES

1. Hodi, F.S., O'Day, S.J., McDermott, D.F. et al. (2010). Improved survival with ipilimumab in patients with metastatic melanoma. *N Engl J Med* 363 (8): 711–723.
2. Institute CR (2024). *Introducing the CRI Cancer Immunotherapy Insights & Impact Report [Internet]*. New York: Cancer Research Institute Available from: https://www.cancerresearch.org/blog/introducing-the-cri-cancer-immunotherapy-insights-impact-report.
3. Sharma, P., Hu-Lieskovan, S., Wargo, J.A., and Ribas, A. (2017). Primary, adaptive, and acquired resistance to cancer immunotherapy. *Cell* 168 (4): 707–723.

4. Ribas, A. and Wolchok, J.D. (2018). Cancer immunotherapy using checkpoint blockade. *Science* 359 (6382): 1350–1355.
5. Roybal, K.T., Rupp, L.J., Morsut, L. et al. (2016). Precision tumor recognition by T cells with combinatorial antigen-sensing circuits. *Cell* 164 (4): 770–779.
6. Tang, L., Pan, S., Wei, X. et al. (2023). Arming CAR-T cells with cytokines and more: innovations in the fourth-generation CAR-T development. *Mol Ther* 31 (11): 3146–3162.
7. Mullard, A. (2024). In vivo CAR T cells move into clinical trials. *Nat Rev Drug Discov* 23 (10): 727–730.
8. Tapia-Galisteo, A., Alvarez-Vallina, L., and Sanz, L. (2023). Bi- and trispecific immune cell engagers for immunotherapy of hematological malignancies. *J Hematol Oncol* 16 (1): 83.
9. Jose, J., Hooper, J.D., and Souza-Fonseca-Guimaraes, F. (2025). Highlights of 2024. Broadening anti-cancer immunotherapy modalities with antibody-drug conjugates: emerging insights from clinical studies. *Immunol Cell Biol* 103 (6): 530–534.
10. Wang, R., Hu, B., Pan, Z. et al. (2025). Antibody-drug conjugates (ADCs): current and future biopharmaceuticals. *J Hematol Oncol* 18 (1): 51.
11. Lin, D., Shen, Y., and Liang, T. (2023). Oncolytic virotherapy: basic principles, recent advances and future directions. *Signal Transduct Target Ther* 8 (1): 156.
12. Kelly, E. and Russell, S.J. (2007). History of oncolytic viruses: genesis to genetic engineering. *Mol Ther* 15 (4): 651–659.
13. Gujar, S., Pol, J.G., Kumar, V. et al. (2024). Tutorial: design, production and testing of oncolytic viruses for cancer immunotherapy. *Nat Protoc* 19 (9): 2540–2570.
14. Chehelgerdi, M. and Chehelgerdi, M. (2023). The use of RNA-based treatments in the field of cancer immunotherapy. *Mol Cancer* 22 (1): 106.
15. Hunter, T.L., Bao, Y., Zhang, Y. et al. (2025). In vivo CAR T cell generation to treat cancer and autoimmune disease. *Science* 388 (6753): 1311–1317.
16. Breedveld, F.C. (2000). Therapeutic monoclonal antibodies. *Lancet* 355 (9205): 735–740.
17. Nisonoff, A. and Rivers, M.M. (1961). Recombination of a mixture of univalent antibody fragments of different specificity. *Arch Biochem Biophys* 93: 460–462.
18. Kohler, G. and Milstein, C. (1975). Continuous cultures of fused cells secreting antibody of predefined specificity. *Nature* 256 (5517): 495–497.
19. Ridgway, J.B., Presta, L.G., and Carter, P. (1996). 'Knobs-into-holes' engineering of antibody CH3 domains for heavy chain heterodimerization. *Protein Eng* 9 (7): 617–621.
20. Topp, M.S., Gokbuget, N., Stein, A.S. et al. (2015). Safety and activity of blinatumomab for adult patients with relapsed or refractory B-precursor acute lymphoblastic leukaemia: a multicentre, single-arm, phase 2 study. *Lancet Oncol* 16 (1): 57–66.
21. Brinkmann, U. and Kontermann, R.E. (2021). Bispecific antibodies. *Science* 372 (6545): 916–917.
22. Hoffmann, P., Hofmeister, R., Brischwein, K. et al. (2005). Serial killing of tumor cells by cytotoxic T cells redirected with a CD19-/CD3-bispecific single-chain antibody construct. *Int J Cancer* 115 (1): 98–104.
23. Chan, A.C., Martyn, G.D., and Carter, P.J. (2025). Fifty years of monoclonals: the past, present and future of antibody therapeutics. *Nat Rev Immunol* 25 (10): 745–765.
24. Sun, Y., Yu, X., Wang, X. et al. (2023). Bispecific antibodies in cancer therapy: target selection and regulatory requirements. *Acta Pharm Sin B* 13 (9): 3583–3597.
25. Li, C.L., Ma, X.Y., and Yi, P. (2024). Bispecific antibodies, immune checkpoint inhibitors, and antibody-drug conjugates directing antitumor immune responses: challenges and prospects. *Cell Biochem Funct* 42 (8): e70011.
26. Xu, T., Ying, T., Wang, L. et al. (2017). A native-like bispecific antibody suppresses the inflammatory cytokine response by simultaneously neutralizing tumor necrosis factor-alpha and interleukin-17A. *Oncotarget* 8 (47): 81860–81872.

27. Tapia-Galisteo, A., Compte, M., Alvarez-Vallina, L., and Sanz, L. (2023). When three is not a crowd: trispecific antibodies for enhanced cancer immunotherapy. *Theranostics* 13 (3): 1028–1041.
28. Moore, G.L., Chen, H., Karki, S., and Lazar, G.A. (2010). Engineered Fc variant antibodies with enhanced ability to recruit complement and mediate effector functions. *MAbs* 2 (2): 181–189.
29. Wang, L., Hoseini, S.S., Xu, H. et al. (2019). Silencing Fc domains in T cell-engaging bispecific antibodies improves T-cell trafficking and antitumor potency. *Cancer Immunol Res* 7 (12): 2013–2024.
30. Kellner, C., Otte, A., Cappuzzello, E. et al. (2017). Modulating cytotoxic effector functions by Fc engineering to improve cancer therapy. *Transfus Med Hemother* 44 (5): 327–336.
31. Mossner, E., Brunker, P., Moser, S. et al. (2010). Increasing the efficacy of CD20 antibody therapy through the engineering of a new type II anti-CD20 antibody with enhanced direct and immune effector cell-mediated B-cell cytotoxicity. *Blood* 115 (22): 4393–4402.
32. Ying, T., Gong, R., Ju, T.W. et al. (2014). Engineered Fc based antibody domains and fragments as novel scaffolds. *Biochim Biophys Acta* 1844 (11): 1977–1982.
33. Curran, E. and Stock, W. (2019). Taking a "BiTE out of ALL": blinatumomab approval for MRD-positive ALL. *Blood* 133 (16): 1715–1719.
34. Kantarjian, H., Stein, A., Gokbuget, N. et al. (2017). Blinatumomab versus chemotherapy for advanced acute lymphoblastic leukemia. *N Engl J Med* 376 (9): 836–847.
35. Garfall, A.L., Nooka, A.K., van de Donk, N.W.C.J. et al. (2024). Long-term follow-up from the phase 1/2 MajesTEC-1 trial of teclistamab in patients with relapsed/refractory multiple myeloma. *J Clin Oncol* 42: 7540.
36. Carretero-Iglesia, L., Hall, O.J., Berret, J. et al. (2024). ISB 2001 trispecific T cell engager shows strong tumor cytotoxicity and overcomes immune escape mechanisms of multiple myeloma cells. *Nat Cancer* 5 (10): 1494–1514.
37. Strebhardt, K. and Ullrich, A. (2008). Paul Ehrlich's magic bullet concept: 100 years of progress. *Nat Rev Cancer* 8 (6): 473–480.
38. Fu, Z., Li, S., Han, S. et al. (2022). Antibody drug conjugate: the "biological missile" for targeted cancer therapy. *Signal Transduct Target Ther* 7 (1): 93.
39. Yang, X., Pan, Z., Choudhury, M.R. et al. (2020). Making smart drugs smarter: the importance of linker chemistry in targeted drug delivery. *Med Res Rev* 40 (6): 2682–2713.
40. Wang, Z., Li, H., Gou, L. et al. (2023). Antibody-drug conjugates: recent advances in payloads. *Acta Pharm Sin B* 13 (10): 4025–4059.
41. McCombs, J.R. and Owen, S.C. (2015). Antibody drug conjugates: design and selection of linker, payload and conjugation chemistry. *AAPS J* 17 (2): 339–351.
42. Moek, K.L., Giesen, D., Kok, I.C. et al. (2017). Theranostics using antibodies and antibody-related therapeutics. *J Nucl Med* 58 (Suppl 2): 83S–90S.
43. Bross, P.F., Beitz, J., Chen, G. et al. (2001). Approval summary: gemtuzumab ozogamicin in relapsed acute myeloid leukemia. *Clin Cancer Res* 7 (6): 1490–1496.
44. Lambert, J., Pautas, C., Terre, C. et al. (2019). Gemtuzumab ozogamicin for de novo acute myeloid leukemia: final efficacy and safety updates from the open-label, phase III ALFA-0701 trial. *Haematologica* 104 (1): 113–119.
45. Joubert, N., Beck, A., Dumontet, C., and Denevault-Sabourin, C. (2020). Antibody-drug conjugates: the last decade. *Pharmaceuticals (Basel)* 13 (9): 245.
46. Jang, J.Y., Kim, D., Lee, N.K. et al. (2025). Antibody-drug conjugates powered by deruxtecan: innovations and challenges in oncology. *Int J Mol Sci* 26 (13): 6523.
47. Bardia, A., Messersmith, W.A., Kio, E.A. et al. (2021). Sacituzumab govitecan, a Trop-2-directed antibody-drug conjugate, for patients with epithelial cancer: final safety and efficacy results from the phase I/II IMMU-132-01 basket trial. *Ann Oncol* 32 (6): 746–756.

48. Tolaney, S.M., Cardillo, T.M., Chou, C.C. et al. (2025). The mode of action and clinical outcomes of Sacituzumab Govitecan in solid tumors. *Clin Cancer Res* 31 (8): 1390–1399.
49. Rondon, A., Rouanet, J., and Degoul, F. (2021). Radioimmunotherapy in oncology: overview of the last decade clinical trials. *Cancers (Basel)* 13 (21): 570.
50. Chamarthy, M.R., Williams, S.C., and Moadel, R.M. (2011). Radioimmunotherapy of non-Hodgkin's lymphoma: from the 'magic bullets' to 'radioactive magic bullets'. *Yale J Biol Med* 84 (4): 391–407.
51. Larson, S.M., Carrasquillo, J.A., Cheung, N.K., and Press, O.W. (2015). Radioimmunotherapy of human tumours. *Nat Rev Cancer* 15 (6): 347–360.
52. Li, Q., Cheng, Y., Tong, Z. et al. (2024). HER2-targeting antibody drug conjugate FS-1502 in HER2-expressing metastatic breast cancer: a phase 1a/1b trial. *Nat Commun* 15 (1): 5158.
53. Lisberg, A., Lu, S., Hamilton, E.P. et al. (2025). DB-1310, a HER3-targeted ADC, in pts with advanced solid tumors: preliminary results from the phase 1/2a trial. *J Clin Oncol* 43: 3000.
54. Parsonson, A.O., Gandhi, C., Henick, B.S. et al. (2025). DB-1311/BNT324 (a novel B7H3 ADC) in patients with heavily pretreated castrate-resistant prostate cancer (CRPC). *J Clin Oncol* 43: 5015.
55. De Pace N. Sulla Scomparsa di un Enorme Cancro Vegetante del Collo Dell'utero Senza Cura Chirurgica. Ginecologia. 1912; 9: 82–89.
56. Babiker, H.M., Riaz, I.B., Husnain, M., and Borad, M.J. (2017). Oncolytic virotherapy including Rigvir and standard therapies in malignant melanoma. *Oncolytic Virother* 6: 11–18.
57. Pol, J., Kroemer, G., and Galluzzi, L. (2016). First oncolytic virus approved for melanoma immunotherapy. *Oncoimmunology* 5 (1): e1115641.
58. Ressler, J., Silmbrod, R., Stepan, A. et al. (2019). Talimogene laherparepvec (T-VEC) in advanced melanoma: complete response in a heart and kidney transplant patient. A case report. *Br J Dermatol* 181 (1): 186–189.
59. Jiang, S., Chai, H., Tang, Q. et al. (2023). Clinical advances in oncolytic virus therapy for malignant glioma: a systematic review. *Discov Oncol* 14 (1): 183.
60. Rahman, M.M. and McFadden, G. (2021). Oncolytic viruses: newest frontier for cancer immunotherapy. *Cancers (Basel)* 13 (21): 5452.
61. Liu, J., Wang, X., Li, Z. et al. (2024). Neoadjuvant oncolytic virus orienx010 and toripalimab in resectable acral melanoma: a phase Ib trial. *Signal Transduct Target Ther* 9 (1): 318.
62. Zhong, L., Gan, L., Wang, B. et al. (2025). Hyperacute rejection-engineered oncolytic virus for interventional clinical trial in refractory cancer patients. *Cell* 188 (4): 1119–1136.e23.
63. Tommasi, C., Airo, G., Prattico, F. et al. (2024). Hormone receptor-positive/HER2-positive breast cancer: hormone therapy and anti-HER2 treatment: an update on treatment strategies. *J Clin Med* 13 (7): 1873.
64. Escriva-de-Romani, S., Cejalvo, J.M., Alba, E. et al. (2025). Zanidatamab plus palbociclib and fulvestrant in previously treated patients with hormone receptor-positive, HER2-positive metastatic breast cancer: primary results from a two-part, multicentre, single-arm, phase 2a study. *Lancet Oncol* 26 (6): 745–758.
65. Slamon, D.J., Neven, P., Chia, S. et al. (2018). Phase III randomized study of ribociclib and fulvestrant in hormone receptor-positive, human epidermal growth factor receptor 2-negative advanced breast cancer: MONALEESA-3. *J Clin Oncol* 36 (24): 2465–2472.
66. Epperla, N. and Hamadani, M. (2021). Double-refractory Hodgkin lymphoma: tackling relapse after brentuximab vedotin and checkpoint inhibitors. *Hematology Am Soc Hematol Educ Program* 2021 (1): 247–253.
67. Nieto, Y., Banerjee, P., Kaur, I. et al. (2025). Allogeneic NK cells with a bispecific innate cell engager in refractory relapsed lymphoma: a phase 1 trial. *Nat Med* 31 (6): 1987–1993.
68. Vogel, A., Meyer, T., Sapisochin, G. et al. (2022). Hepatocellular carcinoma. *The Lancet* 400 (10360): 1345–1362.
69. Shen, Y., Bai, X., Zhang, Q. et al. (2025). Oncolytic virus VG161 in refractory hepatocellular carcinoma. *Nature* 641 (8062): 503–511.

70. Bruix, J., Qin, S., Merle, P. et al. (2017). Regorafenib for patients with hepatocellular carcinoma who progressed on sorafenib treatment (RESORCE): a randomised, double-blind, placebo-controlled, phase 3 trial. *Lancet* 389 (10064): 56–66.
71. Wei, J., Yang, Y., Wang, G., and Liu, M. (2022). Current landscape and future directions of bispecific antibodies in cancer immunotherapy. *Front Immunol* 13: 1035276.
72. Albayrak, G., Wan, P.K., Fisher, K., and Seymour, L.W. (2025). T cell engagers: expanding horizons in oncology and beyond. *Br J Cancer* 133: 1241–1249.
73. Cheal, S.M., Chung, S.K., Vaughn, B.A. et al. (2022). Pretargeting: a path forward for radioimmunotherapy. *J Nucl Med* 63 (9): 1302–1315.
74. Jallinoja, V.I.J. and Houghton, J.L. (2021). Current landscape in clinical pretargeted radioimmunoimaging and therapy. *J Nucl Med* 62 (9): 1200–1206.
75. Li, H., Er Saw, P., and Song, E. (2020). Challenges and strategies for next-generation bispecific antibody-based antitumor therapeutics. *Cell Mol Immunol* 17 (5): 451–461.
76. Nejadmoghaddam, M.R., Minai-Tehrani, A., Ghahremanzadeh, R. et al. (2019). Antibody-drug conjugates: possibilities and challenges. *Avicenna J Med Biotechnol* 11 (1): 3–23.
77. Zheng, M., Huang, J., Tong, A., and Yang, H. (2019). Oncolytic viruses for cancer therapy: barriers and recent advances. *Mol Ther Oncolytics* 15: 234–247.
78. Nikkhoi, S.K., Li, G., and Hatefi, A. (2024). Natural killer cell engagers for cancer immunotherapy. *Front Oncol* 14: 1483884.
79. Nolan-Stevaux, O. and Smith, R. (2024). Logic-gated and contextual control of immunotherapy for solid tumors: contrasting multi-specific T cell engagers and CAR-T cell therapies. *Front Immunol* 15: 1490911.
80. de Graaf, J.F., de Vor, L., Fouchier, R.A.M., and van den Hoogen, B.G. (2018). Armed oncolytic viruses: a kick-start for anti-tumor immunity. *Cytokine Growth Factor Rev* 41: 28–39.
81. Wang, L., Chard Dunmall, L.S., Cheng, Z., and Wang, Y. (2022). Remodeling the tumor microenvironment by oncolytic viruses: beyond oncolysis of tumor cells for cancer treatment. *J Immunother Cancer* 10 (5): e004167.
82. Li, Y.R., Lyu, Z., Shen, X. et al. (2025). Boosting CAR-T cell therapy through vaccine synergy. *Trends Pharmacol Sci* 46 (2): 180–199.
83. Borgers, J.S.W., Lenkala, D., Kohler, V. et al. (2025). Personalized, autologous neoantigen-specific T cell therapy in metastatic melanoma: a phase 1 trial. *Nat Med* 31 (3): 881–893.
84. Liu, Y.T. and Sun, Z.J. (2021). Turning cold tumors into hot tumors by improving T-cell infiltration. *Theranostics* 11 (11): 5365–5386.
85. Olawade, D.B., Teke, J., Fapohunda, O. et al. (2024). Leveraging artificial intelligence in vaccine development: a narrative review. *J Microbiol Methods* 224: 106998.

Index

B

N

www.ingramcontent.com/pod-product-compliance
Ingram Content Group UK Ltd.
Pitfield, Milton Keynes, MK11 3LW, UK
UKHW051451290926
15471UKWH00008B/1142

9 781394 383016